A Clinical Approach to Antiarrhythmic Drugs

A Clinical Approach to Antiarrhythmic Drugs

Editor: Duncan Murray

AMERICAN
MEDICAL PUBLISHERS
www.americanmedicalpublishers.com

AMERICAN
MEDICAL PUBLISHERS
www.americanmedicalpublishers.com

Cataloging-in-Publication Data

A clinical approach to antiarrhythmic drugs / edited by Duncan Murray.
p. cm.
Includes bibliographical references and index.
ISBN 978-1-63927-833-6
1. Myocardial depressants. 2. Arrhythmia--Chemotherapy. 3. Cardiovascular system--Diseases--Chemotherapy.
4. Cardiovascular agents. 5. Pharmacy. I. Murray, Duncan.
RM347 .C55 2023
616.128 061--dc23

American Medical Publishers,
41 Flatbush Avenue,
1st Floor, New York,
NY 11217, USA

ISBN 978-1-63927-833-6 (Hardback)

Contents

Preface

Antiarrhythmic drugs, also known as cardiac dysrhythmia medications, are a class of drugs used to treat irregular heart rhythms (cardiac arrhythmias) such as atrial fibrillation, atrial flutter, ventricular tachycardia, and ventricular fibrillation. Amiodarone, flecainide, ibutilide, and lidocaine are a few antiarrhythmic drugs. Most of these drugs can be administered intravenously or orally, depending on the severity of the illness. These drugs have multiple modes of action. For instance, different classes of antiarrhythmic drugs include sodium channel disrupters, potassium channel blockers, beta-blockers, calcium channel blockers, and cardiac glycosides. The side effects of antiarrhythmic medications are possible issues with the liver, kidney, thyroid or lungs, along with tiredness, nausea, and shortness of breath. This book aims to shed light on some of the unexplored aspects of antiarrhythmic drugs and the recent researches in this field. It consists of contributions made by international experts. This book will serve as a reference to a broad spectrum of readers.

After months of intensive research and writing, this book is the end result of all who devoted their time and efforts in the initiation and progress of this book. It will surely be a source of reference in enhancing the required knowledge of the new developments in the area. During the course of developing this book, certain measures such as accuracy, authenticity and research focused analytical studies were given preference in order to produce a comprehensive book in the area of study.

This book would not have been possible without the efforts of the authors and the publisher. I extend my sincere thanks to them. Secondly, I express my gratitude to my family and well-wishers. And most importantly, I thank my students for constantly expressing their willingness and curiosity in enhancing their knowledge in the field, which encourages me to take up further research projects for the advancement of the area.

Editor

1

Transgenic Rabbit Models in Proarrhythmia Research

István Baczkó[1†], Tibor Hornyik[1,2,3†], Michael Brunner[2,3,4], Gideon Koren[5] and Katja E. Odening[2,3,6,7*]*

[1] Department of Pharmacology and Pharmacotherapy, University of Szeged, Szeged, Hungary, [2] Department of Cardiology and Angiology I, Heart Center, University of Freiburg, Freiburg, Germany, [3] Faculty of Medicine, University of Freiburg, Freiburg, Germany, [4] Department of Cardiology and Medical Intensive Care, St. Josefskrankenhaus, Freiburg, Germany, [5] Cardiovascular Research Center, Division of Cardiology, Rhode Island Hospital, Alpert Medical School of Brown University, Providence, RI, United States, [6] Translational Cardiology, Department of Cardiology, Inselspital, Bern University Hospital, Bern, Switzerland, [7] Institute of Physiology, University of Bern, Bern, Switzerland

***Correspondence:**
István Baczkó
baczko.istvan@med.u-szeged.hu
Katja E. Odening
katja.odening@uniklinik-freiburg.de;
Katja.odening@pyl.unibe.ch

[†]These authors have contributed equally to this work

Drug-induced proarrhythmia constitutes a potentially lethal side effect of various drugs. Most often, this proarrhythmia is mechanistically linked to the drug's potential to interact with repolarizing cardiac ion channels causing a prolongation of the QT interval in the ECG. Despite sophisticated screening approaches during drug development, reliable prediction of proarrhythmia remains very challenging. Although drug-induced long-QT-related proarrhythmia is often favored by conditions or diseases that impair the individual's repolarization reserve, most cellular, tissue, and whole animal model systems used for drug safety screening are based on normal, healthy models. In recent years, several transgenic rabbit models for different types of long QT syndromes (LQTS) with differences in the extent of impairment in repolarization reserve have been generated. These might be useful for screening/prediction of a drug's potential for long-QT-related proarrhythmia, particularly as different repolarizing cardiac ion channels are impaired in the different models. In this review, we summarize the electrophysiological characteristics of the available transgenic LQTS rabbit models, and the pharmacological proof-of-principle studies that have been performed with these models—highlighting the advantages and disadvantages of LQTS models for proarrhythmia research. In the end, we give an outlook on potential future directions and novel models.

Keywords: transgenic LQTS rabbit, drug-induced proarrhythmia, proarrhythmia safety screening, K^+-channel blocker, long QT syndrome, cardiac repolarization reserve

INTRODUCTION: PROARRHYTHMIA AND DRUG DEVELOPMENT

Proarrhythmia—the triggering of arrhythmias following drug therapy—has been known for many decades as being caused by "anti"-arrhythmic cardiac drugs (Selzer and Wray, 1964; Echt et al., 1991; Waldo et al., 1996). This rare but lethal side-effect of drug therapy, however, is not restricted to anti-arrhythmic drugs, but occurs with a variety of other, non-cardiac drugs (Woosley et al., 1993; Wysowski and Bacsanyi, 1996; Darpo, 2001), and therefore is a major concern for patients, physicians, and the pharmaceutical industry. It has been estimated that around 20–60% of novel chemical entities have the potential to modulate the function of cardiac ion channels and therefore, to disturb normal cardiac electrical function (Danker and Moller, 2014). Depending on the nature of the drug-induced effects on ion channels function, proarrhythmia can be associated with prolongation or shortening of the QT interval (long QT syndrome, LQTS or short QT syndrome, SQTS, respectively) and/or with conduction disturbances.

For most drugs, proarrhythmia is assumed to be based on prolongation of cardiac repolarization as a result of drug-induced inhibition of cardiac potassium currents (mostly I_{Kr} current(s)/HERG-channels) (Redfern et al., 2003). This acquired LQTS predisposes to Torsades-de-Pointes (TdP) polymorphic ventricular tachycardia that could lead to ventricular fibrillation and sudden cardiac death (SCD) (Haverkamp et al., 2000; Redfern et al., 2003; Fenichel et al., 2004). Although no less than 2–3% of all marketed drugs have the potential to induce LQTS (Stansfeld et al., 2006), the (documented) incidence of potentially lethal drug-induced TdP is typically very low (1:10,000 for non-cardiovascular drugs) (Yap and Camm, 2003), and therefore very hard to predict reliably (Fenichel et al., 2004). In recent decades, TdP-induced SCD cases were associated with a wide range of commonly used drugs (anti-psychotics, anti-depressants, antihistamines, and antibiotics) (Haverkamp et al., 2000; Redfern et al., 2003; Fenichel et al., 2004) and many of them (such as cisapride, astemizole, terfenadine, grepafloxacin) have been withdrawn from the market (Farkas and Nattel, 2010; Stockbridge et al., 2013; Ferdinandy et al., 2019).

As a response from the regulatory authorities, the International Council for Harmonisation of Technical Requirements for Pharmaceuticals for Human Use (ICH) guidelines [ICH-S7B, 2005 (Food and Drug Administration, 2005b); ICH-E14, 2005 (Food and Drug Administration, 2005a)] were proposed for rigorous safety testing to avoid similar unacceptable human fatalities (SCD) in association with pharmacological therapy of non-life-threatening pathologies. Unfortunately, no "gold"-standard proarrhythmia screening method exist. Therefore, current safety screening in industry rely on combined use of pre-clinical *in vitro* assessment of HERG function, action potential (AP) and *in vivo* ECG (QT) assays, *in silico* computational (Yang et al., 2016; Ortega et al., 2017; Li et al., 2019) risk prediction [integrated risk assessment (IRA) approach], and clinical ECG studies (Food and Drug Administration, 2005a; Food and Drug Administration, 2005b). Usually, different proarrhythmia markers and score systems [see *Proarrhythmia ECG Markers for Temporal Instability of Repolarization (Used in In Vivo and In Vitro Models)*] are employed to try to increase the predictive value of the overall assessment (Hondeghem et al., 2001; Hondeghem and Hoffmann, 2003; Redfern et al., 2003; Lawrence et al., 2005) with moderate to limited success (Park et al., 2018).

Drug-induced I_{Kr}/HERG blockade used to be considered the most important factor responsible for proarrhythmia formation. Therefore, for a long time, safety tests largely focused on detection of HERG-blocking potential of test compounds. As a result, this approach led to elimination of potentially promising drug candidates from the developmental pipeline solely on the basis of their potential to block the HERG channel (Carlsson, 2001; Bouder, 2007; Pugsley et al., 2008). HERG blockade plays an inevitably important role in proarrhythmia formation (Yap and Camm, 2003; Hancox et al., 2008); though, HERG block on its own does not necessarily lead to proarrhythmia since simultaneous reduction in other ion currents—such as in I_{Na} or I_{Ca}—that may have anti-arrhythmic effects could modify the overall proarrhythmic potential of the drug (Van Opstal et al., 2001; Belardinelli et al., 2003; Thomsen et al., 2004; Anderson, 2006). On the other hand, compounds without HERG-blocking characteristics may still have proarrhythmic side effect *via* the inhibition of repolarizing ion currents such as the slow delayed rectifier potassium current I_{Ks} or the inward rectifier potassium current I_{K1} (Pugsley et al., 2008; Roden, 2008; Kannankeril et al., 2010; Pollard et al., 2010). Based on the above, pharmaceutical industry has started the Comprehensive *in vitro* Proarrhythmia Assay (CiPA) initiative to work with validated assays, and to fill gaps in the internal proarrhythmia assessment with the overall goal to comply with the ICH-S7B guidelines. This new approach consists of three main elements: 1) systematic measurement of the effect of drug candidates on multiple human cardiac ion currents (I_{Kr}, I_{Ks}, $I_{Na,peak}$, $I_{Na,late}$, I_{K1}, I_{to}, $I_{Ca,L}$) in heterologous expression systems (Kramer et al., 2013; Cavero and Holzgrefe, 2014; Colatsky et al., 2016), 2) *in silico* integration of these ion channel effects, and 3) evaluation of the drug effect on integrated biological systems such as on stem-cell-derived cardiomyocytes (Colatsky et al., 2016; Crumb et al., 2016; Huang et al., 2017). According to a recent survey on current industrial safety screening practice (Authier et al., 2017), 90% of the pharmaceutical companies use cell lines expressing cardiac ion channels, 50–60% of them perform ion channel binding assays, cardiac AP recordings or use human induced pluripotent stem cell-derived cardiomyocytes, and only around one-third of them integrate their electrophysiological results into an *in silico* model in order to better predict the drug effect on AP shape and duration. The CiPA initiative is undoubtedly a promising approach; however, its overall implementation is not sufficient yet.

The other major challenge in proarrhythmia screening derives from the huge inter-individual differences in susceptibility to arrhythmia, which makes the overall risk stratification particularly difficult. Gender, sex hormones, K^+ homeostasis, and—most importantly—certain diseases highly influence the cardiac "repolarization reserve", defined as the ability of cardiomyocytes to maintain sufficient repolarization despite repolarization-prolonging (mostly K^+ channel blocking) effects *via* compensatory increase of non-affected "reserve" outward K^+ currents (Roden, 1998; Varro and Baczko, 2011).

Apart from a decrease in serum K^+ concentration that results in a massive prolongation of cardiac repolarization, cardiovascular and metabolic diseases such as congestive heart failure (Kjekshus, 1990), cardiac hypertrophy, hypertrophic and dilated cardiomyopathy (Decker et al., 2009), ischemia (Dutta et al., 2016), congenital LQTS (El-Sherif and Turitto, 1999), or diabetes mellitus (Mcnally et al., 1999; Whitsel et al., 2005) play the most important role in decreasing repolarization reserve capacity and thereby in increasing susceptibility to proarrhythmia.

Despite the fact that drug-induced TdP occur mostly in patients with reduced cardiac repolarization reserve, current safety assessments rely still mainly on tests performed on healthy animals with intact repolarization or on their tissues/cells (Food and Drug Administration, 2005a; Food and Drug Administration, 2005b). Consequently, new animal models, (i) with increased sensitivity to channel blockers other than only HERG, such as I_{Ks} or I_{K1}, and (ii) representing different degrees of impairment in their cardiac repolarization reserve were suggested to employ in proarrhythmia research (Hornyik et al., 2020).

Sex hormones also can significantly alter the individual's repolarization reserve capacity and therefore affect susceptibility to arrhythmia. Women are at higher risk for drug-induced prolongation of repolarization and drug-induced TdP (Lehmann et al., 1996; Benton et al., 2000; Wolbrette, 2003; Gowda et al., 2004). This is due to sex hormone effects on cardiac ion currents/channels (Yang and Clancy, 2010; Odening and Koren, 2014): estrogen prolongs cardiac repolarization by decreasing I_{Ks} (Drici et al., 1996) and I_{Kr} (Kurokawa et al., 2008; Ando et al., 2011) and by increasing $I_{Ca,L}$ (Odening et al., 2012a; Odening et al., 2012b) and NCX expression (Chen et al., 2011); therefore, estrogen reduces repolarization reserve and favors drug-induced arrhythmia. In contrast, testosterone and progesterone both increase repolarization reserve by increasing I_{Ks} [testosterone (Liu et al., 2003)/progesterone (Furukawa and Kurokawa, 2008)], I_{K1} and I_{Kr} (testosterone) (Liu et al., 2003), decreasing $I_{Ca,L}$ [testosterone (Furukawa and Kurokawa, 2008)/progesterone (Odening et al., 2012a; Odening et al., 2012b)], and upregulating SERCA expression [progesterone (Odening et al., 2012a; Odening et al., 2012b; Moshal et al., 2014)], thereby exerting a protective, "anti-arrhythmic" effect against drug-induced proarrhythmia (Odening et al., 2012a; Odening et al., 2012b). These observations have consequences for proarrhythmia research, as female animal models (or animal models with altered hormonal state) might be particularly sensitive in detecting potential ion channel-blocking properties of drug candidates.

In this review, we first give an overview about currently employed proarrhythmia markers, the importance of the choice of species for proarrhythmia research, and the advantages and disadvantages of currently used *in vivo* proarrhythmia models, followed by a detailed description of novel transgenic LQTS rabbit models. Finally, we provide a brief outlook on possible future directions and novel models in the field.

Proarrhythmia ECG Markers for Temporal Instability of Repolarization (Used in *In Vivo* and *In Vitro* Models)

Based on the clinical observations that TdP mostly occurred in the setting of prolongation of ventricular repolarization/QT prolongation (Haverkamp et al., 2000; Redfern et al., 2003), preclinical and clinical safety tests have for a long time focused on QT prolongation as a surrogate marker for TdP risk (Food and Drug Administration, 2005b). However, it has been known for some time that prolongation of repolarization does not always equally increase pro-arrhythmic risk since numerous drugs that block I_{Kr}/HERG and prolong QT rarely cause TdP—while others causing less pronounced QT prolongation carry a significant pro-arrhythmic risk (Zhang et al., 1999; Yang et al., 2001; Roden, 2004; Thomsen et al., 2004; Shah and Hondeghem, 2005). Indeed, the extent of QT prolongation did not predict serious ventricular arrhythmias and/or SCD in different rabbit and dog experimental models (Amos et al., 2001; Thomsen et al., 2004; Shah and Hondeghem, 2005; Lengyel et al., 2007a; Jacobson et al., 2011) or in patients with (Strasberg et al., 1983; Yi et al., 1998; Maron et al., 2001; Hinterseer et al., 2009; Hinterseer et al., 2010) or without (Eisenberg et al., 1995; Kusano et al., 2001; Paltoo et al., 2001) congenital/structural heart disease. Thus, these safety tests can yield either false positive results, halting the development of a promising new drug (Roden, 2004; Hondeghem et al., 2007) or false negative results, causing harm to patients with increased susceptibility to arrhythmia. Therefore, there is an unmet need for (i) improved identification of patients at elevated risk for drug-induced arrhythmia (Kaab et al., 2003) and (ii) novel ECG markers with better predictive value for pro-arrhythmic drug adverse effects.

A number of different electrophysiological parameters have been investigated as non-invasive prognostic markers for TdP and SCD risk evaluation both in animal experiments and in the clinical setting. These novel markers mostly derive from the original work by Hondeghem *et al.*, suggesting the assessment of AP triangulation, instability, and dispersion (Hondeghem et al., 2001). These markers were later supplemented by evaluation of disturbances in cardiac wavelength (Hondeghem et al., 2007; Hondeghem, 2016). The importance of an increased spatial (transmural, apico-basal, or inter-ventricular) dispersion of repolarization in reentry-based arrhythmia formation was further supported by other studies (Antzelevitch, 2008; Barbhaiya et al., 2013; Guerard et al., 2014). Therefore, $T_{peak-end}$—the length from the beginning of the T wave (T_p) to the end (T_e) on ECG—that reflect the transmural dispersion of repolarization was suggested to use as an indicator of arrhythmic risk, although, no clear consensus about the value of this parameter has been reached so far (Antzelevitch, 2008; Barbhaiya et al., 2013; Meijborg et al., 2014). Of note, dispersion of repolarization was recently identified (experimentally and by computational modeling) as cause for triggered activity/EAD formation, further enhancing the need to assess dynamic dispersion of repolarization noninvasively (Liu et al., 2018).

The temporal instability of cardiac repolarization can be described by different variables characterizing the small beat-to-beat fluctuations in the QT interval as QT variability [for a recent review see (Baumert et al., 2016)]. Beat-to-beat variability of repolarization can be quantified by calculating the short-term variability of the QT (STV_{QT}) (Thomsen et al., 2004). First in the chronic AV-block dog model, then in other animal experimental proarrhythmia models (Thomsen et al., 2004; Lengyel et al., 2007a; Jacobson et al., 2011) and in clinical settings (Hinterseer et al., 2008; Hinterseer et al., 2009; Hinterseer et al., 2010; Oosterhoff et al., 2010), it has been repeatedly shown that STV_{QT} has a higher predictive value for proarrhythmia risk than the overall prolongation of repolarization (QT duration). STV_{QT} has been used in several studies to confirm the safety of different drugs (Oros et al., 2006; Antoons et al., 2010; Varkevisser et al., 2012), to characterize pro-arrhythmic drug effects (Thomsen et al., 2004; Thomsen et al., 2006b; Kristof et al., 2012), and to assess temporal repolarization instability in patients with co-morbidities associated with repolarization disturbances (Orosz et al., 2015a; Orosz et al., 2015b; Orosz et al., 2017).

Based on the above, it is justified and required to assess and validate measures of temporal QT variability in animal experimental models of proarrhythmia.

CURRENT *IN VIVO* MODELS FOR PRE-CLINICAL PROARRHYTHMIA SAFETY SCREENING AND THEIR LIMITATIONS

Choice of Models: Species Differences in Repolarizing Currents

Cardiac electro-mechanical function shows large inter-species variability. These species differences are especially striking in regard to cardiac repolarization that is governed by tightly regulated activities of various inward and outward ion currents.

Small rodents like mice or rats are commonly used animals for studying ischemia-induced arrhythmias (which are often linked to conduction properties), since cardiac conduction properties in these animals are governed by Na^+ currents, Ca^{2+} currents, and connexin function that are very similar to those in human (Derangeon et al., 2012; Kaese and Verheule, 2012). Furthermore, they have the advantage of low cost, short life-cycle, and their genetic manipulation is much easier than that in larger animals (see *Genetically Modified Mouse Models With Reduced Repolarization Reserve*). On the other hand; however, they have limited value in studying (prolonged) repolarization-related arrhythmogenesis: in mice and rats the fast and slow transient outward (I_{to}), and the delayed rectifier ($I_{K,slow1}$ and $I_{K,slow2}$) (Xu et al., 1999; Brunner et al., 2001; Liu et al., 2008) voltage-gated potassium currents play a major role in repolarization—while in dogs, rabbits, and humans the rapid and slow delayed rectifier potassium currents (I_{Kr} and I_{Ks}) are the major determinants of cardiac repolarization (Varro et al., 1993; Nerbonne, 2000; Nerbonne and Kass, 2005; Grandy et al., 2007; Saito et al., 2009; Yang et al., 2014). The exact role of I_{Kr} and I_{Ks} in small rodents is still not well known and controversial (Nerbonne and Kass, 2005; Grandy et al., 2007; Saito et al., 2009; Yang et al., 2014). As a result, the shape of their AP is different compared to larger animals and humans (triangular shape vs. rectangular AP with prominent plateau phase) (Nerbonne and Kass, 2005; Grandy et al., 2007; Saito et al., 2009; Yang et al., 2014), as well as their pharmacological responses to proarrhythmic potassium channel blocking drugs (**Figures 1A, B**).

Acute I_{Kr}-blocker administration, for example, prolongs repolarization in dogs, rabbits, and humans but not in mice or

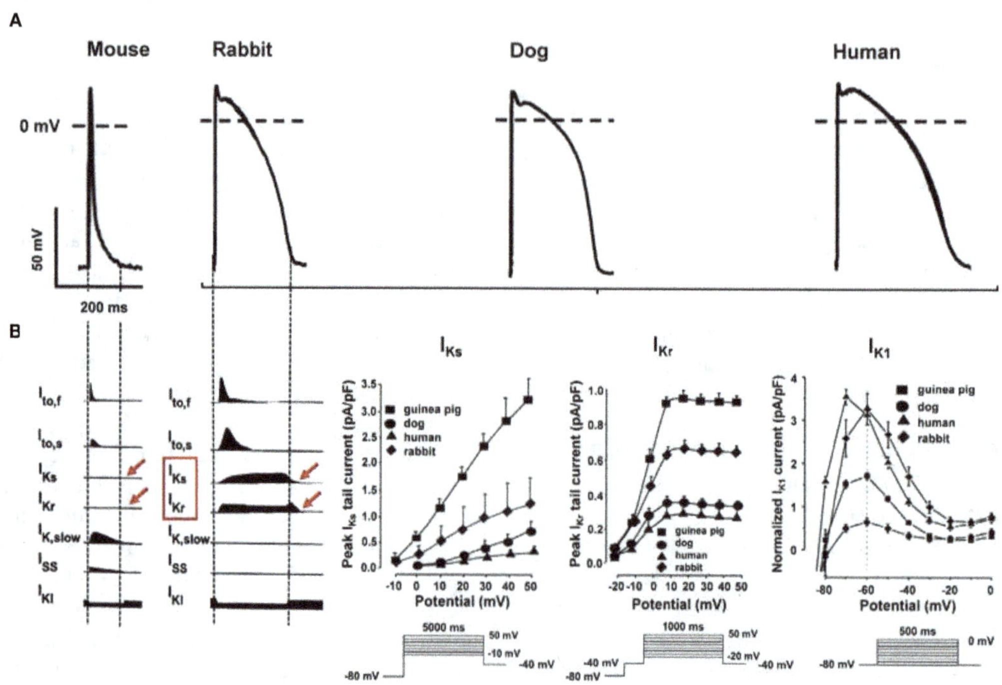

FIGURE 1 | Species differences in repolarizing ion currents. **(A)** Representative action potential (AP) recordings [modified from (Rudy et al., 2008; Blenck et al., 2016)] and **(B)** schematic illustration of the main repolarizing ion currents in mouse, rabbit, dog, and human cardiomyocytes [modified from (Nerbonne et al., 2001)]. Panel **(C)** shows species differences in I_{Ks}, I_{Kr}, and I_{K1} in rabbit, dog, and human.

rats (Varro et al., 2000; Nagy et al., 2009; Jost et al., 2013; Yang et al., 2014). Chronic administration of the I_{Kr}-blocker dofetilide that prolongs repolarization in larger animals and human subjects by blocking HERG channels on the other hand, lengthen repolarization in mice—at least partly—by increasing $I_{Na,L}$ (via phosphoinositide 3-kinase pathway) (Yang et al., 2014). Based on the above, mice and rats have serious limitations in drug-induced proarrhythmia research with little translational potential.

In contrast, the function and gating kinetics of various cardiac potassium channels are very similar in dogs, rabbits, and humans with I_{Kr} and I_{Ks} as main repolarizing ion currents in all three species (Varro et al., 1993; Nerbonne, 2000; Nerbonne and Kass, 2005; Jost et al., 2013), with slight inter-species differences: In humans and dogs—just as in most mammals—I_{to} is formed of two distinct subtypes named as $I_{to,fast}$ and $I_{to,slow}$—with fast and slow recovery from inactivation, determined by Kv3.4 and Kv1.4, respectively (Patel and Campbell, 2005) as opposed to rabbits, where $I_{to,slow}$ is the primary transient Kv current in the left ventricle (Fedida and Giles, 1991), while in the right ventricle $I_{to,fast}$ and its role in LQT1 related arrhythmogenesis has recently been confirmed (Choi et al., 2018). The repolarization capacity of rabbits and dogs is more robust than that in humans due to higher I_{K1}, I_{Kr}, and I_{Ks} current densities (Jost et al., 2013; Husti et al., 2015) (**Figure 1C**).

In summary, the rabbit has a prominent role in arrhythmia research, since: (i) the shape of AP (Varro et al., 1993) and the function and gating kinetics of the underlying cardiac ion channels/currents (Nerbonne, 2000), (ii) the myocardial mechanical function (Jung et al., 2012), (iii) the relative effective heart size relating cardiac mass to the frequency of VF (Panfilov, 2006), and (iv) their responses to pharmacological interventions (Harken et al., 1981) show very close resemblance to human cardiac physiology. Based on the above-described species differences in various ion currents, the rabbit could have advantages over dog models when testing the proarrhythmic potential of drugs with I_{Kr}, I_{Ks}, or I_{K1}-blocking properties since they show very good similarity to human physiology in these currents and are cheaper, easier to handle, and to breed than dogs and can be modified genetically. Dogs or guinea pigs, on the other hand, may be better suited to use for studying arrhythmogenesis in which I_{to}-inhibition plays an important role.

In Vivo Proarrhythmia Models With Reduced Repolarization Reserve

Both drug-induced and genetically modified animal models with impaired repolarization reserve have been generated in various species (such as dogs, mice, and rabbits) and utilized to investigate drug-induced proarrhythmia and its underlying mechanisms [reviewed in (Salama and London, 2007; Lang et al., 2016)]. In addition, animal models with cardiac diseases —e.g. chronic heart failure, hypertrophic cardiomyopathy, diabetes mellitus etc.—leading to electrical remodeling-associated alterations of repolarization reserve can be used for proarrhythmia research. These models have the advantage that they mimic some of the diseases that also predispose human patients to drug-induced arrhythmias.

One main shortcoming of drug-induced animal models, however, is the fact that drugs have to be administered continuously to sustain the drug-induced reduction of repolarization reserve, thus impeding detailed investigation of (long-term) proarrhythmia in free-moving, non-anesthetized animals.

One main short-coming of genetically modified mouse models—the only genetic models with reduced repolarization reserve available until 2008—are the pronounced species differences in cardiac electrophysiology with different ion currents conveying cardiac repolarization in human and murine cardiomyocytes (Varro et al., 1993; Nerbonne, 2000; Nerbonne and Kass, 2005; Jost et al., 2013) as highlighted in the subchapter above.

High cost and need for special technical expertise for example are considered as main shortcomings for the generation of disease-related animal models with cardiac electrical remodeling.

Drug-Induced Animal Models With Reduced Repolarization Reserve

One frequently used drug-induced model is the methoxamine-sensitized rabbit model: anesthetized rabbits are sensitized with the selective α-adrenoceptor-agonist methoxamine, which makes them particularly prone to develop drug-induced ventricular tachycardia when exposed to HERG/I_{Kr}-blocking drugs (Carlsson, 2008; Carlsson et al., 2009). The choice of the anesthetic regimen, however, strongly influences the extent of proarrhythmia development in this model—as the different anesthetics all have different intrinsic cardiac ion channel-blocking properties (Carlsson, 2008; Inaba et al., 2011), indicating the importance of the degree of ion channel blockade in these "mixed" drug-induced models. Pro- and anti-arrhythmic properties of various different drugs have been tested and classified as having a low, intermediate, or high pro-arrhythmic potential for drug-induced TdP using this model (Diness et al., 2008; Carlsson et al., 2009; Jacobson et al., 2011; Mow et al., 2015; Varkevisser et al., 2015). However, as the model depends on α-adrenoceptor sensitization, the full extent of pro-arrhythmic potential of drugs that concomitantly block I_{Kr} and α-adrenoceptors (such as quinidine, cisapride, quinolone) may not be fully appreciated by this model (Carlsson, 2008; Mow et al., 2015).

Other frequently employed drug-induced rabbit models are based on the *ex vivo* blockade of HERG/I_{Kr} by E-4031 (Choi et al., 2002; Maruyama et al., 2011; Parikh et al., 2012; Lau et al., 2015) or by dofetilide (Farkas et al., 2006; Dhein et al., 2008; Orosz et al., 2014), thus generating a drug-induced rabbit model representing LQT2 characteristics. Similar to the genetic reduction of I_{Kr} in congenital LQT2, the drug-blockade of I_{Kr} by E-4031 or dofetilide leads to a high propensity for arrhythmia development in *ex vivo* Langendorff-perfused rabbit hearts—particularly when perfused with low K^+ and Mg^{2+} solutions (Maruyama et al., 2011; Milberg et al., 2011). Similarly, QTc prolongation and arrhythmia susceptibility is particularly high

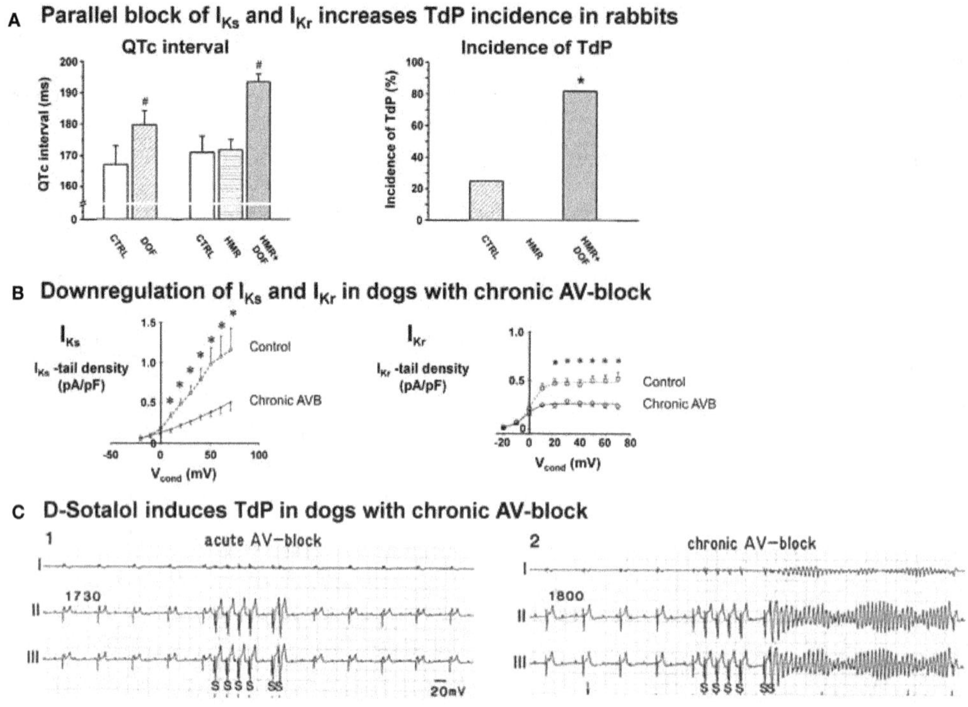

FIGURE 2 | Pro-arrhythmia detection with acquired LQT rabbit and chronic AV-block dog models. **(A)** Left panel: The QTc interval was significantly prolonged by the I_{Kr} blocker dofetilide and was further prolonged by the combination of dofetilide and the I_{Kr} blocker HMR1556 given in any order, while I_{Ks} block alone did not prolong the QTc in anesthetized rabbits. Right panel: I_{Kr} block caused TdP in some of the animals, I_{Ks} block alone did not induce TdP in anesthetized rabbits. Importantly, combined acute pharmacological block of I_{Ks} and I_{Kr}, given in any order, caused a significant increase in TdP incidence. #$p < 0.05$ vs. baseline control in the same group; *$p < 0.05$ vs. dofetilide. N=7-11 animals/group. CTRL: Control, DOF: Dofetilide, HMR: HMR-1556. Modified from (Lengyel et al., 2007a). **(B)** In right ventricular cardiomyocytes isolated from dogs with chronic AV-block and marked myocardial hypertrophy, I_{Ks} tail current density was reduced by approximately 55% (n=9), while I_{Kr} tail current density was reduced by 45% (n=14) compared to those isolated from control animals. *$p < 0.05$ vs. control myocytes. Modified from (Volders et al., 1999). **(C)** Standard bipolar ECG lead recordings illustrating a marked difference in the arrhythmogenic response to administration of the selective I_{Kr} blocker D-sotalol in dogs with acute (left panel) and chronic AV-block (right panel). The pacing protocol involved a basic pacing cycle length (CL) of 1730 ms in acute AV block, and 1800 ms spontaneous idioventricular CL in chronic AV-block. Arrhythmia provocation included a short/long/short sequence at 600 ms CL for 4 beats followed by 2 paced beats with 1200 and 350 ms cycle lengths. No TdP was observed in acute AV-block dogs, while 60% of animals with chronic AV-block exhibited TdP. Modified from (Vos et al., 1998).

when HERG/I_{Kr} blockade is combined with KvLQT1/I_{Ks} blockade by HMR-1556 (Lengyel et al., 2007a) (**Figure 2A**).

Genetically Modified Mouse Models With Reduced Repolarization Reserve

Despite apparent differences between human and mouse electrophysiology—e.g., different ion currents conveying cardiac repolarization in human and murine cardiomyocytes, a different shape of the AP, and a magnitude-faster heart rate in mice [reviewed in (Nerbonne, 2000); (Salama and London, 2007); (Baczko et al., 2016)], the first transgenic and knock-out animal models of LQTS were mouse models (London et al., 1998). The reason for this was that genetic manipulation has for a long time nearly exclusively been feasible in mice and not in other larger mammals such as rabbits. Transgenic models based on mutations in human potassium channel genes or knock-out/knock-in models of mouse potassium channel genes could only partially mimic the characteristics of human patients with impaired repolarization reserve [reviewed in detail in (Nerbonne et al., 2001); (Lang et al., 2016); (Ziupa et al., 2019)], while genetically modified mouse models with mutations in the sodium channel gene (SCN5A; LQT3) more closely mimic the human long QT disease phenotype with AP duration (APD) and QT prolongation as well as spontaneous life-threatening ventricular arrhythmia (Nuyens et al., 2001; Fabritz et al., 2003), since *SCN5A* drives the majority of depolarizing Na^+ currents in both human and murine cardiomyocytes (Derangeon et al., 2012).

None of these mouse models, however, have been systematically used for proarrhythmia research—mainly due to the fact that I_{Kr} current (the most frequent target for drugs inducing proarrhythmia) plays no major role in cardiac repolarization in mice.

Animal Models With Structural/Electrical Remodeling and Reduced Repolarization Reserve

Several experimental animal models of different species exist that are characterized by impaired repolarization reserve associated with cardiac structural and/or electrical remodeling. The most thoroughly characterized of these is the canine cardiac volume overload model with chronic atrioventricular block (Vos et al., 1995). Three months following AV-node ablation, these dogs exhibit severe bradycardia and eccentric, biventricular myocardial hypertrophy without heart failure (Vos et al., 1998). Importantly, the model is characterized by heterogeneous prolongation of APD at baseline and further APD-prolongation and early afterdepolarization (EAD) development upon administration of I_{Kr}-blocker *d*-sotalol, indicating increased susceptibility to drug-induced TdP (Vos et al., 1998) (**Figure 2C**). A significant downregulation of potassium currents, including I_{Ks}—a key player in ventricular repolarization reserve in mammals including humans (Varro et al., 2000; Volders et al., 2003; Jost et al., 2005)—was observed in both left and right ventricular cardiomyocytes isolated from dogs with chronic AV block (Volders et al., 1999) (**Figure 2B**). In addition, I_{Kr} density was reduced by 45% in right ventricular myocytes, while left ventricular (LV) I_{Kr} density was unchanged (Volders et al., 1999).

The ability of the model to detect drug-induced TdP was validated (Takahara et al., 2006) with several drugs such as the H_1 antihistamine terfenadine (Monahan et al., 1990), the antipsychotic drug sertindole (Thomsen et al., 2003), and the D_2 dopamine receptor antagonist sulpiride (Sugiyama et al., 2002). Moreover, with this model, it was demonstrated for the antibiotics moxifloxacin and azithromycin that QT prolongation does not necessarily cause TdP (Thomsen et al., 2006a). An important advantage of this model is an improved proarrhythmia reproducibility within the same experimental animal (Verduyn et al., 2001). There are, however, some disadvantages that may prevent this model from becoming widely used for proarrhythmia research: it is a relatively expensive, time consuming (at least 3 months have to pass before ventricular hypertrophy and increased susceptibility to arrhythmia develops) and low throughput method that requires special technical expertise for performing AV-node ablation (Vos et al., 1998).

In diabetes, a moderate remodeling-associated QT prolongation has been shown (Giunti et al., 2007), and diabetes has been associated with increased risk of SCD (Gill et al., 2009), indicating the patients' higher susceptibility to proarrhythmia. Similarly, in rabbit and dog models of diabetes mellitus, a mild prolongation of repolarization and a decreased repolarization reserve due to downregulation of I_{Ks} and I_{to} (reversible by insulin treatment) were observed (Lengyel et al., 2007b; Lengyel et al., 2008). The authors are not aware, however, of any published studies using experimental diabetes animal models in species with repolarization relevant to human (i.e. not mice or rats) for testing pro-arrhythmic effects of drugs in this "patient" cohort.

TRANSGENIC LQTS RABBIT MODELS WITH IMPAIRED REPOLARIZATION RESERVE (LQTS)

Since cardiac electrophysiological characteristics of the rabbit is much closer to humans than that of mice or rats (Varro et al., 1993; Nerbonne, 2000; Nerbonne and Kass, 2005; Jost et al., 2013),—similar potassium currents (mainly I_{Kr} and I_{Ks}) convey the cardiac repolarization in rabbits and humans—transgenic LQTS rabbit models were generated as soon as it became technically feasible (Bosze et al., 2016) to better mimic pathophysiology of (human) LQTS patients with decreased repolarization reserve, who are most vulnerable to the development of drug-induced arrhythmias.

Generation of Transgenic LQTS Rabbit Models

To generate transgenic LQTS rabbit models with impaired repolarization reserve, the so-called "dominant-negative" transgenic strategy, which describes the fact that the co-assembly of mutated and normal channel subunits completely disrupts the overall ion channel function, was utilized to decrease the expression of functionally normal repolarizing potassium channel proteins. All available transgenic LQTS rabbit models have been engineered by beta-myosin heavy chain promoter-driven cardio-selective over-expression of mutated human genes encoding for voltage-gated K^+ channels such as *KCNQ1*/KvLQT1 (KvLQT1-Y315S, LQT1), *KCNH2*/HERG (HERG-G628S, LQT2), or *KCNE1*/minK (KCNE1-G52R) (Brunner et al., 2008; Major et al., 2016).

To generate the transgenic founder animals, the pronuclear microinjection technique was used. Superovulation was induced in wild-type (WT) rabbits using hormonal stimulation with FSH and GnRH-analogues, and inseminated oocytes were microinjected with transgenic mutant DNA-constructs and re-implanted into foster mothers (Brunner et al., 2008; Major et al., 2016). Mating of the resulting transgenic F0 founders with female WT rabbits resulted in vertical transmission with 50% transgenic and 50% WT offspring. To generate double-transgenic LQT2–5 rabbits, LQT2 male and LQT5 female rabbits were cross-bred (Hornyik et al., 2020).

Electrophysiological Characteristics and Arrhythmogenic Mechanisms in the Transgenic LQTS Models

In LQT1 or LQT2 rabbit cardiomyocytes the repolarizing potassium currents I_{Ks} (LQT1) or I_{Kr} (LQT2), respectively, are completely eliminated. This results in a prolongation of APD on the cellular and whole heart levels and a prolongation of ventricular refractoriness and QT interval duration *in vivo* (Brunner et al., 2008; Odening et al., 2010). This prolongation of APD/QT is particularly pronounced at slower heart rates, leading to a steeper QT/RR ratio—particularly in LQT2 (Brunner et al., 2008) (**Figures 3A–C**). Moreover, these models demonstrate an increased temporal instability of QT duration with an increased STV_{QT} (Hornyik et al., 2020) and spontaneous polymorphic VT in LQT2 [158] (**Figure 3D**).

In transgenic LQT5 rabbit cardiomyocytes, in contrast, the biophysical properties of I_{Ks} and I_{Kr} are altered with accelerated deactivation kinetics (Major et al., 2016)—but overall I_{Ks} and I_{Kr} current densities are not reduced. Consequently, these rabbits exhibit only a partial phenotype with no significant prolongation of whole heart APD (Major et al., 2016; Hornyik et al., 2020), and

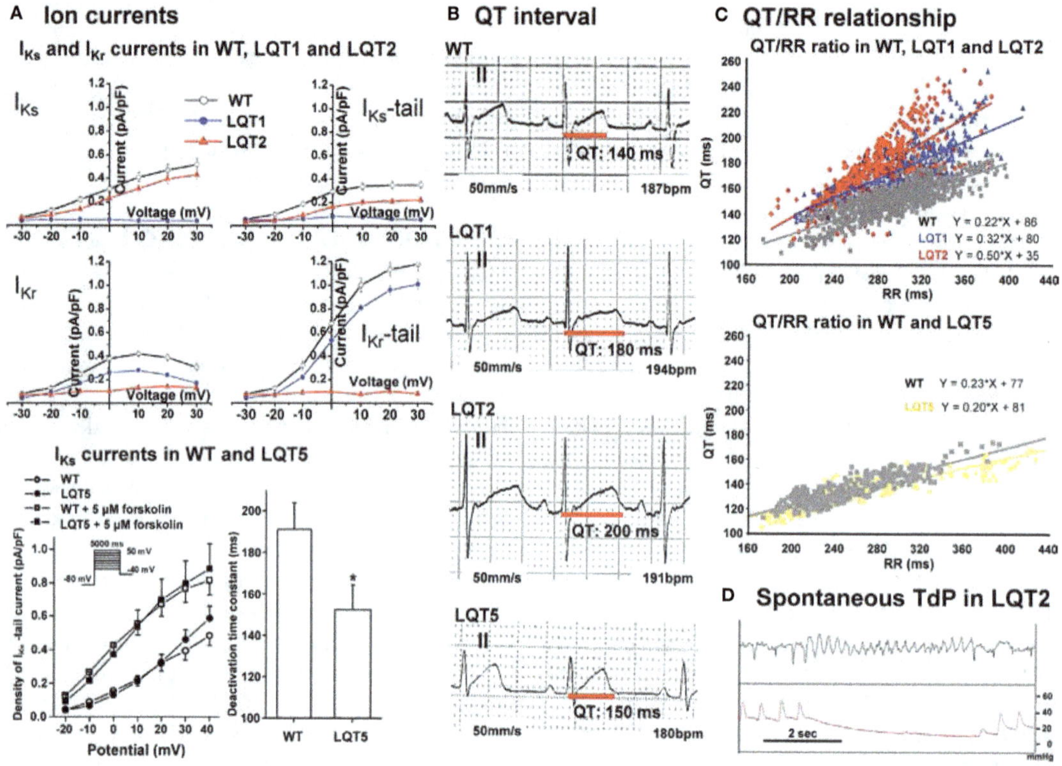

FIGURE 3 | Baseline electrical characteristics of transgenic LQTS rabbits. **(A)** Upper panel: IV-curves of I_{Ks} steady (left)/tail (right) and I_{Kr} steady (left)/tail (right) in cardiomyocytes isolated from wild-type (WT), LQT1, and LQT2 rabbit hearts, indicating loss of I_{Ks} in LQT1 and loss of I_{Kr} in LQT2 [modified from (Brunner et al., 2008)]. Lower panel: IV-curves of I_{Ks} in absence and presence of 5 μM forskolin in WT or transgenic LQT5 rabbit ventricular myocytes. Bar diagrams illustrate a reduced deactivation time constant in transgenic LQT5 ventricular myocytes [modified from (Major et al., 2016)]. **(B)** Representative ECG tracings indicating differences in QT interval in WT, LQT1, LQT2, and LQT5 rabbits [ECG from WT, LQT1 and LQT2 modified from (Brunner et al., 2008)]. **(C)** QT/RR relationship assessed with telemetric ECG in free moving rabbits: WT, LQT1, and LQT2 in upper panel [modified from (Brunner et al., 2008)], in lower panel in WT and LQT5 [modified from (Hornyik et al., 2020)]. **(D)** ECG and blood pressure tracing of LQT2 rabbit with spontaneous ventricular torsade-de-pointes (TdP) tachycardia [modified from (Brunner et al., 2008)]. $^{*}p < 0.05$ vs. WT.

only a very slightly prolonged QT interval at baseline without changes in QT/RR ratio (Major et al., 2016; Hornyik et al., 2020) (**Figures 3A–C**), but exhibit an increased short-term beat-to-beat variability of the QT (Major et al., 2016). Due to their reduced repolarization reserve, the phenotype can be augmented by the I_{Kr}-blocking drug dofetilide, which further increased short-term variability of QT and promoted drug-induced VT (Major et al., 2016).

Studies in transgenic LQT1 and LQT2 rabbits highlight the major role of an enhanced (spatial and temporal) dispersion of repolarization in LQTS-related arrhythmogenesis: in LQT2 rabbit hearts, an increased spatial dispersion of APD was observed throughout left and right ventricles (Brunner et al., 2008; Odening et al., 2013) (**Figure 4A**). Dispersion of repolarization can also occur in a dynamic spatio-temporal fashion with pronounced beat-to-beat alternations and "out-of-phase" heterogeneities between adjacent regions, the so-called "discordant alternans". In transgenic LQT2 rabbit hearts, this discordant alternans developed at physiological heart rates and preceded VT/VF formation (Ziv et al., 2009). VT/VF were easily inducible with LV epicardial stimulation (Brunner et al., 2008), and, importantly, LQT2 rabbits even developed spontaneous polymorphic VT and SCD (Brunner et al., 2008; Odening et al., 2012b), thus representing the first transgenic animal models mimicking the complete electrical phenotype of LQT2. Transgenic LQT1 rabbits with a more homogeneously prolonged APD without substantial dispersion of repolarization within the LV at physiological/normal heart rates, in contrast, developed no spontaneous VT or SCD (Brunner et al., 2008). When LQT1 hearts were further stressed, however, by continuous tachypacing or AV-ablation to induce cardiac tachymyopathy (Lau et al., 2015), or complete AV-block (Kim et al., 2015), respectively, APD dispersion increased, spatially discordant alternans developed and VT/VF was easily inducible or occurred spontaneously. Transgenic LQT5 rabbits demonstrated an increased apico-basal APD heterogeneity compared to healthy WT hearts at baseline—despite their overall "normal" APD (Hornyik et al., 2020).

In addition to increased temporal instability and regional heterogeneity of repolarization that form the electrical "substrate" that facilitates re-entry formation, an increased sympathetic nervous system activity serves as "trigger" for

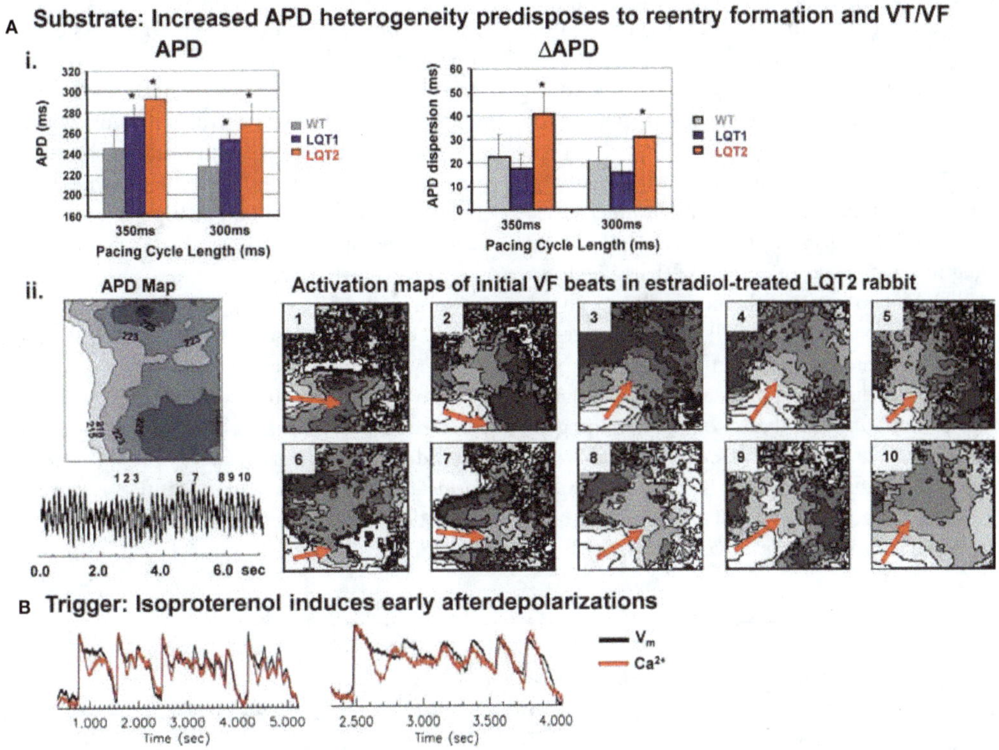

FIGURE 4 | Mechanisms of arrhythmogenesis in transgenic LQT2 rabbits. **(A)** Upper panel (i): Bar graphs of action potential durations (APD) and dispersion of APD (ΔAPD) in Langendorff-perfused hearts of WT, LQT1, and LQT2 rabbits indicate longer APD and increased APD dispersion in LQT2 hearts, *$p < 0.05$ [modified from (Brunner et al., 2008)]. Lower panel (ii): optical mapping APD map (left; indicated are isochrones of APD, in ms) and activation maps (right) of initial beats of ventricular tachycardia/fibrillation (VF) in an estradiol-treated LQT2 heart indicate reentry formation (indicated by red arrows) in line with the regional APD heterogeneities [modified from (Odening et al., 2012b)]. **(B)** Representative trace of Ca^{2+} oscillations and early afterdepolariaztion (EAD) in estradiol-treated LQT2 rabbit heart after AV-node ablation and bolus application of isoproterenol (140 nM). Black line indicates changes in voltage fluorescence signal (Vm); red line indicates changes in Ca^{2+} signal [modified from (Odening et al., 2012b)].

EADs in long QT-related arrhythmogenesis (Antzelevitch, 2007; Brunner et al., 2008; Ziv et al., 2009). In LQT2 cardiomyocytes, beta-adrenergic stimulation related EADs developed during sudden sympathetic surge (**Figure 4B**), while continuous perfusion with beta-agonist isoproterenol prevented EAD formation (Brunner et al., 2008; Liu et al., 2012; Odening et al., 2012b). In LQT1 cardiomyocytes, in contrast, continuous beta-adrenergic stimulation facilitated the occurrence of EADs (Liu et al., 2012). Different time courses in sympathetic activation of cardiac ion currents may explain why different sympathetic modes (sudden surge vs. continuous activation) are associated with arrhythmia formation in different genotypes of LQTS: upon sympathetic stimulation, beta-1 receptor mediated activation of $I_{Ca,L}$—that may elicit EADs—is faster than the activation of I_{Ks}—that shortens APD in LQT2 and acts as anti-arrhythmic mechanism upon continuous adrenergic stimulation in LQT2. In addition, different modes of arrhythmia initiation and maintenance in different LQTS genotypes were identified. While in LQT2, reentry formation played an important role (Brunner et al., 2008), in LQT1 hearts, a novel mechanistic concept of LQTS-related arrhythmogenesis was identified: arrhythmia was initiated by focal excitations arising particularly from the RV and was maintained by multiple shifting excitation foci and bi-excitability (Kim et al., 2015).

Similarly, as in the LQT5 rabbit models, the phenotype and proarrhythmia could be augmented by ion channel blocking drugs and endogenous factors (as highlighted in the following subchapters).

Pro-Arrhythmic Effects of Endogenous Factors (Hormones and Metabolites) in Transgenic LQTS Rabbit Models With Impaired Repolarization Reserve

Pronounced sex differences in arrhythmic risk have been identified in patients with congenital and acquired, drug-induced LQTS with a higher risk for cardiac arrhythmic events in women after puberty than men (Lehmann et al., 1996; Locati et al., 1998; Benton et al., 2000; Wolbrette, 2003; Gowda et al., 2004; Yang and Clancy, 2011). Moreover, while the risk for long QT-related arrhythmia is reduced during pregnancy (Seth et al., 2007), it is particularly high risk during the postpartum (particularly in LQT2 patients) (Sauer et al., 2007). In addition, more pronounced QT-prolongation and arrhythmias are observed during luteal than follicular phases of the menstrual cycle (Rodriguez et al., 2001), strongly suggesting that changing sex hormone levels may affect LQTS-related arrhythmogenesis. This has consequences for proarrhythmia research, as female animal models might be particularly sensitive in detecting potential ion channel-blocking properties of drug candidates.

In transgenic LQT2 rabbits, spontaneous ventricular arrhythmia and SCD also often occurred during postpartum (Brunner et al., 2008; Odening et al., 2012b), suggesting the existence of similar arrhythmia-triggering mechanisms as in human LQTS patients. In these models, estradiol exerted a pro-arrhythmic effect with an increased incidence of lethal polymorphic TdP due to changes in APD dispersion and increased EAD formation upon pro-arrhythmic sympathetic stimuli, while progesterone had an anti-arrhythmic, protective effect that was based on a shortening of cardiac refractoriness, a reduced formation of EAD, and stabilizing Ca^{2+} effects (decreased $I_{Ca,L}$ density, increased SERCA expression) (Odening et al., 2012b). These studies suggest that progesterone-based therapies may be considered as novel anti-arrhythmic approaches in female LQTS patients; and might be considered as therapeutic add-on in cases of severe drug-induced long-QT related proarrhythmia (Odening et al., 2012b). As estradiol-treated hearts are particularly sensitive to proarrhythmia, their use in proarrhythmia research, in contrast, might increase sensitivity to identify candidates with a pro-arrhythmic potential.

Similarly, the postpartum-related hormones oxytocin and prolactin decreased I_{Ks} current densities, thereby prolonging the APD/QT further and predisposing the heart to arrhythmias (Odening et al., 2019).

Hormones as well as other endogenous factors such as certain metabolites may impact on repolarization reserve: it has been demonstrated that (genetic) metabolic disturbances such as propionic acidemia can also cause acquired LQTS (Kakavand et al., 2006; Baumgartner et al., 2007; Jameson and Walter, 2008), thus rendering patients at increased risk for additional drug-induced proarrhythmia. Using rabbit models of LQTS, we could identify a propionic acid-induced reduction of I_{Ks} current densities as underlying mechanism (Bodi et al., 2016).

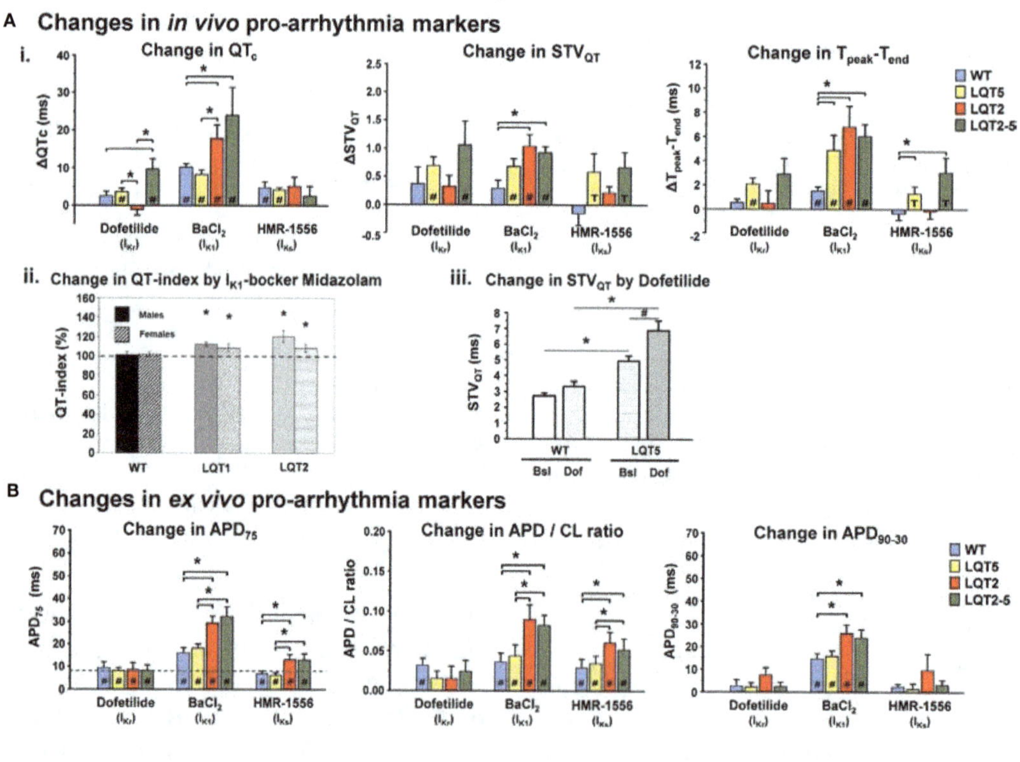

FIGURE 5 | Pro-arrhythmic drug-effects in transgenic LQTS rabbit models: changes in pro-arrhythmia markers. **(A)** Changes in *in vivo* pro-arrhythmia markers. (i.) Bar graphs show changes in QTc, STV_{QT}, and T_{peak}-T_{end} in anaesthetized animals after i.m. injection of I_{Kr}, I_{K1}, and I_{Ks}-blockers dofetilide, $BaCl_2$, HMR-1556, respectively in WT, LQT2, LQT5, and LQT2–5 rabbits [modified from (Hornyik et al., 2020)]. *p < 0.05 inter-genotype comparison, #p < 0.05 vs. baseline, T trend p < 0.1 vs. baseline. (ii.) I_{K1}-blocker midazolam-induced change in heart-rate corrected QT-index in free-moving male (solid bars) and female (hatched bars) WT, LQT1, and LQT2 rabbits is also shown. The dashed line represents the mean QT indexes in free-moving rabbits obtained with the genotype-specific correction formula (=100%) [modified from (Odening et al., 2008)]. *p < 0.05 vs. free-moving rabbits of the same genotype. (iii.) Bar graphs indicate I_{Kr}-blocker dofetilide-induced increase in STV_{QT} in WT and LQT5 animals [modified from (Major et al., 2016)]. Bsl, baseline; Dof, dofetilide.*p < 0.05 inter-genotype comparison, #p < 0.05 vs. baseline. **(B)** Changes in *ex vivo* pro-arrhythmia markers. Bar graphs of changes in action potential duration (ΔAPD75), action potential duration/stimulation cycle length ratio (ΔAPD/CL ratio and action potential triangulation (ΔAPD90-30) after 10 min perfusion with I_{Kr}, I_{K1} and I_{Ks}-blockers dofetilide, $BaCl_2$ and HMR-1556, respectively in WT, LQT2, LQT5, and LQT2–5 rabbits. *p < 0.05 inter-genotype comparison, #p < 0.05 vs. baseline [modified from (Hornyik et al., 2020)].

Transgenic LQTS Rabbit Models for Better Detection of Drug-Induced Ventricular Arrhythmias

Drug-induced proarrhythmia is based on regionally heterogeneous prolongation of cardiac repolarization caused by various groups of drugs blocking multiple ion channels. As it most-often occurs in patients with reduced repolarization reserve (see above), the use of various transgenic LQTS rabbit models (Brunner et al., 2008; Major et al., 2016) with increased sensitivities to potassium channel blocking effects and different degrees of impairment in their cardiac repolarization reserve, is expected to provide more reliable, and more thorough detection of (multi-channel-based) drug-induced ventricular arrhythmias.

Indeed, it has been shown that LQT1 rabbits lacking I_{Ks} and LQT5 rabbits with impaired I_{Ks} function were particularly sensitive in identifying I_{Kr}-blocking properties of drugs; while transgenic LQT2 rabbits lacking I_{Kr} demonstrated a particularly high sensitivity to I_{Ks}- or I_{K1}-blocking drugs (Volders et al., 2003; Jost et al., 2005; Odening et al., 2010; Odening et al., 2013; Hornyik et al., 2020) as further outlined in the following subchapters.

Investigation of Drug-Induced Changes in Proarrhythmia Markers in Transgenic LQTS Rabbit Models

Drug-induced arrhythmia is a relatively rare event, and arrhythmia development as "hard endpoint" cannot be directly studied—especially during "first-in-human" clinical trials. Therefore, model systems with increased susceptibility for proarrhythmia are employed for safety testing and changes in various proarrhythmia markers are monitored to assess the pro-arrhythmic potential of the investigated/applied drug.

Several biomarkers have been suggested to use for proarrhythmia screening that reflect changes in various aspects of repolarization such as: (i) duration (QTc, APD), (ii) spatial ($T_{peak-end}$, APD dispersion), and (iii) temporal dispersion (STV_{QT}, QT/RR steepness, APD restitution) of repolarization (for more details, see previous sections). These were also employed in the different transgenic LQTS rabbit models.

Transgenic LQT2 rabbits demonstrated a high sensitivity to I_{Ks}- or I_{K1}-blocking anesthetic agents such as isoflurane (I_{Ks}) or the anxiolytic sedative midazolam (I_{K1}) as demonstrated by a particularly pronounced prolongation of QT and heart-rate corrected QT index as compared to healthy rabbits (Odening et al., 2008) (**Figure 5A**). In addition, a pronounced increase in *in vivo* ECG proarrhythmia markers (QT, STV_{QT}, and $T_{peak-end}$) and *ex vivo* monophasic AP related proarrhythmia markers (APD, AP triangulation and APD restitution steepness) indicated higher susceptibility also to other I_{K1} and I_{Ks} blocking compounds ($BaCl_2$ and HMR-1556) in transgenic LQT2 and double-transgenic LQT2–5 rabbits (Hornyik et al., 2020) (**Figures 5A, B**).

LQT1 and LQT5 models; on the other hand, were especially sensitive to I_{Kr} blockade (dofetilide, E4031, and erythromycin), as demonstrated *in vivo* by a pronounced increase in QTc, STV_{QT}, and $T_{peak-end}$ and *ex vivo* by a prolongation of APD and (in LQT1) APD dispersion (Odening et al., 2010; Ziupa et al., 2014; Major et al., 2016).

Investigation of *Ex Vivo* Susceptibility to Arrhythmia in Isolated Transgenic LQTS Rabbit Hearts

The direct assessment of *ex vivo* arrhythmia development in isolated Langendorff-perfused transgenic LQTS rabbit hearts were first performed by Hornyik et al., using different provocation factors—such as bradycardia, low $[K^+]_o$, and/or application of K^+-channel blockers—that are also crucial in drug-induced proarrhythmia formation in the clinical setting (Hornyik et al., 2020). It was shown that the application of I_{K1}-blocker $BaCl_2$ alone already significantly increased the incidence and duration of ventricular extra beats in LQT2 and LQT2–5 hearts (**Figure 6A**). When the pre-existing temporal, beat-to-beat-QT-instability, and the prolonged, regionally heterogeneous repolarization were even further aggravated by lowering the $[K^+]_o$, the sensitivity for re-entry formation was increased, leading to significantly longer duration and higher incidence of more malignant type of ventricular arrhythmias (VT and VF) in LQT2 and LQT2–5 but not in healthy WT hearts (**Figure 6A**). In LQT5 hearts with less pronounced reduction of repolarization reserve, only less severe types of ventricular arrhythmias (bigeminy) were detected. These observations of a higher sensitivity of transgenic LQTS hearts to potassium channel blocking drugs than normal WT hearts suggests that the use of different transgenic LQTS rabbits might help in more reliably detect drug-induced proarrhythmia.

Investigation of *In Vivo* Susceptibility to Arrhythmia of Transgenic LQTS Rabbits

High *in vivo* susceptibility to arrhythmia of transgenic LQTS rabbit models were demonstrated as early as the first characterizations of the models were performed.

In transgenic LQT2 rabbit models, exhibiting regionally heterogeneous prolongation of repolarization, VT and VF easily occurred spontaneously resulting in high SCD rates (Brunner et al., 2008). In addition, a further reduction of repolarization reserve by the I_{Ks}-blocker isoflurane or by the I_{to}-/I_{Ks}-blocker propofol led to increased proarrhythmia with a variety of arrhythmic events such as AV 2:1 blocks, T-wave alternans, PVCs, bigeminy, and lethal TdP occurring even during short episodes of anesthesia (Odening et al., 2008) (**Figure 6B**).

Transgenic LQT1 rabbits with normal/physiological heart rates and/or without organic heart diseases exhibited relatively homogenous prolongation of repolarization in the LV without substantial increase in APD dispersion; therefore, no spontaneous arrhythmias and SCD were detected (Brunner et al., 2008). When the repolarization reserve of LQT1 rabbits were further challenged by continuous tachypacing or AV-ablation to induce cardiac tachymyopathy (Lau et al., 2015), or complete AV-block (Kim et al., 2015), respectively, however, significant APD dispersion and discordant alternans developed and VT/VF was easily inducible and even occurred spontaneously (Lau et al., 2015). The model also demonstrated the development of pseudo-AV blocks and drug-induced TdP

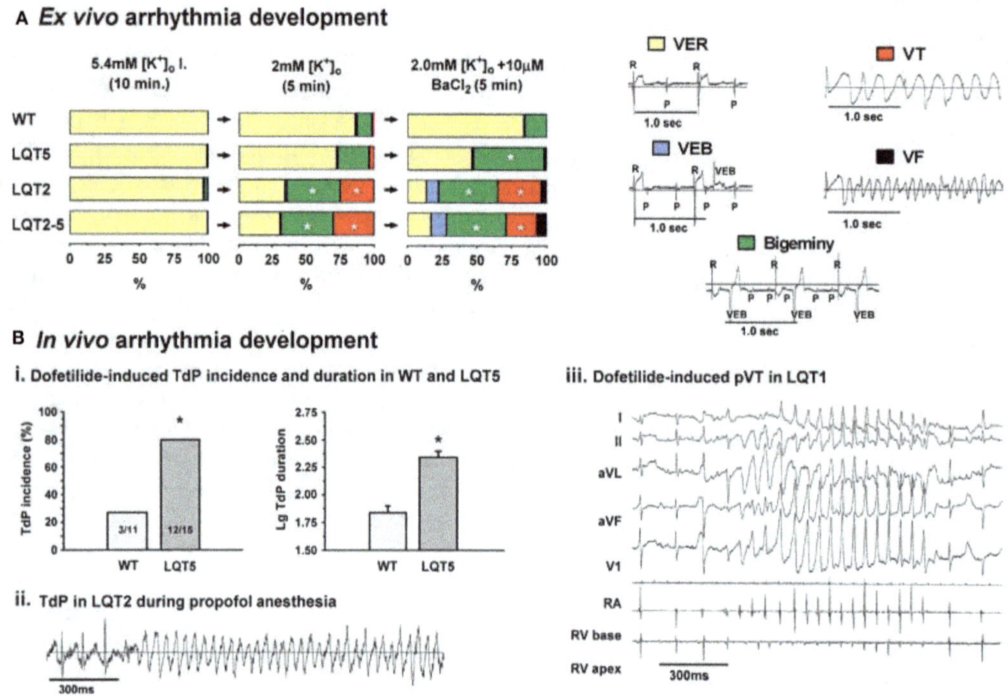

FIGURE 6 | Pro-arrhythmic drug-effects in transgenic LQTS rabbit models: arrhythmia development. **(A)** *Ex vivo* arrhythmia development. Graphs indicating the duration (% of perfusion time) of arrhythmias provoked by perfusing the hearts with low $[K^+]_o$ (2 mM) KH, or with combined low $[K^+]_o$ (2 mM) KH and I_{K1}-blocker $BaCl_2$ (10 µM) in WT, LQT5, LQT2 and LQT2–5 animals. Inlets show representative ECG recordings of ventricular escape rhythm (VER), ventricular extra beats (VEB), bigeminy, ventricular tachycardia (VT) and ventricular fibrillation (VF) [modified from (Hornyik et al., 2020)]. $^*p < 0.05$ inter-genotype comparison. **(B)** *In vivo* arrhythmia development. (i.) Bar graphs of dofetilide-induced incidence (in %) and log duration of torsade de pointes (TdP) tachycardia in WT and LQT5 rabbits [modified from (Major et al., 2016)]. $^*p < 0.05$ inter-genotype comparison. (ii.) Episode of polymorphic TdP tachycardia in female LQT2 rabbit during propofol anesthesia (acquired with telemetric ECG) [modified from (Odening et al., 2008)]. (iii.) Episode of dofetilide-induced pVT in male LQT1 rabbit during episode of alternating AV 2:1/3:1 block [modified from (Odening et al., 2010)].

upon I_{Kr}-blockade by dofetilide and E4031 (Odening et al., 2010; Ziupa et al., 2014; Major et al., 2016; Ziupa et al., 2019) (**Figure 6B**).

The recently generated LQT5 model with slight reduction in I_{Ks} function similarly demonstrated more pronounced I_{Kr}-blocker dofetilide induced TdP formation *in vivo* than healthy WT rabbits (Major et al., 2016) (**Figure 6B**).

Limitations of the Currently Available Models and Outlook

As the "dominant-negative" transgenic strategy was used to generate the LQTS rabbits, instead of a rabbit gene "knock-out"/human transgene "knock in" approach; these models are genetically distinct from LQTS patients. Newly emerging genetic engineering techniques such as CRISPR-cas [as described in details in (Bosze et al., 2016)] may help to develop novel—also genetically closer—animal models for these human diseases. As currently available models demonstrate a LQTS phenotype, however, with different degrees of reduction in repolarization reserve and increased susceptibility to arrhythmia both spontaneously and particularly upon drug-induced ion channel blockade, they could still represent valuable models for proarrhythmia safety testing in the context of reduced repolarization reserve.

Furthermore, compensatory electro-mechanical adaptation of cardiomyocytes in response to the altered function ("cardiac remodeling") can also show species differences that could influence their arrhythmia sensitivity. In transgenic LQTS mice, for example, the observed compensatory upregulation of non-affected potassium currents limit their use in identifying repolarizing prolonging—potentially pro-arrhythmic—agents, as opposed to transgenic LQTS rabbits, in which parallel decrease in reciprocal repolarizing current(s) was seen (Brunner et al., 2008) that even further increased the sensitivity of these models to detect drug-induced proarrhythmia. Currently, very little is known about the nature and extent of these compensatory remodeling processes in human diseases with impaired cardiac repolarization reserve; therefore, it is not known, which animal model mimics most accurately human pathophysiology from this aspect.

In spite of similarities in cardiac ion channels in rabbits and humans, cardiac repolarization is still conveyed through ion channels with slightly different biophysiological characteristics in each species; therefore, caution has to be applied when translating findings based on data from experimental animal models into humans.

Current animal models focus on the detection of repolarization prolonging pro-arrhythmic effects. Drug-induced proarrhythmia may, however, also occur upon pathologically pronounced acceleration/shortening of cardiac repolarization (Malik, 2016). Here, novel models such as the transgenic short QT syndrome rabbit model (Odening et al., 2019), may be particularly useful for the detection of these pro-arrhythmic drug properties.

Further improvement of current *in silico* proarrhythmia screening capabilities by integrating experimental *in vivo*, whole heart, cellular, and ion channel data into computational models are highly warranted (Sager et al., 2014; Colatsky et al., 2016), and could potentially lead to better assessment of mutation-specific aspects of a wide range of cardiac channelopathies, since currently available animal models mimicking cardiac channelopathies are very limited.

Importantly, the future use of patient-specific and/or disease-specific human induced pluripotent stem cell derived cardiomyocytes (iPSC-CM) has the potential to become a relevant additional patient/disease-specific *in vitro* safety screening platform to test the pro-arrhythmic potential of novel drug candidates (Mehta et al., 2013; Sager et al., 2014; Colatsky et al., 2016).

AUTHOR CONTRIBUTIONS

IB wrote the manuscript and designed the figures. TH wrote the manuscript and designed the figures. MB and GK generated the LQT1 and LQT2 rabbits and edited the manuscript. KO wrote the manuscript and designed the figures.

FUNDING

This work was supported by a grant from the German Heart Foundation (F/02/14) and grants from the German Research Foundation (OD 86/6-1, and BR 2107/4-1) to KO and the Hungarian National Research, Development and Innovation Office (NKFIH K128851) and Ministry of Human Capacities (EFOP-3.6.2-16-2017-00006) to IB.

REFERENCES

Amos, G. J., Abrahamsson, C., Duker, G., Hondeghem, L., Palmer, M., and Carlsson, L. (2001). Potassium and calcium current blocking properties of the novel antiarrhythmic agent H 345/52: implications for proarrhythmic potential. *Cardiovasc. Res.* 49, 351–360. doi: 10.1016/S0008-6363(00)00259-5

Anderson, M. E. (2006). QT interval prolongation and arrhythmia: an unbreakable connection? *J. Intern. Med.* 259, 81–90. doi: 10.1111/j.1365-2796.2005.01580.x

Ando, F., Kuruma, A., and Kawano, S. (2011). Synergic effects of beta-estradiol and erythromycin on hERG currents. *J. Membr. Biol.* 241, 31–38. doi: 10.1007/s00232-011-9360-z

Antoons, G., Oros, A., Beekman, J. D., Engelen, M. A., Houtman, M. J., Belardinelli, L., et al. (2010). Late na(+) current inhibition by ranolazine reduces torsades de pointes in the chronic atrioventricular block dog model. *J. Am. Coll. Cardiol.* 55, 801–809. doi: 10.1016/j.jacc.2009.10.033

Antzelevitch, C. (2007). Role of spatial dispersion of repolarization in inherited and acquired sudden cardiac death syndromes. *Am. J. Physiol. Heart Circ. Physiol.* 293, H2024–H2038. doi: 10.1152/ajpheart.00355.2007

Antzelevitch, C. (2008). Drug-induced spatial dispersion of repolarization. *Cardiol. J.* 15, 100–121.

Authier, S., Pugsley, M. K., Koerner, J. E., Fermini, B., Redfern, W. S., Valentin, J. P., et al. (2017). Proarrhythmia liability assessment and the comprehensive in vitro Proarrhythmia Assay (CiPA): An industry survey on current practice. *J. Pharmacol. Toxicol. Methods* 86, 34–43. doi: 10.1016/j.vascn.2017.02.021

Baczko, I., Jost, N., Virag, L., Bosze, Z., and Varro, A. (2016). Rabbit models as tools for preclinical cardiac electrophysiological safety testing: Importance of repolarization reserve. *Prog. Biophys. Mol. Biol.* 121, 157–168. doi: 10.1016/j.pbiomolbio.2016.05.002

Barbhaiya, C., Po, J. R., Hanon, S., and Schweitzer, P. (2013). Tpeak - Tend and Tpeak - Tend /QT ratio as markers of ventricular arrhythmia risk in cardiac resynchronization therapy patients. *Pacing Clin. Electrophysiol.* 36, 103–108. doi: 10.1111/pace.12031

Baumert, M., Porta, A., Vos, M. A., Malik, M., Couderc, J. P., Laguna, P., et al. (2016). QT interval variability in body surface ECG: measurement, physiological basis, and clinical value: position statement and consensus guidance endorsed by the European Heart Rhythm Association jointly with the ESC Working Group on Cardiac Cellular Electrophysiology. *Europace* 18, 925–944. doi: 10.1093/europace/euv405

Baumgartner, D., Scholl-Burgi, S., Sass, J. O., Sperl, W., Schweigmann, U., Stein, J. I., et al. (2007). Prolonged QTc-intervals and decreased left ventricular contractility in patients with propionic acidemia. *J. Pediatr.* 150, 192–197. doi: 10.1016/j.jpeds.2006.11.043

Belardinelli, L., Antzelevitch, C., and Vos, M. A. (2003). Assessing predictors of drug-induced torsade de pointes. *Trends Pharmacol. Sci.* 24, 619–625. doi: 10.1016/j.tips.2003.10.002

Benton, R. E., Sale, M., Flockhart, D. A., and Woosley, R. L. (2000). Greater quinidine-induced QTc interval prolongation in women. *Clin. Pharmacol. Ther.* 67, 413–418. doi: 10.1067/mcp.2000.105761

Blenck, C. L., Harvey, P. A., Reckelhoff, J. F., and Leinwand, L. A. (2016). The Importance of Biological Sex and Estrogen in Rodent Models of Cardiovascular Health and Disease. *Circ. Res.* 118, 1294–1312. doi: 10.1161/CIRCRESAHA.116.307509

Bodi, I., Grunert, S. C., Becker, N., Stoelzle-Feix, S., Spiekerkoetter, U., Zehender, M., et al. (2016). Mechanisms of acquired Long QT syndrome in patients with propionic academia. *Heart Rhythm.* 13, 1335–1345. doi: 10.1016/j.hrthm.2016.02.003

Bosze, Z., Major, P., Baczko, I., Odening, K. E., Bodrogi, L., Hiripi, L., et al. (2016). The potential impact of new generation transgenic methods on creating rabbit models of cardiac diseases. *Prog. Biophys. Mol. Biol.* 121, 123–130. doi: 10.1016/j.pbiomolbio.2016.05.007

Bouder, F. (2007). A case study of long QT regulation: A regulatory tennis game across the Atlantic. *J. Risk Res.* 10, 385–412. doi: 10.1080/13669870701270903

Brunner, M., Guo, W., Mitchell, G. F., Buckett, P. D., Nerbonne, J. M., and Koren, G. (2001). Characterization of mice with a combined suppression of I(to) and I(K,slow). *Am. J. Physiol. Heart Circ. Physiol.* 281, H1201–H1209. doi: 10.1152/ajpheart.2001.281.3.H1201

Brunner, M., Peng, X., Liu, G. X., Ren, X. Q., Ziv, O., Choi, B. R., et al. (2008). Mechanisms of cardiac arrhythmias and sudden death in transgenic rabbits with long QT syndrome. *J. Clin. Invest.* 118, 2246–2259. doi: 10.1172/JCI33578

Carlsson, L., Andersson, B., Linhardt, G., and Lofberg, L. (2009). Assessment of the ion channel-blocking profile of the novel combined ion channel blocker AZD1305 and its proarrhythmic potential versus dofetilide in the methoxamine-sensitized rabbit in vivo. *J. Cardiovasc. Pharmacol.* 54, 82–89. doi: 10.1097/FJC.0b013e3181ac62c9

Carlsson, L. (2001). Drug-induced torsade de pointes: the perspectives of industry. *Eur. Heart J. Suppl.* 3, K114–K120. doi: 10.1016/S1520-765X(01)90016-1

Carlsson, L. (2008). The anaesthetised methoxamine-sensitised rabbit model of torsades de pointes. *Pharmacol. Ther.* 119, 160–167. doi: 10.1016/j.pharmthera.2008.04.004

Cavero, I., and Holzgrefe, H. (2014). Comprehensive in vitro Proarrhythmia Assay, a novel in vitro/in silico paradigm to detect ventricular proarrhythmic liability: a visionary 21st century initiative. *Expert Opin. Drug Saf.* 13, 745–758. doi: 10.1517/14740338.2014.915311

Chen, G., Yang, X., Alber, S., Shusterman, V., and Salama, G. (2011). Regional genomic regulation of cardiac sodium-calcium exchanger by oestrogen. *J. Physiol.* 589, 1061–1080. doi: 10.1113/jphysiol.2010.203398

Choi, B. R., Burton, F., and Salama, G. (2002). Cytosolic Ca2+ triggers early afterdepolarizations and Torsade de Pointes in rabbit hearts with type 2 long QT syndrome. *J. Physiology-London* 543, 615–631. doi: 10.1113/jphysiol.2002.024570

Choi, B. R., Li, W., Terentyev, D., Kabakov, A. Y., Zhong, M., Rees, C. M., et al. (2018). Transient Outward K(+) Current (Ito) Underlies the Right Ventricular Initiation of Polymorphic Ventricular Tachycardia in a Transgenic Rabbit Model of Long-QT Syndrome Type 1. *Circ. Arrhythm. Electrophysiol.* 11, e005414. doi: 10.1161/CIRCEP.117.005414

Colatsky, T., Fermini, B., Gintant, G., Pierson, J. B., Sager, P., Sekino, Y., et al. (2016). The Comprehensive in Vitro Proarrhythmia Assay (CiPA) initiative - Update on progress. *J. Pharmacol. Toxicol. Methods* 81, 15–20. doi: 10.1016/j.vascn.2016.06.002

Crumb, W. J.Jr., Vicente, J., Johannesen, L., and Strauss, D. G. (2016). An evaluation of 30 clinical drugs against the comprehensive in vitro proarrhythmia assay (CiPA) proposed ion channel panel. *J. Pharmacol. Toxicol. Methods* 81, 251–262. doi: 10.1016/j.vascn.2016.03.009

Danker, T., and Moller, C. (2014). Early identification of hERG liability in drug discovery programs by automated patch clamp. *Front. Pharmacol.* 5, 203. doi: 10.3389/fphar.2014.00203

Darpo, B. (2001). Spectrum of drugs prolonging QT interval and the incidence of torsades de pointes. *Eur. Heart J. Suppl.* 3, K70–K80. doi: 10.1016/S1520-765X(01)90009-4

Decker, J. A., Rossano, J. W., Smith, E. O., Cannon, B., Clunie, S. K., Gates, C., et al. (2009). Risk factors and mode of death in isolated hypertrophic cardiomyopathy in children. *J. Am. Coll. Cardiol.* 54, 250–254. doi: 10.1016/j.jacc.2009.03.051

Derangeon, M., Montnach, J., Baro, I., and Charpentier, F. (2012). Mouse Models of SCN5A-Related Cardiac Arrhythmias. *Front. Physiol.* 3, 210. doi: 10.3389/fphys.2012.00210

Dhein, S., Perlitz, F., and Mohr, F. W. (2008). An in vitro model for assessment of drug-induced torsade de pointes arrhythmia : effects of haloperidol and dofetilide on potential duration, repolarization inhomogeneities, and torsade de pointes arrhythmia. *Naunyn Schmiedebergs Arch. Pharmacol.* 378, 631–644. doi: 10.1007/s00210-008-0329-0

Diness, T. G., Yeh, Y. H., Qi, X. Y., Chartier, D., Tsuji, Y., Hansen, R. S., et al. (2008). Antiarrhythmic properties of a rapid delayed-rectifier current activator in rabbit models of acquired long QT syndrome. *Cardiovasc. Res.* 79, 61–69. doi: 10.1093/cvr/cvn075

Drici, M. D., Burklow, T. R., Haridasse, V., Glazer, R. I., and Woosley, R. L. (1996). Sex hormones prolong the QT interval and downregulate potassium channel expression in the rabbit heart. *Circulation* 94, 1471–1474. doi: 10.1161/01.CIR.94.6.1471

Dutta, S., Minchole, A., Zacur, E., Quinn, T. A., Taggart, P., and Rodriguez, B. (2016). Early afterdepolarizations promote transmural reentry in ischemic human ventricles with reduced repolarization reserve. *Prog. Biophys. Mol. Biol.* 120, 236–248. doi: 10.1016/j.pbiomolbio.2016.01.008

Echt, D. S., Liebson, P. R., Mitchell, L. B., Peters, R. W., Obias-Manno, D., Barker, A. H., et al. (1991). Mortality and morbidity in patients receiving encainide, flecainide, or placebo. The Cardiac Arrhythmia Suppression Trial. *N. Engl. J. Med.* 324, 781–788. doi: 10.1056/NEJM199103213241201

Eisenberg, S. J., Scheinman, M. M., Dullet, N. K., Finkbeiner, W. E., Griffin, J. C., Eldar, M., et al. (1995). Sudden cardiac death and polymorphous ventricular tachycardia in patients with normal QT intervals and normal systolic cardiac function. *Am. J. Cardiol.* 75, 687–692. doi: 10.1016/S0002-9149(99)80654-7

El-Sherif, N., and Turitto, G. (1999). The long QT syndrome and torsade de pointes. *Pacing Clin. Electrophysiol.* 22, 91–110. doi: 10.1111/j.1540-8159.1999.tb00305.x

Fabritz, L., Kirchhof, P., Franz, M. R., Nuyens, D., Rossenbacker, T., Ottenhof, A., et al. (2003). Effect of pacing and mexiletine on dispersion of repolarisation and arrhythmias in DeltaKPQ SCN5A (long QT3) mice. *Cardiovasc. Res.* 57, 1085–1093. doi: 10.1016/S0008-6363(02)00839-8

Farkas, A. S., and Nattel, S. (2010). Minimizing repolarization-related proarrhythmic risk in drug development and clinical practice. *Drugs* 70, 573–603. doi: 10.2165/11535230-000000000-00000

Farkas, A. S., Acsai, K., Toth, A., Dezsi, L., Orosz, S., Forster, T., et al. (2006). Importance of extracardiac alpha1-adrenoceptor stimulation in assisting dofetilide to induce torsade de pointes in rabbit hearts. *Eur. J. Pharmacol.* 537, 118–125. doi: 10.1016/j.ejphar.2006.03.014

Fedida, D., and Giles, W. R. (1991). Regional variations in action potentials and transient outward current in myocytes isolated from rabbit left ventricle. *J. Physiol.* 442, 191–209. doi: 10.1113/jphysiol.1991.sp018789

Fenichel, R. R., Malik, M., Antzelevitch, C., Sanguinetti, M., Roden, D. M., Priori, S. G., et al. (2004). Drug-induced torsades de pointes and implications for drug development. *J. Cardiovasc. Electrophysiol.* 15, 475–495. doi: 10.1046/j.1540-8167.2004.03534.x

Ferdinandy, P., Baczko, I., Bencsik, P., Giricz, Z., Gorbe, A., Pacher, P., et al. (2019). Definition of hidden drug cardiotoxicity: paradigm change in cardiac safety testing and its clinical implications. *Eur. Heart J.* 40, 1771–1777. doi: 10.1093/eurheartj/ehy365

Food, and Drug Administration, H.H.S (2005a). International Conference on Harmonisation; guidance on E14 Clinical Evaluation of QT/QTc Interval Prolongation and Proarrhythmic Potential for Non-Antiarrhythmic Drugs; availability. Notice. *Fed. Regist.* 70, 61134–61135.

Food, and Drug Administration, H.H.S (2005b). International Conference on Harmonisation; guidance on S7B Nonclinical Evaluation of the Potential for Delayed Ventricular Repolarization (QT Interval Prolongation) by Human Pharmaceuticals; availability. Notice. *Fed. Regist.* 70, 61133–61134.

Furukawa, T., and Kurokawa, J. (2008). Non-genomic regulation of cardiac ion channels by sex hormones. *Cardiovasc. Hematol. Disord. Drug Targets* 8, 245–251. doi: 10.2174/187152908786786160

Gill, G. V., Woodward, A., Casson, I. F., and Weston, P. J. (2009). Cardiac arrhythmia and nocturnal hypoglycaemia in type 1 diabetes–the 'dead in bed' syndrome revisited. *Diabetologia* 52, 42–45. doi: 10.1007/s00125-008-1177-7

Giunti, S., Bruno, G., Lillaz, E., Gruden, G., Lolli, V., Chaturvedi, N., et al. (2007). Incidence and risk factors of prolonged QTc interval in type 1 diabetes: the EURODIAB Prospective Complications Study. *Diabetes Care* 30, 2057–2063. doi: 10.2337/dc07-0063

Gowda, R. M., Khan, I. A., Punukollu, G., Vasavada, B. C., Sacchi, T. J., and Wilbur, S. L. (2004). Female preponderance in ibutilide-induced torsade de pointes. *Int. J. Cardiol.* 95, 219–222. doi: 10.1016/j.ijcard.2003.04.034

Grandy, S. A., Trepanier-Boulay, V., and Fiset, C. (2007). Postnatal development has a marked effect on ventricular repolarization in mice. *Am. J. Physiol. Heart Circ. Physiol.* 293, H2168–H2177. doi: 10.1152/ajpheart.00521.2007

Guerard, N., Jordaan, P., and Dumotier, B. (2014). Analysis of unipolar electrograms in rabbit heart demonstrated the key role of ventricular apicobasal dispersion in arrhythmogenicity. *Cardiovasc. Toxicol.* 14, 316–328. doi: 10.1007/s12012-014-9254-2

Hancox, J. C., Mcpate, M. J., El Harchi, A., and Zhang, Y. H. (2008). The hERG potassium channel and hERG screening for drug-induced torsades de pointes. *Pharmacol. Ther.* 119, 118–132. doi: 10.1016/j.pharmthera.2008.05.009

Harken, A. H., Simson, M. B., Haselgrove, J., Wetstein, L., Harden, W., and Barlow, C. H. (1981). Early ischemia after complete coronary ligation in the rabbit, dog, pig, and monkey. *Am. J. Physiol.* 241, H202–H210. doi: 10.1152/ajpheart.1981.241.2.H202

Haverkamp, W., Breithardt, G., Camm, A. J., Janse, M. J., Rosen, M. R., Antzelevitch, C., et al. (2000). The potential for QT prolongation and pro-arrhythmia by non-anti-arrhythmic drugs: clinical and regulatory implications. Report on a Policy Conference of the European Society of Cardiology. *Cardiovasc. Res.* 47, 219–233. doi: 10.1016/S0008-6363(00)00119-X

Hinterseer, M., Thomsen, M. B., Beckmann, B. M., Pfeufer, A., Schimpf, R., Wichmann, H. E., et al. (2008). Beat-to-beat variability of QT intervals is increased in patients with drug-induced long-QT syndrome: a case control pilot study. *Eur. Heart J.* 29, 185–190. doi: 10.1093/eurheartj/ehm586

Hinterseer, M., Beckmann, B. M., Thomsen, M. B., Pfeufer, A., Dalla Pozza, R., Loeff, M., et al. (2009). Relation of increased short-term variability of QT interval to congenital long-QT syndrome. *Am. J. Cardiol.* 103, 1244–1248. doi: 10.1016/j.amjcard.2009.01.011

Hinterseer, M., Beckmann, B. M., Thomsen, M. B., Pfeufer, A., Ulbrich, M., Sinner, M. F., et al. (2010). Usefulness of short-term variability of QT intervals as a predictor for electrical remodeling and proarrhythmia in patients with nonischemic heart failure. *Am. J. Cardiol.* 106, 216–220. doi: 10.1016/j.amjcard.2010.02.033

Hondeghem, L. M., and Hoffmann, P. (2003). Blinded test in isolated female rabbit heart reliably identifies action potential duration prolongation and proarrhythmic drugs: importance of triangulation, reverse use dependence, and instability. *J. Cardiovasc. Pharmacol.* 41, 14–24. doi: 10.1097/00005344-200301000-00003

Hondeghem, L. M., Carlsson, L., and Duker, G. (2001). Instability and triangulation of the action potential predict serious proarrhythmia, but action potential duration prolongation is antiarrhythmic. *Circulation* 103, 2004–2013. doi: 10.1161/01.CIR.103.15.2004

Hondeghem, L. M., De Clerck, F., and Camm, J. (2007). Short patent lives jeopardize drug and patient safety. *J. Cardiovasc. Pharmacol.* 50, 353–357. doi: 10.1097/FJC.0b013e3181514032

Hondeghem, L. M. (2016). Disturbances of cardiac wavelength and repolarization precede Torsade de Pointes and ventricular fibrillation in Langendorff perfused rabbit hearts. *Prog. Biophys. Mol. Biol.* 121, 3–10. doi: 10.1016/j.pbiomolbio.2016.03.004

Hornyik, T., Castiglione, A., Franke, G., Perez-Feliz, S., Major, P., Hiripi, L., et al. (2020). Transgenic LQT2, LQT5 and LQT2-5 rabbit models with decreased repolarization reserve for prediction of drug-induced ventricular arrhythmias. *Br. J. Pharmacol.* doi: 10.1111/bph.15098

Huang, H., Pugsley, M. K., Fermini, B., Curtis, M. J., Koerner, J., Accardi, M., et al. (2017). Cardiac voltage-gated ion channels in safety pharmacology: Review of the landscape leading to the CiPA initiative. *J. Pharmacol. Toxicol. Methods* 87, 11–23. doi: 10.1016/j.vascn.2017.04.002

Husti, Z., Tabori, K., Juhasz, V., Hornyik, T., Varro, A., and Baczko, I. (2015). Combined inhibition of key potassium currents has different effects on cardiac repolarization reserve and arrhythmia susceptibility in dogs and rabbits. *Can. J. Physiol. Pharmacol.* 93, 535–544. doi: 10.1139/cjpp-2014-0514

Inaba, H., Hayami, N., Ajiki, K., Kunishima, T., Watanabe, H., Tsutsui, K., et al. (2011). Deep anesthesia suppresses ventricular tachyarrhythmias in rabbit model of the acquired long QT syndrome. *Circ. J.* 75, 89–93. doi: 10.1253/circj.CJ-10-0478

Jacobson, I., Carlsson, L., and Duker, G. (2011). Beat-by-beat QT interval variability, but not QT prolongation per se, predicts drug-induced torsades de pointes in the anaesthetised methoxamine-sensitized rabbit. *J. Pharmacol. Toxicol. Methods* 63, 40–46. doi: 10.1016/j.vascn.2010.04.010

Jameson, E., and Walter, J. (2008). Cardiac arrest secondary to long QT(C) in a child with propionic acidemia. *Pediatr. Cardiol.* 29, 969–970. doi: 10.1007/s00246-007-9160-5

Jost, N., Virag, L., Bitay, M., Takacs, J., Lengyel, C., Biliczki, P., et al. (2005). Restricting excessive cardiac action potential and QT prolongation: a vital role for IKs in human ventricular muscle. *Circulation* 112, 1392–1399. doi: 10.1161/CIRCULATIONAHA.105.550111

Jost, N., Virag, L., Comtois, P., Ordog, B., Szuts, V., Seprenyi, G., et al. (2013). Ionic mechanisms limiting cardiac repolarization reserve in humans compared to dogs. *J. Physiol.* 591, 4189–4206. doi: 10.1113/jphysiol.2013.261198

Jung, B., Odening, K. E., Dall'armellina, E., Foll, D., Menza, M., Markl, M., et al. (2012). A quantitative comparison of regional myocardial motion in mice, rabbits and humans using in-vivo phase contrast CMR. *J. Cardiovasc. Magn. Reson* 14, 87. doi: 10.1186/1532-429X-14-87

Kaab, S., Hinterseer, M., Nabauer, M., and Steinbeck, G. (2003). Sotalol testing unmasks altered repolarization in patients with suspected acquired long-QT-syndrome - a case-control pilot study using i.v. sotalol. *Eur. Heart J.* 24, 649–657. doi: 10.1016/S0195-668X(02)00806-0

Kaese, S., and Verheule, S. (2012). Cardiac electrophysiology in mice: a matter of size. *Front. Physiol.* 3, 345. doi: 10.3389/fphys.2012.00345

Kakavand, B., Schroeder, V. A., and Di Sessa, T. G. (2006). Coincidence of long QT syndrome and propionic acidemia. *Pediatr. Cardiol.* 27, 160–161. doi: 10.1007/s00246-005-1129-7

Kannankeril, P., Roden, D. M., and Darbar, D. (2010). Drug-induced long QT syndrome. *Pharmacol. Rev.* 62, 760–781. doi: 10.1124/pr.110.003723

Kim, T. Y., Kunitomo, Y., Pfeiffer, Z., Patel, D., Hwang, J., Harrison, K., et al. (2015). Complex excitation dynamics underlie polymorphic ventricular tachycardia in a transgenic rabbit model of long QT syndrome type 1. *Heart Rhythm.* 12, 220–228. doi: 10.1016/j.hrthm.2014.10.003

Kjekshus, J. (1990). Arrhythmias and mortality in congestive heart failure. *Am. J. Cardiol.* 65, 42I–48I. doi: 10.1016/0002-9149(90)90125-K

Kramer, J., Obejero-Paz, C. A., Myatt, G., Kuryshev, Y. A., Bruening-Wright, A., Verducci, J. S., et al. (2013). MICE models: superior to the HERG model in predicting Torsade de Pointes. *Sci. Rep.* 3, 2100. doi: 10.1038/srep02100

Kristof, A., Husti, Z., Koncz, I., Kohajda, Z., Szel, T., Juhasz, V., et al. (2012). Diclofenac prolongs repolarization in ventricular muscle with impaired repolarization reserve. *PloS One* 7, e53255. doi: 10.1371/journal.pone.0053255

Kurokawa, J., Tamagawa, M., Harada, N., Honda, S., Bai, C. X., Nakaya, H., et al. (2008). Acute effects of oestrogen on the guinea pig and human IKr channels and drug-induced prolongation of cardiac repolarization. *J. Physiol.* 586, 2961–2973. doi: 10.1113/jphysiol.2007.150367

Kusano, K. F., Hata, Y., Yumoto, A., Emori, T., Sato, T., and Ohe, T. (2001). Torsade de pointes with a normal QT interval associated with hypokalemia: a case report. *Jpn. Circ. J.* 65, 757–760. doi: 10.1253/jcj.65.757

Lang, C. N., Koren, G., and Odening, K. E. (2016). Transgenic rabbit models to investigate the cardiac ion channel disease long QT syndrome. *Prog. Biophys. Mol. Biol.* 121, 142–156. doi: 10.1016/j.pbiomolbio.2016.05.004

Lau, E., Kossidas, K., Kim, T. Y., Kunitomo, Y., Ziv, O., Song, Z., et al. (2015). Spatially Discordant Alternans and Arrhythmias in Tachypacing-Induced Cardiac Myopathy in Transgenic LQT1 Rabbits: The Importance of IKs and Ca2+ Cycling. *PloS One* 10, e0122754. doi: 10.1145/2818302

Lawrence, C. L., Pollard, C. E., Hammond, T. G., and Valentin, J. P. (2005). Nonclinical proarrhythmia models: predicting Torsades de Pointes. *J. Pharmacol. Toxicol. Methods* 52, 46–59. doi: 10.1016/j.vascn.2005.04.011

Lehmann, M. H., Hardy, S., Archibald, D., Quart, B., and Macneil, D. J. (1996). Sex difference in risk of torsade de pointes with d,l-sotalol. *Circulation* 94, 2535–2541. doi: 10.1161/01.CIR.94.10.2535

Lengyel, C., Varro, A., Tabori, K., Papp, J. G., and Baczko, I. (2007a). Combined pharmacological block of I(Kr) and I(Ks) increases short-term QT interval variability and provokes torsades de pointes. *Br. J. Pharmacol.* 151, 941–951. doi: 10.1038/sj.bjp.0707297

Lengyel, C., Virag, L., Biro, T., Jost, N., Magyar, J., Biliczki, P., et al. (2007b). Diabetes mellitus attenuates the repolarization reserve in mammalian heart. *Cardiovasc. Res.* 73, 512–520. doi: 10.1016/j.cardiores.2006.11.010

Lengyel, C., Virag, L., Kovacs, P. P., Kristof, A., Pacher, P., Kocsis, E., et al. (2008). Role of slow delayed rectifier K+-current in QT prolongation in the alloxan-induced diabetic rabbit heart. *Acta Physiol. (Oxf)* 192, 359–368. doi: 10.1111/j.1748-1716.2007.01753.x

Li, Z., Mirams, G. R., Yoshinaga, T., Ridder, B. J., Han, X., Chen, J. E., et al. (2019). General Principles for the Validation of Proarrhythmia Risk Prediction Models: An Extension of the CiPA In Silico Strategy. *Clin. Pharmacol. Ther.* 107, 102–111. doi: 10.1002/cpt.1647

Liu, X. K., Katchman, A., Whitfield, B. H., Wan, G., Janowski, E. M., Woosley, R. L., et al. (2003). In vivo androgen treatment shortens the QT interval and increases the densities of inward and delayed rectifier potassium currents in orchiectomized male rabbits. *Cardiovasc. Res.* 57, 28–36. doi: 10.1016/S0008-6363(02)00673-9

Liu, G. X., Zhou, J., and Koren, G. (2008). Single-channel properties of I K,slow1 and I K,slow2 in mouse ventricular myocytes. *Pflugers Arch.* 456, 541–547. doi: 10.1007/s00424-007-0436-7

Liu, G. X., Choi, B. R., Ziv, O., Li, W., De Lange, E., Qu, Z., et al. (2012). Differential conditions for early after-depolarizations and triggered activity in cardiomyocytes derived from transgenic LQT1 and LQT2 rabbits. *J. Physiol.* 590, 1171–1180. doi: 10.1113/jphysiol.2011.218164

Liu, W., Kim, T. Y., Huang, X., Liu, M. B., Koren, G., Choi, B. R., et al. (2018). Mechanisms linking T-wave alternans to spontaneous initiation of ventricular arrhythmias in rabbit models of long QT syndrome. *J. Physiol.* 596, 1341–1355. doi: 10.1113/JP275492

Locati, E. H., Zareba, W., Moss, A. J., Schwartz, P. J., Vincent, G. M., Lehmann, M. H., et al. (1998). Age- and sex-related differences in clinical manifestations in patients with congenital long-QT syndrome: findings from the International LQTS Registry. *Circulation* 97, 2237–2244. doi: 10.1161/01.CIR.97.22.2237

London, B., Jeron, A., Zhou, J., Buckett, P., Han, X., Mitchell, G. F., et al. (1998). Long QT and ventricular arrhythmias in transgenic mice expressing the N terminus and first transmembrane segment of a voltage-gated potassium channel. *Proc. Natl. Acad. Sci. U. S. A* 95, 2926–2931. doi: 10.1073/pnas.95.6.2926

Major, P., Baczko, I., Hiripi, L., Odening, K. E., Juhasz, V., Kohajda, Z., et al. (2016). A novel transgenic rabbit model with reduced repolarization reserve: long QT syndrome caused by a dominant-negative mutation of the KCNE1 gene. *Br. J. Pharmacol.* 173, 2046–2061. doi: 10.1111/bph.13500

Malik, M. (2016). Drug-Induced QT/QTc Interval Shortening: Lessons from Drug-Induced QT/QTc Prolongation. *Drug Saf.* 39, 647–659. doi: 10.1007/s40264-016-0411-3

Maron, B. J., Leyhe, M. J.3rd, Casey, S. A., Gohman, T. E., Lawler, C. M., Crow, R. S., et al. (2001). Assessment of QT dispersion as a prognostic marker for sudden death in a regional nonreferred hypertrophic cardiomyopathy cohort. *Am. J. Cardiol.* 87, 114–115, A119. doi: 10.1016/S0002-9149(00)01285-6

Maruyama, M., Lin, S. F., Xie, Y. F., Chua, S. K., Joung, B., Han, S., et al. (2011). Genesis of Phase 3 Early Afterdepolarizations and Triggered Activity in Acquired Long-QT Syndrome. *Circulation-Arrhythmia Electrophysiol.* 4, 103–10+. doi: 10.1161/CIRCEP.110.959064

Mcnally, P. G., Lawrence, I. G., Panerai, R. B., Weston, P. J., and Thurston, H. (1999). Sudden death in type 1 diabetes. *Diabetes Obes. Metab.* 1, 151–158. doi: 10.1046/j.1463-1326.1999.00025.x

Mehta, A., Chung, Y., Sequiera, G. L., Wong, P., Liew, R., and Shim, W. (2013). Pharmacoelectrophysiology of viral-free induced pluripotent stem cell-derived human cardiomyocytes. *Toxicol. Sci.* 131, 458–469. doi: 10.1093/toxsci/kfs309

Meijborg, V. M., Conrath, C. E., Opthof, T., Belterman, C. N., De Bakker, J. M., and Coronel, R. (2014). Electrocardiographic T wave and its relation with ventricular repolarization along major anatomical axes. *Circ. Arrhythm. Electrophysiol.* 7, 524–531. doi: 10.1161/CIRCEP.113.001622

Milberg, P., Frommeyer, G., Kleideiter, A., Fischer, A., Osada, N., Breithardt, G., et al. (2011). Antiarrhythmic effects of free polyunsaturated fatty acids in an experimental model of LQT2 and LQT3 due to suppression of early afterdepolarizations and reduction of spatial and temporal dispersion of repolarization. *Heart Rhythm.* 8, 1492–1500. doi: 10.1016/j.hrthm.2011.03.058

Monahan, B. P., Ferguson, C. L., Killeavy, E. S., Lloyd, B. K., Troy, J., and Cantilena, L. R.Jr. (1990). Torsades de pointes occurring in association with terfenadine use. *JAMA* 264, 2788–2790. doi: 10.1001/jama.1990.03450210088038

Moshal, K. S., Zhang, Z., Roder, K., Kim, T. Y., Cooper, L., Patedakis Litvinov, B., et al. (2014). Progesterone modulates SERCA2a expression and function in rabbit cardiomyocytes. *Am. J. Physiol. Cell Physiol.* 307, C1050–C1057. doi: 10.1152/ajpcell.00127.2014

Mow, T., Frederiksen, K., and Thomsen, M. B. (2015). Assessment of anti-arrhythmic activity of antipsychotic drugs in an animal model: influence of non-cardiac alpha(1)-adrenergic receptors. *Eur. J. Pharmacol.* 748, 10–17. doi: 10.1016/j.ejphar.2014.12.012

Nagy, N., Szuts, V., Horvath, Z., Seprenyi, G., Farkas, A. S., Acsai, K., et al. (2009). Does small-conductance calcium-activated potassium channel contribute to cardiac repolarization? *J. Mol. Cell Cardiol.* 47, 656–663. doi: 10.1016/j.yjmcc.2009.07.019

Nerbonne, J. M., and Kass, R. S. (2005). Molecular physiology of cardiac repolarization. *Physiol. Rev.* 85, 1205–1253. doi: 10.1152/physrev.00002.2005

Nerbonne, J. M., Nichols, C. G., Schwarz, T. L., and Escande, D. (2001). Genetic manipulation of cardiac K(+) channel function in mice: what have we learned, and where do we go from here? *Circ. Res.* 89, 944–956. doi: 10.1161/hh2301.100349

Nerbonne, J. M. (2000). Molecular basis of functional voltage-gated K+ channel diversity in the mammalian myocardium. *J. Physiol.* 525 Pt 2, 285–298. doi: 10.1111/j.1469-7793.2000.t01-1-00285.x

Nuyens, D., Stengl, M., Dugarmaa, S., Rossenbacker, T., Compernolle, V., Rudy, Y., et al. (2001). Abrupt rate accelerations or premature beats cause life-threatening arrhythmias in mice with long-QT3 syndrome. *Nat. Med.* 7, 1021–1027. doi: 10.1038/nm0901-1021

Odening, K. E., and Koren, G. (2014). How do sex hormones modify arrhythmogenesis in long QT syndrome? Sex hormone effects on arrhythmogenic substrate and triggered activity. *Heart Rhythm.* 11, 2107–2115. doi: 10.1016/j.hrthm.2014.06.023

Odening, K. E., Hyder, O., Chaves, L., Schofield, L., Brunner, M., Kirk, M., et al. (2008). Pharmacogenomics of anesthetic drugs in transgenic LQT1 and LQT2 rabbits reveal genotype-specific differential effects on cardiac repolarization. *Am. J. Physiol. Heart Circ. Physiol.* 295, H2264–H2272. doi: 10.1152/ajpheart.00680.2008

Odening, K. E., Kirk, M., Brunner, M., Ziv, O., Lorvidhaya, P., Liu, G. X., et al. (2010). Electrophysiological studies of transgenic long QT type 1 and type 2 rabbits reveal genotype-specific differences in ventricular refractoriness and His conduction. *Am. J. Physiol. Heart Circ. Physiol.* 299, H643–H655. doi: 10.1152/ajpheart.00074.2010

Odening, K. E., Choi, B. R., and Koren, G. (2012a). Sex hormones and cardiac arrest in long QT syndrome: does progesterone represent a potential new antiarrhythmic therapy? *Heart Rhythm.* 9, 1150–1152. doi: 10.1016/j.hrthm.2012.02.028

Odening, K. E., Choi, B. R., Liu, G. X., Hartmann, K., Ziv, O., Chaves, L., et al. (2012b). Estradiol promotes sudden cardiac death in transgenic long QT type 2 rabbits while progesterone is protective. *Heart Rhythm.* 9, 823–832. doi: 10.1016/j.hrthm.2012.01.009

Odening, K. E., Jung, B. A., Lang, C. N., Cabrera Lozoya, R., Ziupa, D., Menza, M., et al. (2013). Spatial correlation of action potential duration and diastolic dysfunction in transgenic and drug-induced LQT2 rabbits. *Heart Rhythm.* 10, 1533–1541. doi: 10.1016/j.hrthm.2013.07.038

Odening, K. E., Bodi, I., Franke, G., Rieke, R., Ryan De Medeiros, A., Perez-Feliz, S., et al. (2019). Transgenic short-QT syndrome 1 rabbits mimic the human disease phenotype with QT/action potential duration shortening in the atria and ventricles and increased ventricular tachycardia/ventricular fibrillation inducibility. *Eur. Heart J.* 40, 842–853. doi: 10.1093/eurheartj/ehy761

Oosterhoff, P., Thomsen, M. B., Maas, J. N., Atteveld, N. J., Beekman, J. D., HV, V. A. N. R., et al. (2010). High-rate pacing reduces variability of repolarization and prevents repolarization-dependent arrhythmias in dogs with chronic AV block. *J. Cardiovasc. Electrophysiol.* 21, 1384–1391. doi: 10.1111/j.1540-8167.2010.01824.x

Oros, A., Volders, P. G., Beekman, J. D., Van Der Nagel, T., and Vos, M. A. (2006). Atrial-specific drug AVE0118 is free of torsades de pointes in anesthetized dogs with chronic complete atrioventricular block. *Heart Rhythm.* 3, 1339–1345. doi: 10.1016/j.hrthm.2006.07.017

Orosz, S., Sarusi, A., Csik, N., Papp, J. G., Varro, A., Farkas, S., et al. (2014). Assessment of efficacy of proarrhythmia biomarkers in isolated rabbit hearts with attenuated repolarization reserve. *J. Cardiovasc. Pharmacol.* 64, 266–276. doi: 10.1097/FJC.0000000000000116

Orosz, A., Baczko, I., Nagy, V., Gavaller, H., Csanady, M., Forster, T., et al. (2015a). Short-term beat-to-beat variability of the QT interval is increased and correlates with parameters of left ventricular hypertrophy in patients with hypertrophic cardiomyopathy. *Can. J. Physiol. Pharmacol.* 93, 765–772. doi: 10.1139/cjpp-2014-0526

Orosz, A., Csajbok, E., Czekus, C., Gavaller, H., Magony, S., Valkusz, Z., et al. (2015b). Increased Short-Term Beat-To-Beat Variability of QT Interval in Patients with Acromegaly. *PloS One* 10, e0125639. doi: 10.1371/journal.pone.0125639

Orosz, A., Baczko, I., Nyiraty, S., Korei, A. E., Putz, Z., Takacs, R., et al. (2017). Increased Short-Term Beat-to-Beat QT Interval Variability in Patients with Impaired Glucose Tolerance. *Front. Endocrinol. (Lausanne)* 8, 129. doi: 10.3389/fendo.2017.00129

Ortega, F. A., Grandi, E., Krogh-Madsen, T., and Christini, D. J. (2017). Applications of Dynamic Clamp to Cardiac Arrhythmia Research: Role in Drug Target Discovery and Safety Pharmacology Testing. *Front. Physiol.* 8, 1099. doi: 10.3389/fphys.2017.01099

Paltoo, B., O'donoghue, S., and Mousavi, M. S. (2001). Levofloxacin induced polymorphic ventricular tachycardia with normal QT interval. *Pacing Clin. Electrophysiol.* 24, 895–897. doi: 10.1046/j.1460-9592.2001.00895.x

Panfilov, A. V. (2006). Is heart size a factor in ventricular fibrillation? Or how close are rabbit and human hearts? *Heart Rhythm.* 3, 862–864.

Parikh, A., Mantravadi, R., Kozhevnikov, D., Roche, M. A., Ye, Y. P., Owen, L. J., et al. (2012). Ranolazine stabilizes cardiac ryanodine receptors: A novel mechanism for the suppression of early afterdepolarization and torsades de pointes in long QT type 2. *Heart Rhythm.* 9, 953–960. doi: 10.1016/j.hrthm.2012.01.010

Park, E., Gintant, G. A., Bi, D., Kozeli, D., Pettit, S. D., Pierson, J. B., et al. (2018). Can non-clinical repolarization assays predict the results of clinical thorough QT studies? Results from a research consortium. *Br. J. Pharmacol.* 175, 606–617. doi: 10.1111/bph.14101

Patel, S. P., and Campbell, D. L. (2005). Transient outward potassium current, 'Ito', phenotypes in the mammalian left ventricle: underlying molecular, cellular and biophysical mechanisms. *J. Physiol.* 569, 7–39. doi: 10.1113/jphysiol.2005.086223

Pollard, C. E., Abi Gerges, N., Bridgland-Taylor, M. H., Easter, A., Hammond, T. G., and Valentin, J. P. (2010). An introduction to QT interval prolongation and non-clinical approaches to assessing and reducing risk. *Br. J. Pharmacol.* 159, 12–21. doi: 10.1111/j.1476-5381.2009.00207.x

Pugsley, M. K., Authier, S., and Curtis, M. J. (2008). Principles of safety pharmacology. *Br. J. Pharmacol.* 154, 1382–1399. doi: 10.1038/bjp.2008.280

Redfern, W. S., Carlsson, L., Davis, A. S., Lynch, W. G., Mackenzie, I., Palethorpe, S., et al. (2003). Relationships between preclinical cardiac electrophysiology, clinical QT interval prolongation and torsade de pointes for a broad range of drugs: evidence for a provisional safety margin in drug development. *Cardiovasc. Res.* 58, 32–45. doi: 10.1016/S0008-6363(02)00846-5

Roden, D. M. (1998). Taking the "idio" out of "idiosyncratic": predicting torsades de pointes. *Pacing Clin. Electrophysiol.* 21, 1029–1034. doi: 10.1111/j.1540-8159.1998.tb00148.x

Roden, D. M. (2004). Drug-induced prolongation of the QT interval. *N. Engl. J. Med.* 350, 1013–1022. doi: 10.1056/NEJMra032426

Roden, D. M. (2008). Cellular basis of drug-induced torsades de pointes. *Br. J. Pharmacol.* 154, 1502–1507. doi: 10.1038/bjp.2008.238

Rodriguez, I., Kilborn, M. J., Liu, X. K., Pezzullo, J. C., and Woosley, R. L. (2001). Drug-induced QT prolongation in women during the menstrual cycle. *Jama-Journal Am. Med. Assoc.* 285, 1322–1326. doi: 10.1001/jama.285.10.1322

Rudy, Y., Ackerman, M. J., Bers, D. M., Clancy, C. E., Houser, S. R., London, B., et al. (2008). Systems approach to understanding electromechanical activity in the human heart: a national heart, lung, and blood institute workshop summary. *Circulation* 118, 1202–1211. doi: 10.1161/CIRCULATIONAHA.108.772715

Sager, P. T., Gintant, G., Turner, J. R., Pettit, S., and Stockbridge, N. (2014). Rechanneling the cardiac proarrhythmia safety paradigm: a meeting report from the Cardiac Safety Research Consortium. *Am. Heart J.* 167, 292–300. doi: 10.1016/j.ahj.2013.11.004

Saito, T., Ciobotaru, A., Bopassa, J. C., Toro, L., Stefani, E., and Eghbali, M. (2009). Estrogen contributes to gender differences in mouse ventricular repolarization. *Circ. Res.* 105, 343–352. doi: 10.1161/CIRCRESAHA.108.190041

Salama, G., and London, B. (2007). Mouse models of long QT syndrome. *J. Physiol.* 578, 43–53. doi: 10.1113/jphysiol.2006.118745

Sauer, A. J., Moss, A. J., Mcnitt, S., Peterson, D. R., Zareba, W., Robinson, J. L., et al. (2007). Long QT syndrome in adults. *J. Am. Coll. Cardiol.* 49, 329–337. doi: 10.1016/j.jacc.2006.08.057

Selzer, A., and Wray, H. W. (1964). Quinidine Syncope. Paroxysmal Ventricular Fibrillation Occurring during Treatment of Chronic Atrial Arrhythmias. *Circulation* 30, 17–26. doi: 10.1161/01.CIR.30.1.17

Seth, R., Moss, A. J., Mcnitt, S., Zareba, W., Andrews, M. L., Qi, M., et al. (2007). Long QT syndrome and pregnancy. *J. Am. Coll. Cardiol.* 49, 1092–1098. doi: 10.1016/j.jacc.2006.09.054

Shah, R. R., and Hondeghem, L. M. (2005). Refining detection of drug-induced proarrhythmia: QT interval and TRIaD. *Heart Rhythm.* 2, 758–772. doi: 10.1016/j.hrthm.2005.03.023

Stansfeld, P. J., Sutcliffe, M. J., and Mitcheson, J. S. (2006). Molecular mechanisms for drug interactions with hERG that cause long QT syndrome. *Expert Opin. Drug Metab. Toxicol.* 2, 81–94. doi: 10.1517/17425255.2.1.81

Stockbridge, N., Morganroth, J., Shah, R. R., and Garnett, C. (2013). Dealing with global safety issues : was the response to QT-liability of non-cardiac drugs well coordinated? *Drug Saf.* 36, 167–182. doi: 10.1007/s40264-013-0016-z

Strasberg, B., Welch, W., Palileo, E., Swiryn, S., Bauernfeind, R., and Rosen, K. M. (1983). Familial inducible torsade de pointes with normal QT interval. *Eur. Heart J.* 4, 383–390. doi: 10.1093/oxfordjournals.eurheartj.a061484

Sugiyama, A., Satoh, Y., Shiina, H., Takeda, S., and Hashimoto, K. (2002). Torsadegenic action of the antipsychotic drug sulpiride assessed using in vivo canine models. *J. Cardiovasc. Pharmacol.* 40, 235–245. doi: 10.1097/00005344-200208000-00009

Takahara, A., Sugiyama, A., Ishida, Y., Satoh, Y., Wang, K., Nakamura, Y., et al. (2006). Long-term bradycardia caused by atrioventricular block can remodel the canine heart to detect the histamine H1 blocker terfenadine-induced torsades de pointes arrhythmias. *Br. J. Pharmacol.* 147, 634–641. doi: 10.1038/sj.bjp.0706493

Thomsen, M. B., Volders, P. G., Stengl, M., Spatjens, R. L., Beekman, J. D., Bischoff, U., et al. (2003). Electrophysiological safety of sertindole in dogs with normal and remodeled hearts. *J. Pharmacol. Exp. Ther.* 307, 776–784. doi: 10.1124/jpet.103.052753

Thomsen, M. B., Verduyn, S. C., Stengl, M., Beekman, J. D., De Pater, G., Van Opstal, J., et al. (2004). Increased short-term variability of repolarization predicts d-sotalol-induced torsades de pointes in dogs. *Circulation* 110, 2453–2459. doi: 10.1161/01.CIR.0000145162.64183.C8

Thomsen, M. B., Beekman, J. D., Attevelt, N. J., Takahara, A., Sugiyama, A., Chiba, K., et al. (2006a). No proarrhythmic properties of the antibiotics Moxifloxacin or Azithromycin in anaesthetized dogs with chronic-AV block. *Br. J. Pharmacol.* 149, 1039–1048. doi: 10.1038/sj.bjp.0706900

Thomsen, M. B., Volders, P. G., Beekman, J. D., Matz, J., and Vos, M. A. (2006b). Beat-to-Beat variability of repolarization determines proarrhythmic outcome in dogs susceptible to drug-induced torsades de pointes. *J. Am. Coll. Cardiol.* 48, 1268–1276. doi: 10.1016/j.jacc.2006.05.048

Van Opstal, J. M., Schoenmakers, M., Verduyn, S. C., De Groot, S. H., Leunissen, J. D., Van Der Hulst, F. F., et al. (2001). Chronic amiodarone evokes no torsade de pointes arrhythmias despite QT lengthening in an animal model of acquired long-QT syndrome. *Circulation* 104, 2722–2727. doi: 10.1161/hc4701.099579

Varkevisser, R., Wijers, S. C., Van Der Heyden, M. A., Beekman, J. D., Meine, M., and Vos, M. A. (2012). Beat-to-beat variability of repolarization as a new biomarker for proarrhythmia in vivo. *Heart Rhythm.* 9, 1718–1726. doi: 10.1016/j.hrthm.2012.05.016

Varkevisser, R., Vos, M. A., Beekman, J. D., Tieland, R. G., and Van Der Heyden, M. A. (2015). AV-block and conduction slowing prevail over TdP arrhythmias in the methoxamine-sensitized pro-arrhythmic rabbit model. *J. Cardiovasc. Electrophysiol.* 26, 82–89. doi: 10.1111/jce.12533

Varro, A., and Baczko, I. (2011). Cardiac ventricular repolarization reserve: a principle for understanding drug-related proarrhythmic risk. *Br. J. Pharmacol.* 164, 14–36. doi: 10.1111/j.1476-5381.2011.01367.x

Varro, A., Lathrop, D. A., Hester, S. B., Nanasi, P. P., and Papp, J. G. (1993). Ionic currents and action potentials in rabbit, rat, and guinea pig ventricular myocytes. *Basic Res. Cardiol.* 88, 93–102. doi: 10.1007/BF00798257

Varro, A., Balati, B., Iost, N., Takacs, J., Virag, L., Lathrop, D. A., et al. (2000). The role of the delayed rectifier component IKs in dog ventricular muscle and Purkinje fibre repolarization. *J. Physiol.* 523 Pt 1, 67–81. doi: 10.1111/j.1469-7793.2000.00067.x

Verduyn, S. C., Van Opstal, J. M., Leunissen, J. D., and Vos, M. A. (2001). Assessment of the pro-arrhythmic potential of anti-arrhythmic drugs: an experimental approach. *J. Cardiovasc. Pharmacol. Ther.* 6, 89–97. doi: 10.1177/107424840100600109

Volders, P. G., Sipido, K. R., Vos, M. A., Spatjens, R. L., Leunissen, J. D., Carmeliet, E., et al. (1999). Downregulation of delayed rectifier K(+) currents in dogs with chronic complete atrioventricular block and acquired torsades de pointes. *Circulation* 100, 2455–2461. doi: 10.1161/01.CIR.100.24.2455

Volders, P. G., Stengl, M., Van Opstal, J. M., Gerlach, U., Spatjens, R. L., Beekman, J. D., et al. (2003). Probing the contribution of IKs to canine ventricular repolarization: key role for beta-adrenergic receptor stimulation. *Circulation* 107, 2753–2760. doi: 10.1161/01.CIR.0000068344.54010.B3

Vos, M. A., Verduyn, S. C., Gorgels, A. P., Lipcsei, G. C., and Wellens, H. J. (1995). Reproducible induction of early afterdepolarizations and torsade de pointes arrhythmias by d-sotalol and pacing in dogs with chronic atrioventricular block. *Circulation* 91, 864–872. doi: 10.1161/01.CIR.91.3.864

Vos, M. A., De Groot, S. H., Verduyn, S. C., Van Der Zande, J., Leunissen, H. D., Cleutjens, J. P., et al. (1998). Enhanced susceptibility for acquired torsade de pointes arrhythmias in the dog with chronic, complete AV block is related to cardiac hypertrophy and electrical remodeling. *Circulation* 98, 1125–1135. doi: 10.1161/01.CIR.98.11.1125

Waldo, A. L., Camm, A. J., Deruyter, H., Friedman, P. L., Macneil, D. J., Pauls, J. F., et al. (1996). Effect of d-sotalol on mortality in patients with left ventricular dysfunction after recent and remote myocardial infarction. The SWORD Investigators. Survival With Oral d-Sotalol. *Lancet* 348, 7–12. doi: 10.1016/S0140-6736(96)02149-6

Whitsel, E. A., Boyko, E. J., Rautaharju, P. M., Raghunathan, T. E., Lin, D., Pearce, R. M., et al. (2005). Electrocardiographic QT interval prolongation and risk of primary cardiac arrest in diabetic patients. *Diabetes Care* 28, 2045–2047. doi: 10.2337/diacare.28.8.2045

Wolbrette, D. L. (2003). Risk of proarrhythmia with class III antiarrhythmic agents: sex-based differences and other issues. *Am. J. Cardiol.* 91, 39D–44D. doi: 10.1016/S0002-9149(02)03378-7

Woosley, R. L., Chen, Y., Freiman, J. P., and Gillis, R. A. (1993). Mechanism of the cardiotoxic actions of terfenadine. *JAMA* 269, 1532–1536. doi: 10.1001/jama.1993.03500120070028

Wysowski, D. K., and Bacsanyi, J. (1996). Cisapride and fatal arrhythmia. *N. Engl. J. Med.* 335, 290–291. doi: 10.1056/NEJM199607253350416

Xu, H., Guo, W., and Nerbonne, J. M. (1999). Four kinetically distinct depolarization-activated K+ currents in adult mouse ventricular myocytes. *J. Gen. Physiol.* 113, 661–678. doi: 10.1085/jgp.113.5.661

Yang, P. C., and Clancy, C. E. (2010). Effects of sex hormones on cardiac repolarization. *J. Cardiovasc. Pharmacol.* 56, 123–129. doi: 10.1097/FJC.0b013e3181d6f7dd

Yang, P. C., and Clancy, C. E. (2011). Gender-based differences in cardiac diseases. *J. BioMed. Res.* 25, 81–89. doi: 10.1016/S1674-8301(11)60010-9

Yang, T., Snyders, D., and Roden, D. M. (2001). Drug block of I(kr): model systems and relevance to human arrhythmias. *J. Cardiovasc. Pharmacol.* 38, 737–744. doi: 10.1097/00005344-200111000-00010

Yang, T., Chun, Y. W., Stroud, D. M., Mosley, J. D., Knollmann, B. C., Hong, C., et al. (2014). Screening for acute IKr block is insufficient to detect torsades de pointes liability: role of late sodium current. *Circulation* 130, 224–234. doi: 10.1161/CIRCULATIONAHA.113.007765

Yang, P. C., El-Bizri, N., Romero, L., Giles, W. R., Rajamani, S., Belardinelli, L., et al. (2016). A computational model predicts adjunctive pharmacotherapy for cardiac safety via selective inhibition of the late cardiac Na current. *J. Mol. Cell Cardiol.* 99, 151–161. doi: 10.1016/j.yjmcc.2016.08.011

Yap, Y. G., and Camm, A. J. (2003). Drug induced QT prolongation and torsades de pointes. *Heart* 89, 1363–1372. doi: 10.1136/heart.89.11.1363

Yi, G., Elliott, P., Mckenna, W. J., Prasad, K., Sharma, S., Guo, X. H., et al. (1998). QT dispersion and risk factors for sudden cardiac death in patients with hypertrophic cardiomyopathy. *Am. J. Cardiol.* 82, 1514–1519. doi: 10.1016/S0002-9149(98)00696-1

Zhang, S., Zhou, Z., Gong, Q., Makielski, J. C., and January, C. T. (1999). Mechanism of block and identification of the verapamil binding domain to HERG potassium channels. *Circ. Res.* 84, 989–998. doi: 10.1161/01.RES.84.9.989

Ziupa, D., Beck, J., Franke, G., Perez Feliz, S., Hartmann, M., Koren, G., et al. (2014). Pronounced effects of HERG-blockers E-4031 and erythromycin on APD, spatial APD dispersion and triangulation in transgenic long-QT type 1 rabbits. *PloS One* 9, e107210. doi: 10.1371/journal.pone.0107210

Ziupa, D., Menza, M., Koppermann, S., Moss, R., Beck, J., Franke, G., et al. (2019). Electro-mechanical (dys-)function in long QT syndrome type 1. *Int. J. Cardiol.* 274, 144–151. doi: 10.1016/j.ijcard.2018.07.050

Ziv, O., Morales, E., Song, Y. K., Peng, X., Odening, K. E., Buxton, A. E., et al. (2009). Origin of complex behaviour of spatially discordant alternans in a transgenic rabbit model of type 2 long QT syndrome. *J. Physiol.* 587, 4661–4680. doi: 10.1113/jphysiol.2009.175018

2

Improved Computational Identification of Drug Response Using Optical Measurements of Human Stem Cell Derived Cardiomyocytes in Microphysiological Systems

Karoline Horgmo Jæger[1], Verena Charwat[2], Bérénice Charrez[2], Henrik Finsberg[1], Mary M. Maleckar[1], Samuel Wall[1], Kevin E. Healy[2,3] and Aslak Tveito[1]*

[1] Department of Scientific Computing, Simula Research Laboratory, Oslo, Norway, [2] Department of Bioengineering, College of Engineering, University of California, Berkeley, CA, United States, [3] Department of Materials Science and Engineering, College of Engineering, University of California, Berkeley, CA, United States

***Correspondence:**
Karoline Horgmo Jæger
karolihj@simula.no

Cardiomyocytes derived from human induced pluripotent stem cells (hiPSC-CMs) hold great potential for drug screening applications. However, their usefulness is limited by the relative immaturity of the cells' electrophysiological properties as compared to native cardiomyocytes in the adult human heart. In this work, we extend and improve on methodology to address this limitation, building on previously introduced computational procedures which predict drug effects for adult cells based on changes in optical measurements of action potentials and Ca^{2+} transients made in stem cell derived cardiac microtissues. This methodology quantifies ion channel changes through the inversion of data into a mathematical model, and maps this response to an adult phenotype through the assumption of functional invariance of fundamental intracellular and membrane channels during maturation. Here, we utilize an updated action potential model to represent both hiPSC-CMs and adult cardiomyocytes, apply an IC50-based model of dose-dependent drug effects, and introduce a continuation-based optimization algorithm for analysis of dose escalation measurements using five drugs with known effects. The improved methodology can identify drug induced changes more efficiently, and quantitate important metrics such as IC50 in line with published values. Consequently, the updated methodology is a step towards employing computational procedures to elucidate drug effects in adult cardiomyocytes for new drugs using stem cell-derived experimental tissues.

Keywords: cardiac action potential model, computational inversion, cardiac ion channel blockade, human induced pluripotent stem cell derived cardiomyocytes, computational maturation, computational identification of drug response, voltage sensitive dye

INTRODUCTION

The development of human induced pluripotent stem cells (hiPSCs) opens promising avenues of investigation into a wide variety of fundamental questions in cell physiology and beyond [for recent reviews, see, e.g., (Yoshida and Yamanaka, 2017; Di Baldassarre et al., 2018; Ye et al., 2018)]. One of the more immediately tractable applications of hiPSCs is the creation of specific human cell and tissue samples to augment drug discovery and development pipelines. These pipelines have traditionally relied on animal models in key areas of testing, but are limited by significant physiological differences between animal and human cells [see, e.g., (Mathur et al., 2016; Fine and Vunjak-Novakovic, 2017; Yoshida and Yamanaka, 2017; Ye et al., 2018)]. These differences, both at the genetic and proteomic levels, give rise to distinctly non-human system dynamics, for example, a mouse's heart rate is much more rapid than a human's (~600 bpm vs. ~60 bpm), such that it is often difficult to translate drug effects from one species to another [see, e.g., (Mathur et al., 2016; Fine and Vunjak-Novakovic, 2017; Yoshida and Yamanaka, 2017; Ye et al., 2018)].

By using hiPSC-derived cells, it is possible to measure drug effects directly in human-based systems, and therapeutics can eventually, in principle, be tested and adjusted at the level of the individual patient. This hiPSC-based, patient-centric approach opens up great possibilities for drug development, both in terms of the scope of illnesses approachable, including disorders caused by rare mutations, as well as improved safety by the early identification of drug side effects in *human* cells. Nevertheless, hiPSCs are also associated with a variety of scientific challenges that must be resolved to realize the full potential of the technology [see, e.g., (Mathur et al., 2015; Mathur et al., 2016; Mora et al., 2017; Christensen et al., 2018; Ronaldson-Bouchard et al., 2018; Zhao et al., 2018)].

Maturity of generated cells and tissues is one of these key challenges, a prominent example being the maturation of hiPSC-derived cardiomyocytes (hiPSC-CMs) (Chen et al., 2016). Human cardiomyocytes develop over many years [see (Hille, 2001), ch. 21], and during this period the density of specific ion channels changes significantly, due both to increased area of the cell membrane and proliferation of membrane channels [see, e.g., (Sontheimer et al., 1992; Moody and Bosma, 2005; Bedada et al., 2016)]. Therefore, the physiological response of immature hiPSC-CMs to a drug cannot necessarily be used to infer the properties of the drug, nor the response of adult human cardiomyocytes. Even if it is known exactly how a drug affects an hiPSC-CM, it is difficult to deduce its effect on adult cells; direct interpretation may in fact lead to both false positives and false negatives [see (Liang et al., 2013; Mathur et al., 2015)].

In (Tveito et al., 2018), we used mathematical modeling of cardiac cell dynamics to address these challenges associated with the application of hiPSC-CMs. Such mathematical modeling of the cardiac action potential (AP) remains an active area of research, and sophisticated models have been developed in order to accurately simulate both single cells and cardiac tissue dynamics [see e.g., (CellML Model Repository; Rudy and Silva, 2006; Grandi et al., 2010; O'Hara et al., 2011; Rudy, 2012; Franzone et al., 2014; Qu et al., 2014; Edwards and Louch, 2017; Quarteroni et al., 2017; Tveito et al., 2017)]. We presented an algorithm for inverting experimental measurements of the membrane potential and the cytosolic calcium (Ca^{2+}) concentration in order to obtain parameters for a mathematical model of the hiPSC-CM AP. We then demonstrated how this model of hiPSC-CMs can be mapped to an AP model representing adult cells. We were able to estimate the effect of a drug on essential ion currents for hiPSC-CMs as based on measurements from a microphysiological system (Mathur et al., 2015), and then to map this effect onto the adult cardiomyocyte AP model. The combination of these two methods permitted, in principle, to deduce drug effects on adult human cardiomyocytes as based on measurements of hiPSC-CMs in a microphysiological system.

The overall method developed in (Tveito et al., 2018) is illustrated in **Figure 1**. In this procedure, we take optical measurements using fluorescent dyes in a microphysiological system to define relative traces of the membrane potential and cytosolic Ca^{2+} concentration for cells under normal media conditions and in the presence of drugs. We then define a mathematical model for the control (undrugged) cases by identifying parameters denoted by $p^{\text{hiPSC,C}}$ (hiPSC is for hiPSC-derived, C is for control) in an AP model that matches the experimental waveforms. Using this model of hiPSC-CMs, we then define a maturation matrix Q such that $Qp^{\text{hiPSC,C}} = p^{\text{A,B}}$, where $p^{\text{A,B}}$ (A is for adult, B is for base) are *known* parameters representing a generic AP model of an adult human cardiomyocyte. Here, the matrix Q represents the developmental change in ion channel density and geometry from hiPSC-CMs to adult cardiomyocytes, independent of drug effects on individual channels.

Next, experimental traces of the membrane potential and cytosolic Ca^{2+} concentration are taken for the same cells in the presence of drugs, and these traces are used to define a new parameter-vector $p^{\text{hiPSC,D}}$ (hiPSC-CM, Drug) that matches the data. This new parameterization gives us information about what modeled channels have been altered by the drug. Then, by assuming that the drug affects *every individual ion channel* in the same manner for the hiPSC-CMs and the adult cells, the parameter vector for the adult case is given by $p^{\text{A,D}} = Qp^{\text{hiPSC,D}}$. *Hence, we can find an AP model for adult human cardiomyocytes under the influence of the drug, even though only the effect for hiPSC-CMs has been measured.*

The present report aims to present a number of modifications to improve the accuracy and reliability of these methods. First, using the AP models of Grandi et al. (2010), O'Hara et al. (2011), Paci et al. (2013), Paci et al. (2015), Paci et al. (2017), and Paci et al. (2018) as a basis, we have derived a new AP model to improve representation of experimental data. As our inversion algorithm is based on conducting a huge number of simulations with varying parameter values, it is essential to have a model that is stable with respect to perturbations of the parameters.

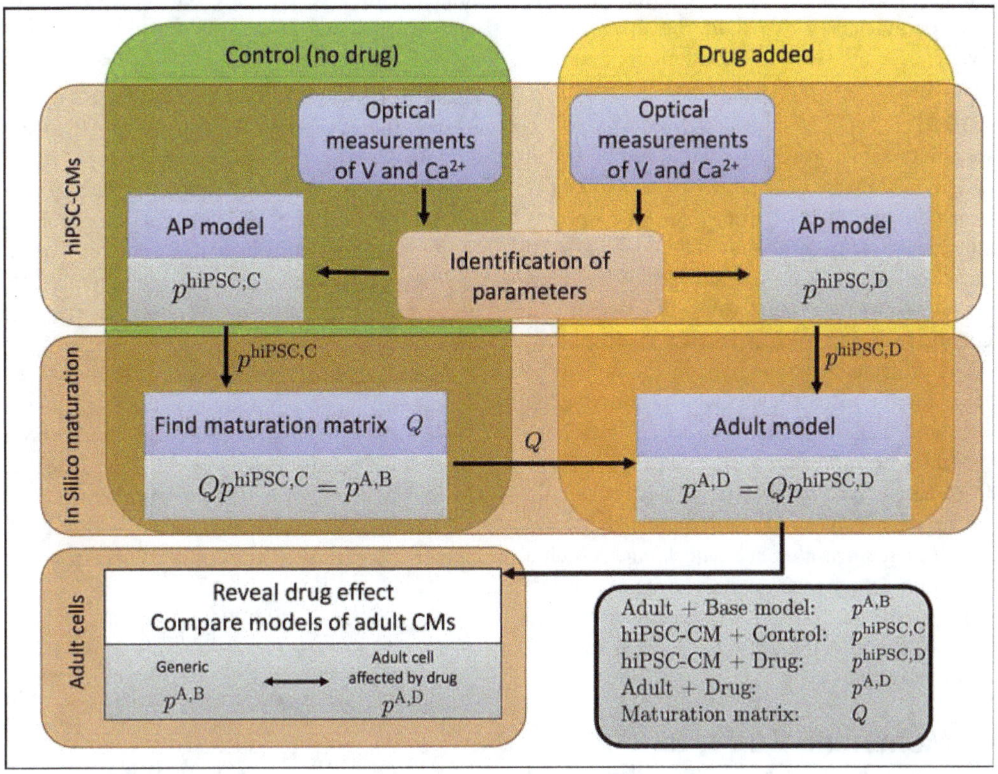

FIGURE 1 | The effect of a drug on adult cardiomyocytes can be identified by the process illustrated. The cytosolic calcium concentration (Ca^{2+}) and the membrane potential (V) are measured in a microphysiological system (Mathur et al., 2015; Mathur et al., 2016) of hiPSC-CMs. Data are collected when no drug has been applied (control, C) and when a drug has been applied (D). The data are used to parameterize a model for both cases, represented by the parameter vectors $p^{\text{hiPSC,C}}$ and $p^{\text{hiPSC,D}}$ for the control and drugged cases, respectively. The control parameter vector $p^{\text{hiPSC,C}}$ is used to define the maturation matrix Q such that $Qp^{\text{hiPSC,C}} = p^{A,B}$, where $p^{A,B}$ is the parameter vector of a generic base model of adult human cardiomyocytes. By comparing the adult parameter vectors for the control and drugged cases, the effect of the drug can be identified.

Therefore, the new model is designed for improved stability. In particular, the model of the intracellular Ca^{2+} dynamics has been modified to avoid instabilities in the balance between the influx and efflux of Ca^{2+} to the sarcoplasmic reticulum (SR).

In addition, our aim has been to create models that can be mapped back and forth between hiPSC-CMs and adult cardiomyocytes. A vital modeling assumption has been that the individual channels are the same in these two cases, and that only channel density should change. However, existing AP models are not derived with such a mapping in mind, and models of identical single channel dynamics vary significantly among models. Therefore, we have derived a new AP model which strictly adheres to the principle that every current (and flux) should be written as a product of the ion channel density and the dynamics of a single channel; identical ion channels are represented by identical mathematical models. Consequently, the mathematical representation of *a single channel* is the same for the hiPSC-CMs and adult cardiomyocytes in the novel AP model presented here.

Finally, we present a new method for inverting experimental data into parameters for the AP model by introducing a continuation-based approach, searching for optimal parameters by gradually moving from known parameters to the parameters we want to identify. Continuation methods are well developed in scientific computing [see e.g., (Keller, 1987; Allgower and Georg, 2012)] and offer significant computational savings to find optimal solutions.

In this manuscript, we first motivate and describe the approaches outlined above. We then evaluate these methods with respect to accuracy using simulated data. Subsequently, the new methods are used to identify the effect of five well-characterized drugs based on optical measurements of hiPSC-CMs. In all cases considered, the predicted effects are consistent with known drug effects, lending credence to the principle that novel drug effects on adult cardiomyocytes could reliably be estimated using measurements of hiPSC-CMs and the described methodology.

METHODS

Here, we offer a detailed presentation of all steps illustrated in **Figure 1**. First, we present the derivation of a new AP model.

Next, we describe the inversion method used in our computations. Finally, we discuss how to characterize the identifiability of the parameters involved in the inversion as based on singular value decomposition (SVD) of model currents.

The Base Model

As noted above, we aim to define an AP model that can be scaled from very early stages of human development (days) to fully developed adult cardiomyocytes. To review, for one specific membrane current, we assume that the only difference between the hiPSC-CM and adult cases is that the number of channels and the membrane area has changed; thus, the density of the specific ion channel carrying the current has changed, but the properties of every individual channel remains the same. The same principle holds for the intracellular Ca^{2+} machinery; the individual channels and buffers remain the same, but both the intracellular volumes and the number of channels change from hiPSC-CMs to adult cardiomyocytes. Our model will, therefore, be based on models of single ion channel dynamics and *only the density of these single channels will change*. When a drug is involved, we assume that the effect of the drug on a *single channel* is the same in the hiPSC-CM and adult cases, and therefore one can use the effect in the hiPSC-CM case to estimate the effect for the adult case.

Modeling the Membrane Currents

The standard model [see, e.g., (Izhikevich, 2007; Plonsey and Barr, 2007; Ermentrout and Terman, 2010; Sterratt et al., 2011)] of the membrane potential of an excitable cell is given by the equation

$$\frac{dv}{dt} = -\sum_x I_x, \tag{1}$$

where v is the membrane potential (in mV), and I_x are the membrane currents through ion channels of different types, as well as pumps and exchangers located on the cell membrane.

These currents are all given in units of A/F, and may be written on the form

$$I_x = \frac{N_x}{AC_m} i_x, \tag{2}$$

where N_x is the number of channels of type x on the cell membrane, A is the area of the cell membrane (in μm^2) and C_m is the specific capacitance of the cell membrane (in pF/μm^2). Furthermore, i_x represents the average current through a single channel of type x (in pA). For voltage-gated ion channels, this average single-channel current is given on the form

$$i_x = g_0^x o_x (v - E_x), \tag{3}$$

where g_0^x is the conductance of a single open channel (in nS), E_x is the equilibrium potential of the channel (in mV), and o_x is the unitless open probability of the channel. Note that in models given on this form, it is common to consider a lumped parameter g_x, given by

$$g_x = \frac{N_x}{AC_m} g_0^x,$$

and parameters of this type are given for each of the ion channels considered in the base model in the **Supplementary Information**. For membrane pumps and exchangers, the single-channel current is given on a similar form. The specific currents included in the model will be described below.

Scaling of the Membrane Currents

As mentioned above, we assume that the specific membrane capacitance and the ion channels responsible for each of the membrane currents are the same during different stages of development for the cell, but that the number of ion channels, N_x, and the membrane area, A, may differ. Therefore, currents can be mapped from one stage of development, S_1, to another stage of development, S_2, simply by adjusting the channel density of the currents.

More specifically, for the formulation (1)–(2), this means that we assume that the parameter C_m and the expressions for the single-channel currents, i_x, are the same for S_1 and S_2, but that the channel density $\frac{N_x}{A}$ can be different. Let $A_x^{S_1}, A_x^{S_2}$ and $N_x^{S_1}, N_x^{S_2}$ denote the membrane area and number of channels of type x for the S_1 and S_2 cases, respectively. Furthermore, let λ_x represent the change of channel density in the sense that

$$\frac{N_x^{S_1}}{A_x^{S_1}} = (1 + \lambda_x) \frac{N_x^{S_2}}{A_x^{S_2}}. \tag{4}$$

Now, the S_1 and S_2 currents are related according to

$$I_x^{S_1} = \frac{N_x^{S_1}}{A_x^{S_1} C_m} i_x = (1 + \lambda_x) \frac{N_x^{S_2}}{A_x^{S_2} C_m} i_x = (1 + \lambda_x) I_x^{S_2}, \tag{5}$$

for each of the currents x.

The Base Model is the Generic Adult Model

Based on these considerations, it is convenient to define *one* default base model from which all other models are derived to simplify a mapping procedure between different development stages.

Defining a base model as representing hiPSC-CMs, from which adult cardiomyocytes subsequently develop, may seem to be a natural choice. However, in the scheme illustrated in **Figure 1**, there is only one fixed model—the generic adult model—while all other models will change depending on the experimental measurements. For simplicity, we, therefore, define the generic adult model to be the *default base model*, and scale all other models relative to this model.

Main Currents Present in Human Cardiomyocytes

Modern models of human cardiomyocytes are complex and the models for the individual currents are based on years of experience using patch-clamp measurements. In the formulation (1), our aim has been to include the main currents present in human cardiomyocytes, but to keep the number of currents as low as feasible in order to keep the base model relatively simple. The experimental inputs in the present methodology are optically-derived, and data based on sensitive dyes are not expected to be able to uncover equally fine details of the dynamics as compared to traditional electrophysiological measurements derived *via* patch clamp. It is, therefore, reasonable to represent the data using simpler models. Our choice of currents is based on the O'Hara et al. (2011) model and the Grandi et al. (2010) model for human adult ventricular cardiomyocytes, in addition to the Paci et al. (2013) model for hiPSC-CMs. Furthermore, we have focused on including currents considered to be critical for depolarization and repolarization of the AP and, therefore, those typically investigated for response to drugs [see, e.g., (Crumb et al., 2016)].

In (Crumb et al., 2016), the fast sodium current, I_{Na}, the late sodium current, I_{NaL}, the L-type Ca^{2+} current, I_{CaL}, the transient outward potassium current, I_{to}, the rapid and slow delayed rectifier potassium currents, I_{Kr} and I_{Ks}, and the inward rectifier potassium current, I_{K1}, were investigated for their drug responses, and we have included each of these currents in our model. In addition, we have included the sodium-potassium pump, I_{NaK}, the sodium-calcium exchanger, I_{NaCa}, the Ca^{2+} pump, I_{pCa}, the background Ca^{2+} current, I_{bCa}, and the background chloride current, I_{bCl}, as they all appear to have a significant effect on the computed AP and Ca^{2+} transient of the Grandi et al. (2010) model. Furthermore, we have included the hyperpolarization-activated cyclic nucleotide-gated funny current, I_{f}. While this current is very small for adult ventricular cardiomyocytes, it is substantial for hiPSC-CMs (Garg et al., 2018). The formulation used for each of the currents is given in the **Supplementary Information**. The formulations are based on those of the currents in the Paci et al. (2013), the Grandi et al. (2010), and the O'Hara et al. (2011) models, and we have chosen formulations that seems to work well for both the hiPSC-CM and adult cases and that are able to provide good fits for our considered data of hiPSC-CMs.

Modeling Intracellular Ca^{2+} Dynamics

In addition to the membrane potential, we also want the base model to represent the dynamics of the intracellular Ca^{2+} concentration. We consider the following five intracellular compartments [based on (Grandi et al., 2010)]:

1. The dyad, representing the small cytosolic subspace between the L-type Ca^{2+} channels and the ryanodine receptors (RyRs),
2. The subsarcolemmal space, representing the remaining part of the cytosolic space that is located close to the membrane,
3. The bulk cytosolic space,
4. The junctional sarcoplasmic reticulum (jSR), representing the part of the SR that is close to the RyR-channels,
5. The network sarcoplasmic reticulum (nSR), representing the remaining part of the SR.

The Ca^{2+} concentrations and volume fractions defined for each of these compartments are given in **Figure 2**. In all compartments except the nSR, we consider both the concentration of free Ca^{2+} and the concentration of Ca^{2+} bound to a buffer. The Ca^{2+} concentration in the extracellular space is assumed to remain constant. The intracellular Ca^{2+} fluxes between compartments are illustrated in **Figure 2**, and the model takes the form

$$
\begin{aligned}
\frac{dc_d}{dt} &= \frac{1}{V_d}(J_{CaL} - J_d^b - J_d^c), & \frac{db_d}{dt} &= \frac{1}{V_d}J_d^b, \\
\frac{dc_{sl}}{dt} &= \frac{1}{V_{sl}}(J_e^{sl} - J_{sl}^c - J_{sl}^b + J_s^{sl}), & \frac{db_{sl}}{dt} &= \frac{1}{V_{sl}}J_{sl}^b, \\
\frac{dc_c}{dt} &= \frac{1}{V_c}(J_{sl}^c + J_d^c - J_c^n - J_c^b), & \frac{db_c}{dt} &= \frac{1}{V_c}J_c^b, \\
\frac{dc_s}{dt} &= \frac{1}{V_s}(J_n^s - J_s^{sl} - J_s^b), & \frac{db_s}{dt} &= \frac{1}{V_s}J_s^b, \\
\frac{dc_n}{dt} &= \frac{1}{V_n}(J_c^n - J_n^s).
\end{aligned}
$$

See Section S2.1 in the **Supplementary Information** for a derivation of these equations.

Definition of Ca^{2+} Fluxes

Every model flux J_x representing the flux through a type of channel can be written on the form

$$J_x = \frac{N_x}{V_{\text{cell}}} j_x,$$

where N_x is the number of channels of type x, V_{cell} is the cell volume (in L) and j_x is the average flux through a single channel of type x (in mmol/ms). Below, we will describe the formulation chosen for the flux through the RyR channels. Definitions of each of the remaining fluxes are specified in the **Supplementary Information**.

Modeling Release From the SR

In our model of Ca^{2+} dynamics, we deviate from previous modeling approaches in two specific ways:

1. Ca^{2+} is released through RyR channels from the SR directly to the subsarcolemmal space (SL) and not to the dyad.
2. Release of Ca^{2+} through the RyR channels is a product of two factors; one factor models the open probability of the RyR channels, whereas the other models the availability of channels that can be opened. We assume that each channel can only process a certain amount of Ca^{2+} before it deactivates.

We will see below that these two modeling assumptions lead to a model that exhibits two key physiological features of Ca^{2+} release from the SR of cardiomyocytes, so-called *high gain* and *graded release* (see Section S2.2 in the **Supplementary Information** for explanations of these terms).

Flux through RyRs (J_s^{sl})

As we will employ the base model for several different parameter combinations, the model for the RyR flux must be stable, in the sense that careful tuning of the model is not requisite to ensure reasonable activation and deactivation of the RyRs.

As outlined above, we let the Ca^{2+} released from the SR enter the SL space rather than the dyad. This is done in order to achieve graded release (see the **Supplementary Information**), in the sense that the amount of Ca^{2+} released from the SR through the RyRs should depend directly upon the amount of Ca^{2+} entering the cell through L-type Ca^{2+} channels. If the model were to be formulated such that Ca^{2+} released from the jSR

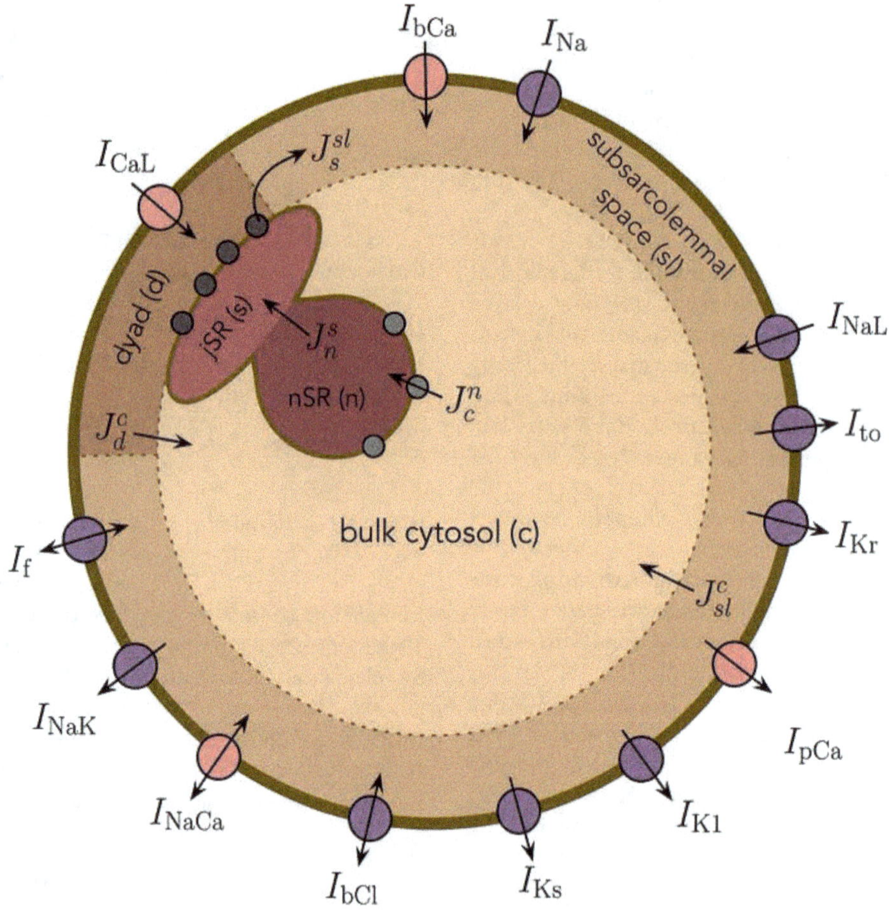

Compartment	Volume fraction	Free Ca^{2+} concentration	Buffered Ca^{2+} concentration
Dyad	$V_d = 0.001$	c_d	b_d
Subsarcolemmal space	$V_{sl} = 0.028$	c_{sl}	b_{sl}
Bulk cytosol	$V_c = 0.917$	c_c	b_c
jSR	$V_s = 0.004$	c_s	b_s
nSR	$V_n = 0.05$	c_n	

FIGURE 2 | Membrane currents, Ca^{2+} fluxes and intracellular compartments of the base model. The volume fractions of the compartments are based on (Grandi et al., 2010).

instead entered the dyad, it would be difficult to distinguish the increase in dyadic Ca^{2+} concentration resulting from L-type Ca^{2+} channel flux as opposed to release via RyRs. Directing the RyR flux into the SL, the concentration change in the dyad is almost exclusively due to the influx through L-type Ca^{2+} channels, and by letting the flux through the RyRs depend on the Ca^{2+} concentration in the dyad, we achieve graded release.

Furthermore, a common modeling approach for the RyRs is to govern inactivation by a decreased jSR concentration [see e.g., (Sobie et al., 2010)]. However, for large variations in parameter values, this may lead to model instabilities, because the jSR concentration depends upon the balance between the flux through the SERCA pumps and the RyRs, which depend upon the balance between the Ca^{2+} fluxes in and out of the cell. In order to avoid an RyR model whose inactivation mechanism depends on the jSR concentration, we instead introduce a new assumption that some RyRs are only able to carry a given amount of Ca^{2+} ions during each AP.

We then assume that a small portion of the RyR channels are always open (type 0), while the remaining channels (type 1) are activated by an increased dyadic Ca^{2+} concentration and are inactivated after they have transported a given amount of Ca^{2+} ions. Therefore, the total flux through the RyRs may be expressed as

$$J_s^{sl} = J_{RyR} + J_{leak}, \tag{6}$$

where J_{RyR} represents the flux through the RyR channels of type 1 and J_{leak} represents the flux through the RyR channels of type 0. We assume that the flux through the two types of RyR channels are given by expressions of the form

$$J_{RyR} = \frac{Mp}{V_{cell}} j_{RyR}, \tag{7}$$

$$J_{leak} = \frac{M_0}{V_{cell}} j_{RyR}, \tag{8}$$

where j_{RyR} denotes the flux through a single open RyR channel (in mmol/ms) and V_{cell} denotes the total cell volume (in L). In addition, M_0 denotes the number of RyR channels that are always open (type 0), M denotes the number of available RyR channels of type 1, and p is the open probability of the channels of type 1. The single channel flux through the RyRs is given by

$$j_{RyR} = \alpha_{RyR,0}(c_s - c_{sl}), \tag{9}$$

where $\alpha_{RyR,0}$ (in L/ms) represents the rate of release. Furthermore, the open probability of the RyR channels of type 1 is modeled by a simple function that increases sigmoidally with the dyadic Ca^{2+} concentration, c_d, based on the model in (Friel, 1995):

$$p = \frac{c_d^3}{c_d^3 + K_{RyR}^3}. \tag{10}$$

We let the total number of RyR channels of type 1 be given by N_{RyR} and the total number of RyR channels of type 0 be given by

$$M_0 = \gamma_{RyR} N_{RyR}. \tag{11}$$

In other words, the total number of RyR channels (of both types) is given by $(1+\gamma_{RyR})N_{RyR}$.

We assume that every RyR of type 1 is able to transport a fixed amount of Z Ca^{2+} ions during an AP. After Z ions have been transported, the channel becomes inactivated. However, we assume that as the dyadic Ca^{2+} concentration, c_d, returns to rest and the open probability, p, consequently decreases, the inactivated channels gradually recover from inactivation. We let the number of available channels of type 1 be governed by

$$\frac{dM}{dt} = -\frac{V_{cell}}{Z} J_{RyR} + \frac{\eta_{RyR}}{p}(N_{RyR} - M). \tag{12}$$

Here, the first term dominates for large values of p, driving M towards zero as more Ca^{2+} is transported through the RyR channels of type 1. Furthermore, for small values of p (i.e., at rest), the second term dominates and drives M towards the maximum value N_{RyR}.

In order to reduce the number of free parameters in the model, we define a scaled variable r, defined as $r = \frac{M}{N_{RyR}}$, and divide both sides of equation (12) by N_{RyR}. The equation then reads

$$\frac{dr}{dt} = -\frac{J_{RyR}}{\beta_{RyR}} + \frac{\eta_{RyR}}{p}(1 - r), \tag{13}$$

where

$$\beta_{RyR} = \frac{N_{RyR}}{V_{cell}} Z. \tag{14}$$

Inserting $M = rN_{RyR}$ into (7) and defining

$$\alpha_{RyR} = \frac{N_{RyR}}{V_{cell}} \alpha_{RyR,0}, \tag{15}$$

we get the following expression for active RyR flux

$$J_{RyR} = p \cdot r \cdot \alpha_{RyR}(c_s - c_{sl}), \tag{16}$$

where we recall that

$$p = \frac{c_d^3}{c_d^3 + K_{RyR}^3}. \tag{17}$$

Moreover, inserting (11) and (15) into (8), we obtain

$$J_{leak} = \gamma_{RyR} \cdot \alpha_{RyR}(c_s - c_{sl}). \tag{18}$$

Scaling the RyR flux

When considering cells of different levels of maturity, we assume that the number of RyRs and the cell volume may be different, but that the function of a single RyR channel is the same for different levels of maturity. We also assume that the ratio between RyR channels of type 0 and 1, γ_{RyR}, and the number of Ca^{2+} ions that each RyR channel of type 1 can transport, Z, is the same for the different maturity levels. Considering the model (13)–(18), this means that the only adjustment necessary between two maturity levels S_1 and S_2 is an adjustment of the density $\frac{N_{RyR}}{V_{cell}}$ in the definition of α_{RyR} and β_{RyR}. We, therefore, introduce a scaling factor λ_{RyR} such that

$$\frac{N_{RyR}^{S_1}}{V_{cell}^{S_1}} = (1 + \lambda_{RyR}) \frac{N_{RyR}^{S_2}}{V_{cell}^{S_2}}, \tag{19}$$

and represent this adjustment of the RyR density in the model by scaling α_{RyR} and β_{RyR} by

$$\alpha_{RyR}^{S_1} = (1 + \lambda_{RyR}) \alpha_{RyR}^{S_2}, \tag{20}$$

$$\beta_{RyR}^{S_1} = (1 + \lambda_{RyR}) \beta_{RyR}^{S_2}, \tag{21}$$

where superscript S_1 and S_2 denote the S_1 and S_2 versions of the parameters, respectively.

Inversion of Optical Measurements

The inversion procedure, used to construct base model representations of data obtained from optical measurements of the AP and Ca^{2+} transient of hiPSC-CMs, is described below. First, in Section *Optical Measurements*, we describe how optical measurements of hiPSC-CMs are obtained. Next, in Section *Definition of Adjustment Factors*, we describe how adjustment factors λ are set up to represent control (non-drugged) cells from different data sets. In Section *IC50 Modeling of Drug Effects*, we describe how the effect of a drug is modeled using IC50 values and corresponding factors, denoted by ε. The aim of the inversion procedure is to find optimal parameter vectors λ and ε so that the model parameterized by λ and ε aligns to the measured data as best possible. This is explained in more detail in Section *Coupled Inversion of Data From Several Doses*. In Section *Properties of the Cost Function*, we describe the cost function constructed to measure the difference between the model and the data. Finally, in Section *A Continuation-Based Minimization Method*, we describe the continuation-based minimization method used to minimize the cost function in our computations.

Optical Measurements

Using previously developed techniques (Mathur et al., 2015), cardiac microphysiological systems derived from a single line of hiPSCs were loaded and matured prior to drug exposure. The resulting tissues consisted of approximately 90% cardiomyoctyes, with a small population of stromal support cells. On the day upon which studies were performed, freshly measured drugs (Nifedipine, Lidocaine, Cisapride, Flecainide, and Verapamil) were dissolved into DMSO or media and serially diluted. Each concentration of the drug to be tested was preheated for 15–20 min in a water bath at 37°C and subsequently sequentially injected in the device. At each dose, after 20 min of exposure, the drug's response on the microtissue was recorded using a Nikon Eclipse TE300 microscope fitted with a QImaging camera. Fluorescent images were acquired at 200 frames per second using filters to capture GCaMP and BeRST-1 fluorescence as previously described. Images were obtained across the entire chip for 6–8 sec at a resolution of 511 x 222 square 1.3 micron pixels. Excitation was paced at 1 Hz, to capture multiple beats for processing.

Fluorescence videos were analyzed using custom Python software utilizing the open source Bio-Formats tool to produce characteristic AP and Ca^{2+} waveforms for each chip and tested drug dose. Briefly, for each analysis, the fluorescent signal was averaged over the entire microtissue. The signal was then smoothed using a 3-point median filter, and five to seven individual action potentials or calcium transients were overlayed by aligning the maximum dF/dt and then averaged into a single transient. For each drug escalation study, we chose the single series with the most continuity between control cases and subsequent drug doses for both AP and Ca^{2+} transient for inversion and mapping analysis.

Definition of Adjustment Factors

In order to make base model representations of control cells from different data sets, we must define adjustment factors λ for a base model parameter set. These adjustment factors represent alterations of the channel densities and geometry of the cells under consideration, as explained above. For example, for each membrane channel type x, the adjustment factor λ_x is defined as

$$\frac{N_x}{A} = (1 + \lambda_x)\frac{N_x^b}{A_b}, \tag{22}$$

where $\frac{N_x}{A}$ is the channel density on the cell membrane for the fitted model and $\frac{N_x^b}{A^b}$ is the channel density in the default base model. We generally consider adjustment factors for the membrane channel densities for all the currents of the model, i.e., λ_{Na}, λ_{NaL}, λ_{CaL}, λ_{to}, λ_{Kr}, λ_{Ks}, λ_{K1}, λ_{NaCa}, λ_{NaK}, λ_{pCa}, λ_{bCl}, λ_{bCa}, and λ_f, although some of the factors are fixed in some cases (see Section *Identifiability of the Currents in the hiPSC-CM Base Model*).

For the density of an intracellular channel type x, the adjustment factor λ_x is similarly defined as

$$\frac{N_x}{V_{cell}} = (1 + \lambda_x)\frac{N_x^b}{V_{cell}^b}, \tag{23}$$

where $\frac{N_x}{V_{cell}}$ and $\frac{N_x^b}{V_{cell}^b}$ are the channel densities for the fitted model and the default base model, respectively. We consider the adjustment factors λ_{RyR} and λ_{SERCA} for intracellular channel densities, and the factors λ_B^d, λ_B^{sl}, λ_B^c and λ_B^s for intracellular calcium buffers (see the **Supplementary Information**). In addition, we consider adjustments to the intracellular diffusion coefficients, λ_d^c, λ_{sl}^c, and λ_n^c (see the **Supplementary Information**). In order to reduce the number of free parameters to be determined in the inversion procedure for different control data, we assume that the buffer concentrations change at the same rate in all intracellular compartments, so that we only consider a single adjustment factor

$$\lambda_B^d = \lambda_B^{sl} = \lambda_B^c = \lambda_B^s := \lambda_B . \tag{24}$$

Similarly, we assume that the intracellular diffusion coefficients change at the same rate, so that

$$\lambda_d^c = \lambda_{sl}^c = \lambda_n^s := \lambda_\alpha . \tag{25}$$

Furthermore, because we wish to avoid ending up with unrealistic values of the surface-to-volume ratio, χ, we assume that the scaling factor for the cell surface-to-volume ratio varies little between data sets and only employ two different values of χ in the computations. We use the value $\chi = 0.6\ \mu m^{-1}$ for adult cells and the value $\chi = 0.9\ \mu m^{-1}$ for hiPSC-CMs, based on the values used in the Grandi et al. AP model for adult cardiomyocytes (Grandi et al., 2010) and the Paci et al. AP model for hiPSC-CMs (Paci et al., 2013). Note here that t-tubules (i.e., invaginations of the cell membrane extending into the center of the cell) are present for adult ventricular cardiomyocytes (Orchard et al., 2009), and this is incorporated into the adult version of χ by increasing the cell surface area by a factor of about two compared to the geometrical surface of the cylinder shape of the cell [see e.g., (Luo and Rudy, 1994)]. For hiPSC-CMs, t-tubules are believed to be absent or underdeveloped [see e.g., (Di Baldassarre et al., 2018; Jiang et al., 2018)], and in our choice of χ for hiPSC-CMs, we have assumed that t-tubules are not present for hiPSC-CMs.

IC50 Modeling of Drug Effects

Following previous modeling of channel blockers [see, e.g., (Brennan et al., 2009; Davies et al., 2012; Zemzemi et al., 2013; Paci et al., 2015)], we model the dose-dependent effect of a drug by scaling the channel conductances according to

$$g_i^D = \frac{1}{1 + \frac{D}{IC50_i}} g_i^C, \tag{26}$$

where g_i^D is the conductance of channel i in the presence of a drug with concentration D, IC50$_i$ is the drug concentration that leads to 50% block of channel i, and g_i^C is the channel conductance in the control case (i.e., in the absence of drugs). Specifically, this means that if the drug concentration D equals the IC50 value, we have $g_i^D = \frac{1}{2} g_i^C$.

It should be mentioned that a drug may certainly affect a channel in a more complex manner than is assumed here. The effect of drugs can realistically be represented by introducing new states in Markov models of the ion channel. In such models, the transition rates between different model states are able to represent the properties of drugs [see e.g., (Clancy et al., 2007; Tveito et al., 2011; Tveito and Lines, 2016; Tveito et al., 2018)]. Although Markov model representations of drug effects are more versatile and realistic than the simple blocking assumption employed here (Tveito et al., 2017), it would greatly increase the complexity of the inversion process, as many more parameters would have to be computed.

From (26), we see that for a given drug dose $D > 0$, the effect of the drug would increase if the IC50 value were decreased, and the effect of the drug would be very small if the IC50 value were much larger than the considered dose. In the continuation-based minimization method applied in our computations (see the section *A Continuation-Based Minimization Method* below), it is most practical to deal with parameters that are small when no change occurs and large when large changes occur. Therefore, we introduce the parameters

$$\varepsilon_i = \frac{1}{IC50_i}. \tag{27}$$

Here, a small value of ε_i represents small effects of a drug while a large value of ε_i represents large effects, and channel blocking is given by

$$g_i^D = \frac{1}{1 + D\varepsilon_i} g_i^C. \tag{28}$$

In our computations, we assume that the considered drugs block either I_{CaL}, I_{NaL}, I_{Kr}, or a combination of these currents, and we therefore only consider the ε-parameters ε_{CaL}, ε_{NaL}, ε_{Kr}.

Coupled Inversion of Data From Several Doses

The control data obtained from different optical experiments tend to vary significantly, and in order to be able to accurately estimate the drug effect from these measurements, the λ-parameters must be tuned so that the control model fits the control data as best possible. In addition, we want the λ parameters to be constructed such that that the scaling (28) for ε_{CaL}, ε_{NaL}, and ε_{Kr} is sufficient to fit the model to the drug doses under consideration. In order to increase the chance of obtaining such a control model, we fit the control parameters, λ, and the drug parameters, ε, simultaneously, instead of first finding the optimal control parameters, λ, by fitting the base model to the control data, and then subsequently finding appropriate drug parameters, ε, for each dose. In addition, all doses are included in the inversion, so that the estimated values of ε are based on *all* the drug doses included in the data set.

In order to illustrate the role of the λ- and ε-parameters more clearly, consider a simplified model consisting of just two currents, and assume that the base model is given by (see the section *Modeling the Membrane Currents*)

$$\frac{dv}{dt} = -g_1 o_1 (v - E_1) - g_2 o_2 (v - E_2). \tag{29}$$

Assume further that we have data from cells with both no drug present and with different doses of a drug (e.g., one low dose and one high dose). We assume that the drug may block any of the two model currents. In the inversion procedure, we try to find optimal values of the four parameters λ_1, λ_2, ε_1, and ε_2 so that the adjusted model of the form

$$\frac{dv}{dt} = -\frac{1 + \lambda_1}{1 + D\varepsilon_1} g_1 o_1 (v - E_1) - \frac{1 + \lambda_2}{1 + D\varepsilon_2} g_2 o_2 (v - E_2) \tag{30}$$

fits the data both for the control case ($D = 0$) and for the considered drug doses. In other words, for a given parameter set λ_1, λ_2, ε_1, and ε_2, we need to compute the solution of the model (30) both for the control case ($D = 0$) and for the considered drug doses and compare the obtained solutions to the corresponding experimental data.

The more general case considered in our computations is conceptually identical; however, as we also consider scaling of parameters that are not assumed to possibly be affected by the drug, we also have some parameters simply scaled by a factor $(1+\lambda_i)$ instead of by $\frac{1+\lambda_i}{1+D\varepsilon_i}$.

Properties of the Cost Function

In order to find the optimal parameters for fitting the model to data, we need to define a cost function that measures the difference between a given model solution and the data. This cost function is defined as

$$H(\lambda, \varepsilon) = \sum_d \sum_j w_{d,j} (H_j(\lambda, \varepsilon, D_d))^2. \tag{31}$$

Here, d runs over each of the considered drug doses, D_d, including the control case ($D_0 = 0$), and j runs over each cost function term, H_j, representing various differences between the data and the model solution. The parameters $w_{d,j}$ represent weights for each of the cost function terms for each of the doses. Each of the cost function terms, H_j, are defined in Section S3.1 of the **Supplementary Information**.

A Continuation-Based Minimization Method

As outlined above, we wish to adjust the base model to data by finding λ- and ε-parameters that minimize a cost function of the form (31), measuring the difference between the input data and the model solution. In order to search for the optimal values of λ and ε, we apply a continuation-based optimization method [see e.g., (Keller, 1987; Allgower and Georg, 2012)]. Briefly, continuation is used to simplify the solution of equations or of optimization problems by introducing a θ-parameterization such that the solution is known for one value of θ. Suppose, for instance, that the parameterization is defined such that the solution is known for $\theta = 0$ and the problem we want to solve is defined by $\theta = 1$. Then the solution at $\theta = 1$ can be found by starting at $\theta = 0$ and carefully step towards the solution at $\theta = 1$. One advantage with this method is that we can start at a solution that we know is correct (at $\theta = 0$) and then take *small steps* towards the goal at $\theta = 1$. For the problem of inverting membrane potential and Ca^{2+} traces, this method has proven to be useful.

Cost function in the continuation case

More specifically, we assume that, for each drug dose, D_d, (including the control case) the data we are trying to invert are given by some vector pair $[v^1(D_d), c^1(D_d)]$, where $v^1(D_d)$ is the membrane potential and $c^1(D_d)$ is the Ca^{2+} concentration. In addition, from the default base model specified by $\lambda = \varepsilon = 0$, we can compute a vector pair (v^0, c^0) for the membrane potential and Ca^{2+} concentration as the starting point of the inversion.

The goal of the continuation method is to compute a path for λ and ε from $\lambda = \varepsilon = 0$, which fit (v^0, c^0) perfectly, to some λ and ε that fit the final data $[v^1(D_d), c^1(D_d)]$ for each of the drug doses, D_d, as best as possible. This is done by defining a cost function of the form

$$\overline{H}(\theta, \lambda, \varepsilon) = \sum_d \sum_j w_{d,j} (\overline{H}_j(\theta, \lambda, \varepsilon, D_d))^2, \tag{32}$$

for the intermediate steps in the algorithm. Here, θ is a parameter that is gradually increased from zero to one. In the definition (32), the terms $\overline{H}_j(\theta, \lambda, \varepsilon, D_d)$ correspond to each of the terms $H_j(\lambda, \varepsilon, D_d)$ defined in Section S3.1 of the **Supplementary Information**. Specifically, the terms take the form

$$\overline{H}_j(\theta, \lambda, \varepsilon, D_d) = \frac{|R_j(v(\lambda, \varepsilon, D_d), c(\lambda, \varepsilon, D_d)) - R_j^{\theta}(D_d)|}{|R_j^{\theta}(D_d)|}, \tag{33}$$

$$R_j^{\theta}(D_d) = (1 - \theta) R_j(v^0, c^0) + \theta R_j(v^1(D_d), c^1(D_d)), \tag{34}$$

where $R_j(v,c)$ represent different characteristics of the AP or Ca^{2+} transient, e.g., the AP duration at some percentage or the upstroke velocity (see Section S3.1 of the **Supplementary Information**[1]). In the case $\theta = 0$, $R_j^{\theta}(D_d)$ is equal to the terms defined by the default model ($\lambda = \varepsilon = 0$) for all the doses D_d. Therefore, $\overline{H}(0, 0, 0, D_d) = 0$,[2] so the optimal solution for $\theta = 0$ is $\lambda = \varepsilon = 0$. In the case $\theta = 1$, the terms $R_j^{\theta}(D_d)$ are equal to the characteristics computed for the data we wish to invert. In other words, $\overline{H}(1, \lambda, \varepsilon) = H(\lambda, \varepsilon)$, where $H(\lambda, \varepsilon)$ is defined in (31). For the intermediate values of θ, the characteristics $R_j^{\theta}(D_d)$ represent weighted averages of characteristics of the model used as a staring point for the inversion ($\lambda = \varepsilon = 0$) and the data we are trying to invert. Therefore, we expect the optimal values of λ and ε to gradually move from zero to the optimal values for the data as θ is increased from zero to one.

The minimization algorithm

In the minimization algorithm, we find the optimal solution in M iterations. We define $\theta_m = \Delta\theta \cdot m$ for $m = 0,\dots,M$, where $\Delta\theta = 1/M$. For $m = 1,\dots,M$, we assume that the optimal values $\lambda(\theta_{m-1})$ and $\varepsilon(\theta_{m-1})$ have been computed, and we want to find $\lambda(\theta_m)$ and $\varepsilon(\theta_m)$ by finding the minimum of $\overline{H}(\theta_m, \lambda, \varepsilon)$. Since the step in θ is small, we assume that the changes in λ and ε are also relatively small. We use the Nelder-Mead algorithm (Nelder and Mead, 1965) to minimize $\overline{H}(\theta_m, \lambda, \varepsilon)$, and we use $\lambda(\theta_{m-1})$ and $\varepsilon(\theta_{m-1})$ as suggestions for the starting vectors to find $\lambda(\theta_m)$ and $\varepsilon(\theta_m)$. However, in order to increase the chance of finding the true optimal value in every iteration, we start the Nelder-Mead algorithm from several randomly chosen starting vectors in the vicinity of $\lambda(\theta_{m-1})$ and $\varepsilon(\theta_{m-1})$. **Figure S3** in the **Supplementary Information** illustrates the development of the ε-values in an inversion aiming to characterize a drug.

Technical specifications

In the applications presented below, we use $M = 20$, and in each iteration m, we draw 63 guesses (as the specific computer used for these simulations has 64 cores) for the starting vectors for the Nelder-Mead algorithm from $[\lambda(\theta_{m-1}) - 0.2, \lambda(\theta_{m-1}) + 0.2]$ and $[\frac{\varepsilon(\theta_{m-1})}{5}, 5 \cdot \varepsilon(\theta_{m-1})]$ for λ and ε, respectively. In the first 15 iterations, we use five iterations of the Nelder-Mead algorithm for each guess, and for the last five iterations we use 25 iterations of the Nelder-Mead algorithm. For each new parameter set, we generally run the simulation for 15 AP cycles using 1 Hz pacing before measuring the AP and Ca^{2+} transient, unless otherwise specified. The choice of 15 AP cycles is selected as a compromise between the desire of minimizing the computational efforts required for each cost function evaluation and the desire of reaching new stable steady state values for the state variables following a parameter change. Presently, each cost function evaluation requires about 14 sec of computing time for a data set including four doses in addition to the control case.

Identifiability of the Base Model Based on Singular Value Decomposition of Currents

In the inversion procedure outlined above, we try to find the optimal adjustment factors λ and ε for the model so that the AP and cytosolic Ca^{2+} transient in the model solution match measurements of the AP and Ca^{2+} transient as best possible. An important element to consider in this process is whether the identified adjustment factors found by the inversion procedure are the only combination of adjustment factors that fit the data, or whether other adjustment factors might exist which fit the data equally well.

In order to investigate the identifiability of the adjustment factors for the currents in the base model, we apply a method based on singular value decomposition [see, e.g., (Liesen and Mehrmann, 2015; Lyche, 2017)] of the currents. This approach is described in detail in (Jæger et al., 2019a). In short, the identifiability of the currents is investigated by collecting the model currents at time points $t_n = n\Delta t$, for $n = 1, \dots, N_t$ into a

[1]Note that this does not apply to the regularization terms of the cost function. These terms are assumed to be the same for all values of θ.

[2]Note that this relies on either the flux balance term $H_{Ca,b}$ being zero for the default base model or on the weight for this term being zero (see Section S3.1.8 in the Supplementary information).

matrix $A \in R^{N_t,N_c}$, where N_c is the number of model currents. Then, the singular value decomposition of the matrix

$$A = USV^T$$

is computed. Here, the matrices $U \in R^{N_t,N_t}$ and $V \in R^{N_c,N_c}$ are unitary matrices, and the matrix $S \in R^{N_t,N_c}$ is a diagonal matrix with singular values σ_i along the diagonal. The columns u_i and v_i of U and V, respectively, are the associated singular vectors.

From the properties of the singular value decomposition it can be shown that perturbations of the adjustment factors along singular vectors v_i associated with large singular values σ_i are expected to result in significant changes in the AP, whereas perturbations of the adjustment factors along singular vectors v_i associated with small singular values are, accordingly, expected to result in small changes in the AP.

In (Jæger et al., 2019a) it was shown that this expected result seemed to hold in the case of three well-known AP models of adult ventricular cardiomyocytes. In addition, it was demonstrated how this analysis could be used to define an *identifiability index* for individual model currents. This index was defined for each current $j=1,...,N_c$ as

$$k(e_j) = ||e_j - P_N e_j||_2, \tag{35}$$

where $e_j \in R^{N_c}$ is the vector that is one in element number j and zero elsewhere. Moreover, $P_N e_j \in R^{N_c}$ is the projection of e_j onto the unidentifiable space spanned by the singular vectors v_i associated with small singular values (or small perturbation effects). In other words, if $k(e_j)$ is close to zero, almost the entire current I_j is in the unidentifiable space, and we cannot be sure that the value of the associated adjustment factors λ_j or ε_j are the only values that fit the data (i.e., result in the same AP). On the other hand, if $k(e_j)$ is close to one, we expect that other values of λ_j or ε_j would not fit the data as well as the currently assumed values, as perturbations of the adjustment factors would result in large changes in the AP.

Note that this approach only aims to determine the identifiability of the adjustment factors for the membrane currents. The analysis could be extended to include other state variables than just the membrane potential (e.g., the Ca^{2+} concentrations). In this case, the identifiability of the remaining adjustment factors might also be suggested. However, at this stage primary focus is on identifying drug effects on membrane ion channels, so we are principally interested in ensuring that the adjustment factors for the currents are unique.

RESULTS

Below, we demonstrate a few applications of the method outlined above. First, in the section *The Base Model*, we define the default hiPSC-CM and adult parameterizations of the general base model formulation. We also demonstrate that these models exhibit high gain and graded release of the Ca^{2+} fluxes. In addition, we illustrate the identifiability of the model currents using SVD analysis, as described above. This analysis is used to determine which model currents should be fixed in the applications of the inversion procedure. Next, in the section *Identification of Drug Effects on hiPSC-CMs Based on Simulated Data*, we use the inversion procedure to identify drug effects for data generated by simulations. Finally, in the section *Identification of Drug Effects on hiPSC-CMs Based on Optical Measurements*, we apply the inversion procedure to identify drug effects from data obtained from optical measurements of hiPSC-CMs.

The Base Model

Here, we set up the default adult and hiPSC-CM base model formulations used in the inversion procedure in the following sections.

Base Model Approximation of the Grandi Model

The adult base model is fitted to approximate the Grandi et al. model using the inversion procedure described above. The upper right panel of **Figure 3** shows the AP and Ca^{2+} transient of the Grandi et al. (2010) model for healthy adult ventricular cardiomyocytes and the AP and Ca^{2+} transient of the adult version of the base model. In the lower right panels, we compare a number of major ionic currents in the base model to those in the Grandi et al. (2010) or the O'Hara et al. (2011) models.

In the inversion, the cost function includes all the terms specified in Section S3.1 of the **Supplementary Information**, except for the regularization terms. For the cost function terms involving information about currents and fluxes, we have included I_{Na}, I_{CaL}, I_{to}, I_{Kr}, I_{Ks}, I_{K1}, I_{NaCa}, I_{pCa}, and I_{bCa}, as well as the fluxes J_{RyR} and J_{SERCA} (see Section S3.1.7 of the **Supplementary Information**). All terms measuring the difference in membrane potential or Ca^{2+} concentration are given the weight $w_j = 1$ and the terms measuring differences in the currents are given the weight $w_j = 0.5$. The initial conditions for the parameters included in the inversion are specified in **Table S9** of the **Supplementary Information.**

As mentioned above, we define the *default* base model as the adult base model because this model will remain fixed, whereas the hiPSC-CM models will change depending on experimental data. The parameter values obtained in the inversion procedure therefore define the default base model and are specified in Section S1 of the **Supplementary Information.**

Default Base Model for hiPSC-CMs

The left panel of **Figure 3** shows the solution of the default base model for hiPSC-CMs fitted to optical measurements of the AP and Ca^{2+} transient. In this case, the cost function consists of the terms H_{APD30}, H_{APD50}, H_{APD80}, H_{CaD20}-H_{CaD80}, H_{int30}, H_{dvdt}, H_{dcdt}, H_{Ca}, $H_{Ca,b}$, $H_{I^{max}_{Na}}$, $H_{I^{max}_{CaL}}$, $H_{I^{max}_{Kr}}$, $H_{I^{max}_{Ks}}$, $H_{I^{max}_{K1}}$, $H_{I^{max}_{to}}$, $H_{I^{max}_{f}}$ (see the **Supplementary Information**), where the information about the currents is obtained from the Paci et al. model (Paci et al., 2013) which is based on patch-clamp recordings of the ionic currents of hiPSC-CMs from (Ma et al., 2011). The terms H_{CaD20}-H_{CaD75} are given the weight 0.5, and H_{APD80} and H_{CaD80} are given the weight 5. Furthermore, $H_{I^{max}_{Na}}$, $H_{I^{max}_{Ks}}$, $H_{I^{max}_{K1}}$, $H_{I^{max}_{to}}$, and $H_{I^{max}_{f}}$ are given the weight 0.5 and $H_{I^{max}_{CaL}}$ and $H_{I^{max}_{Kr}}$ are given the weight 5. The remaining terms are given the weight 1.

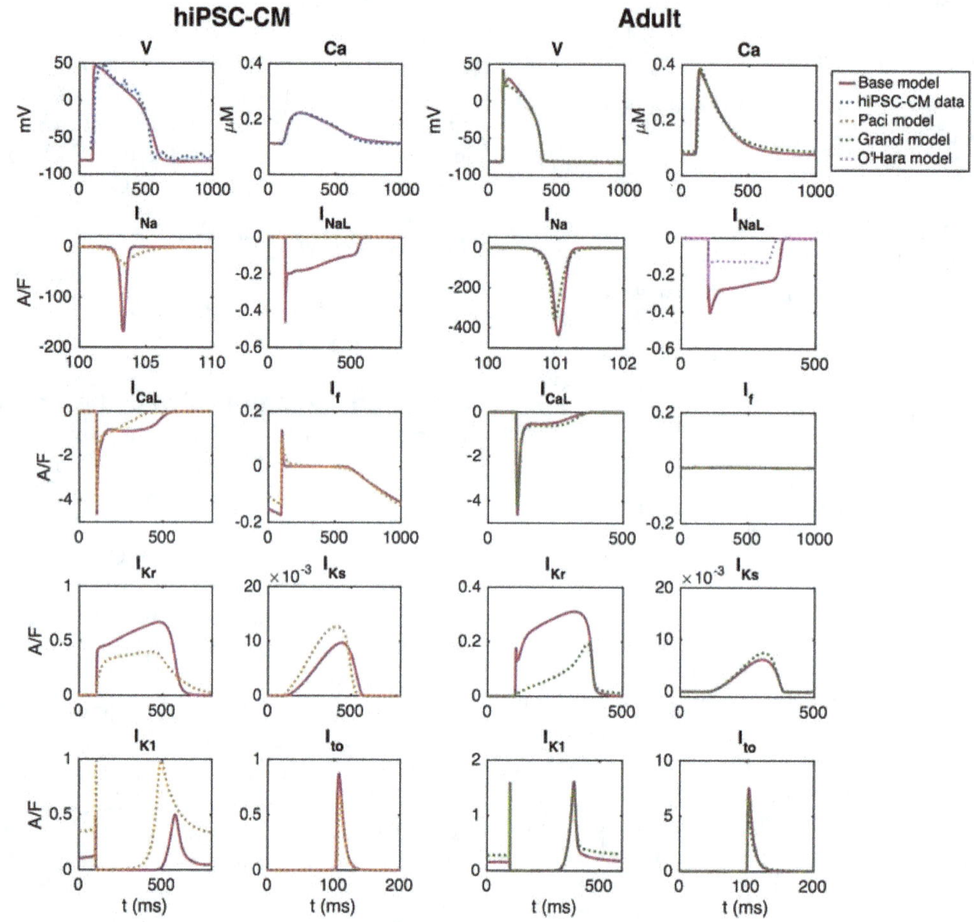

FIGURE 3 | AP, cytosolic Ca^{2+} transient and major ionic currents in the hiPSC-CM and adult versions of the base model. In the left panel, the base model is adjusted to fit data obtained from optical measurements of the AP and Ca^{2+} transient of hiPSC-CMs. In the right panel, the base model is adjusted to approximate the Grandi et al. (2010) model of adult cardiomyocytes.

TABLE 1 | Values defining the maturation map between the default hiPSC-CM and adult base models illustrated in **Figure 3**.

λ_{Na}	2.00	λ_{NaK}	-0.16	λ_{sl}^{c}	−0.14
λ_{NaL}	-0.08	λ_{CaL}	-0.53	λ_{n}^{s}	−0.10
λ_{Kr}	-0.54	λ_{bCa}	3.90	λ_{d}^{c}	−0.61
λ_{Ks}	0.68	λ_{pCa}	-0.85	λ_{B}^{c}	−0.56
λ_{K1}	2.23	λ_{NaCa}	-0.69	λ_{B}^{d}	−0.72
λ_{to}	8.45	λ_{RyR}	-0.20	λ_{B}^{sl}	−0.60
λ_{f}	-0.99	λ_{SERCA}	-0.53	λ_{B}^{s}	−0.58
λ_{bCl}	42.43	λ_{χ}	-0.33		

The adult parameters, p^A, are related to the hiPSC-CM parameters, p^{hiPSC}, by the relation $p^A = (1+\lambda)p^{hiPSC}$. See the sections Modeling the Membrane Currents, Modeling Intracellular Ca^{2+} Dynamics *and Section S2.1 in the* ***Supplementary Information*** *for more detailed definitions of each of the λ-values.*

The mapping between hiPSC-CMs and adult cardiomyocytes returned by the inversion procedure are reported in **Table 1**. Note that these factors represent the default hiPSC-CM base model to be used as a starting point for the inversion of the remaining control data sets. In other words, the specific adjustment factors between the hiPSC-CM and adult models will differ for each new data set. Note also that in our applications of the inversion procedure, we consider data from stimulated hiPSC-CMs, and therefore, the hiPSC-CMs are not required to be spontaneously beating. The default hiPSC-CM version of the base model in **Figure 3** is not spontaneously beating, and whether the model fitted to a specific data set is spontaneously beating or not will depend on the fitted parameter values. In **Figure S4** in the Supplementary material, we report how some of the AP and Ca^{2+} transient features depend on the pacing frequency for the default hiPSC-CM and adult base models and compare the results to those of the Grandi et al. (2010), O'Hara et al. (2011), Paci et al. (2013), and Kernik et al. (2019) models for adult and hiPSC-derived cardiomyocytes.

High Gain and Graded Release of the Base Model

As mentioned above, the base model formulation of Ca^{2+} release is designed to exhibit both high gain and graded release. This has proved impossible to achieve using common pool models [see, e.g., (Rice et al., 1999; Dupont et al., 2016)], as discussed in more detail in the **Supplementary Information**. The Ca^{2+} release model we have designed differs from the classical common pool models in two ways: first, release of Ca^{2+} from the SR is not directed into the dyad (d), but rather directly to the subsarcolemmal (SL) space (see **Figure 2**), and, second; the release mechanism is formulated in terms of both an availability rate and open probability for the RyRs [see (16)].

In **Figure 4**, we show that this model exhibits high gain and graded release both when the hiPSC-CM and adult parameters are applied. In the figure, we report the peak of the J_{CaL} and J_{RyR} fluxes as well as the integrated fluxes for simulations in which the membrane potential is fixed at specific values. The remaining state variables of the model start at the default initial conditions corresponding to the default resting membrane potential of the model, and the simulations record the J_{CaL} and J_{RyR} fluxes resulting from the clamped membrane potential.

We observe that for most values of v, the J_{RyR} flux is considerably larger than the J_{CaL} flux, indicating high gain. Furthermore, a small J_{CaL} flux seems to be associated with a small J_{RyR} flux, whereas a large J_{CaL} flux is associated with a large J_{RyR} flux, indicating graded release.

Identifiability of the Currents in the hiPSC-CM Base Model

In order to investigate the identifiability of the individual model currents, we apply the singular value decomposition analysis from (Jæger et al., 2019a) described in the section *Identifiability of the Base Model Based on Singular Value Decomposition of Currents.*

In **Figure 5**, titles above each plot indicate the value of each of the singular values of the current matrix, A. The upper plots below the singular values show the singular vectors corresponding to each of the singular values. Here, each letter corresponds to a single current specified in the table on the right-hand side. The below left plots show the values of the cost function (31) evaluated using the default base model for hiPSC-CMs as data and a perturbed model as the model solution. In the perturbed model, the maximum conductances are perturbed with λ-values [see (5)] equal to $\omega \cdot v_i$, where v_i is the considered singular vector and ω is varied between zero and one. The cost function includes the terms H_{APD30}, H_{APD50}, H_{APD80}, and H_{Int30} with weight 1 for all terms except H_{APD80}, which is given the weight 5 (see the **Supplementary Information** for definitions). The maximum values of H are given in the top of the plots. The right plots show the solutions resulting from the perturbations for a few selections of ω.

In (Jæger et al., 2019a) it was shown that perturbations of the maximum conductances along singular vectors corresponding to large singular values generally resulted in large perturbation effects, whereas perturbations along singular vectors corresponding to small singular values generally resulted in small perturbation effects for the Ten Tusscher and Panfilov, (2006), the Grandi et al. (2010) and the O'Hara et al. (2011) AP models. **Figure 5** shows correspondence to this result for the hiPSC-CM base model; the main discrepancy is observed for σ_2, which corresponds to a singular vector consisting almost exclusively of the fast sodium current, I_{Na}. The perturbation

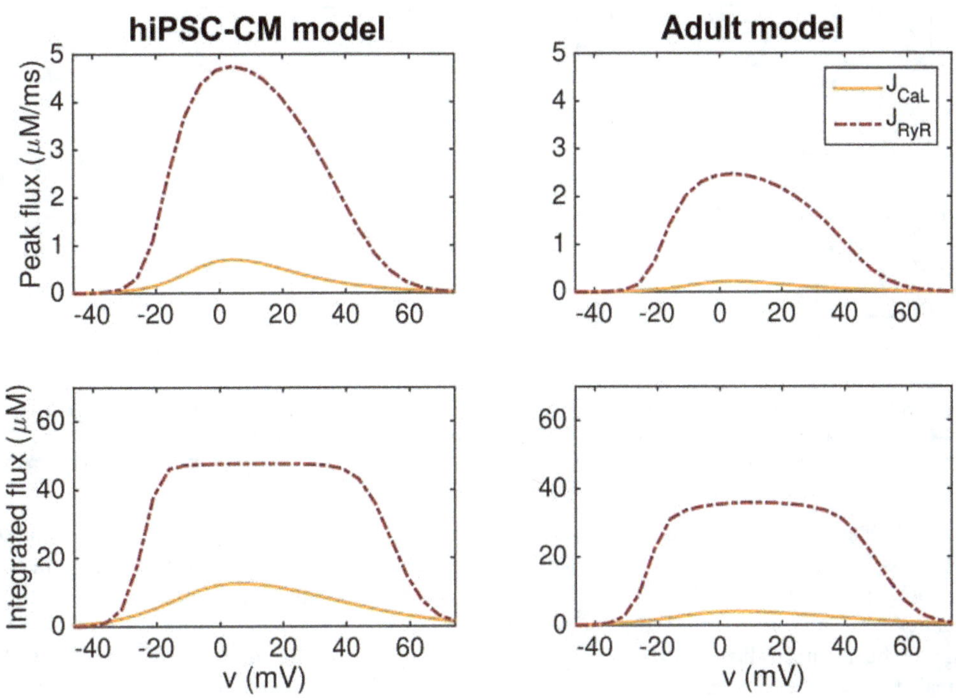

FIGURE 4 | Graded release for the hiPSC-CM (left) and adult (right) versions of the base model. In the upper panel, we report the peak of the J_{CaL} and J_{RyR} fluxes for simulations in which the membrane potential is fixed at specific values between −50 mV and 80 mV. In the lower panel, we show the fluxes integrated with respect to time from t = 0 ms to t = 100 ms. After 100 ms, both J_{CaL} and J_{RyR} have roughly returned to their resting levels.

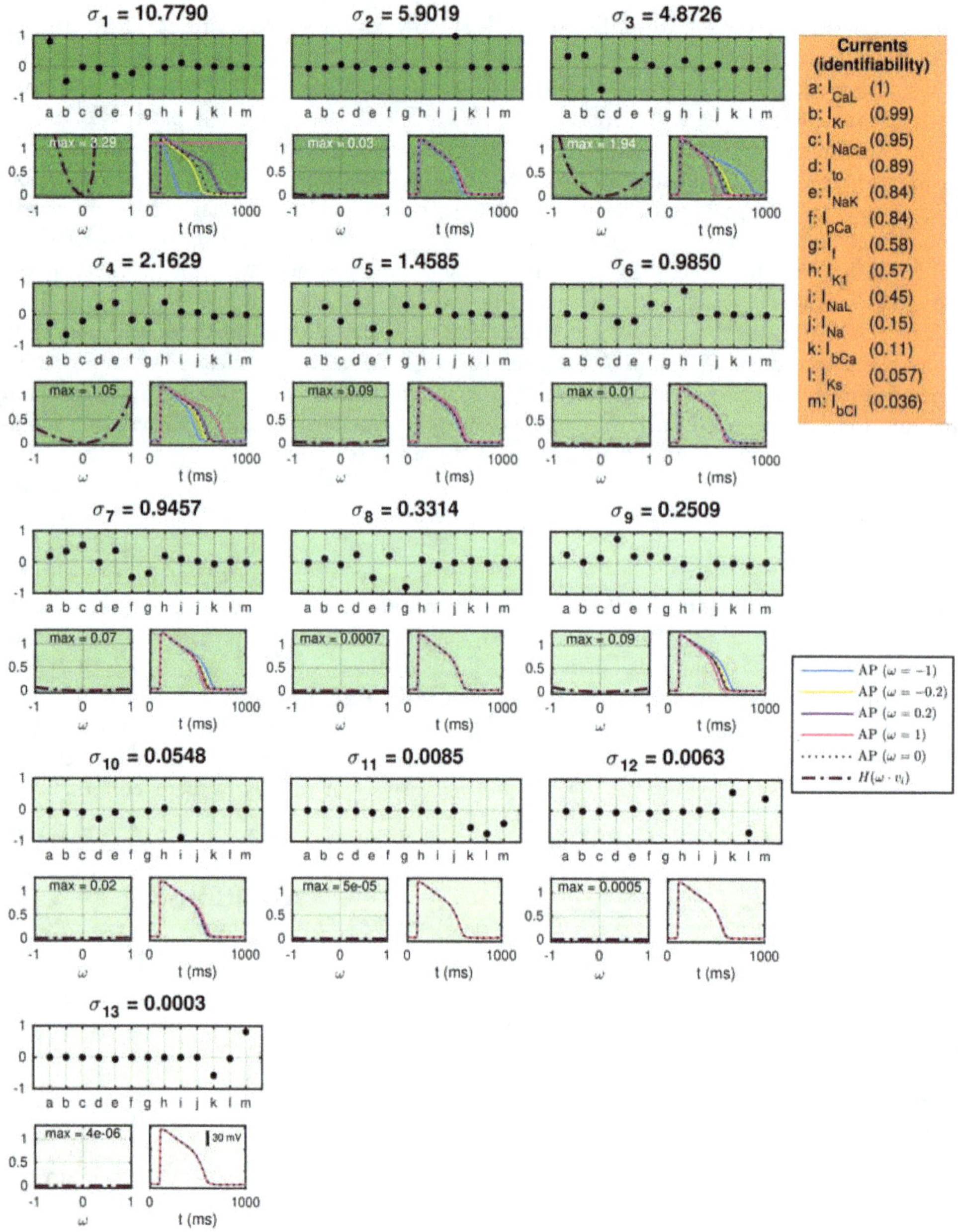

FIGURE 5 | SVD analysis of the currents in the default base model for hiPSC-CMs. The titles above each plot give the singular values of the current matrix A, and the upper plots show the corresponding singular vectors. The below plots show how a perturbation of the currents corresponding to the singular vector affects the computed AP for a few examples (right) and measured by a cost function (left). The identifiability index (35) of each current is given in the orange panel.

effects may be very small for this singular value because the upstroke velocity, physiologically governed by I_{Na}, is not included in the cost function [cf. (Jæger et al., 2019a)].

In order to quantify the identifiability of the individual currents, we compute the identifiability index, k, defined in (35). The unidentifiable space is defined as the space spanned by the singular vectors v_i whose maximum value of $H(\omega v_i)$ for $0 \le \omega \le 1$ is smaller than 0.05. The computed values of the identifiability index for each of the model currents are given in the orange box on the right-hand side of **Figure 5**. A value of k close to 1 indicates a high degree of identifiability, while a value of k close to 0 indicates an unidentifiable current.

From the indices in **Figure 5**, we see that I_{CaL}, I_{Kr}, and I_{NaCa} are highly identifiable, but that the currents I_{NaL}, I_{Na}, I_{bCa}, I_{Ks}, and I_{bCl} has an identifiability index below 0.5. As a consequence, we fix the conductance of I_{Na}, I_{bCa}, I_{Ks}, and I_{bCl} in the applications of the inversion procedure presented below. In addition, we are aware that the I_{NaL} current might be hard to identify, and that estimated drug effects for this current are associated with a level of uncertainty [see also (Poulet et al., 2015)].

Identification of Drug Effects on hiPSC-CMs Based on Simulated Data

Our first application of the inversion procedure is to identify drug effects as based on simulated data. To generate these data, we set $\lambda_{CaL} = \lambda_{NaL} = \lambda_{Kr} = 0.1$ in the default hiPSC-CM base model. In addition, we apply a set of ε-values to represent five specific drugs—Nifedipine, Lidocaine, Cisapride, Flecainide, and Verapamil. We assume that Nifedipine is a pure I_{CaL}-blocker with an IC50 value of 10 nM, that Lidocaine is a pure I_{NaL}-blocker with an IC50 value of 10 μM, and that Cisapride is a pure I_{Kr}-blocker with an IC50 value of 10 nM. Furthermore, Flecainide is assumed to block a combination of all three currents with IC50 values of 25 μM, 20 μM and 10 μM for I_{CaL}, I_{NaL}, and I_{Kr}, respectively. Verapamil is assumed to block I_{CaL} with an IC50 value of 200 nM and I_{Kr} with an IC50 value of 500 nM. Both when the data is generated and in the inversion procedure, we record the sixth generated AP following each parameter change.

Figure 6 shows the result of the inversion procedure using the λ-values λ_{CaL}, λ_{NaL}, and λ_{Kr} and the ε-values ε_{CaL}, ε_{NaL}, and ε_{Kr} as free parameters in the inversion procedure. The left panel shows the ε-values used to generate the data (yellow) and the corresponding ε-values returned by the inversion procedure (pink). The center and right panels show the AP and Ca^{2+} transient, respectively, for the control case and for each of the drug doses included in the data sets. The solid lines show the simulated data and the dotted lines show the solutions generated by the model using the λ- and ε-values returned by the inversion procedure. Note that to clearly see differences in the Ca^{2+} transient amplitude, the Ca^{2+} transients are adjusted so that the Ca^{2+} transient amplitude is preserved, but the minimum Ca^{2+} concentration is set to zero. We observe that the inversion

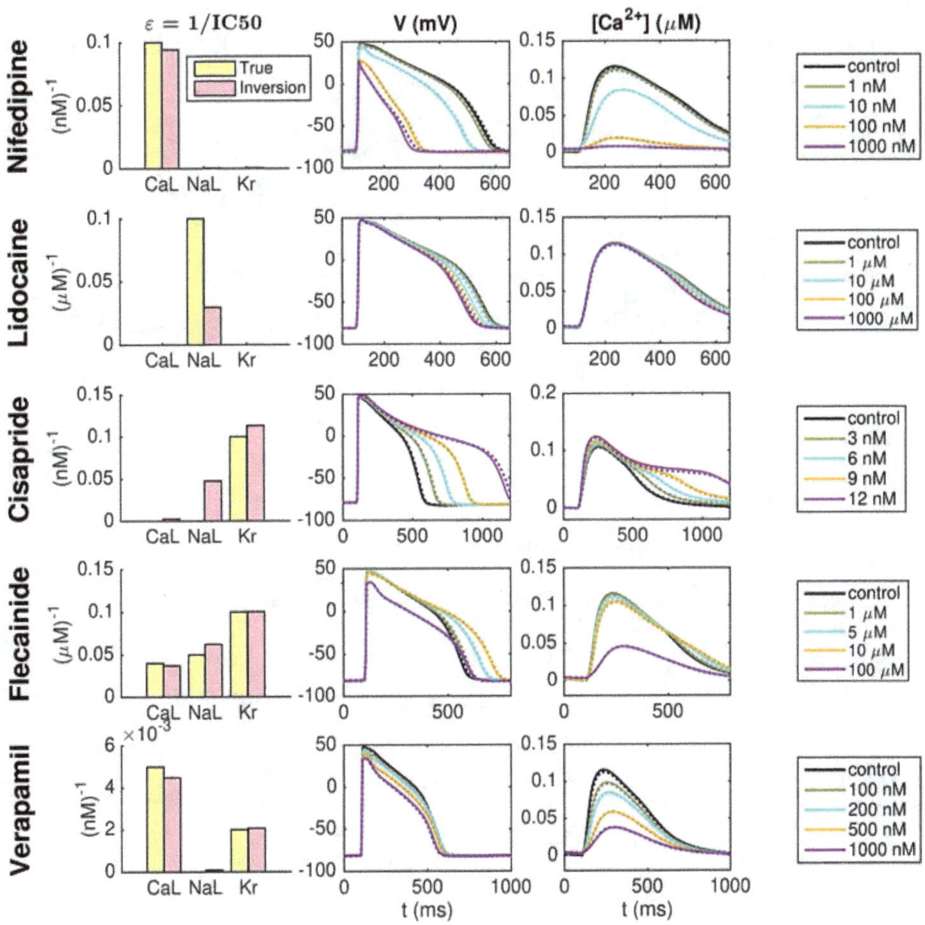

FIGURE 6 | Identification of drug effects for five drugs based on simulated data. The λ-values λ_{CaL}, λ_{NaL}, and λ_{Kr} and the ε-values ε_{CaL}, ε_{NaL}, and ε_{Kr} are allowed to vary in the inversion. The left panel shows the ε-values used to generate the simulated drug data (yellow) and the corresponding ε-values estimated by the inversion procedure (pink). The center and right panels show the AP and Ca^{2+} transients, respectively, for each of the drug doses included in the data sets. Solid lines represent the simulated data and dotted lines show the fitted model solutions returned by the inversion procedure. Note that to clearly see changes in the Ca^{2+} transient amplitude, the Ca^{2+} transients are adjusted so that the Ca^{2+} transient amplitude is preserved, but the minimum value is set to zero in all cases.

procedure is able to identify the correct ε-values accurately, excepting the ε-value for Lidocaine, which is predicted to be considerably lower than the value used to generate the data.

Identification of Drug Effects on hiPSC-CMs Based on Optical Measurements

Below, we present use of the inversion procedure to identify drug effects on hiPSC-CMs from optical measurements of the AP and Ca^{2+} transient.

Nifedipine

Figure 7 shows the result of the inversion procedure applied to data from optical measurements of hiPSC-CMs exposed to the drug Nifedipine. The data includes the control case with no drug present and four different drug doses (3 nM, 30 nM, 300 nM, and 3,000 nM). The left panel of **Figure 7A** shows the membrane potential and Ca^{2+} traces obtained from optical measurements, and the center panel shows the corresponding solutions of the hiPSC-CM version of the base model fitted to the optical measurements. Note that the values of the data are mapped so that the maximum and minimum values of the membrane potential and Ca^{2+} concentration match those of the fitted hiPSC-CM model. Panel C of **Figure 7** compares the experimentally measured data and the fitted model for each of the doses. We observe that the model seems to fit the data quite well for most of the doses, but that the Ca^{2+} transient appears to last a bit longer in the model than in the data for the highest considered drug doses.

The dose-dependent effect of the drug on the I_{CaL}, I_{NaL}, and I_{Kr} currents are modeled using IC50 values (see Section *IC50 Modeling of Drug Effects*). The values of $\varepsilon_i = \frac{1}{IC50_i}$ for i = CaL, NaL, and Kr are given in **Figure 7B**. A large value of ε_i corresponds to a large drug effect on the current i, and a small value of ε_i corresponds to a small drug effect on the current i.

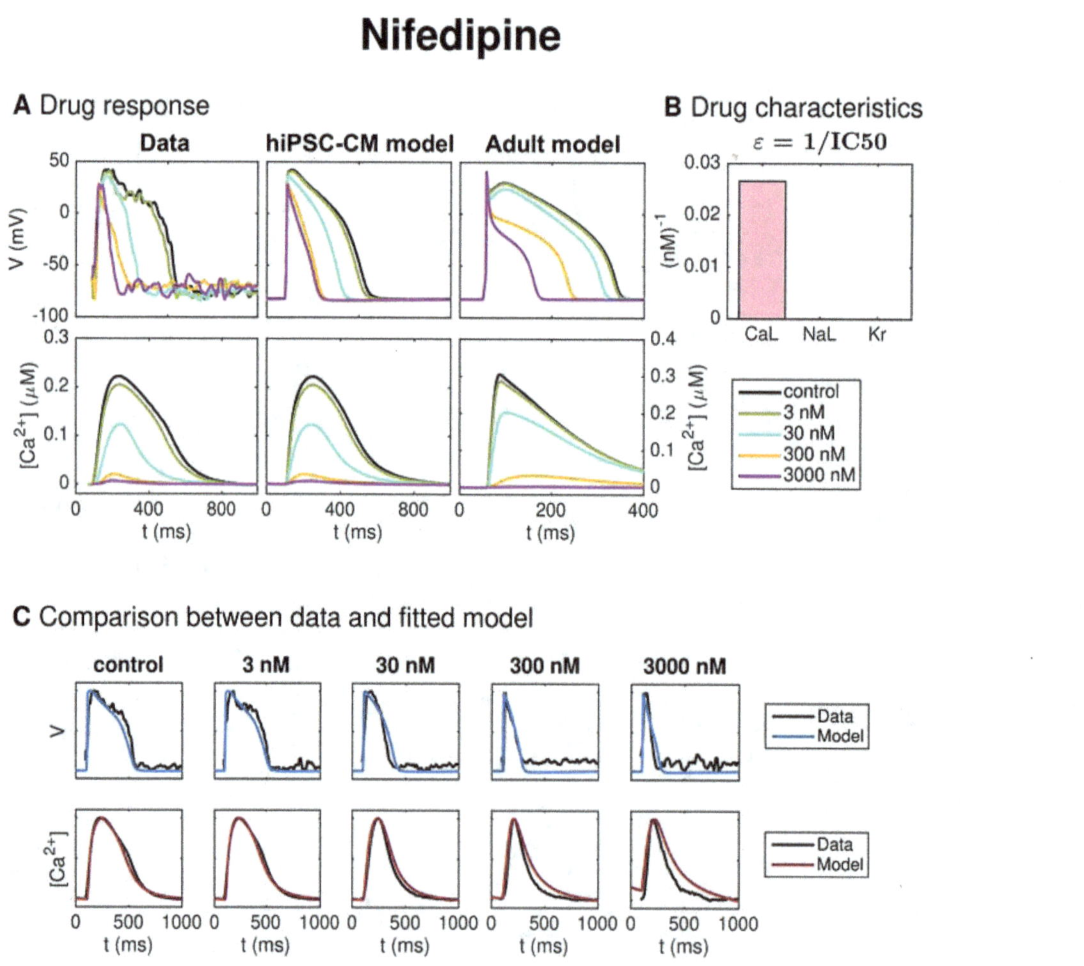

FIGURE 7 | Identification and mapping of drug effects for the drug Nifedipine based on optical measurements of the AP and Ca^{2+} transient of hiPSC-CMs. **(A)** AP and Ca^{2+} transient in the control case and for four drug doses for the data (left) and the fitted hiPSC-CM model (center). The predicted drug effects for adult cardiomyocytes are given in the right panel (note that the scaling of the axes is adjusted for the adult case). Note also that, to clearly see differences in the Ca^{2+} transient amplitude, the displayed Ca^{2+} concentrations are adjusted so that the Ca^{2+} transient amplitude is preserved, but the resting concentration is set to zero in each case. **(B)** Drug effect on I_{CaL}, I_{NaL} and I_{Kr} in the form of ε-values estimated by the inversion procedure. **(C)** Comparison between the measured membrane potential and Ca^{2+} traces and the fitted model solutions for each of the doses in the data set.

From **Figure 7B**, we observe that the inversion procedure predicts that Nifedipine primarily blocks I_{CaL}.

The IC50 values corresponding to the estimated ε-values for I_{CaL}, I_{NaL} and I_{Kr} are given and compared to literature values in **Table 2** for all the five considered drugs of this section (see the *Discussion* section for a discussion of these results).

Lidocaine

Figure 8 shows similar results for inversion of measurements of hiPSC-CMs exposed to the drug Lidocaine. In panel A, we observe that the AP duration is reduced by the drug, and in panel B, we observe that the inversion procedure predicts that the drug primarily blocks the I_{NaL} current.

Cisapride

Figure 9 shows the result of the inversion procedure applied to a data set for hiPSC-CMs exposed to the drug Cisapride. In panel A, we observe that the drug increases the AP duration. In panel B, we observe that the inversion procedure predicts that Cisapride primarily blocks the I_{Kr} current.

Flecainide

Figure 10 shows the result for the inversion procedure applied to optical measurements of hiPSC-CMs exposed to the drug Flecainide. In panel A, we observe that the drug causes increased AP duration. In panel C, we observe that the fitted model fits the data quite well, excepting that the AP duration at high percentages of repolarization is longer for the data than for the model for the highest considered dose. In addition, the shape of the Ca^{2+} transient for the low doses is not entirely captured in the model. In panel B, we observe that the inversion procedure estimates that the drug primarily blocks I_{Kr} and, to some degree, I_{CaL}.

Verapamil

Figure 11 shows the result of the inversion procedure applied to measurements of hiPSC-CMs exposed to the drug Verapamil. In panel A, we observe that the drug leads to decreased AP duration. Panel B shows that the inversion procedure predicts that Verapamil primarily blocks I_{CaL} and, to some extent, I_{Kr}.

Mapping of Drug Effects From hiPSC-CMs to Adult Cells

The rightmost plots of panel A of **Figures 7–11** show the predicted drug effects for adult cells for each of the drugs considered. More specifically, the plots show the solution of the adult base model exposed to each drug's effect (ε-values) as estimated by the inversion procedure for each of the drug doses included in the data set. To review, this represents the predicted drug response for an adult AP and Ca^{2+} transient exposed to each of the drugs, based on the optical measurements of the AP and Ca^{2+} transient as obtained in a microphysiological system of hiPSC-CMs. The predictions are made by first using the inversion procedure to estimate the effect of the drug on the I_{CaL}, I_{NaL}, and I_{Kr} currents in the hiPSC-CM case and then mapping the corresponding drug effects to an adult cell using the determined maturation map based on the assumptions of differences in the channel densities and geometry between hiPSC-CMs and adult cardiomyocytes (see the *Methods* section).

DISCUSSION

Here, we have presented an improved version of the methods presented in (Tveito et al., 2018) for estimating drug effects for adult human cardiomyocytes based on optical measurements of the AP and Ca^{2+} transient of hiPSC-CMs in a microphysiological system. First, we introduce a new base model formulation for representing both adult cells and hiPSC-CMs via different parameter sets. A model for intracellular Ca^{2+} dynamics is updated to a formulation constructed for stability with respect to parameter changes. In addition, we use IC50-based modeling of dose-dependent drug effects and find optimal parameters by running a coupled inversion of both the control data and the drug data for several different doses. The cost function measuring

TABLE 2 | Comparison between the IC50 values obtained from the inversion procedure and values found in literature.

		Nifedipine	Lidocaine	Cisapride	Flecainide	Verapamil
CaL	**Inversion**	**38 nM**	**3400 μM**	**775 nM**	**9 μM**	**495 nM**
	Literature	12 nM (Kramer et al., 2013) 60 nM (Di Stilo et al., 1998)		11 800 nM (Kramer et al., 2013)	26 μM (Crumb et al., 2016) 27 μM (Kramer et al., 2013)	202 nM (Crumb et al., 2016) 200 nM (Kramer et al., 2013) 100 nM (Mirams et al., 2011)
NaL	**Inversion**	**23 600 nM**	**4.3 μM**	**120 nM**	**47 μM**	**23 000 nM**
	Literature		11 μM (Crumb et al., 2016)		19 μM (Crumb et al., 2016)	
Kr	**Inversion**	**40 200 nM**	**50 000 μM**	**13 nM**	**1.9 μM**	**2150 nM**
	Literature	440 000 nM (Kramer et al., 2013) 275 000 nM (Zhabyeyev et al., 2013)		12 nM (Crumb et al., 2016) 20 nM (Kramer et al., 2013) 6.5 nM (Mohammad et al., 1997)	0.7 μM (Crumb et al., 2016) 1.5 μM (Kramer et al., 2013)	499 nM (Crumb et al., 2016) 250 nM (Kramer et al., 2013) 143 nM (Zhang et al., 1999)

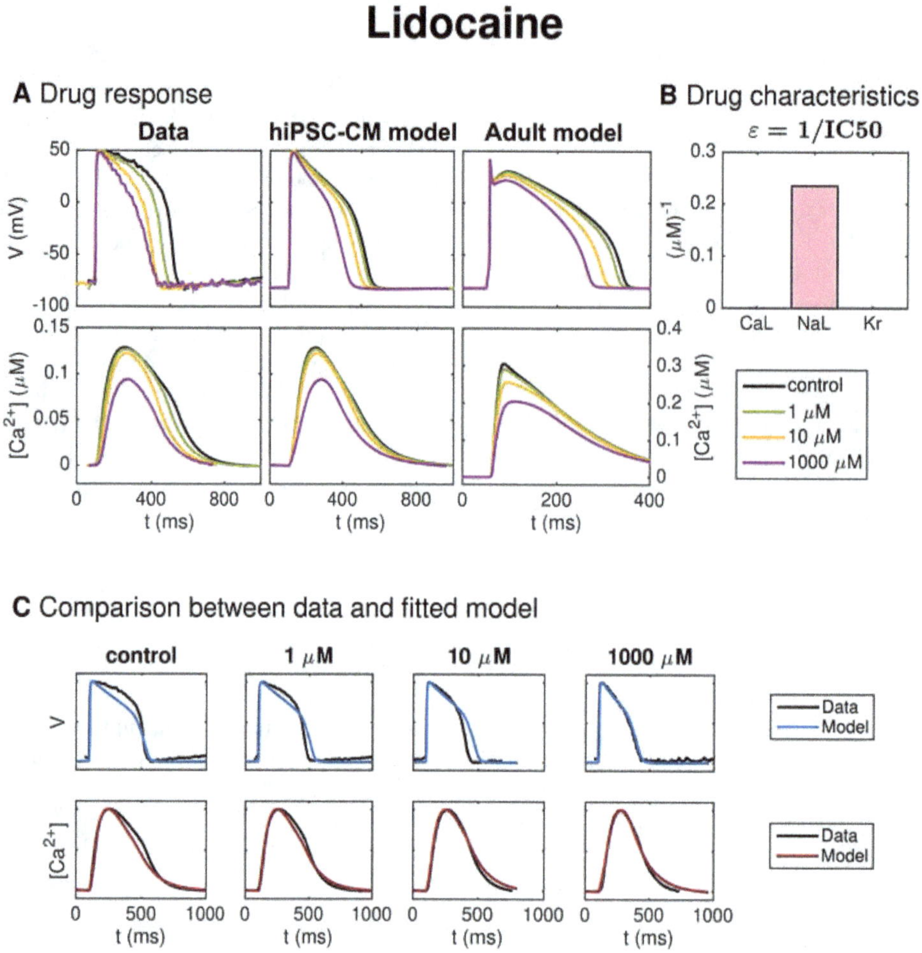

FIGURE 8 | Identification and mapping of drug effects for the drug Lidocaine based on optical measurements of the AP and Ca^{2+} transient of hiPSC-CMs following the same structure as **Figure 7**.

the difference between the data and the model has also been redefined, and we now apply a continuation-based minimization method to minimize the cost function.

Summary of Method Performance and Main Results: Identification of Drug Effects Based on Simulated Data and Optical Measurements of hiPSC-CMs

Figure 6 shows the result of the inversion procedure applied to simulated data. As noted above, we observe that the inversion procedure is able to identify the correct ε-values accurately, excepting the ε-value for Lidocaine, which is predicted to be considerably lower than the value used to generate the data. This suggests that it might be difficult to obtain correct values of ε_{NaL}, as also supported by the low identifiability index for I_{NaL} reported in **Figure 5**. In addition, we observe that the inversion procedure predicts some block of I_{NaL} for the drug Cisapride, even though only I_{Kr} was blocked when the data was generated.

We additionally presented the use of the inversion procedure to identify drug effects on hiPSC-CMs from optical measurements of the AP and Ca^{2+} transients.

Panel C of **Figure 7** compares the experimentally measured data and the fitted model for each of the doses of Nifedipine applied to the microphysiological system. The model fits both the membrane potential and the Ca^{2+} data well for most doses applied, although the Ca^{2+} transient duration is longer in the model than in the data for the highest drug doses considered. Furthermore, in panel B, we observe that the inversion procedure predicts that Nifedipine primarily blocks I_{CaL}. In **Table 2**, we observe that the IC50 value for I_{CaL} is estimated to be 38 nM, in agreement with values found in literature (12 nM–60 nM (Di Stilo et al., 1998; Kramer et al., 2013)]. The IC50 value for I_{NaL} and I_{Kr} are estimated to be 23 600 nM and 40 200 nM, respectively—considerably larger than the doses considered in the data set. We have not found an IC50 value for I_{NaL} for comparison in literature, but the IC50 values found for I_{Kr} support the claim that the IC50 value is much larger than the drug doses included in the data set, although the literature

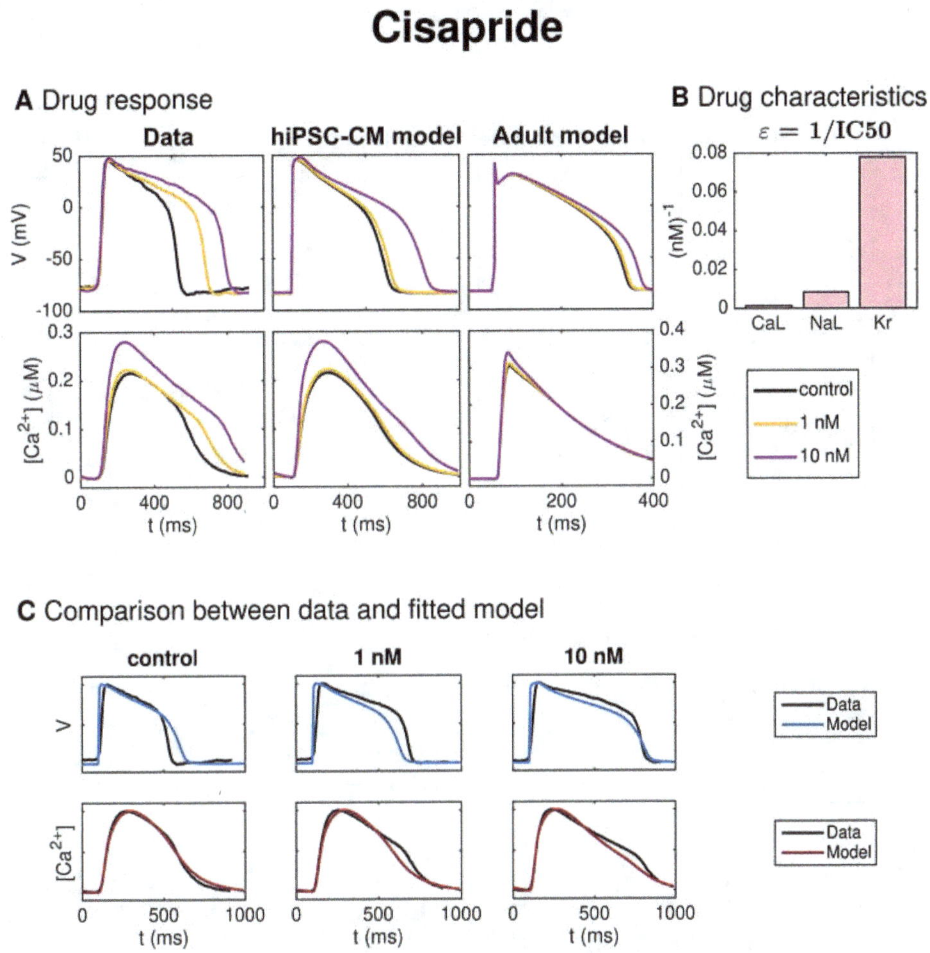

FIGURE 9 | Identification and mapping of drug effects for the drug Cisapride based on optical measurements of the AP and Ca^{2+} transient of hiPSC-CMs following the same structure as **Figure 7**.

values [275,000–440,000 nM (Zhabyeyev et al., 2000; Kramer et al., 2013)] are higher than the value predicted by the inversion procedure.

Figure 8 shows similar results for inversion of measurements of hiPSC-CMs exposed to the drug Lidocaine. The AP duration is reduced by the drug and the inversion procedure predicts that the drug primarily blocks the I_{NaL} current. The IC50 value estimate for I_{NaL} is 4.3 μM (see **Table 2**), in rough agreement with values found in literature [11 μM (Crumb et al., 2016)]. We observe that the model fits the data quite well, but that the AP duration for the drug dose of 10 μM is longer in the model than in the data.

Figure 9 shows the result of the inversion procedure applied to a data set for hiPSC-CMs exposed to the drug Cisapride. Considering the leftmost and center panels of **Figure 9A**, we observe that the prolongation of the AP duration is much more prominent in the data as compared to the fitted hiPSC-CM model for a drug dose of 1 nM. This is also confirmed in **Figure 9C**, where we observe that the model does not fit the membrane potential data for the control case and the 1 nM dose case well. The fit for the largest dose, however, is quite good. In **Figure 9B**, we observe that the inversion procedure predicts that Cisapride primarily blocks I_{Kr}. In **Table 2**, we observe that the IC50 value for I_{Kr} is estimated to be 13 nM, in good agreement with values found in literature [6.5 nM–20 nM (Mohammad et al., 1997; Kramer et al., 2013; Crumb et al., 2016)].

Figure 10 shows the result for the method as applied to measurements of hiPSC-CMs exposed to the drug Flecainide, know to prolong the AP duration. In **Table 2**, we observe that the IC50 value for I_{Kr} predicted by the inversion procedure (1.9 μM) is in quite good agreement with literature values [0.7–1.5 μM (Kramer et al., 2013; Crumb et al., 2016)], but that the predicted IC50 value for I_{CaL} (9 μM) is too low compared to the reported literature values [26–27 μM (Kramer et al., 2013; Crumb et al., 2016)]. In addition, the estimated IC50 value for I_{NaL} (47 μM) is larger than the literature value of 19 μM (Crumb et al., 2016).

In **Figure 11**, the method is applied to measurements of hiPSC-CMs exposed to Verapamil. In panel A, the effect on the AP duration for the smallest dose (100 nM) appears to be more prominent in the data than in the fitted model. This is confirmed

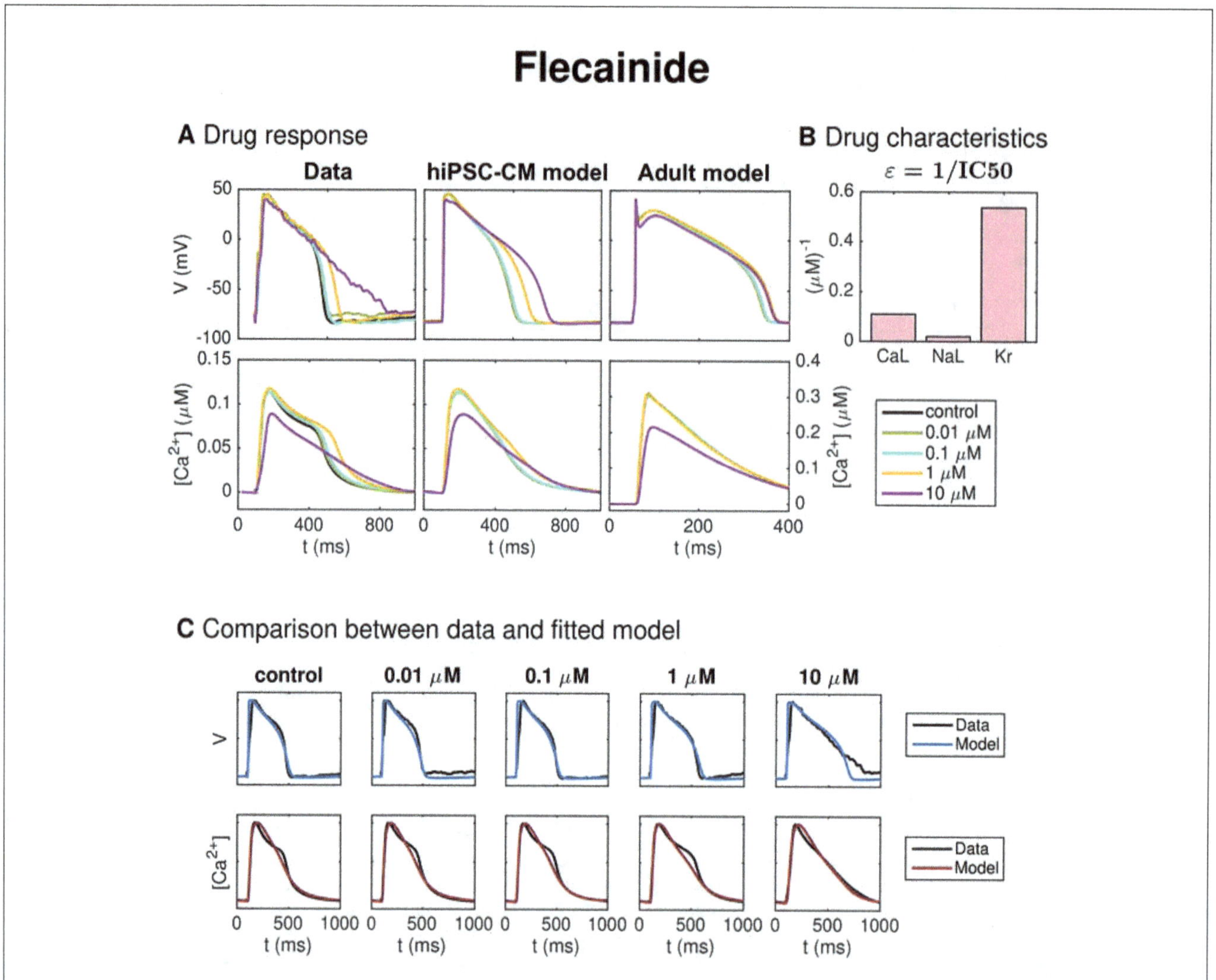

FIGURE 10 | Identification and mapping of drug effects for the drug Flecainide based on optical measurements of the AP and Ca^{2+} transient of hiPSC-CMs following the same structure as **Figure 7**.

in panel C, where we observe that the fitted model seems to fit the Ca^{2+} data considerably better than the membrane potential data. In particular, the AP duration is too short in the control case and too long for the smallest dose of 100 nM. Panel B shows that the inversion procedure predicts that Verapamil primarily blocks I_{CaL} and to some extent I_{Kr}. The predicted IC50 values from **Table 2** (495 nM for I_{CaL} and 2150 nM for I_{Kr}) are both higher than the corresponding values from literature [100–202 nM for I_{CaL} (Mirams et al., 2011; Kramer et al., 2013; Crumb et al., 2016)] and 143–499 nM for I_{Kr} (Zhang et al., 1999; Kramer et al., 2013; Crumb et al., 2016)].

The rightmost plots of panel A of **Figures 7–11** show the predicted drug effects for adult cells for each of the drugs considered. We observe that for some drugs (e.g., Nifedipine and Lidocaine), the drug effects for adult cells are predicted to be approximately as severe as for the hiPSC-CMs. For other drugs, on the other hand, (e.g., Flecainide), the drug effect is predicted to be less severe for the adult cells than for hiPSC-CMs, highlighting the critical importance of maturation phenotype in predictive biophysical models of hiPSC-CMs in pharmacological studies.

Note on Ongoing Complementary Studies

Other recent work has made strong progress in terms of enabling biophysical modeling approaches to assimilate and otherwise make best use of tailored experimental measurements of hiPSC-CMs. For example, in (Gong and Sobie, 2018), the authors address the need to bridge the gap between the effect of drugs on human adult ventricular cardiomyocytes and the effect on animal or hiPSC experimental models often used in drug screening. This work also successfully generated accurate predictions of the effect of ion channel blocking drugs on human adult ventricular cardiomyocytes as based on simulations of hiPSC-CMs via a regression strategy.

Additional recent studies have advanced specific models and methodological approaches for hiPSC-CMs which incorporate experimental variability from multiple data sources [see, e.g., (Kernik et al., 2019)] with the goal of identifying phenotypic

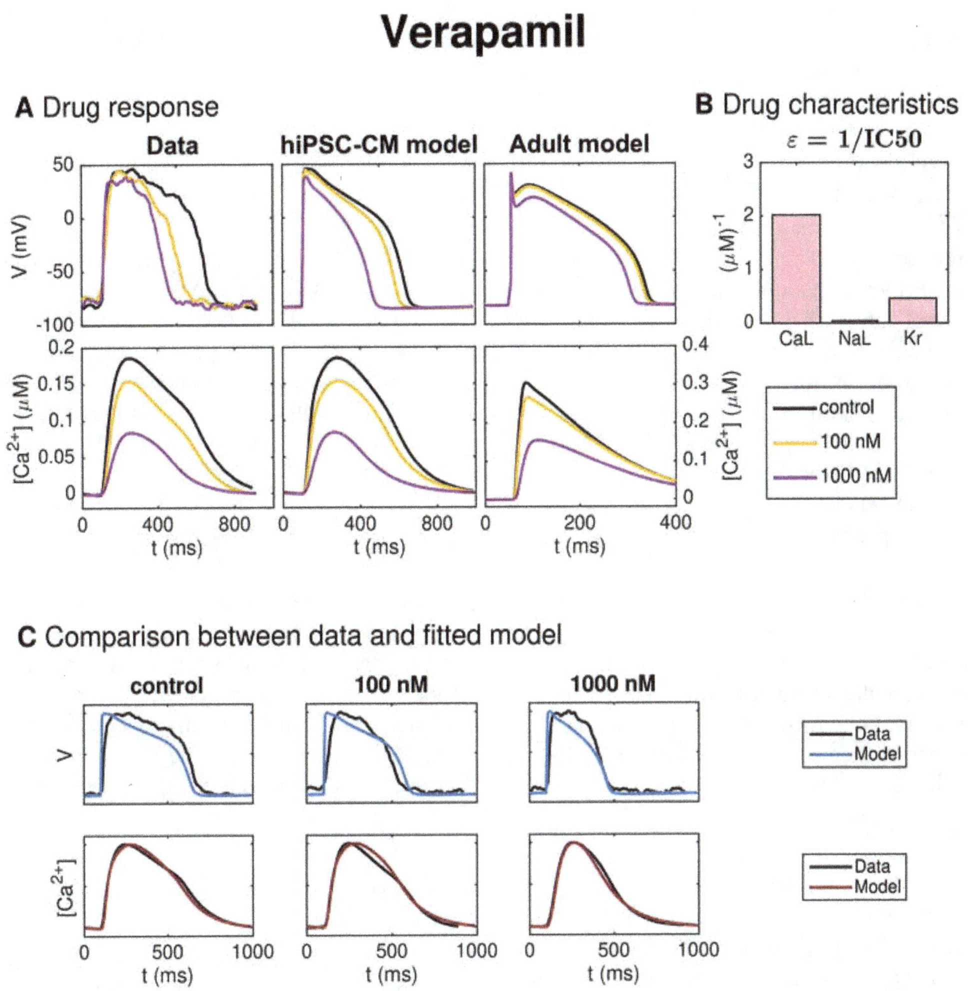

FIGURE 11 | Identification and mapping of drug effects for the drug Verapamil based on optical measurements of the AP and Ca^{2+} transient of hiPSC-CMs, following the same structure as **Figure 7**.

mechanisms and identify key parameter sensitivity. The authors introduce a computational whole-cell electrophysiological model of hiPSC-CMs, composed of single exponential voltage-dependent gating variable rate constants, which are then parameterized to fit experimental measurements of hiPSC-CMs from multiple laboratories (and thus incorporate variability in the single-cell measurements of ionic currents observed experimentally). The authors compare hiPSC-CM and adult cell models to elucidate the primary properties underpinning the phenotype, a mechanistically central goal that was not an aim of our present study.

Limitations and Notes on Future Work

The model for the intracellular Ca^{2+} dynamics in the base model exhibits both high gain and graded release for the hiPSC-CM and adult parameter sets (see **Figure 4**). However, the assumptions underlying the release model are introduced to obtain a stable model, and not necessarily to represent the underlying physiological mechanisms accurately. Future work necessitates assessment of the Ca^{2+} machinery in the base model and potential redevelopment to more accurately represent physiological Ca^{2+} release from the SR, as relevant.

In addition, the intracellular Na^+ and K^+ concentrations are assumed to be constants in the base model formulation. This was done in order to avoid problems with drift of the concentrations following from parameter changes [see, e.g., (Hund et al., 2001; Wilders, 2007; Tveito et al., 2018)]. Moreover, freezing the intracellular Na^+ and K^+ concentrations during an action potential had very limited effects of the computed membrane potential and cytosolic Ca^{2+} concentration. However, in some cases, drugs are believed to lead to significant changes in, e.g., the intracellular Na^+ concentration, which could affect the AP shape [see, e.g., (Brill and Andrew Wasserstrom, 1986; Faber and Rudy, 2000)]. Freezing the Na^+ and K^+ concentrations could therefore potentially make the base model less suitable for detecting such drug effects.

Note also that the terms included in the cost function (31) applied in the inversion procedure may in future work be adapted as required by the specific application under consideration. For example, the cost function could be extended to include information about the frequency dependence of important action potential and Ca^{2+} transient features (see **Figure S4** in the **Supplementary Information**) or to include information about the spontaneous activity of the hiPSC-CMs used in the experiments.

In the construction of the maturation map, we currently assume that the function of a single channel is the same for different levels of maturity and that only the geometry of the cell and the number of channels change with maturation. It is, however, perhaps possible for the function of some channels to change during maturation as well. If the conductance of a channel changes during maturation, the same adjustment factors as we have considered may still be applied, but if the dynamics governing the open probability of the channel change, additional adjustment factors would have to be included in the models for the channel open probability.

In addition, we have only looked at a single dose escalation study for each of the drugs investigated, as well as only tested the method on tissues derived from a single stem cell line. Future work will assess the variability of the inversion methodology in combination with noisy and incomplete experimental data obtained through these systems across a range of biological maturation approaches and starting stem cell lines.

Furthermore, we have only considered data of the drug response for hiPSC-CMs in microphysiological systems, and we have not been able to obtain corresponding data for adult human cardiomyocytes. Drug response data for isolated healthy adult human cardiomyocytes are generally very limited for both technical and ethical reasons (Rodriguez et al., 2015; Sala et al., 2017). We have therefore not been able to validate the predicted adult drug effects against experimental data.

Further validation of the methodology will primarily be based on further analysis of optical data. Hopefully, we will be able to perform analysis of many drugs and also include blind testing for drugs with well-known properties. When more data from patch-clamp measurements become available, that will also be very useful for improvements and validation of our methods.

In future work, we will seek to find ways to estimate the sodium current which is not possible to estimate today because of low time resolution in the optical data. Furthermore, we will combine the base model with the bidomain model [see e.g., (Franzone et al., 2014)] to study extracellular waveforms in the chips, and also the more detailed EMI model [see e.g., (Tveito et al., 2017; Jæger et al., 2019b)] where individual cells can be represented. Hopefully, the spatially resolved models can provide improved accuracy of the inversion process as well as test important considerations such as the effect of tissue composition.

AUTHOR CONTRIBUTIONS

KJ and AT are responsible for the development of the mathematical framework and computer modeling. VC, BC, and KH are responsible for the generation of data provided from microphysiological systems. HF and SW are responsible for the analysis of data from microphysiological systems. KJ, AT, SW, MM, and HF wrote the manuscript text and created the figures. All authors reviewed the manuscript.

FUNDING

We would like to acknowledge the following funding sources: The Research Council of Norway funded INTPART Project 249885, the SUURPh program funded by the Norwegian Ministry of Education and Research, the Peder Sather Center for Advanced Study, NIH-NCATS UH3TR000487, NIH-NHLBI HL130417, and in part by California Institute for Regenerative Medicine DISC2-10090.

REFERENCES

Allgower, E. L., and Georg, K. (2012). *Numerical continuation methods: an introduction* Vol. 13 (Berlin Heidelberg, Germany: Springer Science & Business Media).

Bedada, F. B., Wheelwright, M., and Metzger, J. M. (2016). Maturation status of sarcomere structure and function in human iPSC-derived cardiac myocytes. *Biochim. Biophys. Acta (BBA)-Molecular Cell Res.* 1863 (7), 1829–1838. doi: 10.1016/j.bbamcr.2015.11.005

Brennan, T., Fink, M., and Rodriguez, B. (2009). Multiscale modelling of drug-induced effects on cardiac electrophysiological activity. *Eur. J. Pharmaceut. Sci.* 36 (1), 62–77. doi: 10.1016/j.ejps.2008.09.013

Brill, D. M., and Andrew Wasserstrom, J. (1986). Intracellular sodium and the positive inotropic effect of veratridine and cardiac glycoside in sheep purkinje fibers. *Circ. Res.* 58 (1), 109–119. doi: 10.1161/01.RES.58.1.109

CellML Model Repository. (2019). www.cellml.org/models/.

Chen, I. Y., Matsa, E., and Wu, J. C. (2016). Induced pluripotent stem cells: at the heart of cardiovascular precision medicine. *Nat. Rev. Cardiol.* 13 (6), 333–349. doi: 10.1038/nrcardio.2016.36

Christensen, K., Roudnicky, F., Patsch, C., and Burcin., M. (2018). "Requirements for using iPSC-based cell models for assay development in drug discovery," in *Engineering and Application of Pluripotent Stem Cells*. Eds. U. Martin, R. Zweigerdt and I. Gruh (Cham: Springer International Publishing), 207–220. doi: 10.1007/10_2017_23

Clancy, C. E., Zhu, Z. I., and Rudy, Y. (2007). Pharmacogenetics and anti-arrhythmic drug therapy: A theoretical investigation. *AJP: Heart Circulatory Physiol.* 292 (1), H66–H75. doi: 10.1152/ajpheart.00312.2006

Crumb, W. J., Vicente, J., Johannesen, L., and Strauss, D. G. (2016). An evaluation of 30 clinical drugs against the comprehensive *in vitro* proarrhythmia assay (CiPA) proposed ion channel panel. *J. Pharmacol.*

Toxicol. Methods 81, 251–262. Focused Issue on Safety Pharmacology. doi: 10.1016/j.vascn.2016.03.009

Davies, M. R., Mistry, H. B., Hussein, L., Pollard, C. E., Valentin, J.-P., Swinton, J., et al. (2012). An in silico canine cardiac midmyocardial action potential duration model as a tool for early drug safety assessment. *Am. J. Physiology-Heart Circulatory Physiol* 302, H1466–H1480. doi: 10.1152/ajpheart.00808.2011

Di Baldassarre, A., Cimetta, E., Bollini, S., Gaggi, G., and Ghinassi, B. (2018). Human-induced pluripotent stem cell technology and cardiomyocyte generation: Progress and clinical applications. *Cells* 7 (6), 48. doi: 10.3390/cells7060048

Di Stilo, A., Visentin, S., Cena, C., Gasco, A. M., Ermondi, G., and Gasco, A. (1998). New 1, 4-dihydropyridines conjugated to furoxanyl moieties, endowed with both nitric oxide-like and calcium channel antagonist vasodilator activities. *J. Med. Chem.* 41 (27), 5393–5401. doi: 10.1021/jm9803267

Dupont, G., Falcke, M., Kirk, V., and Sneyd, J. (2016). *Models of calcium signalling* Vol. 43 (Cham, Switzerland: Springer). doi: 10.1007/978-3-319-29647-0

Edwards, A. G., and Louch, W. E. (2017). Species-dependent mechanisms of cardiac arrhythmia: a cellular focus. *Clin. Med. Insights: Cardiol.* 11, 1179546816686061. doi: 10.1177/1179546816686061.

Ermentrout, G. B., and Terman, D. H. (2010). *Mathematical Foundations of Neuroscience* Vol. 35 (New York: Springer-Verlag). doi: 10.1007/978-0-387-87708-2

Faber, G. M., and Rudy, Y. (2000). Action potential and contractility changes in $[Na^+]_i$ overloaded cardiac myocytes: a simulation study. *Biophys. J.* 78 (5), 2392–2404. doi: 10.1016/S0006-3495(00)76783-X

Fine, B., and Vunjak-Novakovic, G. (2017). Shortcomings of animal models and the rise of engineered human cardiac tissue. *ACS Biomaterials Sci. Eng.* 3 (9), 1884–1897. doi: 10.1021/acsbiomaterials.6b00662

Franzone, P. C., Pavarino, L. F., and Scacchi, S. (2014). *Mathematical cardiac electrophysiology* Vol. 13 (Cham, Switzerland: Springer). doi: 10.1007/978-3-319-04801-7

Friel, D. D. (1995). $[Ca^{2+}]_i$ oscillations in sympathetic neurons: an experimental test of a theoretical model. *Biophys. J.* 68 (5), 1752–1766. doi: 10.1016/S0006-3495(95)80352-8

Garg, P., Garg, V., Shrestha, R., Sanguinetti, M. C., Kamp, T. J., and Wu, J. C. (2018). Human induced pluripotent stem cell–derived cardiomyocytes as models for cardiac channelopathies. *Circ. Res.* 123 (2), 224–243. doi: 10.1161/CIRCRESAHA.118.311209

Gong, J. Q. X., and Sobie, E. A. (2018). Population-based mechanistic modeling allows for quantitative predictions of drug responses across cell types. *NPJ Syst. Biol. Appl.* 4 (1), 11. doi: 10.1038/s41540-018-0047-2

Grandi, E., Pasqualini, F. S., and Bers, D. M. (2010). A novel computational model of the human ventricular action potential and Ca transient. *J. Mol. Cell. Cardiol.* 48 (1), 112–121. doi: 10.1016/j.yjmcc.2009.09.019

Hille, B. (2001). *Ion channels of excitable membranes* Vol. 507 (Sinauer Sunderland, MA: Oxford University Press Inc).

Hund, T. J., Kucera, J. P., Otani, N. F., and Rudy, Y. (2001). Ionic charge conservation and long-term steady state in the Luo-Rudy dynamic cell model. *Biophys. J.* 81 (6), 3324–3331. doi: 10.1016/S0006-3495(01)75965-6

Izhikevich, E. M. (2007). *Dynamical Systems in Neuroscience* (Cambridge, MA: MIT Press). doi: 10.7551/mitpress/2526.001.0001

Jæger, K. H., Wall, S., and Tveito, A. (2019a). Detecting undetectables: Can conductances of action potential models be changed without appreciable change in the transmembrane potential? *Chaos: Interdiscip. J. Nonlinear Sci.* 29 (7), 073102. doi: 10.1063/1.5087629

Jæger, K. H., Edwards, A. G., McCulloch, A., and Tveito, A. (2019b). Properties of cardiac conduction in a cell-based computational model. *PloS Comput. Biol.* 15 (5), e1007042. doi: 10.1371/journal.pcbi.1007042

Jiang, Y., Park, P., Hong, S.-M., and Ban, K. (2018). Maturation of cardiomyocytes derived from human pluripotent stem cells: current strategies and limitations. *Molecules Cells* 41 (7), 613. doi: 10.14348/molcells.2018.0143

Keller, H. B. (1987). Lectures on numerical methods in bifurcation problems. *Appl. Math.* 217, 50.

Kernik, D. C., Morotti, S., Di Wu, H., Garg, P., Duff, H. J., Kurokawa, J., et al. (2019). A computational model of induced pluripotent stem-cell derived cardiomyocytes incorporating experimental variability from multiple data sources. *J. Physiol.* 597 (17), 4533–4594. doi: 10.1113/JP277724

Kramer, J., Obejero-Paz, C. A., Myatt, G., Kuryshev, Y. A., Bruening-Wright, A., Verducci, J. S., et al. (2013). MICE models: superior to the HERG model in predicting Torsade de Pointes. *Sci. Rep.* 3, 2100. doi: 10.1038/srep02100

Liang, P., Lan, F., Lee, A. S., Gong, T., Sanchez-Freire, V., Wang, Y., et al. (2013). Drug screening using a library of human induced pluripotent stem cell-derived cardiomyocytes reveals disease specific patterns of cardiotoxicity. *Circulation* 127 (16), 1677–1691. doi: 10.1161/CIRCULATIONAHA.113.001883

Liesen, J., and Mehrmann, V. (2015). *Linear Algebra* (Cham, Switzerland: Springer). doi: 10.1007/978-3-319-24346-7

Luo, C.-H., and Rudy, Y. (1994). A dynamic model of the cardiac ventricular action potential. i. simulations of ionic currents and concentration changes. *Circ. Res.* 74 (6), 1071–1096. doi: 10.1161/01.RES.74.6.1071

Lyche, T. (2017). *Numerical Linear Algebra and Matrix Factorizations* (Oslo, Norway: University of Oslo, lecture notes).

Ma, J., Guo, L., Fiene, S. J., Anson, B. D., Thomson, J. A., Kamp, T. J., et al. (2011). High purity human-induced pluripotent stem cell-derived cardiomyocytes: electrophysiological properties of action potentials and ionic currents. *Am. J. Physiology-Heart Circulatory Physiol.* 301 (5), H2006–H2017. doi: 10.1152/ajpheart.00694.2011

Mathur, A., Loskill, P., Shao, K., Huebsch, N., Hong, S., Marcus, S. G., et al. (2015). Human iPSC-based cardiac microphysiological system for drug screening applications. *Sci. Rep.* 5, 8883. doi: 10.1038/srep08883

Mathur, A., Ma, Z., Loskill, P., Jeeawoody, S., and Healy, K. E. (2016). In vitro cardiac tissue models: current status and future prospects. *Adva. Drug Deliv Rev.* 96, 203–213. doi: 10.1016/j.addr.2015.09.011

Mirams, G. R., Cui, Y., Sher, A., Fink, M., Cooper, J., Heath, B. M., et al. (2011). Simulation of multiple ion channel block provides improved early prediction of compounds' clinical torsadogenic risk. *Cardiovasc. Res.* 91 (1), 53–61. doi: 10.1093/cvr/cvr044

Mohammad, S., Zhou, Z., Gong, Q., and January, C. T. (1997). Blockage of the HERG human cardiac K^+ channel by the gastrointestinal prokinetic agent cisapride. *Am. J. Physiology-Heart Circulatory Physiol.* 273 (5), H2534–H2538. doi: 10.1152/ajpheart.1997.273.5.H2534

Moody, W. J., and Bosma, M. M. (2005). Ion channel development, spontaneous activity, and activity-dependent development in nerve and muscle cells. *Physiol. Rev.* 85 (3), 883–941. doi: 10.1152/physrev.00017.2004

Mora, C., Serzanti, M., Consiglio, A., Memo, M., and Dell'Era, P. (2017). Clinical potentials of human pluripotent stem cells. *Cell Biol. Toxicol.* 33 (4), 351–360. doi: 10.1007/s10565-017-9384-y

Nelder, J. A., and Mead, R. (1965). A simplex method for function minimization. *Comput. J.* 7 (4), 308–313. doi: 10.1093/comjnl/7.4.308

O'Hara, T., Virág, L., Varró, A., and Rudy, Y. (2011). Simulation of the undiseased human cardiac ventricular action potential: Model formulation and experimental validation. *PloS Comput. Biol.* 7 (5), e1002061. doi: 10.1371/journal.pcbi.1002061

Orchard, C. H., Pásek, M., and Brette, F. (2009). The role of mammalian cardiac t-tubules in excitation–contraction coupling: experimental and computational approaches. *Exp. Physiol.* 94 (5), 509–519. doi: 10.1113/expphysiol.2008.043984

Paci, M., Hyttinen, J., Aalto-Setälä, K., and Severi, S. (2013). Computational models of ventricular-and atrial-like human induced pluripotent stem cell derived cardiomyocytes. *Ann. Biomed. Eng.* 41 (11), 2334–2348. doi: 10.1007/s10439-013-0833-3

Paci, M., Hyttinen, J., Rodriguez, B., and Severi, S. (2015). Human induced pluripotent stem cell-derived versus adult cardiomyocytes: an *in silico* electrophysiological study on effects of ionic current block. *Br. J. Pharmacol.* 172 (21), 5147–5160. doi: 10.1111/bph.13282

Paci, M., Passini, E., Severi, S., Hyttinen, J., and Rodriguez, B. (2017). Phenotypic variability in LQT3 human induced pluripotent stem cell-derived cardiomyocytes and their response to anti-arrhythmic pharmacological therapy: an in silico approach. *Heart Rhythm* 14 (11), 1704–1712. doi: 10.1016/j.hrthm.2017.07.026

Paci, M., Pölönen, R.-P., Cori, D., Penttinen, K., Aalto-Setälä, K., Severi, S., et al. (2018). Automatic optimization of an *in silico* model of human iPSC derived cardiomyocytes recapitulating calcium handling abnormalities. *Front. In Physiol.* 9, 709. doi: 10.3389/fphys.2018.00709

Plonsey, R., and Barr, R. C. (2007). *Bioelectricity, A Quantitative Approach* (New York, USA: Springer).

Poulet, C., Wettwer, E., Grunnet, M., Jespersen, T., Fabritz, L., Matschke, K., et al. (2015). Late sodium current in human atrial cardiomyocytes from patients in sinus rhythm and atrial fibrillation. *PloS One* 10 (6), e0131432–e0131432. doi: 10.1371/journal.pone.0131432

Qu, Z., Hu, G., Garfinkel, A., and Weiss, J. N. (2014). Nonlinear and stochastic dynamics in the heart. *Phys. Rep.* 543 (2), 61–162. doi: 10.1016/j.physrep.2014.05.002

Quarteroni, A., Lassila, T., Rossi, S., and Ruiz-Baier, R. (2017). Integrated heart—coupling multiscale and multiphysics models for the simulation of the cardiac function. *Comput. Methods In Appl. Mechanics Eng.* 314, 345–407. doi: 10.1016/j.cma.2016.05.031

Rice, J. J., Jafri, M. S., and Winslow, R. L. (1999). Modeling gain and gradedness of Ca^{2+} release in the functional unit of the cardiac diadic space. *Biophys. J.* 77 (4), 1871–1884. doi: 10.1016/S0006-3495(99)77030-X

Rodriguez, B., Carusi, A., Abi-Gerges, N., Ariga, R., Britton, O., Bub, G., et al. (2015). Human-based approaches to pharmacology and cardiology: an interdisciplinary and intersectorial workshop. *Europace* 18 (9), 1287–1298. doi: 10.1093/europace/euv320

Ronaldson-Bouchard, K., Ma, S. P., Yeager, K., Chen, T., Song, L., Sirabella, D., et al. (2018). Advanced maturation of human cardiac tissue grown from pluripotent stem cells. *Nature* 556 (7700), 239. doi: 10.1038/s41586-018-0016-3

Rudy, Y., and Silva, J. R. (2006). Computational biology in the study of cardiac ion channels and cell electrophysiology. *Q. Rev. Biophys.* 39 (01), 57–116. doi: 10.1017/S0033583506004227

Rudy, Y. (2012). From genes and molecules to organs and organisms: Heart. *Compr. Biophys.* 9, 268–327. doi: 10.1016/B978-0-12-374920-8.00924-3

Sala, L., Bellin, M., and Mummery, C. L. (2017). Integrating cardiomyocytes from human pluripotent stem cells in safety pharmacology: has the time come? *Br. J. Pharmacol.* 174 (21), 3749–3765. doi: 10.1111/bph.13577

Sobie, E. A., Jafri, M. S., and Lederer, W. J. (2010). "Models of cardiac Ca^{2+}-induced Ca^{2+} release and Ca^{2+} sparks," in *Understanding Calcium Dynamics. Experiments and Theory., chapter 6.* Eds. M. Falcke and D. Malchow (Berlin Heidelberg, Germany: Springer-Verlag, Berlin Heidelberg), 97–118. doi: 10.1007/978-3-540-44878-5_6

Sontheimer, H., Ransom, B. R., and Waxman, S. G. (1992). Different Na^+ currents in P0- and P7-derived hippocampal astrocytes *in vitro*: evidence for a switch in Na^+ channel expression *in vivo*. *Brain Res.* 597 (1), 24–29. doi: 10.1016/0006-8993(92)91501-5

Sterratt, D., Graham, B., Gillies, A., and Willshaw, D. (2011). *Principles of Computational Modelling in Neuroscience* (New York, USA: Cambridge University Press).

Ten Tusscher, K. H. W. J., and Panfilov, A. V. (2006). Cell model for efficient simulation of wave propagation in human ventricular tissue under normal and pathological conditions. *Phys. In Med. Biol.* 51 (23), 6141. doi: 10.1088/0031-9155/51/23/014

Tveito, A., and Lines, G. T. (2016). *Computing Characterizations of Drugs for Ion Channels and Receptors Using Markov Models* Vol. 111 (Cham, Switzerland: Springer-Verlag, Lecture Notes). doi: 10.1007/978-3-319-30030-6

Tveito, A., Lines, G. T., Li, P., and McCulloch, A. (2011). Defining candidate drug characteristics for long-QT (LQT3) syndrome. *Math. Biosci. Eng.* 8 (3), 861–873. doi: 10.3934/mbe.2011.8.861

Tveito, A., Jæger, K. H., Kuchta, M., Mardal, K.-A., and Rognes, M. E. (2017). A cell-based framework for numerical modeling of electrical conduction in cardiac tissue. *Front. In Phys.* 5, 48. doi: 10.3389/fphy.2017.00048

Tveito, A., Jæger, K. H., Huebsch, N., Charrez, B., Edwards, A. G., Wall, S., et al. (2018). Inversion and computational maturation of drug response using human stem cell derived cardiomyocytes in microphysiological systems. *Sci. Rep.* 8 (1), 17626. doi: 10.1038/s41598-018-35858-7

Tveito, A., Maleckar, M. M., and Lines, G. T. (2018). Computing optimal properties of drugs using mathematical models of single channel dynamics. *Comput. Math. Biophys.* 6 (1), 41–64. doi: 10.1515/cmb-2018-0004

Wilders, R. (2007). Computer modelling of the sinoatrial node. *Med. Biol. Eng. Comput.* 45 (2), 189–207. doi: 10.1007/s11517-006-0127-0

Ye, L., Ni, X., Zhao, Z.-A., Lei, W., and Hu, S. (2018). The application of induced pluripotent stem cells in cardiac disease modeling and drug testing. *J. Cardiovasc. Trans. Res.* 11 (5), 366–374. doi: 10.1007/s12265-018-9811-3

Yoshida, Y., and Yamanaka, S. (2017). Induced pluripotent stem cells 10 years later. *Circ. Res.* 120 (12), 1958–1968. doi: 10.1161/CIRCRESAHA.117.311080

Zemzemi, N., Bernabeu, M. O., Saiz, J., Cooper, J., Pathmanathan, P., Mirams, G. R., et al. (2013). Computational assessment of drug-induced effects on the electrocardiogram: from ion channel to body surface potentials. *Br. J. Pharmacol.* 168 (3), 718–733. doi: 10.1111/j.1476-5381.2012.02200.x

Zhabyeyev, P., Missan, S., Jones, S. E., and McDonald, T. F. (2000). Low-affinity block of cardiac K^+ currents by nifedipine. *Eur. J. Pharmacol.* 401 (2), 137–143. doi: 10.1016/S0014-2999(00)00413-1

Zhang, S., Zhou, Z., Gong, Q., Makielski, J. C., and January, C. T. (1999). Mechanism of block and identification of the verapamil binding domain to HERG potassium channels. *Circ. Res.* 84 (9), 989–998. doi: 10.1161/01.RES.84.9.989

Zhao, Z., Lan, H., El-Battrawy, I., Li, X., Buljubasic, F., Sattler, K., et al. (2018). et al. Ion channel expression and characterization in human induced pluripotent stem cell-derived cardiomyocytes. *Stem Cells Int.* 2018, 6067096. doi: 10.1155/2018/6067096

3

Novel Na^+/Ca^{2+} Exchanger Inhibitor ORM-10962 Supports Coupled Function of Funny-Current and Na^+/Ca^{2+} Exchanger in Pacemaking of Rabbit Sinus Node Tissue

Zsófia Kohajda[1,2†], *Noémi Tóth*[2†], *Jozefina Szlovák*[2], *Axel Loewe*[3], *Gergő Bitay*[2], *Péter Gazdag*[2], *János Prorok*[2], *Norbert Jost*[1,2], *Jouko Levijoki*[4], *Piero Pollesello*[4], *Julius Gy. Papp*[1,2], *András Varró*[1,2*] *and Norbert Nagy*[1,2]

[1] *MTA-SZTE Research Group of Cardiovascular Pharmacology, Hungarian Academy of Sciences, Szeged, Hungary,* [2] *Department of Pharmacology and Pharmacotherapy, Faculty of Medicine, University of Szeged, Szeged, Hungary,* [3] *Institute of Biomedical Engineering, Karlsruhe Institute of Technology (KIT), Karlsruhe, Germany,* [4] *Orion Pharma, Espoo, Finland*

Correspondence:
András Varró
varro.andras@med.u-szeged.hu

†*These authors have contributed equally to this work*

Background and Purpose: The exact mechanism of spontaneous pacemaking is not fully understood. Recent results suggest tight cooperation between intracellular Ca^{2+} handling and sarcolemmal ion channels. An important player of this crosstalk is the Na^+/Ca^{2+} exchanger (NCX), however, direct pharmacological evidence was unavailable so far because of the lack of a selective inhibitor. We investigated the role of the NCX current in pacemaking and analyzed the functional consequences of the I_f-NCX coupling by applying the novel selective NCX inhibitor ORM-10962 on the sinus node (SAN).

Experimental Approach: Currents were measured by patch-clamp, Ca^{2+}-transients were monitored by fluorescent optical method in rabbit SAN cells. Action potentials (AP) were recorded from rabbit SAN tissue preparations. Mechanistic computational data were obtained using the Yaniv *et al.* SAN model.

Key Results: ORM-10962 (ORM) marginally reduced the SAN pacemaking cycle length with a marked increase in the diastolic Ca^{2+} level as well as the transient amplitude. The bradycardic effect of NCX inhibition was augmented when the funny-current (I_f) was previously inhibited and *vice versa,* the effect of I_f was augmented when the Ca^{2+} handling was suppressed.

Conclusion and Implications: We confirmed the contribution of the NCX current to cardiac pacemaking using a novel NCX inhibitor. Our experimental and modeling data support a close cooperation between I_f and NCX providing an important functional consequence: these currents together establish a strong depolarization capacity providing important safety factor for stable pacemaking. Thus, after individual inhibition of I_f or NCX, excessive bradycardia or instability cannot be expected because each of these currents may compensate for the reduction of the other providing safe and rhythmic SAN pacemaking.

Keywords: Na^+/Ca^{2+} exchanger, funny-current, ORM-10962, pacemaking, sinus-node

INTRODUCTION

Computational modeling as well as experimental results established previously that the normal pacemaker function is not only regulated by the hyperpolarization-activated funny current (I_f) (DiFrancesco, 1981) but is also regulated by the intracellular Ca^{2+} handling (Lakatta and DiFrancesco, 2009; Yaniv et al., 2013a; Yaniv et al., 2015; Sirenko et al., 2016). Lakatta and co-workers suggested that the sinus node (SAN) cells operate by a rhythmic clock-like oscillator system where the sarcoplasmic reticulum serves as a Ca^{2+}-clock, which rhythmically discharges diastolic local Ca^{2+} releases (LCRs), and activates the forward (inward) Na^+/Ca^{2+} exchanger (NCX) current to accelerate the diastolic depolarization and facilitates the membrane-clock (M-clock) (Yaniv et al., 2015). Recent experimental results further suggest that these clocks work tightly coupled since the M-clock regulates the Ca^{2+} influx and efflux while the NCX also regulates the diastolic depolarization forming a coupled-clock system. Therefore, NCX may have crucial importance in the clock-like oscillator system since the NCX-mediated inward current is directly translated to membrane potential changes *via* the operation of forward mode of the exchanger. This hypothesis was repeatedly challenged and the pivotal role of Ca^{2+} clock was questioned by other authors (Noble et al., 2010; Himeno et al., 2011; DiFrancesco and Noble, 2012).

As early as 1983, Irishawa and Morad showed in elegant experiments that full inhibition of I_f current by caesium did not significantly influence SAN spontaneous activity arguing for mechanisms other than I_f (Noma et al., 1983). On the other hand, other studies suggest a fundamental role of the exchanger in normal automaticity. A low-sodium bath solution inhibited spontaneous action potentials (AP) firing in guinea-pig SAN cells *via* suppressing normal function of NCX (Sanders et al., 2006). Other studies reported that depletion of SR store by application of ryanodine markedly disturbed the normal pacemaker activity in rabbit SAN cells (Bogdanov et al., 2001). Mouse genetic models revealed that partial atrial NCX1 knock out (≈90%) caused severe bradycardia and other rhythm disorders (Herrmann et al., 2013), while complete atrial NCX knock-out completely suppressed the atrial depolarization exerting ventricular escape rhythm on the ECG (Groenke et al., 2013). The application of KB-R7943, a non-selective NCX inhibitor, also suppressed spontaneous beating in guinea-pig SAN cells (Sanders et al., 2006) however it has also marked effect on the Ca^{2+}-currents. The supposed crucial role of NCX in the normal pacemaker function of SAN could not be directly investigated experimentally so far due to the lack of a selective NCX inhibitor. Recently, two novel NCX inhibitors were synthesized: ORM-10103 and ORM-10962, both showing improved selectivity without influencing I_{CaL} function (Jost et al., 2013; Kohajda et al., 2016; Oravecz et al., 2017).

Abbreviations: AP, action potential; APD, action potential duration; CL, cycle length; CLV, cycle length variability; DD, diastolic depolarization; DI, diastolic interval; DOF, dofetilide; NCX, sodium-calcium exchanger; I_f, funny-current; IVA, ivabradine; ORM, ORM-10962; RYA, ryanodine; SAN, sinoatrial-node.

In this study we confirmed the contributing role of NCX to spontaneous pacemaking by its direct pharmacological inhibition *via* the novel, selective inhibitor ORM-10962. Our data suggest that a strong crosstalk between I_f and NCX also exists in multicellular level, which was described and discussed by the Lakatta group earlier in single cell level (Yaniv et al., 2015). In addition, however, extending these earlier findings, we show that the effect of individual I_f and NCX inhibition is minimal whereas a combined inhibition acts synergistically, providing an important safety margin for secure spontaneous activity of the SAN.

MATERIALS AND METHODS

Ethical Statement

All experiments were conducted in compliance with the *Guide for the Care and Use of Laboratory Animals* (USA NIH publication No 85-23, revised 1996) and conformed to Directive 2010/63/EU of the European Parliament. The protocols were approved by the Review Board of the Department of Animal Health and Food Control of the Ministry of Agriculture and Rural Development, Hungary (XIII./1211/2012).

Animals

The measurements were performed in right atrial tissue obtained from young New-Zealand white rabbits from both genders weighing 2.0–2.5 kg.

Voltage-Clamp Measurements

Cell Preparations

For measuring I_f pacemaker current, we isolated single cells from the SAN region of rabbit heart by enzymatic dissociation. The animals were sacrificed by concussion after receiving 400 IU/kg heparin intravenously. The chest was opened and the heart was quickly removed and placed into cold (4°C) solution with the following composition (mM): NaCl 135, KCl 4.7, KH_2PO_4 1.2, $MgSO_4$ 1.2, 4-(2-hydroxyethyl)-1-piperazineethanesulfonic acid (HEPES) 10, $NaHCO_3$ 4.4, glucose 10, $CaCl_2$ 1.8, (pH 7.2 with NaOH). The heart was mounted on a modified, 60 cm high Langendorff column and perfused with oxygenated and prewarmed (37°C) solution mentioned above. After washing out of blood (3–5 min) the heart was perfused with nominally Ca-free solution until the heart stopped beating (approx. 3–4 min). The digestion was performed by perfusion with the same solution supplemented with 1.8 mg/ml (260 U/ml) collagenase (type II, Worthington). After 10–12 min, the heart was removed from the cannula. The right atrium was cut and the crista terminalis and SAN region were excised and cut into small strips. Strips were placed into enzyme free solution containing 1 mM $CaCl_2$ and equilibrated at 37°C for 10 min. After 10 min with gentle agitation, the cells were separated by filtering through a nylon mesh. Sedimentation was used for harvesting cells. The supernatant was removed and replaced by HEPES-buffered Tyrode's solution. The cells were stored at room temperature in the Tyrode's solution.

Measurement of Pacemaker Current (Funny Current)

For the measurement of the I_f current, the method of Verkerk et al. (2009) was adapted and applied. The current was recorded in HEPES-buffered Tyrode's solution while the composition of the pipette solution was the following (in mM): KOH 110, KCl 40, K_2ATP 5, $MgCl_2$ 5, EGTA 5, HEPES 10, and GTP 0.1 (pH was adjusted to 7.2 by aspartic acid). The current was activated by hyperpolarizing voltage pulses to −120 mV from a holding potential of −30 mV. The pacemaker current was identified as ivabradine (IVA) sensitive current. The experiments were performed at 37°C.

Fluorescent Optical Measurements

Isolated, spontaneously beating SAN cells were used for measurements. Ca^{2+} transients were measured by Fluo-4 AM fluorescent dye. Isolated cells were loaded with 5 μM dye for 20 min in room temperature in dark. Loaded cells were mounted in a low volume imaging chamber (RC47FSLP, Warner Instruments) and continuously superfused with normal Tyrode solution. Fluorescence measurements were performed on the stage of an Olympus IX 71 inverted fluorescence microscope. The dye was excited at 480 nm and the emitted fluorescence was detected at 535 nm. Optical signals were sampled at 1 kHz and recorded by a photon counting photomultiplier module (Hamamatsu, model H7828). Amplitudes of the Ca^{2+} transients were calculated as differences between systolic and diastolic values. To measure Ca^{2+} changes the cells were damaged by a patch pipette at the end of the experiment to obtain maximal fluorescence (F_{max}). Ca^{2+} was calibrated using the following formula: $K_d(F-F_{min})/(F_{max}-F)$. K_d of the Fluo-4 AM was 335 nM.

Action Potential Measurements With Standard Microelectrode Technique

We have chosen multicellular preparations for action potential measurements for three reasons: 1) all of the ion channels remained intact (current density, kinetics) because of the lack of enzymatic dissociation, thus providing more precise estimates of the ratio between the currents, 2) since the SAN cells are surrounded with atrial cells having a more negative resting membrane potential, the electrotonic coupling may intimately influence the SAN cells. It may have great importance since the I_f current markedly increases as the membrane potential drops to more negative values (Morad and Zhang, 2017), (3) the action potential frequency was very stable with a cycle-length variability lower than 5 ms.

SAN regions obtained from right atria were mounted in a tissue chamber superfused with oxygenated Locke's solution at 37°C. A conventional microelectrode technique was performed as previously described (Kormos et al., 2014; Kohajda et al., 2016; Oravecz et al., 2017). In the case of SAN, the action potentials were empirically found in the right atrium. SAN action potentials were verified by the maximum upstroke speed, which had to be lower than 15 V/s, the resting membrane potential (>−60 mV), and a clear diastolic depolarization (DD). Efforts were made to maintain the same impalement throughout each experiment. If impalement became dislodged, however, electrode adjustment was attempted and, if the action potential characteristics of the re-established impalement deviated by less than 5% from those of the previous measurement, the experiment was continued. When this 5% limit was exceeded, the experiment was terminated and all data were excluded from the analyses.

Action potential durations were measured at 90, 50, and 25% of repolarization. The maximal diastolic potential was defined as the most negative potential reached during the repolarization. The take off potential is the most negative point of the AP upstroke. DD was defined as the interval between the maximal diastolic potential and take off potential. The DD slope was calculated as $\Delta V_m/\Delta t$ between these points. The cycle length was calculated as the peak-to-peak interval between two consecutive APs. The phase 0 depolarization velocity was defined as the maximum of the first derivative of the AP during the upstroke.

Modeling

To complement the experiments, we performed mechanistic computational modeling using the Yaniv *et al.* model of rabbit SAN cells (Yaniv et al., 2013b). The differential equations of the model were solved using a forward Euler scheme. Simulation results were analyzed when the system had converged to a cyclic steady-state.

Statistical Analysis

All data are expressed as mean ± standard error (SEM). Statistical analysis was performed with Student's *t*-test and ANOVA with Bonferroni *post-hoc* test. The results were considered statistically significant when $p < 0.05$. In the case of action potential experiments, all recordings were obtained from different hearts.

Materials

With the exception of ORM-10962 (ORM) (from Orion Pharma, Espoo, Finland), and Fluo-4 AM (Thermo Fisher Scientific, Waltham, MA, USA), all chemicals were purchased from Sigma-Aldrich Fine Chemicals (St. Louis, MO, USA). ORM was dissolved in dimethyl-sulfoxide (DMSO) to obtain a 1 mM stock solution. This stock solution was diluted to reach the desired final concentration (DMSO concentration not exceeding 0.1%) in the bath.

RESULTS

ORM-10962 Has No Effect on Funny Current

Figure 1 shows the measurement of I_f in isolated SAN cells by applying the whole cell configuration of the patch clamp method. The selectivity of ORM on Na^+-, Ca^{2+}-, and major K^+ currents was tested in a previous study from our laboratory (Kohajda et al., 2016). However, its potential effect on the I_f current was not investigated in that previous study. As **Figures 1A, C** show a slowly developed current at negative hyperpolarizing membrane potential (from −30 to −120 mV), which was not altered by application of 1 μM ORM (**Figure 1B**). In contrast, it was markedly inhibited by 10 μM IVA (69.3 ± 3.4%), a well known inhibitor of I_f.

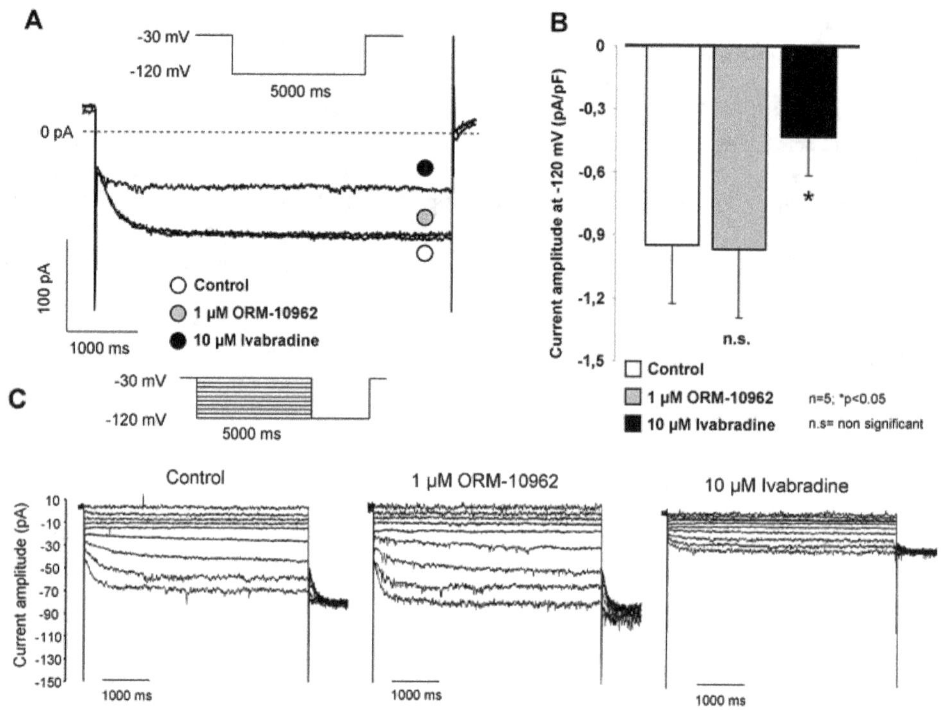

FIGURE 1 | Investigation of the possible effect of ORM-10962 (ORM) on funny current (I_f) in isolated sinus node (SAN) cells. The hyperpolarization activated I_f was elicited by 5,000 ms long rectangle pulse potentials to −120 mV from a holding potential of −30 mV. As representative current traces indicate, the current amplitude after ORM application (gray circle) was identical with the control (open circle). The considerable effect of 10 μM ivabradine (IVA) verified that the elicited current was indeed I_f **(A, B)**. Original traces in panel **(C)** represent the absence of ORM effects on current-voltage relationship of I_f by applying hyperpolarization pulses from −120 mV to −30 mV with 10 mV increments.

Na^+/Ca^{2+} Exchanger Inhibition Exerted Moderate Bradycardic Effect on Sinus Node Tissue

Figure 2 summarizes the effect of selective NCX inhibition by ORM on the spontaneous automaticity in SAN. Following application of 1 μM ORM a moderate but significant lengthening effect on the CL was observed (455.6 ± 32 ms *vs.* 493.0 ± 38 ms; Δ = 8.1 ± 1.8% $p < 0.05$, n = 16/16 hearts; **Figures 2A–C**) without any influence on the action potential duration (APD) (94.3 ± 6.7 ms *vs.* 96.7 ± 5.9 ms; **Figure 2D**). The slope of the diastolic depolarization phase was significantly reduced after ORM application (15.7 ± 3.1 mV/s *vs.* 10.9 ± 2.8 mV/s; n = 14/14; $p < 0.05$ **Figure 2E**) while the CL variability remained unchanged (7.6 ± 1.2 ms *vs.* 8.1 ± 1.3 ms; **Figure 2F**). The slope of phase 0 AP depolarization was identical during control and ORM experiments (11.2 ± 2.7 V/s *vs.* 12.5 ± 2.3 V/s). The preparations maintained the stable frequency in the time control experiments when DMSO was applied (440 ± 36.1 ms *vs.* 445 ± 37.6; n = 4). In the computational SAN action potential model (Yaniv et al., 2013b), we identified the degree of NCX current suppression required to obtain a similar CL increase as was experimentally measured. Forty-one percent of NCX inhibition was required to obtain 8% CL increase which was equal with the CL change observed experimentally (**Figure 2G**).

Na^+/Ca^{2+} Exchanger Inhibition Slightly Increased the Diastolic Ca^{2+} Level in Isolated Sinus Node Cells

The diastolic Ca^{2+} level increased in isolated SAN cells after ORM treatment (70 ± 11 nM *vs.* 130 ± 24 nM; $p < 0.05$, n = 10; **Figures 3A, B**), the effect was similar than was predicted by the Yaniv et al. SAN model (**Figure 3D**). In contrast to the model prediction, we found considerable increase in the transient amplitude (312 ± 37 nM *vs.* 568 ± 85 nM; $p < 0.05$, n = 10 **Figure 3C**), which was nearly doubled (82.1 ± 22%) in response to ORM application compared to the control value.

The Concomitant Application of Ivabradine and ORM-10962 Revealed Coupled Frequency Control Between Funny Current and Na^+/Ca^{2+} Exchanger Measured in Sinus Node Tissue

In the next set of experiments, IVA and ORM were subsequently applied to study a possible coupling between I_f and NCX.

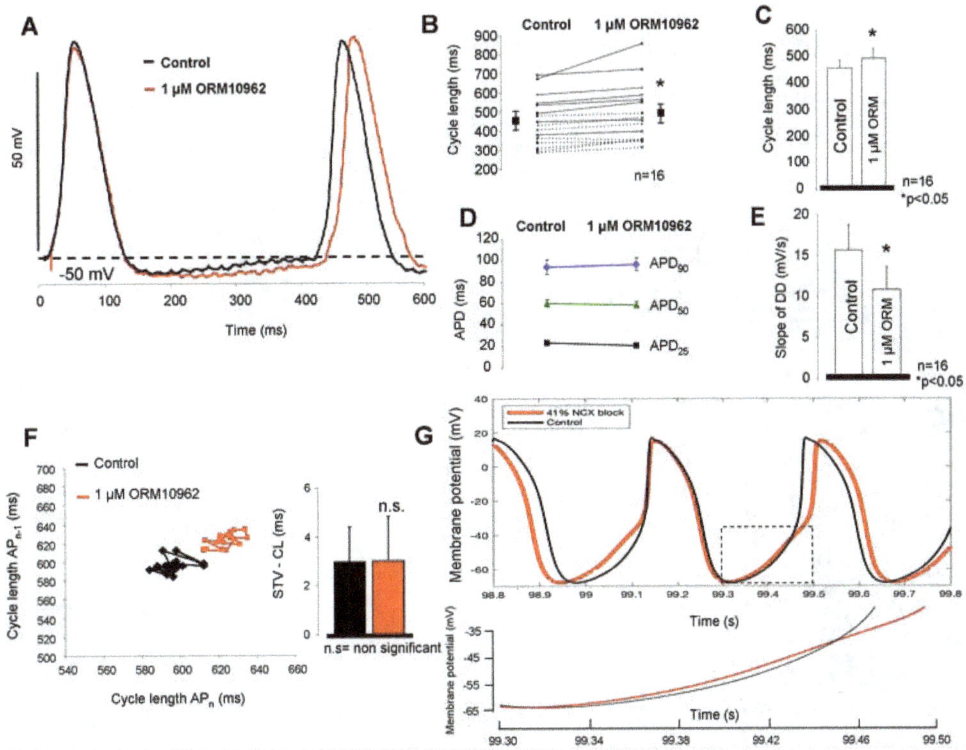

FIGURE 2 | Estimation of the effect of selective Na+/Ca2+ exchanger (NCX) inhibition on sinus node (SAN) tissue. As representative action potential traces **(A)** as well as individual experiments **(B)** and bar graphs **(C)** indicate, application of 1 μM ORM-10962 (ORM) exerted a slight but statistically significant bradycardic effect on SAN tissue. The action potential duration (APD) did not change during the experiment **(D)**, however the slope of the spontaneous depolarization was considerably decreased **(E)**. 30 consecutive cycles were analyzed to estimate the pacing rate variability. Poincaré-plot and bar graphs depict that ORM did not alter the short-term cycle length (CL) variability **(F)**. The Yaniv SAN cell model predicts 41% NCX inhibition to meet with the observed bradycardic effect of 1 μM ORM. The inset illustrates the reduced slope during late diastolic depolarization (DD) when 41% NCX inhibition was applied (red curve) **(G)**.

The effect of 1 μM ORM was substantially larger when I_f was previously inhibited (**Figures 4A, B**). Ca^{2+} transient measurements from spontaneously contracting SAN cells showed identical amplitudes (327 ± 23 nM *vs.* 337 ± 42 nM; n = 12) as well as diastolic Ca^{2+} levels (89 ± 22 nM *vs.* 85 ± 13 nM; n = 12) between control and 3 μM IVA (**Figure 4C**). A clear, gradual increase of ORM effect on the CL was observed with combined increasing concentration of IVA (1 μM ORM effect in the presence of 0 μM IVA: 8.1 ± 1.88%; in the presence of 0.5 μM IVA: 9.6 ± 2.3%; in the presence of 3 μM IVA: 17.1 ± 2.5%; **Figure 4D**). The ORM effect in the presence of 0.5 μM IVA did not differ significantly from the control, where 0 μM IVA was applied (8.1 ± 1.88% *versus* 9.6 ± 2.3%). In contrast, ORM effect was significantly larger on the CL in the presence of 3 μM IVA, compared with the control where IVA was not applied (8.1 ± 1.88% *versus* 17.1 ± 2.5%; $p < 0.05$, ANOVA, Bonferroni *post hoc* test). IVA significantly increased the CL both in 0.5 and in 3 μM concentrations ($p < 0.05$, ANOVA, Bonferroni *post hoc* test). In **Figure 4E**, we compare modeling and experimental results. In the Yaniv et al. model, based on a previous study (Bois et al., 1996), I_f inhibition was varied between 0%/20%/60% block (corresponding to 0, 0.5, and 3 μM IVA). Larger, 85% inhibition was only set in the model, since experimental application of 10 μM IVA is not feasible because of the marked I_{Kr} inhibition which can also reduce automaticity. The NCX inhibition was 41% in all cases. As **Figure 4E** shows, the modeling results do not match the experiments quantitatively, however they show a similar tendency (when I_f block increases, the same NCX inhibition causes larger CL prolongation) with markedly steeper correlation.

Figure 4F shows original modeling traces in the presence of 20% (left panel), 60% (middle panel), and 85% (right panel) I_f inhibition when NCX inhibition was 41% in all cases. The action potential modeling demonstrates an increased CL prolongation effect of NCX inhibition as I_f suppression becomes stronger, however, in contrast to the model prediction the steepness of NCX inhibition-induced CL increase was considerable flatter during experiments.

I_{Kr} Inhibition-Induced Bradycardia Did Not Facilitate the Effect of Selective Na^+/Ca^{2+} Exchanger Inhibition on Cycle Length in Sinus Node Tissue

We investigated how bradycardia induced by a mechanism which does not directly involve the inward depolarizing

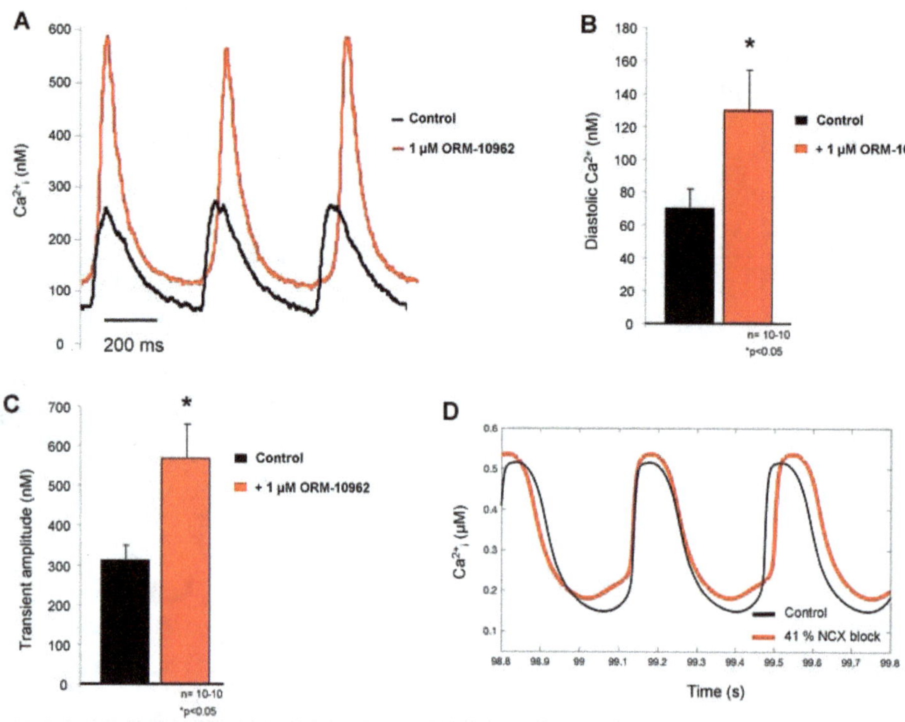

FIGURE 3 | (A) Representative Ca^{2+} transient traces from spontaneously contracting isolated sinus node (SAN) cells under control conditions (black trace) and after 1 µM ORM-10962 (ORM) application (red trace). As original fluorescent data as well as bar graphs indicate, a slight but significant increase of the diastolic Ca^{2+} level **(B)** with increased transient amplitude **(C)** was observed. In line with experimental data, the Yaniv SAN cell model predicted similar diastolic Ca^{2+} gain after 41% Na+/Ca2+ exchanger (NCX) inhibition **(D)**, however the increase of transient amplitude is much more pronounced during the experimental results.

currents (I_f and NCX) would influence the effect of NCX inhibition. Full I_{Kr} block induced by 100 nM dofetilide (DOF) markedly increased the CL of SAN AP (control: 489.3 ± 31 ms → 100 nM dofetilide: 649.1 ± 40.2 ms). This degree of increase of CL was due to the lengthening of APD without changing the DI. The subsequent application of 1 µM ORM exerted a similar effect (1 µM ORM-10962: 679.6 ± 52.6 ms; n = 7/7 hearts; **Figures 5A, B**), compared with results obtained after individual administration presented in **Figure 2** (7.2 ± 1.8% *vs.* 8.1 ± 1.8%, **Figure 5F**). It is important that the effect of DOF on CL was nearly similar to 3 µM IVA (32.9 ± 6.7% *vs.* 20.9 ± 4.1%). However, the major difference was that the DOF-mediated increase in CL was practically entirely an APD increase-induced effect (APD_{90}: 94.4 ± 3 ms *vs.* 187 ± 7.1 ms; $p < 0.05$, n = 7; diastolic interval (DI): 338.3 ± 39 ms *vs.* 352.7 ± 44.6 ms, n = 7) while the IVA influenced only the DI without affecting the APD_{90} (**Figures 5C–E**). In contrast, both NCX inhibition by ORM and I_f inhibition by IVA increased the CL due to lengthening of the time of the DI by decreasing its slope. When ORM was applied in combination with DOF the increase of the CL was not additive.

Suppression of Ca^{2+} Increases the Effect of I_f Inhibition on Cycle Length in Sinus Node Tissue

In the next set of experiments, we investigated the potential effect of suppression of SR Ca^{2+} release on the effect of IVA (**Figure 6A**). The aim was to minimize the depolarizing activity of the Ca^{2+} release-induced augmentation of the forward NCX by application of 5 µM ryanodine (RYA) after the control recording. This caused a significant CL prolongation (437.8 ± 20.3 ms *vs.* 499.8 ± 10.4 ms; $p < 0.05$, n = 6/6). The subsequently applied 1 µM ORM-10962 marginally but statistically significantly increased the CL (499.8 ± 10.4 ms *vs.* 520.8 ± 29.9 ms; $p < 0.05$; n = 6/6). However, further 3 µM IVA markedly and significantly augmented the CL of the SAN preparations (520.8 ± 29.9 ms *vs.* 726.6 ± 39.8 ms; $p < 0.05$, n = 6/6; **Figure 6B**). In the **Figure 6C** we compared the IVA effects under normal condition (i.e., in the absence of any other inhibitors—20.9 ± 4.1%) and in the presence of RYA+ORM. As bar graphs in **Figure 6C** show, the IVA exerted markedly larger CL prolongation in the presence of RYA+ORM (42.4 ± 5.7%, $p < 0.05$, Student's T-test).

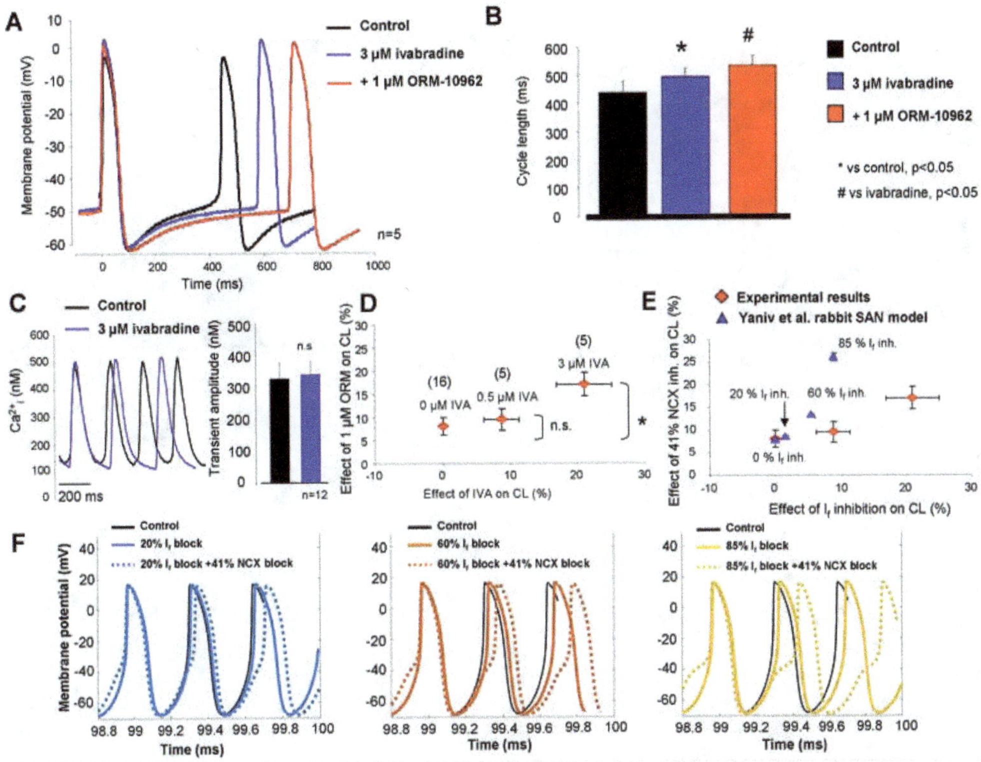

FIGURE 4 | Combined inhibition of Na+/Ca2+ exchanger (NCX) and I_f in sinus node (SAN). As original SAN action potentials and bar graphs report **(A, B)**, 1 μM ORM-10962 (ORM) (red trace) exerted an increased effect after 0.3 μM ivabradine (IVA) pretreatment (blue trace). Panel **(C)** represent Ca^{2+} transients measured from isolated SAN cells under control condition (black trace) and in the presence of 3 μM IVA (blue trace). We found identical Ca^{2+} levels as a result of IVA treatment. In panel **(D)**, the dose dependent effect of IVA (abscissa) on SAN cycle length (CL) was plotted against the effect of consecutive application of 1 μM ORM on CL (ordinate). As was previously described in **Figures 2A–C**, 1 μM ORM has ≈8% effect without IVA. In the presence of 0.5 and 3 μM IVA, the ORM-induced reduction of pacing rate was gradually increased. The numbers in parentheses indicate the corresponding n. The experimental results (red) are compared with the Yaniv SAN cell model (blue) in panel **(E)**. Based on a previous study, 0.5 and 3 μM IVA were represented by 20 and 60% funny current (I_f) inhibition in the presence of constant 41% NCX inhibition. Panel **(F)** represents the modeling results of combined I_f-NCX block. In the three panels, I_f was inhibited by varying degrees (straight lines) and combined with 41% NCX inhibition (dotted lines) yielding an increasing NCX inhibition effect on CL as I_f inhibition increases.

Decrease of $[Ca^{2+}]_o$ Increases the Effect of Funny Current Inhibition on Cycle Length in Sinus Node Tissue

We further tested the coupling between Ca^{2+} handling and I_f on CL control. Reduced $[Ca^{2+}]_o$ (0.9 mM) external solution was selected to achieve this goal since in this concentration, the CL was only slightly reduced (10.3 ± 3.7%). We found that the reduced extracellular Ca^{2+} slightly increased the CL which was further increased after application of 3 μM IVA (control: 469 ± 39.5 ms → 0.9 mM $[Ca^{2+}]_o$: 515.8 ± 40.8 ms → 3 μM IVA: 777 ± 58.7 ms; $p < 0.05$, n = 6/6 hearts, **Figures 7A, B**). We compared again the effects of IVA on the CL under normal condition (i.e., 1.8 $[Ca^{2+}]_o$) and in the presence of low external Ca^{2+} (0.9 mM $[Ca^{2+}]_o$). As bar graphs in **Figure 7C** demonstrates the IVA has markedly improved effect when extracellular Ca^{2+} is low compared with normal Ca^{2+} settings (51.1 ± 5.1% *versus* 20.99 ± 4.1%, $p < 0.05$; Student's t-test). **Figure 7D** represents Ca^{2+} transient measurements from spontaneously contracting isolated cells. We can observe that the application of 0.9 mM $[Ca^{2+}]_o$ significantly decreased the transient amplitude (295 ± 52 nM *vs.* 185 ± 32 nM; $p < 0.05$, n = 8) which may reflect decreased Ca^{2+} influx, SR Ca^{2+} release which may decrease the NCX current and thus attenuate the compensating capacity of NCX. The diastolic Ca^{2+} also significantly decreased (127 ± 33 *vs.* 64 ± 10 nM; $p < 0.05$, n = 8). We addressed this question by using mechanistic modeling (Yaniv et al., 2013b). Left column of **Figure 7E** represents action potentials (upper traces), NCX and I_f current kinetics (middle traces), and global Ca^{2+} transients (lower traces) under normal condition. Upon application of 0.9 mM $[Ca^{2+}]_o$ (right column) the CL slightly reduced, the integral of NCX current under the late phase of DD decreased while the magnitude of I_f current did not changed. The amplitude of the global transient decreased in similar extent as was obtained from SAN cell experiments.

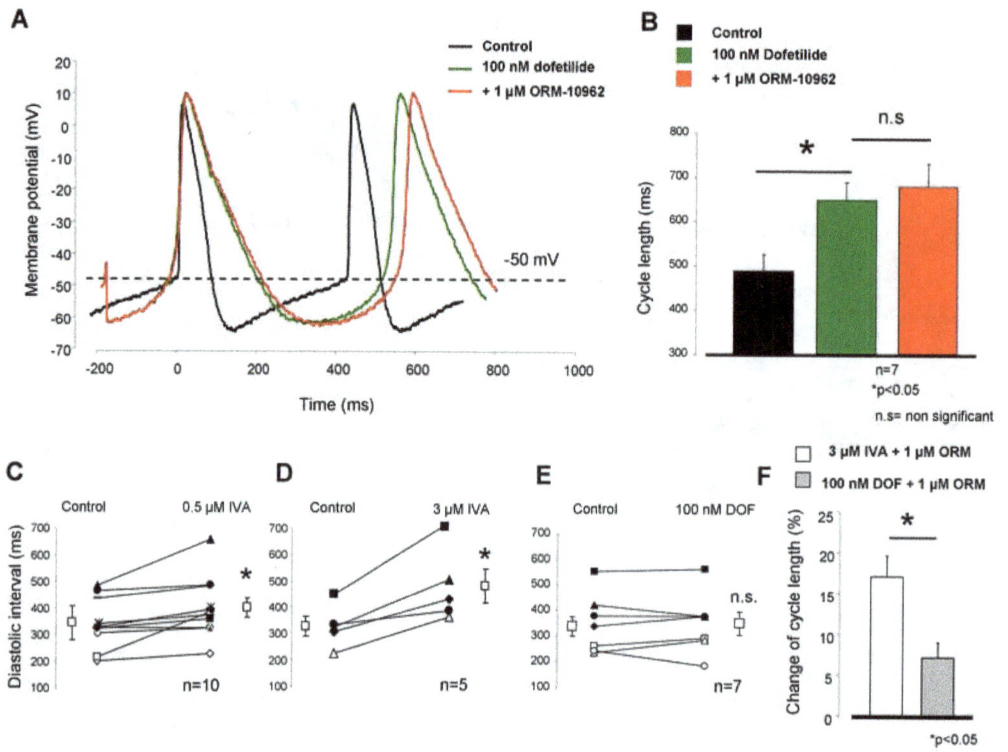

FIGURE 5 | Sinus node (SAN) frequency was decreased by complete I_{Kr} inhibition by 100 nM dofetilide administration. The control cycle length (CL) (black trace) largely increased after dofetilide (green trace). However, the effect of 1 μM ORM-10962 (ORM) did not change compared with the individual effect (red trace, panels **A, B, F**). The main difference between ivabradine (IVA) and dofetilide (DOF)-induced bradycardia is that 0.5 and 3 μM IVA markedly increased the diastolic interval **(C, D)**, which remained unchanged in the case of I_{Kr} inhibition by DOF **(E)**.

Concomitant Inhibition of Na^+/Ca^{2+} Exchanger and Funny Current Increases the Cycle Length Variability in Sinus Node Tissue

The short term CL variability (CLV) was calculated by the analysis of CLs of N = 30 consecutive action potentials by applying the following formula:

$$STV = \Sigma(CL;i+1-CL;i)/\left(n_{beats} x \sqrt{2}\right).$$

One micrometer of ORM-10962 and 3 μM IVA individually prolong the CL without considerable influence on the CL variability (see the area covered in **Figures 8A, B**). The subsequent application of 5 μM RYA (**Figure 8C**, green line) and 5 μM RYA + 1 μM ORM-10962 (**Figure 8C**, red line) showed a tendency to increase the CL variability, however it proved not to be statistically significant. In contrast, additionally adding 3 μM IVA markedly and statistically significantly enhanced the variability parallel with the CL increase, when the Ca^{2+} release and NCX activity were suppressed (**Figure 8C**, blue line). As **Figures 8D, E** show, the CL variability exerts similar results as the CL measurements: individual inhibition of NCX (2.53 ± 0.8 ms *vs.* 2.71 ± 0.9 ms; n = 16/16; red line) and I_f (3.6 ± 0.9 ms *vs.* 5.19 ± 0.7 ms; n = 5/5; blue line) or Ca^{2+} handling suppression (3.03 ± 0.87 ms *vs.* 7.0 ± 2.73 ms, n = 7/7; green line) do not alter significantly the CLV while the variability was largely increased if IVA was administrated in the presence of reduced Ca^{2+} cycling activity (7.0 ± 2.73 ms *vs.* 15.29 ± 5.6 ms; orange line).

DISCUSSION

The aim of this study was to verify and estimate the possible contribution of NCX function in SAN automaticity by direct selective pharmacological inhibition. Furthermore, we evaluated the functional consequences of the previously mentioned (Yaniv et al., 2015) I_f-NCX coupling in multicellular tissue level. In this study, we provided evidence for the first time regarding the essential role of NCX in spontaneous automaticity of the SAN by selective pharmacological inhibition. In addition, we described its functional interaction with I_f. This interaction between the DD currents is based on the following experimental results: i) 3 μM IVA has moderate effects on CL (~21%) and CLV (Δ ~ 2 ms), ii) 1 μM ORM has marginal effects on CL (~8%) and no change on CLV, iii) Ca^{2+} cycling suppression by 1 μM ORM + 5 μM RYA has moderate effects on CL (~19%) and CLV (Δ ~ 4 ms), iv) increasing I_f inhibition augments the effect of a

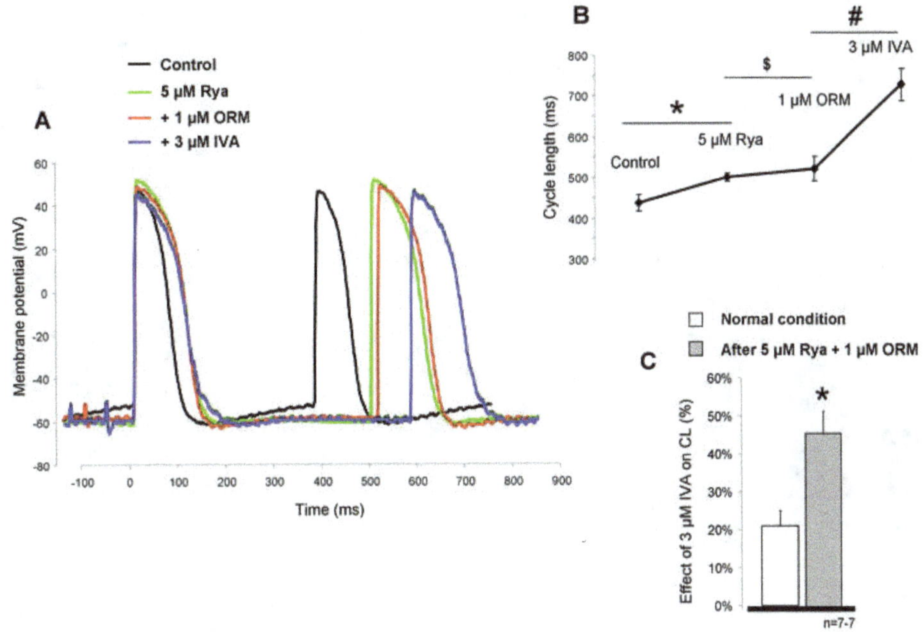

FIGURE 6 | The potential influence of Ca^{2+} handling suppression by 5 µM ryanodine (RYA) (green line) and 1 µM ORM-10962 (red line) on the effect of funny current (I_f) reduction was investigated. As representative curves panel **(A)** and diagram panel **(B)** report, both drugs increased the cycle length (CL) of the action potential. Statistical analysis was achieved by ANOVA. * means RYA compared to control, $ means ORM-10962 (ORM) compared to RYA, and # means ivabradine (IVA) compared to ORM. Comparison of the effect of 3 µM IVA on the CL under normal condition (i.e., without any other inhibitors) and after 5 µM RYA + 1µM ORM shows that the same dose of IVA has markedly increased effect when the contribution of Na+/Ca2+ exchanger (NCX) is reduced by concomitant application of RYA and ORM panel **(C)**.

fixed ORM dose (1 µM) on CL (~ 8 to 17%), v) the effect of 3 uM IVA is enhanced when Ca^{2+} cycling was previously suppressed (from ~ 20 to 42%).

ORM-10962 Does Not Inhibit the Funny Current

The effectiveness and selectivity of ORM-10962, a novel, potent NCX inhibitor was investigated in detail in our previous studies (Kohajda et al., 2016; Oravecz et al., 2017). In these studies, it was shown that ORM inhibited both forward and reverse mode NCX with an IC_{50} values of 55 and 67 nM without changing the I_{Ca}, I_{Na}, I_{K1}, I_{Kr}, I_{Ks}, I_{to}, and $I_{Na/K}$ pump currents even at high (1 µM) concentrations. However, the I_f current was not investigated. The present study demonstrates that 1 µM ORM did not influence I_f (**Figure 1**) in the presence of high Ca^{2+} buffering, which means that ORM is a suitable tool for the evaluation of NCX in SAN automaticity, however the indirect effects related with ORM-induced Ca^{2+} elevation (without Ca^{2+} buffering) may influence the I_f indirectly (Mattick et al., 2007).

Na^+/Ca^{2+} Exchanger Inhibition Slightly Decreases Sinus Node Firing Rate

We found slight, but statistically significant reduction in the spontaneous firing rate in SAN tissue which is the consequence of the reduced rate of the DD (**Figure 2**). This result is a direct evidence and verification for the contribution of the inward NCX in rhythm generation. Previous studies (Yaniv et al., 2013a; Yaniv et al., 2015) reported that not only the increase of CL, but the parallel increase of pacing variability reports the uncoupling of the I_f-NCX and the destabilization of the DD. Since in our experiments the CL slightly increased while the pacing rate variability did not change, we conclude that the individual NCX inhibition did not cause considerable uncoupling of I_f-NCX.

The rate of forward NCX inhibition by using 1 µM ORM was estimated to ≈90% by applying conventional ramp protocol in the presence of ≈160 nM $[Ca^{2+}]_i$ in canine ventricular myocytes in our previous study (Kohajda et al., 2016). The actual ratio of inhibited NCX which corresponds with the observed CL changes was calculated to 41% by using the Yaniv SAN cell model (Yaniv et al., 2013b). It is important to note, that in our previous study (Oravecz et al., 2017) we have demonstrated that the extent of NCX inhibition (*via* ORM-10962) is decreased when the intracellular Ca^{2+} is intact (i.e., in the presence of Ca^{2+} transient). The underlying mechanism could be asymmetrical block between two modes, autoregulation of the Ca^{2+}_i or by preserved inducibility of forward NCX by elevated Ca^{2+}_i.

Na^+/Ca^{2+} Exchanger Inhibition Markedly Increases the Ca^{2+}_I Level

The selective NCX inhibition caused similar diastolic Ca^{2+} changes compared to the Yaniv model predicted, however, in

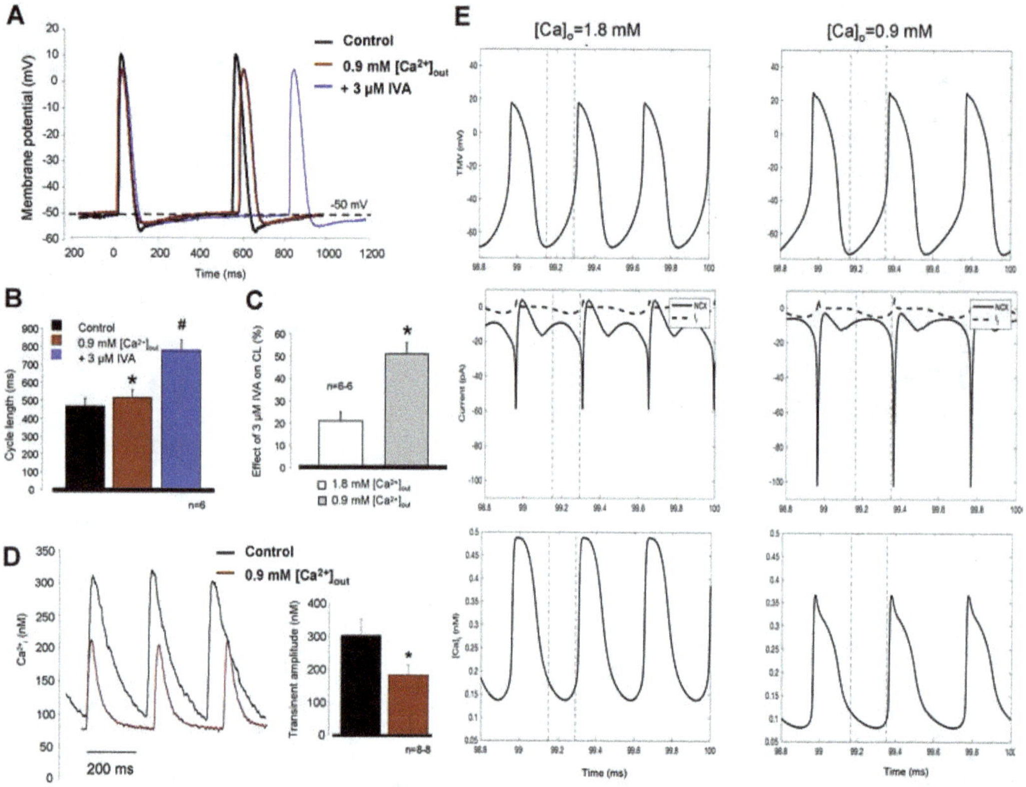

FIGURE 7 | Decreased extracellular Ca^{2+} solution (0.9 mM) was used to suppress the intracellular Ca^{2+} cycling and therefore Na+/Ca2+ exchanger (NCX). The effect of hypocalcemic solution on the cycle length (CL) was marginal (**A, B**, brown trace) however the subsequently applied 3 µM ivabradine (IVA) (blue trace) caused considerable prolongation in the CL. Comparison of the IVA effect in the presence of normal (1.8 mM—white column) *versus* low (0.9 mM—gray column) $CaCl_2$ on panel **(C)** demonstrates nearly doubled effect of IVA on the CL in response of Ca^{2+} reduction **(C)**. * means 0.9 mM $[Ca^{2+}]_o$ compared to control, # means IVA *versus* 0.9 mM $[Ca^{2+}]_o$. Original traces measured from isolated sinus node (SAN) cells in panel **(D)** demonstrate that 0.9 mM $[Ca^{2+}]_o$ (brown trace) significantly decreased the transient amplitude without significant action on diastolic Ca^{2+} levels. **(E)** Modeling simulation of action potentials (upper traces), NCX currents (middle traces, solid lines), I_f currents (middle traces, dashed lines), and global Ca^{2+} transients (lower traces) in the present of normal (1.8 mM), external Ca^{2+} (left column), and 0.9 mM $[Ca^{2+}]_o$ (right column). The results indicate decreased transient amplitude coupled with smaller NCX current in the late diastolic depolarization (DD) with maintained I_f current magnitude in the presence of 0.9 mM $[Ca^{2+}]_o$.

contrast with modeling, we found markedly increased Ca^{2+} transient amplitude which is generally expected after decreased rate of Ca^{2+} extrusion (**Figure 3**). The observed quantitative discrepancy between experiments and modeling may indicate that the extent of NCX inhibition in the experiments could be larger than 41%.

We can speculate that the increasing intracellular Ca^{2+} is known to facilitate the inactivation of the L-type Ca^{2+} current as a part of the autoregulation (Eisner et al., 1998; Eisner et al., 2000). The gain of the $[Ca^{2+}]_i$ may indirectly shortens the CL which means two parallel, counteracting effect of selective NCX inhibition: the inhibition of the inward NCX current may reduce the actual frequency by suppressing its contribution in the DD, however it is partially compensated for the CL abbreviating effect of increased $[Ca^{2+}]_i$. Furthermore, the I_f may also contribute in the limitation of the ORM effect: i) a theoretical possibility exists that ORM-induced Ca^{2+} elevation may increase the I_f, however this was ruled out by a previous work (Zaza et al., 1991). ii) It was reported that SAN myocytes express Ca^{2+}-activated adenylate cyclase isoform, which might raise cAMP (and I_f) in response to NCX blockade (Mattick et al., 2007).

The Moderate Bradycardic Effect of Na^+/Ca^{2+} Exchanger Inhibition May Be Explained by Funny Current-Na^+/Ca^{2+} Exchanger Coupling

However, one may speculate after considering the crucial role of NCX in the coupled-clock theory, why the NCX inhibition-induced "bradycardia" exerted a relatively low influence. Using genetic mouse models Gao *et al.* claimed that partial ablation of NCX (≈70–80%) using an αMHC-inducible "Cre" transgenic line, has also a slight effect on the baseline spontaneous AP firing frequency (Gao et al., 2013). In line with this, it was found that even a small NCX fraction is able to generate sufficient inward current to provide appropriate depolarization current which is

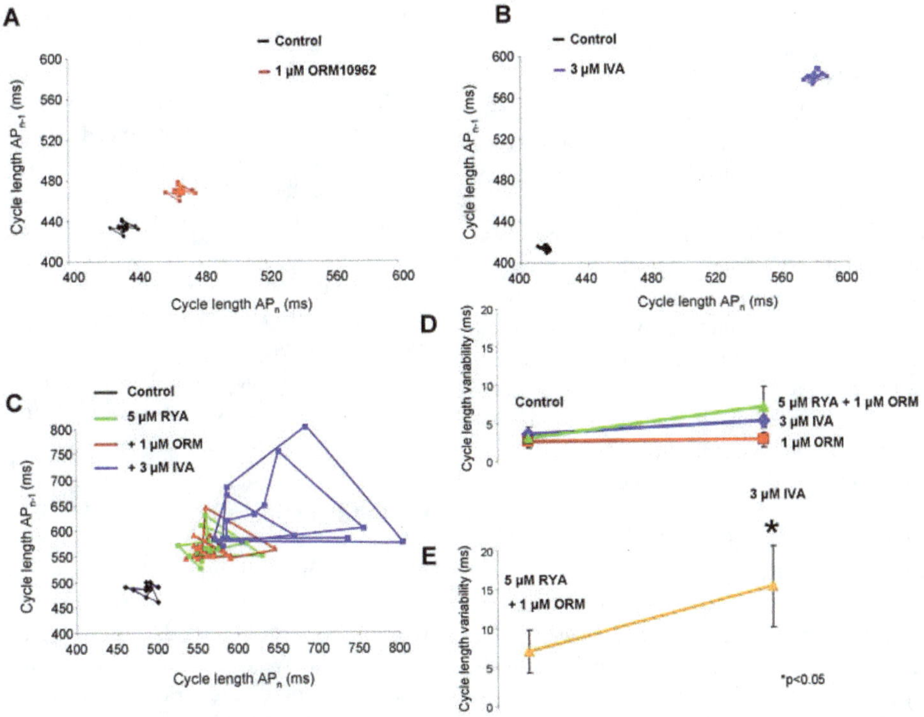

FIGURE 8 | The effect of suppression of diastolic depolarization (DD) currents [Na+/Ca2+ exchanger (NCX) and I_f] on short time cycle length (CL) variability. When 1 μM ORM-10962 panel **(A)** or 3 μM ivabradine (IVA) panel **(B)** were applied, the variability did not change significantly. Instead, the CL was prolonged. Comparison of the effect of 1 μM ORM-10962 (ORM) (red line), 5 μM ryanodine (RYA) (blue line), and 5 μM RYA + 1 μM ORM (green line) on the CL variability shows that these compound do not change the variability significantly panel **(D)**. In contrast IVA administration after the application of RYA+ORM caused considerably increased variability panel **(E)** as the Poincaré-plot (panel **C,** blue line) shows.

able to maintain normal SAN cell activity (Groenke et al., 2013). Our and these previous results highlight the possibility that a functional coupling between I_f and NCX represents a potency to compensate for the NCX inhibition-induced reduction of the pacing frequency.

In accordance with this theory our and previous results indicate a relatively moderate effect of IVA on the CL when it is administrated at 3 μM (**Figure 4A**) or at 10 μM (Yaniv et al., 2012). At the same time, caesium was unable to stop SAN beating even though it has a large effect on I_f (Noma et al., 1983). These inconsistent results can be explained by the voltage-dependent block of IVA or caesium (DiFrancesco, 1995), or by proposing an insulator function of the I_f to protect the SAN cells from the strong negative electrical sink of the connected atrial tissue (Morad and Zhang, 2017). However, a functional coupling between I_f and NCX (Bois et al., 1996; Lakatta et al., 2010; Yaniv et al., 2013a) providing redundant pacemaking systems could also explain—or at least contribute to—the observed results. This phenomenon, which could be very similar to the repolarization reserve (Biliczki et al., 2002; Herrmann et al., 2007; Lengyel et al., 2007; Nagy et al., 2009), may be also able to reduce the effects of the individual inhibition of NCX or I_f explaining the relatively small extent of IVA or NCX effects.

Indeed, we found that the effect of 1 μM ORM gradually increased as the rate of I_f block was enhanced (**Figure 4**). In line with this, the Yaniv model provided similar but steeper tendency, when we represented the 0.5, 1, and 3 μM IVA doses by 20, 60, and 80% I_f block based on previous results (Bois et al., 1996). While 10 μM IVA was not used experimentally due to selectivity problems, 85% I_f inhibition could be computed in the Yaniv model. The detailed modeling results are depicted in **Figures 4E, F**. Consistent with experimental results, the effect of 41% NCX inhibition on CL is increased as I_f inhibition becomes stronger. However, the modeling predicts a much steeper increase in the CL in the presence of enhancing I_f block. The underlying mechanism of this discrepancy could be the markedly higher Ca^{2+} increase measured during experiments which could limit the bradycardic effect of NCX inhibition. A previous study reported a decreased SR Ca^{2+} content after I_f inhibition by IVA (Yaniv et al., 2013a) demonstrating an indirect suppression of NCX during I_f inhibition. Our Ca^{2+} measurements (**Figure 4C**) indicate unchanged Ca^{2+} release after application of IVA, which may indicate that the underlying mechanism of increased ORM effect may be rather related with the increased sensitivity of DD when it is already inhibited by the I_f block.

I_{Kr} Inhibition Mediated Bradycardia Does Not Alter the Effect of Na^+/Ca^{2+} Exchanger Inhibition

It is possible to decelerate spontaneous frequency without major direct influence on I_f or NCX. The SAN rate was reduced by 100% I_{Kr} block (**Figure 5**) in which the developed decrease in the firing rate was mainly achieved by APD prolongation without or minimal change in diastolic interval—instead of I_f block, which markedly increases the diastolic interval without effect on APD. This also means that despite the bradycardia, I_f is intact during these experiments. In line with this, NCX inhibition provided a similar effect to the one which was experienced when NCX was inhibited individually in **Figure 2**. This observation could be explained by an I_f dependent compensation of NCX reduction. At the same time it also means that the mechanism of the bradycardia is important regarding the effect of NCX inhibition. It seems possible that I_f mediated bradycardia and concomitant increase in diastolic interval may be important in the I_f-NCX interaction.

Suppression of $Ca^{2+}{}_i$ Augments the Effect of Funny Current Inhibition

Assuming that a mutual interaction between I_f and NCX exists, this crosstalk should work in the opposite direction as well, i.e., a disturbance in the Ca^{2+} cycling should affect I_f. The suppression of the Ca^{2+} handling by the subsequent application of ryanodine and ORM together caused ≈20% increase in the CL in line with previous results (Bucchi et al., 2003). Under this condition, the effect of 3 μM IVA was considerably larger compared with normal settings (≈45% *vs.* 20%, see **Figure 6C**). In line with this, we found similar augmentation of IVA effect (21% *vs.* 51%) when Ca^{2+} handling was suppressed by low extracellular Ca^{2+} (**Figure 7**). Experimental as well as modeling simulations suppose that the Ca^{2+} handling and thus the NCX current suppression decreases the flux of the depolarizing NCX current, increases the length of DD, thus, the suppressed net current underlying the DD provides improved effect for I_f inhibition.

Funny Current-Na^+/Ca^{2+} Exchanger Coupling Controls Cycle Length Variability

Previous studies (Yaniv et al., 2013a; Yaniv et al., 2015) reported that the I_f-NCX coupling not only controls the current CL but it may have a crucial role in maintaining the normal rhythm of the SAN. Therefore, the increase of the CL variability could be a further indicator of the integrity of I_f-NCX axis appearing after a considerable CL increase reporting significant I_f-NCX uncoupling. Our results support this assumption indicating that after individual inhibition of I_f or NCX, not only the excessive CL increase is restricted but the SAN rhythm is also maintained. However, when both of I_f and NCX are suppressed, besides the marked CL increase, a perturbation in the rhythm also appeared indicating the exhausted capacity of the I_f-NCX to depolarize the membrane during the DD (**Figure 8**). Since we could not reach complete inhibition of I_f and NCX in our experiments, we cannot estimate precisely the relative importance of these currents in the normal SAN rhythm. However, it seems possible that these currents contribute in the "depolarization reserve" (Herrmann et al., 2007) not only to the control of the current CL but also to the maintenance of the normal pacing rhythm as a consequence of the strong depolarizing of the I_f-NCX crosstalk.

Proposed Mechanism

We suggest that the observed NCX-I_f interplay is the consequence of the increased susceptibility of DD to any intervention when the DD was previously inhibited by another compound (Rocchetti et al., 2000; Zaza and Lombardi, 2001; Monfredi et al., 2014). This means that the bradycardic effect of NCX inhibition is larger when I_f was previously inhibited (independently from the Ca^{2+} handling). *Vice versa*, when the NCX was previously suppressed (as a consequence of reduced Ca^{2+} release) the decreased DD current density is more sensitive to changes, which increases the bradycardic effect of IVA.

CONCLUSION

In the present study, we provide direct pharmacological evidence regarding the role of NCX in pacemaker mechanism by its selective inhibition with the novel, highly selective compound ORM-10962. We found that individual inhibitions of NCX or I_f cause only moderate bradycardia and rhythm disturbance. However, combined suppression of these currents acted synergistically and supports the hypothesis of mutual crosstalk between NCX and I_f in SAN even in multicellular tissue having important functional consequences. This means that individual inhibition of DD currents may have moderated effect on CL and variability under normal conditions because the underlying currents may be able to compensate each other. This important crosstalk may provide a considerable safety margin for SAN pacemaking.

STUDY LIMITATIONS

Our study has three important limitations. 1) The action potentials measured in our experiments do not represent the characteristics of the core SAN cells. These cells are much more "follower" cells, having AP waveforms largely influenced by the cell-to-cell coupling. 2) The applied inhibitors (IVA, ORM, RYA) are not able to cause complete block of ion channels in the applied concentrations. Therefore, the described phenomena indicate only partial effects and not able to estimate the absolute contribution of NCX during the DD. 3) Since our aim was to explore ion current cooperation, our results represent ion channel function independent from the autonomic nervous system. The activation of the sympathetic or parasympathetic nervous system—or modulation of the β_1/M_2 receptors—intimately changes the cAMP, PKA, CaMKII levels which have effects on the DD currents, therefore the discussed I_f-NCX coupling cannot be directly extrapolated to *in vivo* systems. The ion current crosstalk characterization during intact autonomic control requires further experiments.

AUTHOR CONTRIBUTIONS

ZK performed ion current measurements and data analysis. NT performed fluorescent optical measurements, action potential measurements and data analysis. JS performed ion current measurements and data analysis. AL performed the computational modeling and data analysis, contributed to conception of the study as well as manuscript preparation and funding for the computational study. PG performed ion current measurements, GB and JP performed action potential measurements. NJ organized the database and ensured the financial support of the study. JL and PP contributed to the development of ORM-10962. JGYP contributed to manuscript preparation, AV and NN ensured the financial support of the study, contributed conception and design of the study, data analysis and visualization, and manuscript preparation. All authors contributed to manuscript revision, read and approved the submitted version.

FUNDING

This work was supported by grants from the National Research Development and Innovation Office (NKFIH PD-125402 (for NN), FK-129117 (for NN), GINOP-2.3.2-15-2016-00006, the LIVE LONGER EFOP-3.6.2-16-2017-00006 project, the János Bolyai Research Scholarship of the Hungarian Academy of Sciences (for NN), the UNKP-18-4-SZTE-76 New National Excellence Program of the Ministry for Innovation and Technology (for NN), the EFOP 3.6.3 VEKOP-16-2017-00009 (for NT), the Hungarian Academy of Sciences and by the Orion Pharma (ORM-10962).

ACKNOWLEDGMENTS

We are grateful to Prof. Dr. David Eisner (University of Manchester, UK) for his help and suggestions for the manuscript. We gratefully acknowledge financial support by the Deutsche Forschungsgemeinschaft (DFG, German Research Foundation) - Project-ID 258734477 - SFB 1173 (to AL). The publication of this study was supported by the University of Szeged Open Access Fund (4309).

REFERENCES

Biliczki, P., Virag, L., Iost, N., Papp, J. G., and Varro, A. (2002). Interaction of different potassium channels in cardiac repolarization in dog ventricular preparations: role of repolarization reserve. *Br. J. Pharmacol.* 137 (3), 361–368. doi: 10.1038/sj.bjp.0704881

Bogdanov, K. Y., Vinogradova, T. M., and Lakatta, E. G. (2001). Sinoatrial nodal cell ryanodine receptor and Na(+)-Ca(2+) exchanger: molecular partners in pacemaker regulation. *Circ. Res.* 88 (12), 1254–1258. doi: 10.1161/hh1201.092095

Bois, P., Bescond, J., Renaudon, B., and Lenfant, J. (1996). Mode of action of bradycardic agent, S 16257, on ionic currents of rabbit sinoatrial node cells. *Br. J. Pharmacol.* 118 (4), 1051–1057. doi: 10.1111/j.1476-5381.1996.tb15505.x

Bucchi, A., Baruscotti, M., Robinson, R. B., and DiFrancesco, D. (2003). I(f)-dependent modulation of pacemaker rate mediated by cAMP in the presence of ryanodine in rabbit sino-atrial node cells. *J. Mol. Cell Cardiol.* 35 (8), 905–913. doi: 10.1016/s0022-2828(03)00150-0

DiFrancesco, D., and Noble, D. (2012). The funny current has a major pacemaking role in the sinus node. *Heart Rhythm.* 9 (2), 299–301. doi: 10.1016/j.hrthm.2011.09.021

DiFrancesco, D. (1981). A new interpretation of the pace-maker current in calf Purkinje fibres. *J. Physiol.* 314, 359–376. doi: 10.1113/JPHYSIOL.1981.SP013713

DiFrancesco, D. (1995). Cesium and the pacemaker current. *J. Cardiovasc. Electrophysiol.* 6 (12), 1152–1155.

Eisner, D. A., Trafford, A. W., Diaz, M. E., Overend, C. L., and O'Neill, S. C. (1998). The control of Ca release from the cardiac sarcoplasmic reticulum: regulation versus autoregulation. *Cardiovasc. Res.* 38 (3), 589–604. doi: 10.1016/s6363(98)00062-5

Eisner, D. A., Choi, H. S., Diaz, M. E., O'Neill, S. C., and Trafford, A. W. (2000). Integrative analysis of calcium cycling in cardiac muscle. *Circ. Res.* 87 (12), 1087–1094. doi: 10.1161/01.res.87.12.1087

Gao, Z., Rasmussen, T. P., Li, Y., Kutschke, W., Koval, O. M., Wu, Y., et al. (2013). Genetic inhibition of Na^+-Ca^{2+} exchanger current disables fight or flight sinoatrial node activity without affecting resting heart rate. *Circ. Res.* 112 (2), 309–317. doi: 10.1161/CIRCRESAHA.111.300193

Groenke, S., Larson, E. D., Alber, S., Zhang, R., Lamp, S. T., Ren, X., et al. (2013). Complete atrial-specific knockout of sodium-calcium exchange eliminates sinoatrial node pacemaker activity. *PloS One* 8 (11), e81633. doi: 10.1371/journal.pone.0081633

Herrmann, S., Stieber, J., Stockl, G., Hofmann, F., and Ludwig, A. (2007). HCN4 provides a 'depolarization reserve' and is not required for heart rate acceleration in mice. *EMBO J.* 26 (21), 4423–4432. doi: 10.1038/sj.emboj.7601868

Herrmann, S., Lipp, P., Wiesen, K., Stieber, J., Nguyen, H., Kaiser, E., et al. (2013). The cardiac sodium-calcium exchanger NCX1 is a key player in the initiation and maintenance of a stable heart rhythm. *Cardiovasc. Res.* 99 (4), 780–788. doi: 10.1093/cvr/cvt154

Himeno, Y., Toyoda, F., Satoh, H., Amano, A., Cha, C. Y., Matsuura, H., et al. (2011). Minor contribution of cytosolic Ca2+ transients to the pacemaker rhythm in guinea pig sinoatrial node cells. *Am. J. Physiol. Heart Circ. Physiol.* 300 (1), H251–H261. doi: 10.1152/ajpheart.00764.2010

Jost, N., Nagy, N., Corici, C., Kohajda, Z., Horvath, A., Acsai, K., et al. (2013). ORM-10103, a novel specific inhibitor of the Na+/Ca2+ exchanger, decreases early and delayed afterdepolarizations in the canine heart. *Br. J. Pharmacol.* 170 (4), 768–778. doi: 10.1111/bph.12228

Kohajda, Z., Farkas-Morvay, N., Jost, N., Nagy, N., Geramipour, A., Horvath, A., et al. (2016). The effect of a novel highly selective inhibitor of the Sodium/Calcium exchanger (NCX) on cardiac arrhythmias in In Vitro and In Vivo experiments. *PloS One* 11 (11), e0166041. doi: 10.1371/journal.pone.0166041

Kormos, A., Nagy, N., Acsai, K., Vaczi, K., Agoston, S., Pollesello, P., et al. (2014). Efficacy of selective NCX inhibition by ORM-10103 during simulated ischemia/reperfusion. *Eur. J. Pharmacol.* 740, 539–551. doi: 10.1016/j.ejphar.2014.06.033

Lakatta, E. G., and DiFrancesco, D. (2009). What keeps us ticking: a funny current, a calcium clock, or both? *J. Mol. Cell Cardiol.* 47 (2), 157–170. doi: 10.1016/j.yjmcc.2009.03.022

Lakatta, E. G., Maltsev, V. A., and Vinogradova, T. M. (2010). A coupled system of intracellular Ca^{2+} clocks and surface membrane voltage clocks controls the timekeeping mechanism of the heart's pacemaker. *Circ. Res.* 106 (4), 659–673. doi: 10.1161/CIRCRESAHA.109.206078

Lengyel, C., Varro, A., Tabori, K., Papp, J. G., and Baczko, I. (2007). Combined pharmacological block of I(Kr) and I(Ks) increases short-term QT interval variability and provokes torsades de pointes. *Br. J. Pharmacol.* 151 (7), 941–951. doi: 10.1038/sj.bjp.0707297

Mattick, P., Parrington, J., Odia, E., Simpson, A., Collins, T., and Terrar, D. (2007). Ca^{2+}-stimulated adenylyl cyclase isoform AC1 is preferentially expressed in guinea-pig sino-atrial node cells and modulates the I(f) pacemaker current. *J.7 Physiol.* 582 (Pt 3), 1195–1203. doi: 10.1113/jphysiol.2007.133439

Monfredi, O., Lyashkov, A. E., Johnsen, A. B., Inada, S., Schneider, H., Wang, R., et al. (2014). Biophysical characterization of the underappreciated and important relationship between heart rate variability and heart rate. *Hypertension* 64 (6), 1334–1343. doi: 10.1161/HYPERTENSIONAHA.114.03782

Morad, M., and Zhang, X. H. (2017). Mechanisms of spontaneous pacing: sinoatrial nodal cells, neonatal cardiomyocytes, and human stem cell derived cardiomyocytes. *Can. J. Physiol. Pharmacol.* 95 (10), 1100–1107. doi: 10.1139/cjpp-2016-0743

Nagy, N., Szuts, V., Horvath, Z., Seprenyi, G., Farkas, A. S., Acsai, K., et al. (2009). Does small-conductance calcium-activated potassium channel contribute to cardiac repolarization? *J. Mol. Cell Cardiol.* 47 (5), 656–663. doi: 10.1016/j.yjmcc.2009.07.019

Noble, D., Noble, P. J., and Fink, M. (2010). Competing oscillators in cardiac pacemaking: historical background. *Circ. Res.* 106 (12), 1791–1797. doi: 10.1161/CIRCRESAHA.110.218875

Noma, A., Morad, M., and Irisawa, H. (1983). Does the "pacemaker current" generate the diastolic depolarization in the rabbit SA node cells? *Pflugers Arch.* 397 (3), 190–194. doi: 10.1007/bf00584356

Oravecz, K., Kormos, A., Gruber, A., Marton, Z., Kohajda, Z., Mirzaei, L., et al. (2017). Inotropic effect of NCX inhibition depends on the relative activity of the reverse NCX assessed by a novel inhibitor ORM-10962 on canine ventricular myocytes. *Eur. J. Pharmacol.* 818, 278–286. doi: 10.1016/j.ejphar.2017.10.039

Rocchetti, M., Malfatto, G., Lombardi, F., and Zaza, A. (2000). Role of the input/output relation of sinoatrial myocytes in cholinergic modulation of heart rate variability. *J. Cardiovasc. Electrophysiol.* 11 (5), 522–530. doi: 10.1111/j.1540-8167.2000.tb00005.x

Sanders, L., Rakovic, S., Lowe, M., Mattick, P. A., and Terrar, D. A. (2006). Fundamental importance of Na+-Ca2+ exchange for the pacemaking mechanism in guinea-pig sino-atrial node. *J. Physiol.* 571 (Pt 3), 639–649. doi: 10.1113/jphysiol.2005.100305

Sirenko, S. G., Maltsev, V. A., Yaniv, Y., Bychkov, R., Yaeger, D., Vinogradova, T., et al. (2016). Electrochemical Na+ and Ca2+ gradients drive coupled-clock regulation of automaticity of isolated rabbit sinoatrial nodal pacemaker cells. *Am. J. Physiol. Heart Circ. Physiol.* 311 (1), H251–H267. doi: 10.1152/ajpheart.00667.2015

Verkerk, A. O., den Ruijter, H. M., Bourier, J., Boukens, B. J., Brouwer, I. A., Wilders, R., et al. (2009). Dietary fish oil reduces pacemaker current and heart rate in rabbit. *Heart Rhythm.* 6 (10), 1485–1492. doi: 10.1016/j.hrthm.2009.07.024

Yaniv, Y., Maltsev, V. A., Ziman, B. D., Spurgeon, H. A., and Lakatta, E. G. (2012). The "funny" current (I(f)) inhibition by ivabradine at membrane potentials encompassing spontaneous depolarization in pacemaker cells. *Molecules* 17 (7), 8241–8254.

Yaniv, Y., Sirenko, S., Ziman, B. D., Spurgeon, H. A., Maltsev, V. A., and Lakatta, E. G. (2013a). New evidence for coupled clock regulation of the normal automaticity of sinoatrial nodal pacemaker cells: bradycardic effects of ivabradine are linked to suppression of intracellular Ca(2)(+) cycling. *J. Mol. Cell Cardiol.* 62, 80–89. doi: 10.1016/j.yjmcc.2013.04.026

Yaniv, Y., Stern, M. D., Lakatta, E. G., and Maltsev, V. A. (2013b). Mechanisms of beat-to-beat regulation of cardiac pacemaker cell function by Ca(2)(+) cycling dynamics. *Biophys. J.* 105 (7), 1551–1561. doi: 10.1016/j.bpj.2013.08.024

Yaniv, Y., Lakatta, E. G., and Maltsev, V. A. (2015). From two competing oscillators to one coupled-clock pacemaker cell system. *Front. Physiol.* 6, 28. doi: 10.3389/fphys.2015.00028

Zaza, A., and Lombardi, F. (2001). Autonomic indexes based on the analysis of heart rate variability: a view from the sinus node. *Cardiovasc. Res.* 50 (3), 434–442. doi: 10.1016/s0008-6363(01)00240-1

Zaza, A., Maccaferri, G., Mangoni, M., and DiFrancesco, D. (1991). Intracellular calcium does not directly modulate cardiac pacemaker (if) channels. *Pflugers Arch.* 419 (6), 662–664. doi: 10.1007/BF00370312

4

Late Sodium Current Inhibitors as Potential Antiarrhythmic Agents

Balázs Horváth[1,2]*, *Tamás Hézső*[1], *Dénes Kiss*[1], *Kornél Kistamás*[1], *János Magyar*[1,3], *Péter P. Nánási*[1,4] *and Tamás Bányász*[1]

[1] Department of Physiology, Faculty of Medicine, University of Debrecen, Debrecen, Hungary, [2] Faculty of Pharmacy, University of Debrecen, Debrecen, Hungary, [3] Division of Sport Physiology, University of Debrecen, Debrecen, Hungary, [4] Department of Dental Physiology and Pharmacology, Faculty of Dentistry, University of Debrecen, Debrecen, Hungary

Correspondence:
Balázs Horváth
horvath.balazs@med.unideb.hu

Based on recent findings, an increased late sodium current ($I_{Na,late}$) plays an important pathophysiological role in cardiac diseases, including rhythm disorders. The article first describes what is $I_{Na,late}$ and how it functions under physiological circumstances. Next, it shows the wide range of cellular mechanisms that can contribute to an increased $I_{Na,late}$ in heart diseases, and also discusses how the upregulated $I_{Na,late}$ can play a role in the generation of cardiac arrhythmias. The last part of the article is about $I_{Na,late}$ inhibiting drugs as potential antiarrhythmic agents, based on experimental and preclinical data as well as in the light of clinical trials.

Keywords: voltage gated sodium channel, late sodium current, arrhythmias, antiarrhythmic drugs, sodium channel inhibitors

INTRODUCTION

During the non-pacemaker action potential (AP) in the heart, depolarization of the cell membrane opens voltage gated sodium channels (Na_v) for a short period of time (Scanley et al., 1990; Mitsuiye and Noma, 2002) giving rise to the early sodium current peak ($I_{Na,early}$). This $I_{Na,early}$ causes the upstroke of the non-pacemaker AP. Through the course of the AP Na_v channels may recover from inactivation and reopen, generating a sustained current component, called late sodium current ($I_{Na,late}$). $I_{Na,late}$ flows throughout the plateau phase of the AP therefore it significantly contributes to AP morphology, even though its magnitude is only a fraction of $I_{Na,early}$ (**Figure 1A**).

If $I_{Na,late}$ is increased, it might play a pathophysiological role in acquired cardiac diseases (**Figure 1B**) such as myocardial ischemia (Maier and Sossalla, 2013) and heart failure (Coppini et al., 2013; Pourrier et al., 2014). In the cardiomyocytes, an upregulated $I_{Na,late}$ hinders repolarization and causes a larger sodium entry, therefore increasing intracellular sodium concentration ($[Na^+]_i$). An increased $[Na^+]_i$, in turn, leads to a larger intracellular calcium content. These factors together can possibly cause contractile dysfunction (Sossalla et al., 2011), disturbed myocardial energetics (Liu and O'Rourke, 2008) and cardiac arrhythmias (Antzelevitch et al., 2014).

ELECTROPHYSIOLOGICAL IDENTIFICATION OF $I_{NA,LATE}$

Mammalian cardiac cells express a wide variety of Na_v isoforms, differing in unit conductance, voltage sensitivity, kinetics, and drug sensitivity. In the majority of cardiac tissues, the dominant isoform of the pore-forming subunit is $Na_v1.5$, which is relatively insensitive to the sodium channel toxin tetrodotoxin (TTX) (Gellens et al., 1992; Catterall et al., 2005). Many of the TTX-sensitive ("non-cardiac") Na_v channels ($Na_v1.1$, $Na_v1.2$, $Na_v1.3$, $Na_v1.4$, and $Na_v1.6$) are also shown to be present in cardiac tissue (Maier et al., 2002; Haufe et al., 2005; Valdivia et al., 2005; Biet et al., 2012; Yang et al., 2012). In nodal tissue $Na_v1.1$ and $Na_v1.6$ are expressed in the largest quantities. Besides the pore-forming subunit, four auxiliary subunits ($ß_1$, $ß_2$, $ß_3$, and $ß_4$) and certain scaffolding proteins also participate in building up the whole complex, which also attaches to the cytoskeleton. These molecules can interact with each other and may modify the kinetics and voltage dependence of the actual channel (Malhotra et al., 2001).

Mechanisms that are discussed in the followings may contribute to the profile of $I_{Na,late}$ during the AP. Understanding these mechanisms better might be helpful in developing new antiarrhythmic therapeutic strategies targeting $I_{Na,late}$.

$I_{Na,late}$ Is Underlain by Different Channel Gating Modes

At the resting membrane potential, the vast majority of $Na_v1.5$ channels are in their closed state. Upon depolarization, $Na_v1.5$ channels open up within 1–2 ms after which they inactivate rapidly (Scanley et al., 1990; Mitsuiye and Noma, 2002). This produces $I_{Na,early}$ and the upstroke of the non-pacemaker cardiac AP. During a sustained depolarization, $Na_v1.5$ channels can reopen with a small probability. In ventricular myocytes, three modes of Nav1.5 channel activity have been characterized in single-channel experiments: transient mode (TM), burst mode (BM), and late scattered mode (LSM) (Maltsev, 2006).

$I_{Na,early}$ is mainly the result of TM activity, while BM and LSM are responsible for the sustained sodium current, $I_{Na,late}$ (**Figure 1A**). The magnitude of the sustained current component is only about 0.5–1 % of $I_{Na,early}$ measured 50 ms after the onset of the depolarizing pulse (Maltsev, 2006). During a sustained depolarization BM openings rapidly decline in the first tens of milliseconds therefore leaving LSM as the gating mode being mainly responsible for $I_{Na,late}$ toward the end of the plateau phase.

Mutations of the channel protein and certain diseases can change the contribution of different $Na_v1.5$ channel activity patterns to the macroscopic current, therefore increasing $I_{Na,late}$ (Bezzina et al., 1999; Valdivia et al., 2005; Wu et al., 2006; Maltsev et al., 2007; Maltsev and Undrovinas, 2008; Song et al., 2008; Maltsev et al., 2009; Xi et al., 2009; Guo et al., 2010; Trenor et al., 2012) (**Figure 1B**). Apparently, each gating mode has a distinct drug sensitivity or drug affinity as well (Belardinelli et al., 2004; Ravens et al., 2004; Belardinelli et al., 2006). Based on this, selective pharmacological targeting of certain gating modes might have potential antiarrhythmic and/or cardioprotective effects (Belardinelli et al., 2006; Hoyer et al., 2011; Morita et al., 2011).

Window Sodium Current

The voltage dependence of the steady state activation and inactivation of most Na_v channels overlaps with each other (Zaza and Rocchetti, 2013). This overlap provides a voltage range ("window") where inactivated Na_v channels are able to recover from inactivation and then might reopen. When the actual membrane potential falls within this "window" of overlap, a sustained current is evoked. Under physiological circumstances this "window current" mechanism likely plays a limited role in $I_{Na,late}$, because the $Na_v1.5$ voltage "window" is around −70 mV, falling quite far from the AP plateau. Additionally, in the window voltage range, the current density is less than 5 % of the maximum current density in healthy myocytes (Maltsev et al., 1998; Wang et al., 2002; Liu et al., 2007). Hence, the "window current" mechanism is unlikely to be a major determinant of $I_{Na,late}$ in healthy myocytes. Mutations of channel proteins or altered regulation in certain diseases may shift either the steady-state

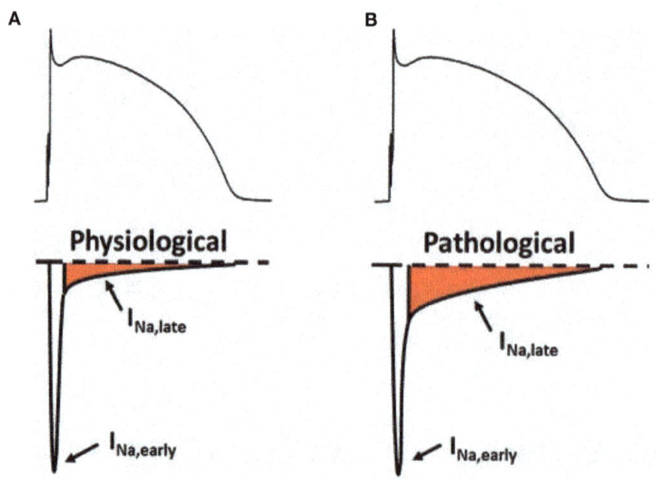

FIGURE 1 | The early and the late component of the sodium current under physiological **(A)** and pathological **(B)** conditions. Upper panels: membrane potential; lower panels: sodium current. $I_{Na,early}$, early (peak) component of the sodium current; $I_{Na,late}$, late (sustained) component of the sodium current.

activation or inactivation curves of Na_V channels to significantly change this voltage window, therefore increasing $I_{Na,late}$ under these pathological conditions (Wang et al., 1996; Ruan et al., 2009).

Non-Equilibrium Channel Gating

During the AP of cardiac myocytes, the membrane potential changes continuously. Na_V channels are incorporated into this dynamic system. It has been proposed by Clancy et al. (2003) that the voltage "history" of the cell membrane can modulate the transition between Na_V channel states, termed "non-equilibrium gating". As a result, recovery from inactivation is also modulated by the dynamics of voltage change. The theory is supported by experimental data showing that the application of repolarizing voltage ramps or AP shape voltage commands evoke a larger $I_{Na,late}$ compared to conventional square pulses or model simulations where "non-equilibrium gating" is not incorporated into the numerical model (Clancy et al., 2003; Magyar et al., 2004; Horvath et al., 2013).

Non-Cardiac Sodium Channel Isoforms in the Heart

Epilepsy (Alekov et al., 2000; Akalin et al., 2003) and certain skeletal muscle diseases (Komajda et al., 1980; Pereon et al., 2003) has been associated with pathological ECG recordings. Therefore it seemed possible that non-cardiac sodium channel mutations might cause electrical alterations in the heart. Later, $Na_V1.1$, $Na_V1.2$, $Na_V1.3$, $Na_V1.4$, $Na_V1.6$, and $Na_V1.8$ isoforms have been identified in cardiac tissue (Maier et al., 2002; Haufe et al., 2005; Valdivia et al., 2005; Biet et al., 2012; Yang et al., 2012). Based on the findings of *Biet et al.*, as much as 44 % of $I_{Na,late}$ is due to non-cardiac sodium channels (Biet et al., 2012) in canine ventricular cardiomyocytes. Furthermore, *Yang et al.* have shown that in mice and rabbit the TTX-resistant $Na_V1.8$ provides a substantial amount of $I_{Na,late}$ (Yang et al., 2012). Based on these experimental data, isoform specific sodium channel modulators might provide a valid approach in pharmacological antiarrhythmic therapy (See *Non-Cardiac Sodium Channel Inhibitors as Potential Antiarrhythmic Agent* for further details).

ROLE OF $I_{NA,LATE}$ IN CARDIAC PHYSIOLOGY

Role of $I_{Na,late}$ in Cardiac Electrical Activity

Contribution of $I_{Na,late}$ to cardiac APs was questioned because of its small density. However, the plateau phase of the cardiac AP is shaped by a delicate balance between minuscule inward and outward current fluxes. Therefore even a small change in these currents may significantly alter the duration of the AP (Horvath et al., 2006). Inhibition of $I_{Na,late}$ substantially shortens the cardiac AP in the conductive system (Coraboeuf et al., 1979) and in ventricular cells (Kiyosue and Arita, 1989) as well, indicating that $I_{Na,late}$ significantly contributes to determining the duration of the non-pacemaker AP in cardiac myocytes. Recent AP voltage clamp experiments show that the density of $I_{Na,late}$ is of similar magnitude as the major potassium currents in guinea pig (Horvath et al., 2013) and rabbit (Hegyi et al., 2018) ventricular myocytes. There is a characteristic interspecies difference in the shape of $I_{Na,late}$ as shown in the case of guinea pig, canine, and human ventricular myocytes (Horvath et al., 2020).

The sustained sodium current is also an important factor in determining electrophysiological properties of sinoatrial node cells (Maier et al., 2003; Lei et al., 2004). Tetrodotoxin, applied in lower than 1 μM concentrations, reduces the rate of spontaneous depolarization in sinoatrial node cells (Huang et al., 2015), clearly indicating that non-cardiac Na_V isoforms also contribute to cardiac automaticity.

Cardiac Purkinje cells have the largest rate-dependence of their AP duration (APD) among cardiomyocytes with fast response APs. Purkinje cell APs are longer at lower stimulation rates, while shorter at higher rates than APs of ventricular cells. It has been shown that $I_{Na,late}$ contributes to this feature by possessing much slower decay and recovery kinetics in Purkinje cells than in ventricular cells. As a result Purkinje cell $I_{Na,late}$ is significantly larger at low heart rates, while smaller at high heart rates compared to ventricular cells. This unique feature predisposes Purkinje cells to serve as triggers in generating arrhythmias (Li et al., 2017).

$I_{Na,late}$ plays a role in forming the atrial AP as well (Burashnikov and Antzelevitch, 2013; Luo et al., 2014). $I_{Na,late}$ is expected to be larger in atria than in ventricles because $I_{Na,\ early}$ density is greater in atrial cells under similar conditions (Li et al., 2002; Burashnikov et al., 2007), suggesting a higher sodium channel expression in atrial cells. On the other hand, an overall more positive membrane potential, and a more negative steady-state inactivation voltage of the sodium current (Li et al., 2002; Burashnikov et al., 2007) in the atrial cells reduce the availability of the sodium channels (Burashnikov and Antzelevitch, 2008). In one set of experiments by Luo et al. maximum $I_{Na,late}$ density has been reported to be greater in rabbit left atrial myocytes than in ventricular cells (Luo et al., 2014) and in a different investigation the two cell types seemed to be similar in this matter (Persson et al., 2007). APs are shorter in the atria compared to the ventricles reducing the amount of Na^+ influx through $I_{Na,late}$ in the former (Burashnikov and Antzelevitch, 2013).

$I_{Na,late}$ Plays a Significant Role in the Sodium Homeostasis of Cardiomyocytes

$[Na^+]_i$ is set by a dynamic equilibrium of the influx of Na^+ into the cell and efflux of Na^+ to the interstitial space. The $[Na^+]_i$ of non-paced ventricular myocytes is around 4–8 mM in guinea-pig, rabbit, and canine; and about twice as high in rat and mouse (9–14 mM) (Despa and Bers, 2013). In non-paced human myocytes $[Na^+]_i$ is thought to be in the 4–10 mM range.

Na^+ can enter into the cell through Na^+ channels, Na^+/Ca^{2+} exchanger (NCX) and Na^+/H^+ exchanger (NHE). Na^+ leaves the cell mainly via the Na^+/K^+ pump (NKP), but the reverse mode NCX is also responsible for a moderate Na^+ efflux during the first few milliseconds of the cardiac AP. Furthermore, Na^+/HCO_3^- cotransport, Na^+/Mg^{2+} exchange, and $Na^+/K^+/2Cl^-$ cotransport can play a role in the sodium homeostasis of cardiomyocytes to a small extent (Despa and Bers, 2013). It also has to be mentioned that Na^+ concentrations between the cytosol and intracellular organelles are continuously balanced.

Upon pacing, $[Na^+]_i$ increases with increasing stimulation frequency, caused by the larger Na^+ entry through Na^+ channels and NCX. In paced, single cardiac cells approximately 25 % of the Na^+ entry is mediated by Na_v channels (Despa and Bers, 2013). The Na^+ entry through Na_v channels is about equally distributed between $I_{Na,early}$ and $I_{Na,late}$ (Makielski and Farley, 2006; Zaza and Rocchetti, 2013; Despa and Bers, 2013; Shryock et al., 2013), however this contribution can change at different heart rates (see *Heart Rate and AP Duration Influences $I_{Na,late}$* for details). The higher Na^+ influx into paced cells is matched by an increased efflux through an elevated NKP activity. This is mainly caused by the increased $[Na^+]_i$ itself, but nitric oxide-, and phospholemman-dependent mechanisms can also add to this effect (Despa and Bers, 2013).

Na^+ and Ca^{2+} Homeostasis Is Linked in Cardiomyocytes

The Direct Connection Between Na^+ and Ca^{2+} Homeostasis: Na^+/Ca^{2+} Exchanger

The NCX is a secondarily active transporter that carries 1 Ca^{2+} and 3 Na^+ at the same time (Janvier and Boyett, 1996; Fujioka et al., 2000; Sipido et al., 2007; Despa and Bers, 2013; Ginsburg et al., 2013). The NCX function is determined by the relation of the actual membrane voltage and the sum of the actual electrochemical gradients of Ca^{2+} and Na^+. The main role of NCX is to remove Ca^{2+} from the cells by utilizing the potential energy present in the form of Na^+ gradient ("forward mode"). Besides this mode, in the first few milliseconds of the AP, NCX mediates Na^+ extrusion from the cell and Ca^{2+} entry into the cytosol ("reverse mode").

$I_{Na,late}$ Facilitates Ca^{2+} Influx via L-Type Calcium Channels

Being an inward current, $I_{Na,late}$ depolarizes the membrane, causing an increased membrane potential throughout the plateau phase and a longer AP. The more time the membrane spends in a depolarized state (above +40 mV) the higher the possibility that L-type calcium channels can open or re-open. It is well documented with AP voltage clamp technique that the L-type calcium current is flowing throughout the AP plateau (Linz and Meyer, 1998; Linz and Meyer, 2000; Banyasz et al., 2003; Fulop et al., 2004; Banyasz et al., 2012). Therefore a longer AP inevitably results in a larger Ca^{2+} entry to the myocyte.

Heart Rate and AP Duration Influences $I_{Na,late}$

Heart rate determines the magnitude of $I_{Na,late}$. Like many electrophysiological characteristics of cardiac cells (Banyasz et al., 2009), $I_{Na,late}$ is reverse-rate dependent, so the faster the stimulation rate the smaller the current density will be (Nagatomo et al., 2002; Wu et al., 2011). However, with increasing heart rate the density of $I_{Na,early}$ and maximum rate of depolarization during the AP upstroke (V_{max}; an AP parameter determined by $I_{Na,early}$) does not decrease that much (Nagatomo et al., 2002). This is because recovery of $I_{Na,late}$ is much slower than $I_{Na,early}$ (Carmeliet, 2006). At higher heart rates this feature of the two sodium current components also results in a decreasing contribution of $I_{Na,late}$ to the overall Na^+ influx. Under these conditions, the more frequent AP upstrokes cause a greater Na^+ entry through $I_{Na,early}$, and there is a reduction of $I_{Na,late}$ density because of the very slow $I_{Na,late}$ recovery kinetics. Moreover, rate-dependent changes of the AP length also influence Na^+ entry. At high heart rates APs are shorter, therefore $I_{Na,late}$ is active for a shorter time, accounting for a further reduction of Na^+ influx through the already smaller $I_{Na,late}$. At the same time, extrusion of Na^+ by the NKP is reduced at high pacing rates (Despa and Bers, 2013) leading to a rate-dependent $[Na^+]_i$ loading in isolated cells. It must also be noted that this phenomenon is largely offset or may not occur at all during β-adrenergic stimulation because it augments NKP activity through phospholemman (Cheung et al., 2010).).

As it is described in the previous section, APD influences $I_{Na,late}$: the shorter the AP the smaller the Na^+ flux through $I_{Na,late}$ is. Therefore under any conditions that result in a shorter AP the contribution of $I_{Na,late}$ to the overall Na^+ influx will be smaller. This fact, together with significant differences in heart rate underlies differences in $I_{Na,late}$ between species having short APs (e.g.: rats or mice) and long APs (guinea pig, rabbit, pig, human, etc.). In rats and mice both $I_{Na,late}$ and Na^+ influx driven by $I_{Na,late}$ should be much smaller than in species having long APs.

Modulation of $I_{Na,late}$

Cytosolic Ca^{2+} Modulates $I_{Na,late}$ in a Complex Way

Ca^{2+} is the key player in the excitation-contraction coupling of cardiac cells and it also regulates many other cellular functions including sarcolemmal transport mechanisms. Na_v channels are regulated by the individual and cooperative actions of Ca^{2+}, calmodulin (CaM), and Ca^{2+}-CaM dependent protein kinase II (CaMKII) as well (Bers and Grandi, 2009; Maier, 2011; Scheuer, 2011). Signaling through the Ca^{2+}—CaM—CaMKII pathway is thought to facilitate the sodium current, especially $I_{Na,late}$ (Maltsev et al., 2008; Maltsev et al., 2009; Bers and Grandi, 2009).

Na_v Channels, Ca^{2+} and CaM

Motifs with Ca^{2+} binding (EF hand) as well as CaM binding (IQ motifs) capabilities are present in the $Na_v1.5$ channel structure. Some groups have shown that Ca^{2+} alone can regulate sodium channels (Wingo et al., 2004), while other results support that Ca^{2+} is not capable of regulating Na_v channels directly; the regulation is mediated via Ca^{2+}-CaM complex (Tan et al., 2002; Kim et al., 2004). Besides the exact regulatory mechanism, the general agreement is that when Ca^{2+} is elevated the SSI curve shifts toward more positive voltages (Sarhan et al., 2012), although this is a largely negligible effect at physiologically relevant Ca^{2+} concentrations in wild type channels. However, under conditions when Ca^{2+} or CaM sensing regions are mutated or when the Ca^{2+} sensitivity of Na_v channels are severely altered, diverse functional disturbances may arise leading to an increased $I_{Na,late}$.

Ca^{2+}-CaM Dependent Protein Kinase II (CaMKII)

Besides the direct regulation of Na_v channels, the Ca^{2+}-CaM complex activates CaMKIIδ_C that also modulates these channels (Zhang and Brown, 2004; Anderson, 2005; Bers and Grandi, 2009). The active CaMKII is a Ser/Thr kinase that can phosphorylate $Na_v1.5$ channels on at least three amino acid residues (Grandi and Herren, 2014). While there is an ongoing debate about the exact role of these phosphorylation sites in channel gating, all the studies agree on that activation of CaMKII increases $I_{Na,late}$.

Complex Modulation by β-Adrenergic Stimulation

In a meticulous set of AP voltage clamp experiments, Hegyi et al. (Hegyi et al., 2018) showed how different downstream elements of the β-adrenergic pathway regulate $I_{Na,late}$ in rabbit ventricular myocytes. Protein kinase A, CaMKII, Epac, nitrosylation, as well as reactive oxygen species (ROS) contributed to the upregulation of $I_{Na,late}$ during different phases of the ventricular AP.

Cellular Metabolites

ROS and H_2O_2 increase $I_{Na,late}$ (Song et al., 2004; Song et al., 2006; Sossalla et al., 2008). Some results suggest that CaMKII can be involved in $I_{Na,late}$ facilitation observed in the presence of oxygen free radicals (Wagner et al., 2011), because ROS can also activate CaMKII (Erickson et al., 2008). See (Wagner et al., 2013) for a detailed review.

Acidosis also modulates Na_v channels (Murphy et al., 2011; Jones et al., 2011; Jones et al., 2013a; Jones et al., 2013b). Acidosis caused a rightward shift in steady-state activation, but not in steady-state inactivation in isolated canine ventricular myocytes therefore reducing $I_{Na,late}$ (Murphy et al., 2011).

Many studies have found that hypoxia increases $I_{Na,late}$ (Ju et al., 1996; Carmeliet, 1999; Harnmarstrom and Gage, 2002; Wang et al., 2007; Shimoda and Polak, 2011; Tang et al., 2012). Following a 15 minute hypoxic period, *Wang et al.* reported an increased BM channel activity, a plausible explanation of the increased $I_{Na,late}$.

Intermediary lipid metabolites shown to increase $I_{Na,late}$. Na_v channels treated with lysophosphatidylcholine exhibited a sustained BM channel activity (Burnashev et al., 1991; Undrovinas et al., 1992), while palmitoylcarnitine induced a slowly inactivating sodium current (Wu and Corr, 1994). According to more recent data, poly-unsaturated fatty acids (docosahexaenoic acid and eicosapentaenoic acid) reduce both $I_{Na,early}$ and $I_{Na,late}$ (Pignier et al., 2007). According to the authors, the reduction is caused by a decreased overlap between the steady-state activation and inactivation voltage range.

Nitric oxide (NO) has been shown to enhance $I_{Na,late}$ (Ahern et al., 2000). The neural NO synthase (nNOS) belongs to the huge macromolecular complex of $Na_v1.5$, with caveolin-3 and α1-syntrophin among some additional proteins (Cheng et al., 2013).

Other Mechanisms

Transcriptional Regulation

The possible promoter regions and their role in the regulation of human SCN5A gene transcription has already been reported. (Yang et al., 2004; van Stuijvenberg et al., 2010) Recent studies have shown that the zinc-finger transcription factor, GATA4 (Tarradas et al., 2017), and the myocyte enhancing factor-2C (MEF2C) enhances SCN5A transcription (Zhou et al., 2018). However, most likely many other transcription factors are involved in the transcriptional regulation of the SCN5A gene.

Glycosylation

Some amino acid motifs found in the $Na_v1.5$ protein are subject to N-glycosylation. Carbohydrates account for an about 5 % of the total mass of Na_v channels in the rat heart (Cohen and Levitt, 1993). The lack of channel glycosylation caused shifts toward positive voltages in both steady state activation and inactivation curves when naturally sialic-acid deficient channels were used (Zhang et al., 1999), or when these carbohydrate residues were removed by enzymatic treatment (Ufret-Vincenty et al., 2001) Glycosylation also seem to be involved in channel trafficking (Mercier et al., 2015; Cortada and Brugada, 2019)

Protein Kinase C

Upon protein kinase C activation, Na^+ channels are internalized from the plasma membrane (Hallaq et al., 2012). For the process, both channel phosphorylation on S1503 and ROS are required (Liu et al., 2017).

Phosphorylation on Tyrosine Residues

The "Fyn" tyrosine kinase phosphorylates $Na_v1.5$ channels on the Y1495 Tyr residue, located in the III–IV linker domain. This tyrosine residue helps with anchoring Ca^{2+}/CaM to the inactivation gate of the channel (Sarhan and Van Petegem, 2009). When Fyn phosphorylates the channel on Y1495, it increases the window voltage range by shifting the steady-state inactivation toward more positive potentials (Ahern et al., 2005), therefore resulting in an enhanced $I_{Na,late}$.

Arginine Methylation

There are three known arginine residues in $Na_v1.5$ (R513, R526, and R680), that are subject to methylation (Beltran-Alvarez et al., 2011). These residues are found in the domain I and domain II linker region. There are two known mutations of these arginines (namely R526H and R680H) that cause Brugada (Kapplinger et al., 2010) and LQT3 syndromes (Wang et al., 2007), respectively.

Mechanosensitivity

Mechanical stimuli also affect channel gating in $Na_v1.5$ channels. *Beyder et al.* investigated this phenomenon both in an expression system (Beyder et al., 2010) and in isolated mouse ventricular cells (Beyder et al., 2012). The pressure ramp applied by the authors caused a 235 % increase in LSM $Na_v1.5$ channel openings suggesting that $I_{Na,late}$ is enhanced by mechanical stress. Similar mechanical effects can modify certain signal transduction mechanisms like nNOS and CaMKII (Jian et al., 2014), which can, in turn, increase $I_{Na,late}$.

THE ROLE OF SODIUM HOMEOSTASIS AND ELEVATED $I_{NA,LATE}$ IN CARDIAC ARRHYTHMIAS

The pathophysiology of cardiac arrhythmias is based on the classical concept of "arrhythmic triad"; combination of a proarrhythmic *substrate*, a *trigger*, and the *modulating effect of the autonomic nervous system* (Merchant and Armoundas, 2012). The exact combination depends on etiology, cardiac-, and extracardiac comorbidities. Abnormal $[Na^+]_i$ homeostasis can play a role in creating an arrhythmia-prone substrate as well as in generating a trigger for the rhythm disorder. The discussed mechanisms are summarized on **Figure 2**.

$[Na^+]_i$ Increases in Many Cardiac Pathologies

Compared to non-failing myocytes, $[Na^+]_i$ is about 2–6 mM larger in myocytes from failing hearts (Pieske et al., 2002; Despa et al., 2002; Schillinger et al., 2006; Louch et al., 2010). In a pressure- and volume-overload rabbit HF model, Despa et al. have found an increased TTX-sensitive Na^+ influx (Despa et al., 2002). Interestingly, this larger influx was present not only in electrically stimulated myocytes, but in non-paced cells as well. In paced cells the most plausible candidate of this increased TTX-sensitive Na^+ influx is $I_{Na,late}$. However, the underlying mechanism of this influx is not yet understood completely in resting myocytes.

$I_{Na,late}$ Can Contribute to the Elevated $[Na^+]_i$

Many cardiac diseases are associated with an increased $I_{Na,late}$. The list contains cardiac myocytes originating from end-stage HF (Maltsev et al., 1998; Maltsev et al., 2007) and post-myocardial infarction (Huang et al., 2001) preparations as well as animal HF models (Valdivia et al., 2005; Maltsev et al., 2007). The larger $I_{Na,late}$ can be caused by several pathophysiologic factors including oxidative stress (ROS (Song et al., 2006; Sossalla et al., 2008) and NO (Ahern et al., 2000) mainly by S-nitrosylation of the $Na_v1.5$ channels (Cheng et al., 2013)), hypoxia (Carmeliet, 1999; Tang et al., 2012), mechanical stress (Beyder et al., 2012), and certain ischemic metabolites, for example oxidized lipids (Burnashev et al., 1991). Looking at gating modes in single $Na_v1.5$ channels, enhanced $I_{Na,late}$ is likely underlain by an increased number of BM and LSM openings (Undrovinas et al., 2002; Maltsev, 2006) in HF.

The Ca^{2+}—CaM—CaMKII signal transduction pathway is upregulated in HF (Bers, 2010), and this pathway has been shown to increase $I_{Na,late}$ (Tan et al., 2002; Wagner et al., 2006; Ashpole et al., 2012; Ma et al., 2012). Oxidation activates CaMKII (Wagner et al., 2011) and keeps it constitutively active. The enhanced CaMKII-mediated $Na_v1.5$ phosphorylation, therefore, certainly takes part in increasing $I_{Na,late}$ under oxidative stress. Recent studies have found that $Na_v1.8$ expression is significantly up-regulated, while $Na_v1.5$ is reduced in human left ventricular hypertrophy (Ahmad et al., 2019) and HF (Dybkova et al., 2018).

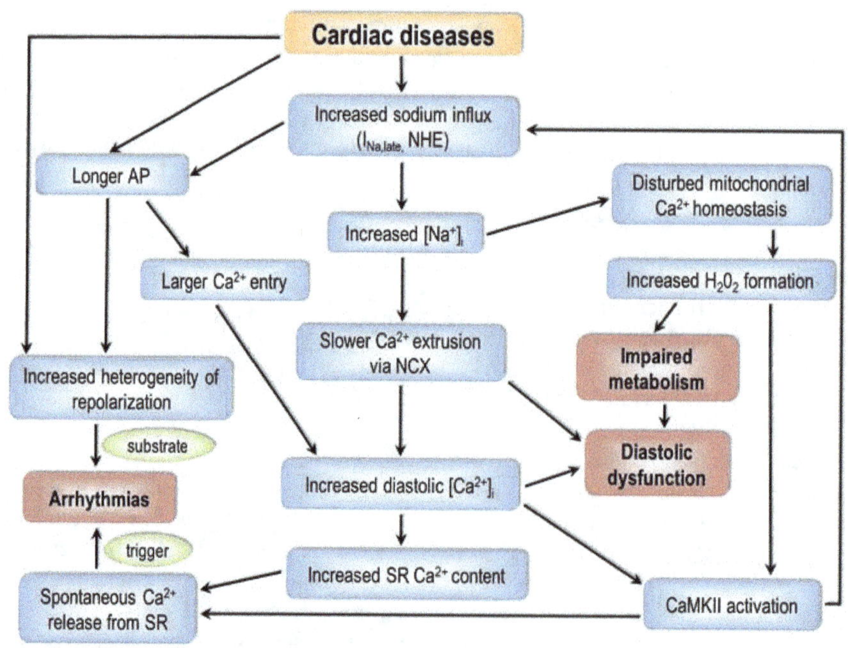

FIGURE 2 | How can an impaired sodium homeostasis of cardiac myocytes lead to arrhythmias? AP, action potential; NHE, Na^+/H^+ exchanger; $[Na^+]_i$, intracellular sodium concentration; NCX, Na^+/Ca^{2+} exchanger; $[Ca^{2+}]_i$, intracellular calcium concentration; SR, sarcoplasmic reticulum; CaMKII, calcium/calmodulin dependent protein kinase II.

The Vicious Circle of CaMKII—$I_{Na,late}$—$[Na^+]_i$—$[Ca^{2+}]_i$—CaMKII

When $[Na^+]_i$ is elevated, it makes the NCX forward mode energetically less favorable, therefore a smaller amount of Ca^{2+} will leave the cell through NCX. This causes an increased $[Ca^{2+}]_i$ load, and therefore further activates CaMKII, leading to enhanced phosphorylation of CaMKII targets such as $Na_v1.5$. This, in turn, increases $I_{Na,late}$, which further elevates $[Na^+]_i$ finally creating an arrhythmogenic vicious circle (Grandi and Herren, 2014). By using genetic (LQT3 mutation) as well as pharmacological (anemone toxin-II, ATX-II) approaches to increase $I_{Na,late}$, and therefore achieve $[Na^+]_i$ loading, Yao et al. described this feedback (Yao et al., 2011). These conditions lead to the vicious circle described above, and as a result, arrhythmias can be generated because of an increase in the CaMKII-dependent phosphorylation of phospholamban and RyRs.

$[Na^+]_i$—Mitochondrial $[Ca^{2+}]$—Oxidative Stress—CaMKII—$I_{Na,late}$—$[Na^+]_i$ Feedback

The mitochondrial NCX dynamically equilibrate concentrations of Ca^{2+} and Na^+ of the mitochondrion and the cytosol. Ca^{2+} in the mitochondrion plays a role in determining the production of ATP and ROS by regulating the expression of enzymes involved in oxidative phosphorylation (Yang et al., 2014). If $[Na^+]_i$ is elevated, it will impair Ca^{2+} accumulation in the mitochondrion at high pacing rates, leading to a decrease in $NADH/NAD^+$ redox potential. This increases H_2O_2 generation in the cells (Liu and O'Rourke, 2008), causing oxidative stress and thereby directly and indirectly (through CaMKII (Erickson et al., 2008)) activating $I_{Na,late}$. Finally, the process leads to a further increase in $[Na^+]_i$ (Wagner et al., 2011). This shows that, similar to an elevated $[Na^+]_i$, CaMKII activation can be caused by and can also lead to an increased ROS production.

Arrhythmogenic Consequences of an Increased $I_{Na,late}$ and $[Na^+]_i$

Many inherited and acquired diseases can lead to a longer ventricular repolarization, presented as long QT (LQT) syndromes (El-Sherif et al., 2019; Locati et al., 2019). The inherited LQT3 syndrome is caused by an increased $I_{Na,late}$ because of a mutant, much slower inactivating $Na_v1.5$ channel. Acquired LQTs include for example heart failure (Maltsev et al., 1998; Maltsev et al., 2007; Coppini et al., 2013), myocardial ischemia and post-infarction state (Huang et al., 2001; Rivera-Fernandez et al., 2016), and type 2 diabetes mellitus (Ninkovic et al., 2016).

Under physiological conditions there is a fine balance between the inward and outward currents during the AP plateau. During the plateau phase the impedance of the membrane is large, therefore even a small change in the delicate balance can lead to a marked change in AP duration. In this setting, the depolarizing drive caused by an increased $I_{Na,late}$ causes a longer AP (Studenik et al., 2001; Horvath et al., 2013), as well as under a longer AP, $I_{Na,late}$ will generate a larger Na^+ influx. Even in normal hearts, both APD and $I_{Na,late}$ is greater in Purkinje fibers and in "M" cells than in the rest of the myocardium contributing to the physiological heterogeneity of repolarization. LQT syndromes increase both the spatial heterogeneity of repolarization (Maltsev et al., 2007) and the temporal variability of repolarization (El-Sherif et al., 2019) and therefore can present an *arrhythmogenic substrate.* This can be further exaggerated by bradycardia, where the APs are already long, and having larger heterogeneity (Szentandrassy et al., 2015). Cardiac diseases can also provide the *proarrhythmic substrate* in the form of temporal repolarization heterogeneity, "repolarization alternans" (Bonatti et al., 2014; Justo et al., 2016) which phenomenon is more pronounced in tachycardia.

The *trigger* is also highly rate-dependent. At low heart rates, where the cardiac APs are already long even under physiological conditions, an augmented $I_{Na,late}$ can further prolong repolarization therefore increasing the probability of early afterdepolarizations (EADs), and the risk for (fatal) ventricular arrhythmias (Wang et al., 1995; Wang et al., 1996; Makita et al., 2002; Hedley et al., 2009; Cardona et al., 2010; Yamamura et al., 2010; Lowe et al., 2012). Severe bradycardia together with an enhanced $I_{Na,late}$ and a long APD may also promote delayed afterdepolarization (DAD)-mediated triggered activities (Song et al., 2008; Coppini et al., 2013; Horvath et al., 2013). These triggered activities seem to heavily depend on an increased $[Ca^{2+}]_i$.

As described previously, an increased $[Na^+]_i$ offsets NCX, decreasing Ca^{2+} removal from the cytosol (Bers, 2002; Nagy et al., 2004; Despa and Bers, 2013). This elevates diastolic $[Ca^{2+}]_i$ and therefore increasing SR Ca^{2+} content; leading to spontaneous Ca^{2+} release events from the Ca^{2+}-overloaded SR (Gyorke and Terentyev, 2008). This can generate DADs and therefore possibly triggering arrhythmias. At high heart rates this can further be aggravated by the two feedback loops involving CaMKII, as described in the previous sections, resulting in an enhanced CaMKII mediated phosphorylation of RyR2 therefore increasing the probability of spontaneous SR Ca^{2+} release events. It must be noted again that *in vivo*, there is no high heart rate without β-adrenergic stimulation. Adrenergic stimulation on one hand further activates CaMKII (Hegyi et al., 2018) but on the other hand, it also reduces or even diminishes $[Na^+]_i$ loading of the cells by enhancing NKP activity (Cheung et al., 2010). This makes the role of $I_{Na,late}$ in DAD-mediated arrhythmias occurring at high heart rates questionable.

In the diseased heart, however, rate-dependent properties of $I_{Na,late}$ and [Na+]i are quite poorly investigated. At high pacing rates, $I_{Na,late}$ decreases in LQT3 ΔKPQ mutant cells (Nagatomo et al., 2002) and an increased $[Na^+]_i$ load was reported in hypertrophied feline cells (Mills et al., 2007) as well as in human cardiomyocytes from failing hearts (Pieske et al., 2002).

Pharmacologically enhanced $I_{Na,late}$ increases repolarization heterogeneity in intact, isolated rabbit and guinea pig hearts (Restivo et al., 2004; Milberg et al., 2005), as well as in canine left ventricular wedge preparations giving rise to TdP (Shimizu and Antzelevitch, 1999a; Shimizu and Antzelevitch, 1999b). ATX-II also induces AF in a wide range of experimental conditions (Lu et al., 2012; Liang et al., 2016). Many gain-of-function SCN5A mutations (including LQT3) have been associated with atrial fibrillation (AF) (Benito et al., 2008). Also, in cases of chronic (permanent) AF, larger $I_{Na,late}$ was found (Sossalla et al., 2010; Poulet et al., 2015). These data suggest that enhancement of $I_{Na,late}$ might play a role in generating or maintaining AF most likely because of $[Na^+]_i$ overload dependent Ca^{2+} overload (Nattel and Dobrev, 2012).

$I_{NA,LATE}$ AS AN ANTIARRHYTHMIC THERAPEUTIC TARGET

Sodium Channel Inhibitors

Natural products of peptide and non-peptide structure can inhibit sodium channels, although these compounds have negligible therapeutical relevance. Clinically relevant small-molecule sodium channel inhibitors include local anesthetics, anticonvulsants, and antiarrhythmic agents such as lidocaine, carbamazepine, phenytoin, lamotrigine, and mexiletine. These small-molecule inhibitors all bind to the so-called "local anesthetic site" of sodium channels where amino acid residues are highly conserved among different Na_v subtypes (de Lera Ruiz and Kraus, 2015). Because of this, the "classic" Na_v blockers are not subtype specific, they inhibit all subtypes to a certain extent. Also, these compounds somewhat inhibit both $I_{Na,early}$ and $I_{Na,late}$, usually having a higher inhibitory effect on $I_{Na,late}$. Therefore most Na_v blockers reduce excitability and impulse propagation (parameters associated with $I_{Na,early}$) together with the plateau sodium current ($I_{Na,late}$).

Selective $I_{Na,late}$ Inhibitors

A few sodium channel blockers differ from the "classic" inhibitors, because they inhibit $I_{Na,late}$ more potently than $I_{Na,early}$. The molecular mechanism of the preferential $I_{Na,late}$ inhibition is still not completely understood. Even though ranolazine was used for most of the experimental and clinical studies, other selective $I_{Na,late}$ inhibitors also exist such as lidocaine, GS-458967, GS-462808, F15845, and GS-6615 (eleclazine). The half-maximal inhibitory concentration (IC_{50}) values of these inhibitors for the late and the early sodium current component are summarized in **Table 1**. For a more thorough data summary on this, see Table 2 in the review of Antzelevitch et al. (2014).

TABLE 1 | IC_{50} values of selective late sodium current inhibitors for the late and the early sodium current component.

Compound	IC_{50} for		Reference
	$I_{Na,late}$	$I_{Na,early}$	
Lidocaine	29 μM	367 μM	Antzelevitch et al., 2014
Ranolazine	17 μM	1329 μM	Belardinelli et al., 2013
	6 μM	294 μM	Undrovinas et al., 2006
GS-458967	333 nM	<15 % block at 333 nM	Koltun et al., 2016a
	130 nM	7.5 % reduction at 10 μM	Belardinelli et al., 2013
GS-462808	1.9 μM	10 % reduction at 10 μM	Koltun et al., 2016b
GS-6615	0.62 μM	51 μM	Zablocki et al., 2016
F15845	3.25 μM	23 % reduction at 10 μM	Vacher et al., 2009

Where the IC_{50} value is missing, inhibition percentage at a given concentration was used instead.

For lidocaine, IC_{50} values of around 25 and 300 μM were determined for $I_{Na,late}$ and $I_{Na,early}$, respectively (Antzelevitch et al., 2014).

In case of ranolazine, the IC_{50} values are 17 μM for $I_{Na,late}$ and 1,329 μM for $I_{Na,early}$ in rabbit (Belardinelli et al., 2013), whereas 6 μM for $I_{Na,late}$ (Antzelevitch et al., 2004; Undrovinas et al., 2006) and 294 μM for $I_{Na,early}$ (Undrovinas et al., 2006) in canine ventricular myocytes.

GS-458967 was found to have an IC_{50} of 333 nM for $I_{Na,late}$ inhibition while exhibiting smaller than 15% block of $I_{Na,early}$ at the same concentration at 1 and 3 Hz pacing frequencies (Koltun et al., 2016a) measured on $Na_v1.5$ channels expressed in HEK-293 cells with automated patch-clamp. In rabbit ventricular cardiomyocytes, the IC_{50} was 130 nM for $I_{Na,late}$, and at 10 μM, GS-458967 caused an approximately 7.5 % reduction in $I_{Na,early}$. (Belardinelli et al., 2013). Unfortunately for the developer, GS-458967 had a high brain penetration and a profound use dependent block on all the various sodium channel isoforms, making the compound prone for possible central nervous system side effects (Koltun et al., 2016a).

GS-462808 has an IC_{50} of 1.9 μM for $I_{Na,late}$ inhibition while blocking 10 % of $I_{Na,early}$ at 10 μM and it is also more cardiac isoform selective than GS-458967 blocking only 8 % of the $Na_v1.1$ peak current. The problem with GS-462808 is that it caused liver lesions during the acute animal toxicity tests (Koltun et al., 2016b).

For GS-6615 the IC_{50} values of 0.62 and 51 μM were reported for $I_{Na,late}$ and $I_{Na,early}$ blockade, respectively, in manual patch-clamp experiments, with practically no effect on $Na_v1.1$ channels (Zablocki et al., 2016).

F15845 has an IC_{50} of 3.25 μM for the inhibition of veratridine-induced $I_{Na,late}$ while blocking 23 % of $I_{Na,early}$ at 10 μM (Vacher et al., 2009). Last experimental data about F15845 were published in 2010, where it prevented ischemia-induced arrhythmias in rats (Pignier et al., 2010). Since then no new results came out regarding this agent.

Selectivity of these specific $I_{Na,late}$ inhibitors is usually voltage-dependent, these blockers have very little effect on $I_{Na,early}$ at more negative (quite unphysiological, for example −120 mV) holding potentials. As the holding potential gets closer to physiological resting membrane potentials, the selectivity of these compounds decrease, they start to inhibit $I_{Na,early}$ more. Also, most inhibitors block the sodium channels in a rate-dependent ("use-dependent") fashion; the blockers are more effective at rapid than at slow heart rates. This is because most inhibitors preferentially bind to the open and/or inactivated channels rather than the closed channel. This effect is especially strong in sodium channel blockers having fast association and dissociation kinetics (Pless et al., 2011) (Vaughan-Williams class Ib agents).

In case of 1 μM GS-458967 for example, $I_{Na,early}$ did not change in rabbit ventricular myocytes held at −120 mV at pacing rates of 0.1, 1, or 3 Hz. When the holding potential was −80 mV, however, 1 μM GS-458967 reduced $I_{Na,early}$ by 48 ± 7%, 50 ± 7%, and 56 ± 8% at rates of 0.1, 1, and 3 Hz, respectively (Belardinelli et al., 2013).

Ranolazine also inhibits sodium channels in a voltage-, and use-dependent fashion, moreover this blockade is also significantly larger in atria compared to ventricles (Zygmunt et al., 2011). With 50 ms long depolarizing pulses and 250 ms diastolic intervals (at 3.33 Hz), the use-dependent block by ranolazine at −120 mV was 21 % in ventricular, versus 32 % in atrial cells, whereas at −100 mV the block was 47 % versus 56 %, respectively. This data suggest that the rate dependency (use-dependency) is very pronounced in case of $I_{Na,early}$ inhibition, but much smaller with $I_{Na,late}$. Therefore, based on the rate-dependent physiological (see *Heart Rate and AP Duration Influences $I_{Na,late}$*) and pharmacological characteristics of $I_{Na,\ early}$ and $I_{Na,late}$, a quite selective inhibition of $I_{Na,late}$ might be achieved at slow heart rates and with long APs, but at fast rates, with short AP duration, sodium channel blockers similarly inhibit both $I_{Na,\ early}$ and $I_{Na,late}$.

At therapeutical plasma concentrations, ranolazine inhibits other ionic currents besides $I_{Na,late}$. This includes I_{Kr} (approximately 40 % inhibition at 6 μM), and $I_{Ca,L}$ (around 25 % inhibition at 6 μM) (Antzelevitch et al., 2004). Consequently, inhibiting $I_{Na,late}$ and applying ranolazine are very far from being identical concepts. When ranolazine is used to inhibit $I_{Na,late}$, effects on other channels must not be forgotten. Besides the previous features, ranolazine is also a weak β-adrenergic antagonist (Letienne et al., 2001) and an inhibitor of fatty acid oxidation (Chaitman, 2006), even though this latter effect only becomes prominent at supratherapeutical plasma concentrations.

Non-Cardiac Sodium Channel Inhibitors as Potential Antiarrhythmic Agents

Riluzole blocks TTX-sensitive sodium channels preferentially, which are associated with damaged neurons (Song et al., 1997). Riluzole also directly inhibits the kainate and NMDA receptors (Debono et al., 1993) as well as potentiates $GABA_A$ receptors (He et al., 2002). In anaesthetized pigs, myocardial damage and arrhythmias induced by coronary occlusion has been reduced by riluzole (Weiss et al., 2013). Riluzole has also been found to be anti-ischemic and antiarrhythmic in a pig model of acute myocardial infarction. (Weiss and Saint, 2010).

Targeting $Na_v1.8$ with specific inhibitors might provide a potential novel approach in the future in antiarrhythmic drug therapy, because recent studies have found that $Na_v1.8$ expression is significantly up-regulated in human left ventricular hypertrophy (Ahmad et al., 2019) and HF (Dybkova et al., 2018). By using $Na_v1.8$-specific blockers [either A-803467 (30 nM) or PF-01247324 (1 μM)] the authors managed to reduce $I_{Na,late}$ and APD in these experiments. Other $Na_v1.8$ specific inhibitors include funapide and VX-150, however these compounds have not been tested in relation to cardiac pathophysiology so far.

Experimental Pathophysiology Studies

Because of the pronounced use-dependent effect of specific $I_{Na,late}$ inhibitors, interpretation of experimental studies conducted on rats and mice (having resting heart rates around 400 bpm) are very difficult. Therefore this review will focus on experimental data originating from larger mammalian species.

Late Sodium Current Inhibition and Ventricular Arrhythmias

As it was demonstrated in the previous sections, $I_{Na,late}$ has quite different characteristics under different heart rates. Therefore it is worthwhile to split the ventricular arrhythmia topic into two subtopics accordingly.

Bradycardia and Long APs

Many *in vitro* experimental studies have shown that at low pacing rates with prolonged APs and increased repolarization heterogeneity (LQT3 syndrome, heart failure, hypertrophic cardiomyopathy), inhibition of $I_{Na,late}$ effectively reduces the burden of arrhythmic episodes [EADs, DADs, triggered APs, Torsade de Pointes (TdP) (Shimizu and Antzelevitch, 1997; Song et al., 2004; Coppini et al., 2013; Belardinelli et al., 2013; Rajamani et al., 2016)].

Ranolazine and GS-458967 has been shown to suppress dofetilide-induced TdP in a canine in vivo model (Antoons et al., 2010; Bossu et al., 2018).

There was one experimental study about the potential antiarrhythmic role of F15845, where it prevented ischemia-induced arrhythmias in rats (Pignier et al., 2010). However the use of a rat model makes it hard to extrapolate this study to humans.

Under the pathological conditions listed above, the fine balance between the inward and outward currents during the AP plateau is shifted toward the depolarizing inward currents, resulting in a longer AP. Therefore, theoretically, any intervention that reduces the depolarizing currents (e.g.: L-type calcium current, NCX current, $I_{Na,late}$) could be effective in bringing the repolarization closer to normal. In this setting, therefore, inhibiting $I_{Na,late}$ will reduce the depolarization drive resulting in a significantly shorter APD and the suppression of arrhythmogenic events such as EADs, even if the magnitude of $I_{Na,late}$ is not increased. Under similar conditions, other interventions such as L-type calcium channel blockade (Abrahamsson et al., 1996) or potassium channel activation (Carlsson et al., 1992) can also shorten APD, reduce repolarization heterogeneity, and suppress the occurrence of arrhythmogenic events even if $I_{Na,late}$ is upregulated. In LQT syndromes $I_{Na,late}$-mediated increase in $Ca^{2+}{}_i$ is just a fraction of the total $Ca^{2+}{}_i$, and even total $Ca^{2+}{}_i$ just contributes to rather than determines the arrhythmogenic events (Carlsson et al., 1996).

Tachycardia-Induced Tachyarrhythmias (VT, VF)

$I_{Na,late}$ blockers seem to effectively prevent or terminate tachycardia-induced ventricular tachycardia, and ventricular fibrillation in healthy animal models in the presence of a β-adrenergic agonist (Alves Bento et al., 2015; Carneiro et al., 2015; Bacic et al., 2017).

However, inhibition of $I_{Na,late}$ does not likely play a crucial role here, based on the following theoretical considerations. To start with, in healthy ventricular tissue at high heart rates $I_{Na,late}$ is quite small, as it was discussed in *Heart Rate and AP Duration Influences $I_{Na,late}$*. Furthermore, at rapid heart rates with β-adrenergic stimulation the major arrhythmogenic mechanism is likely to be the increased L-type calcium current, the increased SR Ca^{2+} content, and the leaky RyR together (Merchant and Armoundas, 2012). The third but similarly important factor is that these VT/VF episodes are likely underlain by a reentry mechanism, therefore heavily depending on the fast conduction provided by $I_{Na,early}$. At high pacing rates the "specific" $I_{Na,late}$ inhibitors will also block a considerable amount of $I_{Na,early}$ as well (see *Selective $I_{Na,late}$ Inhibitors* for details), and this might just be enough to break the reentry circuit (Burashnikov and Antzelevitch, 2017).

Based on the experimental data, $I_{Na,late}$ inhibition seems to be a valid therapeutic approach to tackle ventricular arrhythmias especially at low heart rates. These experimental studies also suggest that $I_{Na,late}$ inhibition mainly affects the arrhythmogenic substrate by making the repolarization less heterogenous (Carneiro et al., 2015), with only low impact on suppressing the triggers (Bossu et al., 2018).

Late Sodium Current Inhibition in AF

GS-458967 was shown to suppress isoproterenol-, and high Ca^{2+}-induced DADs in healthy canine pulmonary-, and superior vena cava preparations (Sicouri et al., 2013). GS-458967 also suppressed autonomically triggered AF in an intact porcine model (Carneiro et al., 2015). In other experimental studies, "classic" sodium channel inhibitors (eg, lidocaine, flecainide) also prevented and terminated AF (Wang et al., 1992; Comtois et al., 2008). However, these agents were used at concentrations causing a suppression of $I_{Na,early}$. Experimental data about ranolazine shows an effective reduction of AF burden (AFB) only at concentrations that potently inhibit both $I_{Na,early}$ (Burashnikov et al., 2007; Kumar et al., 2009; Burashnikov et al., 2014) and I_{Kr} (Burashnikov et al., 2007) Suppressing I_{Kr} reduces the diastolic interval between APs therefore promoting rate-dependent $I_{Na,early}$ inhibition.

Based on these data, *specific* $I_{Na,late}$ blockade alone is not a clear and straightforward approach in AF, except for cases when a longer atrial AP is the pathogenetic factor in the initiation of AF.

Clinical Studies

Ranolazine

So far, ranolazine has been used in the vast majority of clinical studies involving $I_{Na,late}$ blockers. When interpreting these trials, it has to be considered that ranolazine has other effects besides inhibiting $I_{Na,late}$. With the use of ranolazine, the first favorable results from phase 2 clinical trials were published in the 1990s (Cocco et al., 1992; Thadani et al., 1994). In 2006, following the outcome of the MARISA (Chaitman et al., 2004a), CARISA (Chaitman et al., 2004b), and ERICA (Stone et al., 2006) trials, the Food and Drug Administration approved ranolazine as an anti-anginal agent.

The effect of clinical outcome and safety of ranolazine therapy was investigated in more than 6,500 patients with non-ST-elevation acute coronary syndrome in the MERLIN TIMI-36 trial (Morrow et al., 2007). Although cardiovascular death or myocardial infarction has not been significantly reduced by ranolazine when compared to standard therapy; but recurrent ischemia (Morrow et al., 2007) and the incidence of arrhythmias (Scirica et al., 2007) were significantly lower with ranolazine. Treatment with ranolazine, compared to placebo, resulted in significantly lower incidences of arrhythmias. Fewer patients had episodes of ventricular tachycardia lasting more than eight beats [166 (5.3%) versus 265 (8.3%); $p<0.001$], supraventricular tachycardia [1413 (44.7%) versus 1752 (55.0%); $p<0.001$], or new-onset AF [55 (1.7%) versus 75 (2.4%); $p=0.08$]. Moreover, longer than 3 s pauses were less frequent with ranolazine [97 (3.1%) versus 136 (4.3%); $p=0.01$].

In the double-blind HARMONY (ClinicalTrials.gov ID: NCT01522651) phase 2 trial (Reiffel et al., 2015), patients with paroxysmal AF and implanted pacemakers were enrolled, so that AFB could continuously be monitored over the 12 weeks of treatment period. Patients were randomized to placebo, ranolazine alone (750 mg twice a day—BID), dronedarone alone (225 mg BID), or ranolazine (750 mg BID) combined with dronedarone (either 150 mg BID or 225 mg BID). The idea behind the combination was to reduce the dose of dronedarone, and therefore the negative inotropic effect associated with dronedarone. Placebo or the drugs alone did not significantly reduce AFB. In the combination therapies, however, ranolazine with dronedarone 225 mg BID reduced AFB by 59% vs placebo ($p=0.008$), and ranolazine with dronedarone 150 mg BID reduced AFB by 43% ($p=0.072$). Also, patients tolerated both combinations well.

Into the RAFFAELLO phase 2 trial (De Ferrari et al., 2015) patients with persistent AF (7 days to 6 months) were enrolled. Two hours after successful electrical cardioversion participants were randomized to either placebo, or ranolazine 375 mg, 500 mg, or 750 mg BID. Patients were monitored daily by transtelephonic ECG. The primary end-point was the time to first AF recurrence. No dose of the ranolazine prolonged time to AF recurrence significantly compared to placebo. Of the 238 patients who took at least one dose of the study drug, AF recurred in 56.4%, 56.9%, 41.7%, and 39.7% of patients in the placebo and ranolazine 375 mg/500 mg/750 mg groups, respectively. The reduction in overall AF recurrence in the combined 500-mg and 750-mg groups was of borderline significance compared to the placebo group ($p=0.053$) and significant compared to 375-mg group ($p=0.035$).

The RAID clinical trial (NCT01534962) (Zareba et al., 2018) investigated high-risk cardiomyopathy patients who received an implantable cardioverter-defibrillator (ICD). The subjects received either ranolazine (1,000 mg BID) or placebo. The primary endpoints were VT or VF requiring ICD shock or death. Among 1,012 ICD patients the ranolazine versus placebo hazard ratio was 0.84 (95% confidence interval: 0.67 to 1.05; p=0.117) for the primary endpoint. In the ranolazine group the risk of ICD therapies for recurrent VT or VF were significantly lower (hazard ratio: 0.70; 95% confidence interval: 0.51 to 0.96; p=0.028). Other effects of ranolazine treatment however has not been significant. These included individual components of the primary endpoint, quality of life, cardiac hospitalizations, and inappropriate ICD shocks as well.

In a smaller group of participants of the RAND-CFR trial (NCT01754259) (Evaristo et al., 2018) where symptomatic diabetic patients participated with non-flow-limiting coronary artery stenosis with diffuse atherosclerosis and/or microvascular dysfunction, effect of ranolazine on T-wave heterogeneity was evaluated. At physical rest, in the ranolazine group T-wave heterogeneity was 28 % smaller (placebo: 47±6 μV, ranolazine: 39±5 μV, p=0.002), however ranolazine did not differ from the placebo group during exercise. The trial also suggested that reduction in repolarization abnormalities seemed to be independent of alterations in myocardial blood flow.

In a meta-analysis of eight randomized clinical trials (Gong et al., 2017) *Gong et al.* found that ranolazine significantly reduced AF incidence in different clinical settings, such as in acute coronary syndromes, after cardiac surgery and after electrical cardioversion of AF (relative risk=0.67, 95% confidence interval: 0.52–0.87, p=0.002). Moreover, the combined use of ranolazine and amiodarone compared to amiodarone alone showed a 1.23-times higher conversion rate of AF (95% confidence interval: 1.08–1.40), together with a significantly, about 10 h shorter conversion time.

Based on the evidence above, ranolazine may have therapeutic role in the treatment of cardiac rhythm disorders, of both atrial and ventricular origin. For stronger evidence, more phase 3 clinical investigations are necessary.

Eleclazine (GS-6615)

Besides ranolazine, until now eleclazine was the only other selective $I_{Na,late}$ inhibitor drug candidate that made it to phase 3 clinical trials. In the first trial (NCT02300558) eleclazine was tested for safety, tolerability, and its effect on shortening of the QT interval in LQT3 patients. The primary outcome of the study showed that after 24 weeks the mean daytime corrected QT interval was significantly, 8.5 ms shorter than at baseline, and there was only one patient with a serious adverse event (nephrolithiasis). The other trial (LIBERTY-HCM; NCT02291237) targeted HCM patients for the effect of eleclazine on exercise capacity. In this trial, eleclazine has not been proven to be superior to placebo.

The last moment in the development of eleclazine came after results of the phase 2 TEMPO study (NCT02104583) were analyzed. In the trial, subjects with ventricular tachycardia/ventricular fibrillation and ICD participated. Results of the study have shown that the rate of ICD shocks was higher in subjects who received eleclazine compared to the placebo arm. Therefore in late 2016, the further development of eleclazine was terminated for all indications.

CONCLUSIONS

An increased $I_{Na,late}$ is present in many heart diseases. The upregulated $I_{Na,late}$ lengthens the cardiac AP, increases $[Na^+]_i$, and causes Ca^{2+} overload of cardiomyocytes by offsetting the forward mode NCX. The elevated Ca^{2+}, in turn, mainly through CaMKII, can further increase $I_{Na,late}$ in a vicious circle. These pathophysiological mechanisms together may result in impaired cardiac energetics and contractile dysfunction of the heart as well as cardiac arrhythmias. The prolonged AP can serve as a substrate that is prone to rhythm disorders, whereas Ca^{2+} overload can be the trigger. $I_{Na,late}$ seems to possess a pathogenetic role especially in AF and in ventricular arrhythmias occurring under bradycardic conditions.

Multitude of pathophysiology studies have drawn the consequence that selective $I_{Na,late}$ inhibition is a favorable antiarrhythmic tool in many experimental settings. Despite all these studies, the one and only drug on the market that selectively inhibits $I_{Na,late}$ is ranolazine, although it significantly affects other ionic currents as well. Ranolazine has been a safe and effective antianginal medication since 2006 based on large randomized studies. Some recent clinical evidence also proves that ranolazine shows favorable effects in AF and in ventricular arrhythmias. For stronger evidence, more phase 3 clinical investigations are necessary. Targeting $Na_v1.8$ with specific inhibitors is also an interesting novel approach in the future of antiarrhythmic drug therapy.

AUTHOR CONTRIBUTIONS

BH: conception, design and drafting the manuscript TH, DK, KK: writing sections of the manuscript JM, PN, TB: conception and final review of the manuscript. All authors agreed on publishing the manuscript in the current form.

FUNDING

Funding was obtained from the National Research, Development and Innovation Fund for research projects FK-128116 and PD-120794, and the Thematic Excellence Programme ED_18-1-2019-0028. Further funding was obtained from the GINOP-2.3.2-15-2016-00040 and EFOP-3.6.2-16-2017-00006 projects, which are co-financed by the European Union and the European Regional Development Fund. Research of BH and DK was supported by the Ministry of Human Capacities (ÚNKP-19-4-DE-284 to BH, ÚNKP-19-3-II-DE-288 to DK). The work was also supported by the Hungarian Academy of Sciences (János Bolyai Research Scholarship to BH).

REFERENCES

Abrahamsson, C., Carlsson, L., and Duker, G. (1996). Lidocaine and nisoldipine attenuate almokalant-induced dispersion of repolarization and early afterdepolarizations in vitro. *J. Cardiovasc. Electrophysiol.* 7 (11), 1074–1081. doi: 10.1111/j.1540-8167.1996.tb00483.x

Ahern, G. P., Hsu, S. F., Klyachko, V. A., and Jackson, M. B. (2000). Induction of persistent sodium current by exogenous and endogenous nitric oxide. *J. Biol. Chem.* 275 (37), 28810–28815. doi: 10.1074/jbc.M003090200

Ahern, C. A., Zhang, J.-F., Wookalis, M. J., and Horn, R. (2005). Modulation of the Cardiac Sodium Channel NaV1.5 by Fyn, a Src Family Tyrosine Kinase. *Circ. Res.* 96 (9), 991–998. doi: 10.1161/01.RES.0000166324.00524.dd

Ahmad, S., Tirilomis, P., Pabel, S., Dybkova, N., Hartmann, N., Molina, C. E., et al. (2019). The functional consequences of sodium channel NaV 1.8 in human left ventricular hypertrophy. *ESC Heart Fail* 6 (1), 154–163. doi: 10.1002/ehf2.12378

Akalin, F., Tirtir, A., and Yilmaz, Y. (2003). Increased QT dispersion in epileptic children. *Acta Paediatr.* 92 (8), 916–920. doi: 10.1080/08035250310003550

Alekov, A. K., Rahman, M. M., Mitrovic, N., Lehmann-Horn, F., and Lerche, H. (2000). A sodium channel mutation causing epilepsy in man exhibits subtle defects in fast inactivation and activation in vitro. *J. Physiol. (Lond.)* 529 (3), 533–539. doi: 10.1111/j.1469-7793.2000.00533.x

Alves Bento, A. S., Bacic, D., Saran Carneiro, J., Nearing, B. D., Fuller, H., Justo, F. A., et al. (2015). Selective late INa inhibition by GS-458967 exerts parallel suppression of catecholamine-induced hemodynamically significant ventricular tachycardia and T-wave alternans in an intact porcine model. *Heart Rhythm* 12 (12), 2508–2514. doi: 10.1016/j.hrthm.2015.07.025

Anderson, M. E. (2005). Calmodulin kinase signaling in heart: an intriguing candidate target for therapy of myocardial dysfunction and arrhythmias. *Pharmacol. Ther.* 106 (1), 39–55. doi: 10.1016/j.pharmthera.2004.11.002

Antoons, G., Oros, A., Beekman, J. D., Engelen, M. A., Houtman, M. J., Belardinelli, L., et al. (2010). Late na(+) current inhibition by ranolazine reduces torsades de pointes in the chronic atrioventricular block dog model. *J. Am. Coll. Cardiol.* 55 (8), 801–809. doi: 10.1016/j.jacc.2009.10.033

Antzelevitch, C., Belardinelli, L., Zygmunt, A. C., Burashnikov, A., Di Diego, J. M., Fish, J. M., et al. (2004). Electrophysiological effects of ranolazine, a novel antianginal agent with antiarrhythmic properties. *Circulation* 110 (8), 904–910. doi: 10.1161/01.CIR.0000139333.83620.5D

Antzelevitch, C., Nesterenko, V., Shryock, J. C., Rajamani, S., Song, Y., and Belardinelli, L. (2014). The role of late I na in development of cardiac arrhythmias. *Handb. Exp. Pharmacol.* 221, 137–168. doi: 10.1007/978-3-642-41588-3_7

Ashpole, N. M., Herren, A. W., Ginsburg, K. S., Brogan, J. D., Johnson, D. E., Cummins, T. R., et al. (2012). Ca2+/calmodulin-dependent protein kinase II (CaMKII) regulates cardiac sodium channel NaV1.5 gating by multiple phosphorylation sites. *J. Biol. Chem.* 288, 19856–19869. doi: 10.1074/jbc.M111.322537

Bacic, D., Carneiro, J. S., Bento, A. A., Nearing, B. D., Rajamani, S., Belardinelli, L., et al. (2017). Eleclazine, an inhibitor of the cardiac late sodium current, is superior to flecainide in suppressing catecholamine-induced ventricular tachycardia and T-wave alternans in an intact porcine model. *Heart Rhythm.* 14 (3), 448–454. doi: 10.1016/j.hrthm.2016.10.021

Banyasz, T., Fulop, L., Magyar, J., Szentandrassy, N., Varro, A., and Nanasi, P. P. (2003). Endocardial versus epicardial differences in L-type calcium current in canine ventricular myocytes studied by action potential voltage clamp. *Cardiovasc. Res.* 58 (1), 66–75. doi: 10.1016/s0008-6363(02)00853-2

Banyasz, T., Horvath, B., Virag, L., Barandi, L., Szentandrassy, N., Harmati, G., et al. (2009). Reverse rate dependency is an intrinsic property of canine cardiac preparations. *Cardiovasc. Res.* 84 (2), 237–244. doi: 10.1093/cvr/cvp213

Banyasz, T., Horvath, B., Jian, Z., Izu, L. T., and Ye, C.-I. (2012). Profile of L-type Ca2+ current and Na+/Ca2+ exchange current during cardiac action potential in ventricular myocytes. *Heart Rhythm* 9 (1), 134–142. doi: 10.1016/j.hrthm.2011.08.029

Belardinelli, L., Antzelevitch, C., and Fraser, H. (2004). Inhibition of late (sustained/persistent) sodium current: a potential drug target to reduce intracellular sodium-dependent calcium overload and its detrimental effects on cardiomyocyte function. *Eur. Heart J. Suppl.* 6 (I), I3–I7. doi: 10.1093/eurheartj/6.suppl_i.i3

Belardinelli, L., Shryock, J. C., and Fraser, H. (2006). Inhibition of the late sodium current as a potential cardioprotective principle: effects of the late sodium current inhibitor ranolazine. *Heart* 92, 6–14. doi: 10.1136/hrt.2005.078790

Belardinelli, L., Liu, G., Smith-Maxwell, C., Wang, W. Q., El-Bizri, N., Hirakawa, R., et al. (2013). A novel, potent, and selective inhibitor of cardiac late sodium current suppresses experimental arrhythmias. *J. Pharmacol. Exp. Ther.* 344 (1), 23–32. doi: 10.1124/jpet.112.198887

Beltran-Alvarez, P., Pagans, S., and Brugada, R. (2011). The cardiac sodium channel is post-translationally modified by arginine methylation. *J. Proteome Res.* 10 (8), 3712–3719. doi: 10.1021/pr200339n

Benito, B., Brugada, R., Perich, R. M., Lizotte, E., Cinca, J., Mont, L., et al. (2008). A mutation in the sodium channel is responsible for the association of long QT syndrome and familial atrial fibrillation. *Heart Rhythm* 5 (10), 1434–1440. doi: 10.1016/j.hrthm.2008.07.013

Bers, D. M., and Grandi, E. (2009). Calcium/Calmodulin-dependent Kinase II Regulation of Cardiac Ion Channels. *J. Cardiovasc. Pharmacol.* 54 (3), 180–187. doi: 10.1097/FJC.0b013e3181a25078

Bers, D. M. (2002). Cardiac excitation-contraction coupling. *Nature* 415 (6868), 198–205. doi: 10.1038/415198a

Bers, D. M. (2010). CaMKII Inhibition in Heart Failure Makes Jump to Human. *Circ. Res.* 107 (9), 1044–1046. doi: 10.1161/circresaha.110.231902

Beyder, A., Rae, J. L., Bernard, C., Strege, P. R., Sachs, F., and Farrugia, G. (2010). Mechanosensitivity of Na(v)1.5, a voltage-sensitive sodium channel. *J. Physiol. (Lond.)* 588 (24), 4969–4985. doi: 10.1113/jphysiol.2010.199034

Beyder, A., Strege, P. R., Reyes, S., Bernard, C. E., Terzic, A., Makielski, J., et al. (2012). Ranolazine Decreases Mechanosensitivity of the Voltage-Gated Sodium Ion Channel Na(V)1.5 A Novel Mechanism of Drug Action. *Circulation* 125 (22), 2698–U2695. doi: 10.1161/circulationaha.112.094714

Bezzina, C., Veldkamp, M. W., van den Berg, M. P., Postma, A. V., Rook, M. B., Viersma, J. W., et al. (1999). A single Na+ channel mutation causing both long-QT and Brugada syndromes. *Circ. Res.* 85 (12), 1206–1213. doi: 10.1161/01.RES.85.12.1206

Biet, M., Barajas-Martinez, H., Ton, A. T., Delabre, J. F., Morin, N., and Dumaine, R. (2012). About half of the late sodium current in cardiac myocytes from dog ventricle is due to non-cardiac-type Na+ channels. *J. Mol. Cell. Cardiol.* 53 (5), 593–598. doi: 10.1016/j.yjmcc.2012.06.012

Bonatti, R., Silva, A. F., Batatinha, J. A., Sobrado, L. F., Machado, A. D., Varone, B. B., et al. (2014). Selective late sodium current blockade with GS-458967 markedly reduces ischemia-induced atrial and ventricular repolarization alternans and ECG heterogeneity. *Heart Rhythm* 11 (10), 1827–1835. doi: 10.1016/j.hrthm.2014.06.017

Bossu, A., Houtman, M. J. C., Meijborg, V. M. F., Varkevisser, R., Beekman, H. D. M., Dunnink, A., et al. (2018). Selective late sodium current inhibitor GS-458967 suppresses Torsades de Pointes by mostly affecting perpetuation but not initiation of the arrhythmia. *Br. J. Pharmacol.* 175 (12), 2470–2482. doi: 10.1111/bph.14217

Burashnikov, A., and Antzelevitch, C. (2008). Atrial-selective sodium channel blockers: do they exist? *J. Cardiovasc. Pharmacol.* 52 (2), 121–128. doi: 10.1097/FJC.0b013e31817618eb

Burashnikov, A., and Antzelevitch, C. (2013). Role of late sodium channel current block in the management of atrial fibrillation. *Cardiovasc. Drugs Ther.* 27 (1), 79–89. doi: 10.1007/s10557-012-6421-1

Burashnikov, A., and Antzelevitch, C. (2017). Effectiveness of Late INa Versus Peak INa Block in the Setting of Ventricular Fibrillation. *Circ. Arrhythm. Electrophysiol.* 10 (3), e005111. doi: 10.1161/CIRCEP.117.005111

Burashnikov, A., Di Diego, J. M., Zygmunt, A. C., Belardinelli, L., and Antzelevitch, C. (2007). Atrium-selective sodium channel block as a strategy for suppression of atrial fibrillation: differences in sodium channel inactivation between atria and ventricles and the role of ranolazine. *Circulation* 116 (13), 1449–1457. doi: 10.1161/CIRCULATIONAHA.107.704890

Burashnikov, A., Di Diego, J. M., Barajas-Martinez, H., Hu, D., Cordeiro, J. M., Moise, N. S., et al. (2014). Ranolazine effectively suppresses atrial fibrillation in the setting of heart failure. *Circ. Heart Fail* 7 (4), 627–633. doi: 10.1161/CIRCHEARTFAILURE.114.001129

Burnashev, N. A., Undrovinas, A. I., Fleidervish, I. A., Makielski, J. C., and Rosenshtraukh, L. V. (1991). Modulation of cardiac sodium-channel gating by lysophosphatidylcholine. *J. Mol. Cell Cardiol.* 23, 23–30. doi: 10.1016/0022-2828(91)90020-m

Cardona, K., Trenor, B., Rajamani, S., Romero, L., Ferrero, J. M., and Saiz, J. (2010). "Effects of late sodium current enhancement during LQT-related arrhythmias. A simulation study," in *Conference proceedings: Annual International Conference of the IEEE Engineering in Medicine and Biology*

Society. [Buenos Aires: IEEE (Institute of Electrical and Electronics Engineers)] 2010, 3237–3240. doi: 10.1109/iembs.2010.5627184

Carlsson, L., Abrahamsson, C., Drews, L., and Duker, G. (1992). Antiarrhythmic effects of potassium channel openers in rhythm abnormalities related to delayed repolarization. *Circulation* 85 (4), 1491–1500. doi: 10.1161/01.cir.85.4.1491

Carlsson, L., Drews, L., and Duker, G. (1996). Rhythm anomalies related to delayed repolarization in vivo: influence of sarcolemmal Ca++ entry and intracellular Ca++ overload. *J. Pharmacol. Exp. Ther.* 279 (1), 231–239.

Carmeliet, E. (1999). Cardiac ionic currents and acute ischemia: From channels to arrhythmias. *Physiol. Rev.* 79 (3), 917–1017. doi: 10.1152/physrev.1999.79.3.917

Carmeliet, E. (2006). Action potential duration, rate of stimulation, and intracellular sodium. *J. Cardiovasc. Electrophysiol.* 17 Suppl 1, S2–S7. doi: 10.1111/j.1540-8167.2006.00378.x

Carneiro, J. S., Bento, A. S., Bacic, D., Nearing, B. D., Rajamani, S., Belardinelli, L., et al. (2015). The Selective Cardiac Late Sodium Current Inhibitor GS-458967 Suppresses Autonomically Triggered Atrial Fibrillation in an Intact Porcine Model. *J. Cardiovasc. Electrophysiol.* 26 (12), 1364–1369. doi: 10.1111/jce.12824

Catterall, W. A., Goldin, A. L., and Waxman, S. G. (2005). International Union of Pharmacology. XLVII. Nomenclature and structure-function relationships of voltage-gated sodium channels. *Pharmacol. Rev.* 57 (4), 397–409. doi: 10.1124/pr.57.4.4

Chaitman, B. R., Skettino, S. L., Parker, J. O., Hanley, P., Meluzin, J., Kuch, J., et al. (2004a). Anti-ischemic effects and long-term survival during ranolazine monotherapy in patients with chronic severe angina. *J. Am. Coll. Cardiol.* 43 (8), 1375–1382. doi: 10.1016/j.jacc.2003.11.045

Chaitman, B. R., Pepine, C. J., Parker, J. O., Skopal, J., Chumakova, G., Kuch, J., et al. (2004b). Effects of ranolazine with atenolol, amlodipine, or diltiazem on exercise tolerance and angina frequency in patients with severe chronic angina: a randomized controlled trial. *JAMA* 291 (3), 309–316. doi: 10.1001/jama.291.3.309

Chaitman, B. R. (2006). Ranolazine for the treatment of chronic angina and potential use in other cardiovascular conditions. *Circulation* 113 (20), 2462–2472. doi: 10.1161/CIRCULATIONAHA.105.597500

Cheng, J., Valdivia, C. R., Vaidyanathan, R., Balijepalli, R. C., Ackerman, M. J., and Makielski, J. C. (2013). Caveolin-3 suppresses late sodium current by inhibiting nNOS-dependent S-nitrosylation of SCN5A. *J. Mol. Cell Cardiol.* 61, 102–110. doi: 10.1016/j.yjmcc.2013.03.013

Cheung, J. Y., Zhang, X. Q., Song, J., Gao, E., Rabinowitz, J. E., Chan, T. O., et al. (2010). Phospholemman: a novel cardiac stress protein. *Clin. Transl. Sci.* 3 (4), 189–196. doi: 10.1111/j.1752-8062.2010.00213.x

Clancy, C. E., Tateyama, M., Liu, H., Wehrens, X. H., and Kass, R. S. (2003). Non-equilibrium gating in cardiac Na+ channels: an original mechanism of arrhythmia. *Circulation* 107 (17), 2233–2237. doi: 10.1161/01.CIR.0000069273.51375.BD

Cocco, G., Rousseau, M. F., Bouvy, T., Cheron, P., Williams, G., Detry, J. M., et al. (1992). Effects of a new metabolic modulator, ranolazine, on exercise tolerance in angina pectoris patients treated with beta-blocker or diltiazem. *J. Cardiovasc. Pharmacol.* 20 (1), 131–138.

Cohen, S. A., and Levitt, L. K. (1993). Partial characterization of the rH1 sodium channel protein from rat heart using subtype-specific antibodies. *Circ. Res.* 73 (4), 735–742. doi: 10.1161/01.res.73.4.735

Comtois, P., Sakabe, M., Vigmond, E. J., Munoz, M., Texier, A., Shiroshita-Takeshita, A., et al. (2008). Mechanisms of atrial fibrillation termination by rapidly unbinding Na+ channel blockers: insights from mathematical models and experimental correlates. *Am. J. Physiol. Heart Circ. Physiol.* 295 (4), H1489–H1504. doi: 10.1152/ajpheart.01054.2007

Coppini, R., Ferrantini, C., Yao, L., Fan, P., Del Lungo, M., Stillitano, F., et al. (2013). Late sodium current inhibition reverses electromechanical dysfunction in human hypertrophic cardiomyopathy. *Circulation* 127 (5), 575–584. doi: 10.1161/circulationaha.112.134932

Coraboeuf, E., Deroubaix, E., and Coulombe, A. (1979). Effect of tetrodotoxin on action potentials of the conducting system in the dog heart. *Am. J. Physiol.* 236 (4), H561–H567. doi: 10.1152/ajpheart.1979.236.4.H561

Cortada, E., and Brugada, R. (2019). Verges M. N-Glycosylation of the voltage-gated sodium channel beta2 subunit is required for efficient trafficking of NaV1.5/beta2 to the plasma membrane. *J. Biol. Chem.* 294 (44), 16123–16140. doi: 10.1074/jbc.RA119.007903

De Ferrari, G. M., Maier, L. S., Mont, L., Schwartz, P. J., Simonis, G., Leschke, M., et al. (2015). Ranolazine in the treatment of atrial fibrillation: Results of the dose-ranging RAFFAELLO (Ranolazine in Atrial Fibrillation Following An ELectricaL CardiOversion) study. *Heart Rhythm* 12 (5), 872–878. doi: 10.1016/j.hrthm.2015.01.021

de Lera Ruiz, M., and Kraus, R. L. (2015). Voltage-Gated Sodium Channels: Structure, Function, Pharmacology, and Clinical Indications. *J. Med. Chem.* 58 (18), 7093–7118. doi: 10.1021/jm501981g

Debono, M. W., Le Guern, J., Canton, T., Doble, A., and Pradier, L. (1993). Inhibition by riluzole of electrophysiological responses mediated by rat kainate and NMDA receptors expressed in Xenopus oocytes. *Eur. J. Pharmacol.* 235 (2-3), 283–289. doi: 10.1016/0014-2999(93)90147-a

Despa, S., and Bers, D. M. (2013). Na+ transport in the normal and failing heart - Remember the balance. *J. Mol. Cell Cardiol.* 61, 2–10. doi: 10.1016/j.yjmcc.2013.04.011

Despa, S., Islam, M. A., Weber, C. R., Pogwizd, S. M., and Bers, D. M. (2002). Intracellular Na+ Concentration Is Elevated in Heart Failure But Na/K Pump Function Is Unchanged. *Circulation* 105 (21), 2543–2548. doi: 10.1161/01.cir.0000016701.85760.97

Dybkova, N., Ahmad, S., Pabel, S., Tirilomis, P., Hartmann, N., Fischer, T. H., et al. (2018). Differential regulation of sodium channels as a novel proarrhythmic mechanism in the human failing heart. *Cardiovasc. Res.* 114 (13), 1728–1737. doi: 10.1093/cvr/cvy152

El-Sherif, N., Turitto, G., and Boutjdir, M. (2019). Acquired Long QT Syndrome and Electrophysiology of Torsade de Pointes. *Arrhythm. Electrophysiol. Rev.* 8 (2), 122–130. doi: 10.15420/aer.2019.8.3

Erickson, J. R., Joiner, M. L. A., Guan, X., Kutschke, W., Yang, J. Y., Oddis, C. V., et al. (2008). A dynamic pathway for calcium-independent activation of CaMKII by methionine oxidation. *Cell* 133 (3), 462–474. doi: 10.1016/j.cell.2008.02.048

Evaristo, E., Stocco, F. G., Shah, N. R., Cheezum, M. K., Hainer, J., Foster, C., et al. (2018). Ranolazine reduces repolarization heterogeneity in symptomatic patients with diabetes and non-flow-limiting coronary artery stenosis. *Ann. Noninvas. Electrocardiol.* 23 (1), e12480. doi: 10.1111/anec.12480

Fujioka, Y., Hiroe, K., and Matsuoka, S. (2000). Regulation kinetics of Na+-Ca2+ exchange current in guinea-pig ventricular myocytes. *J. Physiol. (Lond.)* 529 (3), 611–624. doi: 10.1111/j.1469-7793.2000.00611.x

Fulop, L., Banyasz, T., Magyar, J., Szentandrassy, N., Varro, A., and Nanasi, P. P. (2004). Reopening of L-type calcium channels in human ventricular myocytes during applied epicardial action potentials. *Acta Physiol. Scand.* 180 (1), 39–47. doi: 10.1046/j.0001-6772.2003.01223.x

Gellens, M. E., George, A. L., Chen, L. Q., Chahine, M., Horn, R., Barchi, R. L., et al. (1992). Primary structure and functional expression of the human cardiac tetrodotoxin-insensitive voltage-dependent sodium-channel. *Proc. Natl. Acad. Sci. U. S. A.* 89 (2), 554–558. doi: 10.1073/pnas.89.2.554

Ginsburg, K. S., Weber, C. R., and Bers, D. M. (2013). Cardiac Na+Ca2 +exchanger: dynamics of Ca2+-dependent activation and deactivation in intact myocytes. *J. Physiol. (Lond.)* 591 (8), 2067–2086. doi: 10.1113/jphysiol.2013.252080

Gong, M., Zhang, Z., Fragakis, N., Korantzopoulos, P., Letsas, K. P., Li, G., et al. (2017). Role of ranolazine in the prevention and treatment of atrial fibrillation: A meta-analysis of randomized clinical trials. *Heart Rhythm* 14 (1), 3–11. doi: 10.1016/j.hrthm.2016.10.008

Grandi, E., and Herren, A. W. (2014). CaMKII-dependent regulation of cardiac Na homeostasis. *Front. Pharmacol.* 5, 41. doi: 10.3389/fphar.2014.00041

Guo, D., Young, L., Wu, Y., Belardinelli, L., Kowey, P. R., and Yan, G.-X. (2010). Increased late sodium current in left atrial myocytes of rabbits with left ventricular hypertrophy: its role in the genesis of atrial arrhythmias. *Am. J. Physiol.-Heart Circ. Physiol.* 298 (5), H1375–H1381. doi: 10.1152/ajpheart.01145.2009

Gyorke, S., and Terentyev, D. (2008). Modulation of ryanodine receptor by luminal calcium and accessory proteins in health and cardiac disease. *Cardiovasc. Res.* 77 (2), 245–255. doi: 10.1093/cvr/cvm038

Hallaq, H., Wang, D. W., Kunic, J. D., George, A. L.Jr., Wells, K. S., and Murray, K. T. (2012). Activation of protein kinase C alters the intracellular distribution and mobility of cardiac Na+ channels. *Am. J. Physiol. Heart Circulatory Physiol.* 302 (3), H782–H789. doi: 10.1152/ajpheart.00817.2010

Harnmarstrom, A. K. M., and Gage, P. W. (2002). Hypoxia and persistent sodium current. *Eur. Biophys. J. Biophys. Lett.* 31 (5), 323–330. doi: 10.1007/s00249-002-0218-2

Haufe, V., Cordeiro, J. M., Zimmer, T., Wu, Y. S., Schiccitano, S., Benndorf, K., et al. (2005). Contribution of neuronal sodium channels to the cardiac fast sodium current I-Na is greater in dog heart Purkinje fibers than in ventricles. *Cardiovasc. Res.* 65 (1), 117–127. doi: 10.1016/j.cardiores.2004.08.017

He, Y., Benz, A., Fu, T., Wang, M., Covey, D. F., Zorumski, C. F., et al. (2002). Neuroprotective agent riluzole potentiates postsynaptic GABA(A) receptor function. *Neuropharmacology* 42 (2), 199–209. doi: 10.1016/s0028-3908(01)00175-7

Hedley, P. L., Jorgensen, P., Schlamowitz, S., Wangari, R., Moolman-Smook, J., Brink, P. A., et al. (2009). The Genetic Basis of Long QT and Short QT Syndromes: A Mutation Update. *Hum. Mutat.* 30 (11), 1486–1511. doi: 10.1002/humu.21106

Hegyi, B., Banyasz, T., Izu, L. T., Belardinelli, L., Bers, D. M., and Chen-Izu, Y. (2018). beta-adrenergic regulation of late Na(+) current during cardiac action potential is mediated by both PKA and CaMKII. *J. Mol. Cell. Cardiol.* 123, 168–179. doi: 10.1016/j.yjmcc.2018.09.006

Horvath, B., Magyar, J., Szentandrassy, N., Birinyi, P., Nanasi, P. P., and Banyasz, T. (2006). Contribution of I-Ks to ventricular repolarization in canine myocytes. *Pflug. Arch. Eur. J. Physiol.* 452 (6), 698–706. doi: 10.1007/s00424-006-0077-2

Horvath, B., Banyasz, T., Jian, Z., Hegyi, B., Kistamas, K., Nanasi, P. P., et al. (2013). Dynamics of the late Na+ current during cardiac action potential and its contribution to afterdepolarizations. *J. Mol. Cell Cardiol.* 64, 59–68. doi: 10.1016/j.yjmcc.2013.08.010

Horvath, B., Hezso, T., Szentandrassy, N., Kistamas, K., Arpadffy-Lovas, T., Varga, R., et al. (2020). Late sodium current in human, canine and guinea pig ventricular myocardium. *J. Mol. Cell. Cardiol.* 139, 14–23. doi: 10.1016/j.yjmcc.2019.12.015

Hoyer, K., Song, Y. J., Wang, D. S., Phan, D., Balschi, J., Ingwall, J. S., et al. (2011). Reducing the Late Sodium Current Improves Cardiac Function during Sodium Pump Inhibition by Ouabain. *J. Pharmacol. Exp. Ther.* 337 (2), 513–523. doi: 10.1124/jpet.110.176776

Huang, B., El-Sherif, T., Gidh-Jain, M., Qin, D., and El-Sherif, N. (2001). Alterations of sodium channel kinetics and gene expression in the postinfarction remodeled myocardium. *J. Cardiovasc. Electrophysiol.* 12 (2), 218–225. doi: 10.1046/j.1540-8167.2001.00218.x

Huang, X., Du, Y., Yang, P., Lin, S., Xi, Y., Yang, Z., et al. (2015). Age-dependent alterations of voltage-gated Na+ channel isoforms in rat sinoatrial node. *Mech. Ageing Dev.* 152, 80–90. doi: 10.1016/j.mad.2015.10.003

Janvier, N. C., and Boyett, M. R. (1996). The role of Na-Ca exchange current in the cardiac action potential. *Cardiovasc. Res.* 32 (1), 69–84. doi: 10.1016/s0008-6363(96)00017-x

Jian, Z., Han, H., Zhang, T., Puglisi, J., Izu, L. T., Shaw, J. A., et al. (2014). Mechanochemotransduction during cardiomyocyte contraction is mediated by localized nitric oxide signaling. *Sci. Signal.* 7 (317), ra27. doi: 10.1126/scisignal.2005046

Jones, D. K., Peters, C. H., Tolhurst, S. A., Claydon, T. W., and Ruben, P. C. (2011). Extracellular Proton Modulation of the Cardiac Voltage-Gated Sodium Channel, Na(v)1.5. *Biophys. J.* 101 (9), 2147–2156. doi: 10.1016/j.bpj.2011.08.056

Jones, D. K., Peters, C. H., Allard, C. R., Claydon, T. W., and Ruben, P. C. (2013a). Proton Sensors in the Pore Domain of the Cardiac Voltage-gated Sodium Channel. *J. Biol. Chem.* 288 (7), 4782–4791. doi: 10.1074/jbc.M112.434266

Jones, D. K., Claydon, T. W., and Ruben, P. C. (2013b). Extracellular Protons Inhibit Charge Immobilization in the Cardiac Voltage-Gated Sodium Channel. *Biophys. J.* 105 (1), 101–107. doi: 10.1016/j.bpj.2013.04.022

Ju, Y. K., Saint, D. A., and Gage, P. W. (1996). Hypoxia increases persistent sodium current in rat ventricular myocytes. *J. Physiol. (Lond.)* 497 (2), 337–347. doi: 10.1113/jphysiol.1996.sp021772

Justo, F., Fuller, H., Nearing, B. D., Rajamani, S., Belardinelli, L., and Verrier, R. L. (2016). Inhibition of the cardiac late sodium current with eleclazine protects against ischemia-induced vulnerability to atrial fibrillation and reduces atrial and ventricular repolarization abnormalities in the absence and presence of concurrent adrenergic stimulation. *Heart Rhythm* 13 (9), 1860–1867. doi: 10.1016/j.hrthm.2016.06.020

Kapplinger, J. D., Tester, D. J., Alders, M., Benito, B., Berthet, M., Brugada, J., et al. (2010). An international compendium of mutations in the SCN5A-encoded cardiac sodium channel in patients referred for Brugada syndrome genetic testing. *Heart Rhythm* 7 (1), 33–46. doi: 10.1016/j.hrthm.2009.09.069

Kim, J., Ghosh, S., Liu, H. J., Tateyama, M., Kass, R. S., and Pitt, G. S. (2004). Calmodulin mediates Ca2+ sensitivity of sodium channels. *J. Biol. Chem.* 279 (43), 45004–45012. doi: 10.1074/jbc.M407286200

Kiyosue, T., and Arita, M. (1989). Late sodium current and its contribution to action potential configuration in guinea pig ventricular myocytes. *Circ. Res.* 64 (2), 389–397. doi: 10.1161/01.res.64.2.389

Koltun, D. O., Parkhill, E. Q., Elzein, E., Kobayashi, T., Notte, G. T., Kalla, R., et al. (2016a). Discovery of triazolopyridine GS-458967, a late sodium current inhibitor (Late INai) of the cardiac NaV 1.5 channel with improved efficacy and potency relative to ranolazine. *Bioorg. Med. Chem. Lett.* 26 (13), 3202–3206. doi: 10.1016/j.bmcl.2016.03.101

Koltun, D. O., Parkhill, E. Q., Elzein, E., Kobayashi, T., Jiang, R. H., Li, X., et al. (2016b). Discovery of triazolopyridinone GS-462808, a late sodium current inhibitor (Late INai) of the cardiac Nav1.5 channel with improved efficacy and potency relative to ranolazine. *Bioorg. Med. Chem. Lett.* 26 (13), 3207–3211. doi: 10.1016/j.bmcl.2016.03.096

Komajda, M., Frank, R., Vedel, J., Fontaine, G., Petitot, J. C., and Grosgogeat, Y. (1980). Intracardiac conduction defects in dystrophia myotonica - electrophysiological study of 12 cases. *Br. Heart J.* 43 (3), 315–320. doi: 10.1136/hrt.43.3.315

Kumar, K., Nearing, B. D., Carvas, M., Nascimento, B. C., Acar, M., Belardinelli, L., et al. (2009). Ranolazine exerts potent effects on atrial electrical properties and abbreviates atrial fibrillation duration in the intact porcine heart. *J. Cardiovasc. Electrophysiol.* 20 (7), 796–802. doi: 10.1111/j.1540-8167.2009.01437.x

Lei, M., Jones, S. A., Liu, J., Lancaster, M. K., Fung, S. S., Dobrzynski, H., et al. (2004). Requirement of neuronal- and cardiac-type sodium channels for murine sinoatrial node pacemaking. *J. Physiol.* 559 (Pt 3), 835–848. doi: 10.1113/jphysiol.2004.068643

Letienne, R., Vie, B., Puech, A., Vieu, S., Le Grand, B., and John, G. W. (2001). Evidence that ranolazine behaves as a weak beta1- and beta2-adrenoceptor antagonist in the rat [correction of cat] cardiovascular system. *Naunyn-Schmiedeberg's Arch. Pharmacol.* 363 (4), 464–471. doi: 10.1007/s002100000378

Li, G. R., Lau, C. P., and Shrier, A. (2002). Heterogeneity of sodium current in atrial vs epicardial ventricular myocytes of adult guinea pig hearts. *J. Mol. Cell. Cardiol.* 34 (9), 1185–1194. doi: 10.1006/jmcc.2002.2053

Li, W., Yu, Y., Hou, J. W., Zhou, Z. W., Guo, K., Zhang, P. P., et al. (2017). Larger rate dependence of late sodium current in cardiac Purkinje cells: A potential link to arrhythmogenesis. *Heart Rhythm* 14 (3), 422–431. doi: 10.1016/j.hrthm.2016.11.036

Liang, F., Fan, P., Jia, J., Yang, S., Jiang, Z., Karpinski, S., et al. (2016). Inhibitions of late INa and CaMKII act synergistically to prevent ATX-II-induced atrial fibrillation in isolated rat right atria. *J. Mol. Cell. Cardiol.* 94, 122–130. doi: 10.1016/j.yjmcc.2016.04.001

Linz, K. W., and Meyer, R. (1998). Control of L-type calcium current during the action potential of guinea-pig ventricular myocytes. *J. Physiol. (Lond.)* 513 (2), 425–442. doi: 10.1111/j.1469-7793.1998.425bb.x

Linz, K. W., and Meyer, R. (2000). Profile and kinetics of L-type calcium current during the cardiac ventricular action potential compared in guinea-pigs, rats and rabbits. *Pflug. Arch.-Eur. J. Physiol.* 439 (5), 588–599. doi: 10.1007/s004240050982

Liu, T., and O'Rourke, B. (2008). Enhancing Mitochondrial Ca2+ Uptake in Myocytes From Failing Hearts Restores Energy Supply and Demand Matching. *Circ. Res.* 103 (3), 279–288. doi: 10.1161/circresaha.108.175919

Liu, H., Sun, H. Y., Lau, C. P., and Li, G. R. (2007). Regulation of voltage-gated cardiac sodium current by epidermal growth factor receptor kinase in guinea pig ventricular myocytes. *J. Mol. Cell Cardiol.* 42 (4), 760–768. doi: 10.1016/j.yjmcc.2006.10.013

Liu, M., Shi, G., Yang, K. C., Gu, L., Kanthasamy, A. G., Anantharam, V., et al. (2017). Role of protein kinase C in metabolic regulation of the cardiac Na(+) channel. *Heart Rhythm* 14 (3), 440–447. doi: 10.1016/j.hrthm.2016.12.026

Locati, E. T., Bagliani, G., Cecchi, F., Johny, H., Lunati, M., and Pappone, C. (2019). Arrhythmias due to Inherited and Acquired Abnormalities of Ventricular Repolarization. *Card. Electrophysiol. Clin.* 11 (2), 345–362. doi: 10.1016/j.ccep.2019.02.009

Louch, W. E., Hougen, K., Mørk, H. K., Swift, F., Aronsen, J. M., Sjaastad, I., et al. (2010). Sodium accumulation promotes diastolic dysfunction in end-stage heart failure following Serca2 knockout. *J. Physiol.* 588 (3), 465–478. doi: 10.1113/jphysiol.2009.183517

Lowe, J. S., Stroud, D. M., Yang, T., Hall, L., Atack, T. C., and Roden, D. M. (2012). Increased late sodium current contributes to long QT-related arrhythmia susceptibility in female mice. *Cardiovasc. Res.* 95 (3), 300–307. doi: 10.1093/cvr/cvs160

Lu, Y. Y., Cheng, C. C., Chen, Y. C., Chen, S. A., and Chen, Y. J. (2012). ATX-II-induced pulmonary vein arrhythmogenesis related to atrial fibrillation and long QT syndrome. *Eur. J. Clin. Invest.* 42 (8), 823–831. doi: 10.1111/j.1365-2362.2012.02655.x

Luo, A., Ma, J., Song, Y., Qian, C., Wu, Y., Zhang, P., et al. (2014). Larger late sodium current density as well as greater sensitivities to ATX II and ranolazine in rabbit left atrial than left ventricular myocytes. *Am. J. Physiol. Heart Circ. Physiol.* 306 (3), H455–H461. doi: 10.1152/ajpheart.00727.2013

Ma, J. H., Luo, A. T., Wu, L., Wan, W., Zhang, P. H., Ren, Z. Q., et al. (2012). Calmodulin kinase II and protein kinase C mediate the effect of increased intracellular calcium to augment late sodium current in rabbit ventricular myocytes. *Am. J. Physiol. Cell Physiol.* 302 (8), C1141–C1151. doi: 10.1152/ajpcell.00374.2011

Magyar, J., Kiper, C. E., Dumaine, R., Burgess, D. E., Banyasz, T., and Satin, J. (2004). Divergent action potential morphologies reveal nonequilibrium properties of human cardiac Na channels. *Cardiovasc. Res.* 64 (3), 477–487. doi: 10.1016/j.cardiores.2004.07.014

Maier, L. S., and Sossalla, S. (2013). The late Na current as a therapeutic target: Where are we? *J. Mol. Cell Cardiol.* 61, 44–50. doi: 10.1016/j.yjmcc.2013.03.001

Maier, S. K., Westenbroek, R. E., Schenkman, K. A., Feigl, E. O., Scheuer, T., and Catterall, W. A. (2002). An unexpected role for brain-type sodium channels in coupling of cell surface depolarization to contraction in the heart. *Proc. Natl. Acad. Sci. United States America* 99 (6), 4073–4078. doi: 10.1073/pnas.261705699

Maier, S. K. G., Westenbroek, R. E., Yamanushi, T. T., Dobrzynski, H., Boyett, M. R., Catterall, W. A., et al. (2003). An unexpected requirement for brain-type sodium channels for control of heart rate in the mouse sinoatrial node. *Proc. Natl. Acad. Sci.* 100 (6), 3507–3512. doi: 10.1073/pnas.2627986100

Maier, L. S. (2011). CaMKII regulation of voltage-gated sodium channels and cell excitability. *Heart Rhythm* 8 (3), 474–477. doi: 10.1016/j.hrthm.2010.09.080

Makielski, J. C., and Farley, A. L. (2006). Na(+) current in human ventricle: implications for sodium loading and homeostasis. *J. Cardiovasc. Electrophysiol.* 17 (Suppl 1), S15–S20. doi: 10.1111/j.1540-8167.2006.00380.x

Makita, N., Horie, M., Nakamura, T., Ai, T., Sasaki, K., Yokoi, H., et al. (2002). Drug-induced Long-QT syndrome associated with a subclinical SCN5A mutation. *Circulation* 106 (10), 1269–1274. doi: 10.1161/01.cir.0000027139.42087.b6

Malhotra, J. D., Chen, C. L., Rivolta, I., Abriel, H., Malhotra, R., Mattei, L. N., et al. (2001). Characterization of sodium channel alpha- and beta-subunits in rat and mouse cardiac myocytes. *Circulation* 103 (9), 1303–1310. doi: 10.1161/01.CIR.103.9.1303

Maltsev, V. A., and Undrovinas, A. (2008). Late sodium current in failing heart: friend or foe? *Prog. Biophys. Mol. Biol.* 96 (1-3), 421–451. doi: 10.1016/j.pbiomolbio.2007.07.010

Maltsev, V. A., Sabbah, H. N., Higgins, R. S., Silverman, N., Lesch, M., and Undrovinas, A. I. (1998). Novel, ultraslow inactivating sodium current in human ventricular cardiomyocytes. *Circulation* 98 (23), 2545–2552. doi: 10.1161/01.CIR.98.23.2545

Maltsev, V. A., Silverman, N., Sabbah, H. N., and Undrovinas, A. I. (2007). Chronic heart failure slows late sodium current in human and canine ventricular myocytes: Implications for repolarization variability. *Eur. J. Heart Fail.* 9 (3), 219–227. doi: 10.1016/j.ejheart.2006.08.007

Maltsev, V. A., Reznikov, V., Undrovinas, N. A., Sabbah, H. N., and Undrovinas, A. (2008). Modulation of late sodium current by Ca2+, calmodulin, and CaMKII in normal and failing dog cardiomyocytes: similarities and differences. *Am. J. Physiol. Heart Circulatory Physiol.* 294 (4), H1597–H1608. doi: 10.1152/ajpheart.00484.2007

Maltsev, V. A., Kyle, J. W., and Undrovinas, A. (2009). Late Na(+) current produced by human cardiac Na(+) channel isoform Na(v)1.5 is modulated by its beta(1) subunit. *J. Physiol. Sci.* 59 (3), 217–225. doi: 10.1007/s12576-009-0029-7

Maltsev, V. A. (2006). Undrovinas AI. A multi-modal composition of the late Na+ current in human ventricular cardiomyocytes. *Cardiovasc. Res.* 69 (1), 116–127. doi: 10.1016/j.cardiores.2005.08.015

Merchant, F. M., and Armoundas, A. A. (2012). Role of substrate and triggers in the genesis of cardiac alternans, from the myocyte to the whole heart: implications for therapy. *Circulation* 125 (3), 539–549. doi: 10.1161/CIRCULATIONAHA.111.033563

Mercier, A., Clement, R., Harnois, T., Bourmeyster, N., Bois, P., and Chatelier, A. (2015). Nav1.5 channels can reach the plasma membrane through distinct N-glycosylation states. *Biochim. Biophys. Acta* 1850 (6), 1215–1223. doi: 10.1016/j.bbagen.2015.02.009

Milberg, P., Reinsch, N., Wasmer, K., Monnig, G., Stypmann, J., Osada, N., et al. (2005). Transmural dispersion of repolarization as a key factor of arrhythmogenicity in a novel intact heart model of LQT3. *Cardiovasc. Res.* 65 (2), 397–404. doi: 10.1016/j.cardiores.2004.10.016

Mills, G. D., Harris, D. M., Chen, X., and Houser, S. R. (2007). Intracellular sodium determines frequency-dependent alterations in contractility in hypertrophied feline ventricular myocytes. *Am. J. Physiol. Heart Circ. Physiol.* 292 (2), H1129–H1138. doi: 10.1152/ajpheart.00375.2006

Mitsuiye, T., and Noma, A. (2002). Inactivation of cardiac Na+ channel simply through open states as revealed by single-channel analysis in guinea pig ventricular myocytes. *Jpn. J. Physiol.* 52 (5), 457–469. doi: 10.2170/jjphysiol.52.457

Morita, N., Lee, J. H., Xie, Y., Sovari, A., Qu, Z., Weiss, J. N., et al. (2011). Suppression of re-entrant and multifocal ventricular fibrillation by the late sodium current blocker ranolazine. *J. Am. Coll. Cardiol.* 57 (3), 366–375. doi: 10.1016/j.jacc.2010.07.045

Morrow, D. A., Scirica, B. M., Karwatowska-Prokopczuk, E., Murphy, S. A., Budaj, A., Varshavsky, S., et al. (2007). Effects of ranolazine on recurrent cardiovascular events in patients with non-ST-elevation acute coronary syndromes: the MERLIN-TIMI 36 randomized trial. *JAMA* 297 (16), 1775–1783. doi: 10.1001/jama.297.16.1775

Murphy, L., Renodin, D., Antzelevitch, C., Di Diego, J. M., and Cordeiro, J. M. (2011). Extracellular proton depression of peak and late Na current in the canine left ventricle. *Am. J. Physiol. Heart Circ. Physiol.* 301 (3), H936–H944. doi: 10.1152/ajpheart.00204.2011

Nagatomo, T., January, C. T., Ye, B., Abe, H., Nakashima, Y., and Makielski, J. C. (2002). Rate-dependent QT shortening mechanism for the LQT3 deltaKPQ mutant. *Cardiovasc. Res.* 54 (3), 624–629. doi: 10.1016/s0008-6363(02)00265-1

Nagy, Z. A., Virag, L., Toth, A., Biliczki, P., Acsai, K., Banyasz, T., et al. (2004). Selective inhibition of sodium-calcium exchanger by SEA-0400 decreases early and delayed afterdepolarization in canine heart. *Br. J. Pharmacol.* 143 (7), 827–831. doi: 10.1038/sj.bjp.0706026

Nattel, S., and Dobrev, D. (2012). The multidimensional role of calcium in atrial fibrillation pathophysiology: mechanistic insights and therapeutic opportunities. *Eur. Heart J.* 33 (15), 1870–1877. doi: 10.1093/eurheartj/ehs079

Ninkovic, V. M., Ninkovic, S. M., Miloradovic, V., Stanojevic, D., Babic, M., Giga, V., et al. (2016). Prevalence and risk factors for prolonged QT interval and QT dispersion in patients with type 2 diabetes. *Acta Diabetol.* 53 (5), 737–744. doi: 10.1007/s00592-016-0864-y

Pereon, Y., Lande, G., Demolombe, S., Tich, S. N. T., Sternberg, D., Le Marec, H., et al. (2003). Paramyotonia congenita with an SCN4A mutation affecting cardiac repolarization. *Neurology* 60 (2), 340–342. doi: 10.1212/01.WNL.0000042093.96309.5A

Persson, F., Andersson, B., Duker, G., Jacobson, I., and Carlsson, L. (2007). Functional effects of the late sodium current inhibition by AZD7009 and lidocaine in rabbit isolated atrial and ventricular tissue and Purkinje fibre. *Eur. J. Pharmacol.* 558 (1-3), 133–143. doi: 10.1016/j.ejphar.2006.11.040

Pieske, B., Maier, L. S., Piacentino, V., Weisser, J., Hasenfuss, G., and Houser, S. (2002). Rate Dependence of [Na+]i and Contractility in Nonfailing and Failing Human Myocardium. *Circulation* 106 (4), 447–453. doi: 10.1161/01.cir.0000023042.50192.f4

Pignier, C., Revenaz, C., Rauly-Lestienne, I., Cussac, D., Delhon, A., Gardette, J., et al. (2007). Direct protective effects of poly-unsaturated fatty acids, DHA and EPA, against activation of cardiac late sodium current. *Basic Res. Cardiol.* 102 (6), 553–564. doi: 10.1007/s00395-007-0676-x

Pignier, C., Rougier, J. S., Vie, B., Culie, C., Verscheure, Y., Vacher, B., et al. (2010). Selective inhibition of persistent sodium current by F 15845 prevents ischaemia-induced arrhythmias. *Br. J. Pharmacol.* 161 (1), 79–91. doi: 10.1111/j.1476-5381.2010.00884.x

Pless, S. A., Galpin, J. D., Frankel, A., and Ahern, C. A. (2011). Molecular basis for class Ib anti-arrhythmic inhibition of cardiac sodium channels. *Nat. Commun.* 2, 351. doi: 10.1038/ncomms1351

Poulet, C., Wettwer, E., Grunnet, M., Jespersen, T., Fabritz, L., Matschke, K., et al. (2015). Late Sodium Current in Human Atrial Cardiomyocytes from Patients in Sinus Rhythm and Atrial Fibrillation. *PloS One* 10 (6), e0131432. doi: 10.1371/journal.pone.0131432

Pourrier, M., Williams, S., McAfee, D., Belardinelli, L., and Fedida, D. (2014). CrossTalk proposal: The late sodium current is an important player in the development of diastolic heart failure (heart failure with a preserved ejection fraction). *J. Physiol.* 592 (Pt 3), 411–414. doi: 10.1113/jphysiol.2013.262261

Rajamani, S., Liu, G., El-Bizri, N., Guo, D., Li, C., Chen, X. L., et al. (2016). The novel late Na(+) current inhibitor, GS-6615 (eleclazine) and its anti-arrhythmic effects in rabbit isolated heart preparations. *Br. J. Pharmacol.* 173 (21), 3088–3098. doi: 10.1111/bph.13563

Ravens, U., Wettwer, E., and Hala, O. (2004). Pharmacological modulation of ion channels and transporters. *Cell Calcium* 35 (6), 575–582. doi: 10.1016/j.ceca.2004.01.011

Reiffel, J. A., Camm, A. J., Belardinelli, L., Zeng, D., Karwatowska-Prokopczuk, E., Olmsted, A., et al. (2015). The HARMONY Trial: Combined Ranolazine and Dronedarone in the Management of Paroxysmal Atrial Fibrillation: Mechanistic and Therapeutic Synergism. *Circ. Arrhythm. Electrophysiol.* 8 (5), 1048–1056. doi: 10.1161/CIRCEP.115.002856

Restivo, M., Caref, E. B., Kozhevnikov, D. O., and El-Sherif, N. (2004). Spatial dispersion of repolarization is a key factor in the arrhythmogenicity of long QT syndrome. *J. Cardiovasc. Electrophysiol.* 15 (3), 323–331. doi: 10.1046/j.1540-8167.2004.03493.x

Rivera-Fernandez, R., Arias-Verdu, M. D., Garcia-Paredes, T., Delgado-Rodriguez, M., Arboleda-Sanchez, J. A., Aguilar-Alonso, E., et al. (2016). Prolonged QT interval in ST-elevation myocardial infarction and mortality: new prognostic scale with QT, Killip and age. *J. Cardiovasc. Med. (Hagerstown)* 17 (1), 11–19. doi: 10.2459/JCM.0000000000000015

Ruan, Y., Liu, N., and Priori, S. G. (2009). Sodium channel mutations and arrhythmias. *Nat. Rev. Cardiol.* 6 (5), 337–348. doi: 10.1038/nrcardio.2009.44

Sarhan, M. F., and Van Petegem, F. (2009). Ahern CA. A Double Tyrosine Motif in the Cardiac Sodium Channel Domain III-IV Linker Couples Calcium-dependent Calmodulin Binding to Inactivation Gating. *J. Biol. Chem.* 284 (48), 33265–33274. doi: 10.1074/jbc.M109.052910

Sarhan, M. F., Tung, C. C., Van Petegem, F., and Ahern, C. A. (2012). Crystallographic basis for calcium regulation of sodium channels. *Proc. Natl. Acad. Sci. U. S. A.* 109 (9), 3558–3563. doi: 10.1073/pnas.1114748109

Scanley, B. E., Hanck, D. A., Chay, T., and Fozzard, H. A. (1990). Kinetic-analysis of single sodium-channels from canine cardiac purkinje-cells. *J. Gen. Physiol.* 95 (3), 411–437. doi: 10.1085/jgp.95.3.411

Scheuer, T. (2011). Regulation of sodium channel activity by phosphorylation. *Semin. Cell Dev. Biol.* 22 (2), 160–165. doi: 10.1016/j.semcdb.2010.10.002

Schillinger, W., Teucher, N., Christians, C., Kohlhaas, M., Sossalla, S., Van Nguyen, P., et al. (2006). High intracellular Na+ preserves myocardial function at low heart rates in isolated myocardium from failing hearts. *Eur. J. Heart Fail.* 8 (7), 673–680. doi: 10.1016/j.ejheart.2006.01.013

Scirica, B. M., Morrow, D. A., Hod, H., Murphy, S. A., Belardinelli, L., Hedgepeth, C. M., et al. (2007). Effect of ranolazine, an antianginal agent with novel electrophysiological properties, on the incidence of arrhythmias in patients with non ST-segment elevation acute coronary syndrome: results from the Metabolic Efficiency With Ranolazine for Less Ischemia in Non ST-Elevation Acute Coronary Syndrome Thrombolysis in Myocardial Infarction 36 (MERLIN-TIMI 36) randomized controlled trial. *Circulation* 116 (15), 1647–1652. doi: 10.1161/CIRCULATIONAHA.107.724880

Shimizu, W., and Antzelevitch, C. (1997). Sodium channel block with mexiletine is effective in reducing dispersion of repolarization and preventing torsade des pointes in LQT2 and LQT3 models of the long-QT syndrome. *Circulation* 96 (6), 2038–2047. doi: 10.1161/01.CIR.96.6.2038

Shimizu, W., and Antzelevitch, C. (1999a). Cellular basis for long QT, transmural dispersion of repolarization, and torsade de pointes in the long QT syndrome. *J. Electrocardiol.* 32 (Suppl), 177–184. doi: 10.1016/s0022-0736(99)90077-8

Shimizu, W., and Antzelevitch, C. (1999b). Cellular and ionic basis for T-wave alternans under long-QT conditions. *Circulation* 99 (11), 1499–1507. doi: 10.1161/01.cir.99.11.1499

Shimoda, L. A., and Polak, J. (2011). Hypoxia. 4. Hypoxia and ion channel function. *Am. J. Physiol. Cell Physiol.* 300 (5), C951–C967. doi: 10.1152/ajpcell.00512.2010

Shryock, J. C., Song, Y. J., Rajamani, S., Antzelevitch, C., and Belardinelli, L. (2013). The arrhythmogenic consequences of increasing late I-Na in the cardiomyocyte. *Cardiovasc. Res.* 99 (4), 600–611. doi: 10.1093/cvr/cvt145

Sicouri, S., Belardinelli, L., and Antzelevitch, C. (2013). Antiarrhythmic effects of the highly selective late sodium channel current blocker GS-458967. *Heart Rhythm.* 10 (7), 1036–1043. doi: 10.1016/j.hrthm.2013.03.023

Sipido, K. R., Bito, V., Antoons, G., Volders, P. G., and Vos, M. A. (2007). "Na/Ca exchange and cardiac ventricular arrhythmias," in *Sodium-Calcium Exchange and the Plasma Membrane Ca2+-Atpase in Cell Function: Fifth International Conference*, vol. 1099 . Eds. A. Herchuelz, M. P. Blaustein, J. Lytton and K. D. Philipson (Annals of the New York Academy of Sciences), 339–348.

Song, J. H., Huang, C. S., Nagata, K., Yeh, J. Z., and Narahashi, T. (1997). Differential action of riluzole on tetrodotoxin-sensitive and tetrodotoxin-resistant sodium channels. *J. Pharmacol. Exp. Ther.* 282 (2), 707–714.

Song, Y., Shryock, J. C., Wu, L., and Belardinelli, L. (2004). Antagonism by ranolazine of the pro-arrhythmic effects of increasing late INa in guinea pig ventricular myocytes. *J. Cardiovasc. Pharmacol.* 44 (2), 192–199. doi: 10.1097/00005344-200408000-00008

Song, Y., Shryock, J. C., Wagner, S., Maier, L. S., and Belardinelli, L. (2006). Blocking late sodium current reduces hydrogen peroxide-induced arrhythmogenic activity and contractile dysfunction. *J. Pharmacol. Exp. Ther.* 318 (1), 214–222. doi: 10.1124/jpet.106.101832

Song, Y., Shryock, J. C., and Belardinelli, L. (2008). An increase of late sodium current induces delayed afterdepolarizations and sustained triggered activity in atrial myocytes. *Am. J. Physiol. Heart Circ. Physiol.* 294 (5), H2031–H2039. doi: 10.1152/ajpheart.01357.2007

Sossalla, S., Wagner, S., Rasenack, E. C., Ruff, H., Weber, S. L., Schondube, F. A., et al. (2008). Ranolazine improves diastolic dysfunction in isolated myocardium from failing human hearts–role of late sodium current and intracellular ion accumulation. *J. Mol. Cell. Cardiol.* 45 (1), 32–43. doi: 10.1016/j.yjmcc.2008.03.006

Sossalla, S., Kallmeyer, B., Wagner, S., Mazur, M., Maurer, U., Toischer, K., et al. (2010). Altered Na(+) currents in atrial fibrillation effects of ranolazine on arrhythmias and contractility in human atrial myocardium. *J. Am. Coll. Cardiol.* 55 (21), 2330–2342. doi: 10.1016/j.jacc.2009.12.055

Sossalla, S., Maurer, U., Schotola, H., Hartmann, N., Didie, M., Zimmermann, W. H., et al. (2011). Diastolic dysfunction and arrhythmias caused by overexpression of CaMKIIdelta(C) can be reversed by inhibition of late Na(+) current. *Basic Res. Cardiol.* 106 (2), 263–272. doi: 10.1007/s00395-010-0136-x

Stone, P. H., Gratsiansky, N. A., Blokhin, A., Huang, I. Z., and Meng, L. (2006). Antianginal efficacy of ranolazine when added to treatment with amlodipine: the ERICA (Efficacy of Ranolazine in Chronic Angina) trial. *J. Am. Coll. Cardiol.* 48 (3), 566–575. doi: 10.1016/j.jacc.2006.05.044

Studenik, C. R., Zhou, Z., and January, C. T. (2001). Differences in action potential and early afterdepolarization properties in LQT2 and LQT3 models of long QT syndrome. *Br. J. Pharmacol.* 132 (1), 85–92. doi: 10.1038/sj.bjp.0703770

Szentandrassy, N., Kistamas, K., Hegyi, B., Horvath, B., Ruzsnavszky, F., Vaczi, K., et al. (2015). Contribution of ion currents to beat-to-beat variability of action potential duration in canine ventricular myocytes. *Pflug. Arch. Eur. J. Physiol.* 467 (7), 1431–1443. doi: 10.1007/s00424-014-1581-4

Tan, H. L., Kupershmidt, S., Zhang, R., Stepanovic, S., Roden, D. M., Wilde, A. A. M., et al. (2002). A calcium sensor in the sodium channel modulates cardiac excitability. *Nature* 415 (6870), 442–447. doi: 10.1038/415442a

Tang, Q., Ma, J. H., Zhang, P. H., Wan, W., Kong, L. H., and Wu, L. (2012). Persistent sodium current and Na+/H+ exchange contributes to the augmentation of the reverse Na+/Ca2+ exchange during hypoxia or acute ischemia in ventricular myocytes. *Pflug. Arch. Eur. J. Physiol.* 463 (4), 513–522. doi: 10.1007/s00424-011-1070-y

Tarradas, A., Pinsach-Abuin, M. L., Mackintosh, C., Llora-Batlle, O., Perez-Serra, A., Batlle, M., et al. (2017). Transcriptional regulation of the sodium channel gene (SCN5A) by GATA4 in human heart. *J. Mol. Cell. Cardiol.* 102, 74–82. doi: 10.1016/j.yjmcc.2016.10.013

Thadani, U., Ezekowitz, M., Fenney, L., and Chiang, Y. K. (1994). Double-blind efficacy and safety study of a novel anti-ischemic agent, ranolazine, versus placebo in patients with chronic stable angina pectoris. Ranolazine Study Group. *Circulation* 90 (2), 726–734. doi: 10.1161/01.CIR.90.2.726

Trenor, B., Cardona, K., Gomez, J. F., Rajamani, S., Ferrero, J. M.Jr., Belardinelli, L., et al. (2012). Simulation and mechanistic investigation of the arrhythmogenic role of the late sodium current in human heart failure. *PloS One* 7 (3), e32659. doi: 10.1371/journal.pone.0032659

Ufret-Vincenty, C. A., Baro, D. J., Lederer, W. J., Rockman, H. A., Quiñones, L. E., and Santana, L. F. (2001). Role of Sodium Channel Deglycosylation in the Genesis of Cardiac Arrhythmias in Heart Failure. *J. Biol. Chem.* 276 (30), 28197–28203. doi: 10.1074/jbc.M102548200

Undrovinas, A. I., Fleidervish, I. A., and Makielski, J. C. (1992). Inward sodium current at resting potentials in single cardiac myocytes induced by the ischemic metabolite lysophosphatidylcholine. *Circ. Res.* 71 (5), 1231–1241. doi: 10.1161/01.RES.71.5.1231

Undrovinas, A. I., Maltsev, V. A., Kyle, J. W., Silverman, N., and Sabbah, H. N. (2002). Gating of the late Na+ channel in normal and failing human myocardium. *J. Mol. Cell Cardiol.* 34 (11), 1477–1489. doi: 10.1006/jmcc.2002.2100

Undrovinas, A. I., Belardinelli, L., Undrovinas, N. A., and Sabbah, H. N. (2006). Ranolazine improves abnormal repolarization and contraction in left ventricular myocytes of dogs with heart failure by inhibiting late sodium current. *J. Cardiovasc. Electrophysiol.* 17 (Suppl 1), S169–S177. doi: 10.1111/j.1540-8167.2006.00401.x

Vacher, B., Pignier, C., Letienne, R., and Verscheure, Y. (2009). Le Grand B. F 15845 inhibits persistent sodium current in the heart and prevents angina in animal models. *Br. J. Pharmacol.* 156 (2), 214–225. doi: 10.1111/j.1476-5381.2008.00062.x

Valdivia, C. R., Chu, W. W., Pu, J. L., Foell, J. D., Haworth, R. A., Wolff, M. R., et al. (2005). Increased late sodium current in myocytes from a canine heart failure model and from failing human heart. *J. Mol. Cell Cardiol.* 38 (3), 475–483. doi: 10.1016/j.yjmcc.2004.12.012

van Stuijvenberg, L., Yildirim, C., Kok, B. G., van Veen, T. A., Varro, A., Winckels, S. K., et al. (2010). Alternative promoter usage and splicing of the human SCN5A gene contribute to transcript heterogeneity. *DNA Cell Biol.* 29 (10), 577–587. doi: 10.1089/dna.2009.0999

Wagner, S., Dybkova, N., Rasenack, E. C. L., Jacobshagen, C., Fabritz, L., Kirchhof, P., et al. (2006). Ca2+/calmodulin-dependent protein kinase II regulates cardiac Na+ channels. *J. Clin. Invest.* 116 (12), 3127–3138. doi: 10.1172/jci26620

Wagner, S., Ruff, H. M., Weber, S. L., Bellmann, S., Sowa, T., Schulte, T., et al. (2011). Reactive oxygen species-activated Ca/calmodulin kinase IIdelta is required for late I(Na) augmentation leading to cellular Na and Ca overload. *Circ. Res.* 108 (5), 555–565. doi: 10.1161/CIRCRESAHA.110.221911

Wagner, S., Rokita, A. G., Anderson, M. E., and Maier, L. S. (2013). Redox regulation of sodium and calcium handling. *Antioxid. Redox Signal.* 18 (9), 1063–1077. doi: 10.1089/ars.2012.4818

Wang, Z., Page, P., and Nattel, S. (1992). Mechanism of flecainide's antiarrhythmic action in experimental atrial fibrillation. *Circ. Res.* 71 (2), 271–287. doi: 10.1161/01.res.71.2.271

Wang, Q., Shen, J., Splawski, I., Atkinson, D., Li, Z., Robinson, J. L., et al. (1995). SCN5A mutations associated with an inherited cardiac arrhythmia, long QT syndrome. *Cell* 80 (5), 805–811. doi: 10.1016/0092-8674(95)90359-3

Wang, D. W., Yazawa, K., George, A. L.Jr., and Bennett, P. B. (1996). Characterization of human cardiac Na+ channel mutations in the congenital long QT syndrome. *Proc. Natl. Acad. Sci. U. S. A.* 93 (23), 13200–13205. doi: 10.1073/pnas.93.23.13200

Wang, D. W., Viswanathan, P. C., Balser, J. R., George, A. L., and Benson, D. W. (2002). Clinical, genetic, and biophysical characterization of SCN5A mutations associated with atrioventricular conduction block. *Circulation* 105 (3), 341–346. doi: 10.1161/hc0302.102592

Wang, W. P., Ma, J. H., Zhang, P. H., and Luo, A. T. (2007). Redox reaction modulates transient and persistent sodium current during hypoxia in guinea pig ventricular myocytes. *Pflug. Arch. Eur. J. Physiol.* 454 (3), 461–475. doi: 10.1007/s00424-007-0219-1

Wang, D. W., Desai, R. R., Crotti, L., Arnestad, M., Insolia, R., Pedrazzini, M., et al. (2007). Cardiac sodium channel dysfunction in sudden infant death syndrome. *Circulation* 115 (3), 368–376. doi: 10.1161/CIRCULATIONAHA.106.646513

Weiss, S. M., and Saint, D. A. (2010). The persistent sodium current blocker riluzole is antiarrhythmic and anti-ischaemic in a pig model of acute myocardial infarction. *PloS One* 5 (11), e14103. doi: 10.1371/journal.pone.0014103

Weiss, S. M., Dahlstrom, J. E., and Saint, D. A. (2013). Riluzole reduces arrhythmias and myocardial damage induced by coronary occlusion in anaesthetized pigs. *Clin. Exp. Pharmacol. Physiol.* 40 (12), 856–863. doi: 10.1111/1440-1681.12175

Wingo, T. L., Shah, V. N., Anderson, M. E., Lybrand, T. P., Chazin, W. J., and Balser, J. R. (2004). An EF-hand in the sodium channel couples intracellular calcium to cardiac excitability. *Nat. Struct. Mol. Biol.* 11 (3), 219–225. doi: 10.1038/nsmb737

Wu, J. Y., and Corr, P. B. (1994). Palmitoyl carnitine modifies sodium currents and induces transient inward current in ventricular myocytes. *Am. J. Physiol.* 266 (3), H1034–H1046. doi: 10.1152/ajpheart.1994.266.3.H1034

Wu, L., Shryock, J. C., Song, Y., and Belardinelli, L. (2006). An increase in late sodium current potentiates the proarrhythmic activities of low-risk QT-prolonging drugs in female rabbit hearts. *J. Pharmacol. Exp. Ther.* 316 (2), 718–726. doi: 10.1124/jpet.105.094862

Wu, L., Ma, J., Li, H., Wang, C., Grandi, E., Zhang, P., et al. (2011). Late sodium current contributes to the reverse rate-dependent effect of IKr inhibition on ventricular repolarization. *Circulation* 123 (16), 1713–1720. doi: 10.1161/CIRCULATIONAHA.110.000661

Xi, Y. T., Wu, G. R., Yang, L., Han, K., Du, Y., Wang, T. Z., et al. (2009). Increased late sodium currents are related to transcription of neuronal isoforms in a pressure-overload model. *Eur. J. Heart Fail.* 11 (8), 749–757. doi: 10.1093/eurjhf/hfp092

Yamamura, K., Muneuchi, J., Uike, K., Ikeda, K., Inoue, H., Takahata, Y., et al. (2010). A novel SCN5A mutation associated with the linker between III and IV domains of Na(v)1.5 in a neonate with fatal long QT syndrome. *Int. J. Cardiol.* 145 (1), 61–64. doi: 10.1016/j.ijcard.2009.04.023

Yang, P., Kupershmidt, S., and Roden, D. M. (2004). Cloning and initial characterization of the human cardiac sodium channel (SCN5A) promoter. *Cardiovasc. Res.* 61 (1), 56–65. doi: 10.1016/j.cardiores.2003.09.030

Yang, T., Atack, T. C., Stroud, D. M., Zhang, W., Hall, L., and Roden, D. M. (2012). Blocking Scn10a Channels in Heart Reduces Late Sodium Current and Is Antiarrhythmic. *Circ. Res.* 111 (3), 322–332. doi: 10.1161/circresaha.112.265173

Yang, K. C., Bonini, M. G., and Dudley, S. C.Jr. (2014). Mitochondria and arrhythmias. *Free Radic. Biol. Med.* 71, 351–361. doi: 10.1016/j.freeradbiomed.2014.03.033

Yao, L., Fan, P., Jiang, Z., Viatchenko-Karpinski, S., Wu, Y., Kornyeyev, D., et al. (2011). Nav1.5-dependent persistent Na+ influx activates CaMKII in rat ventricular myocytes and N1325S mice. *Am. J. Physiol. Cell Physiol.* 301 (3), C577–C586. doi: 10.1152/ajpcell.00125.2011

Zablocki, J. A., Elzein, E., Li, X., Koltun, D. O., Parkhill, E. Q., Kobayashi, T., et al. (2016). Discovery of Dihydrobenzoxazepinone (GS-6615) Late Sodium Current Inhibitor (Late INai), a Phase II Agent with Demonstrated Preclinical Anti-Ischemic and Antiarrhythmic Properties. *J. Med. Chem.* 59 (19), 9005–9017. doi: 10.1021/acs.jmedchem.6b00939

Zareba, W., Daubert, J. P., Beck, C. A., Huang, D. T., Alexis, J. D., Brown, M. W., et al. (2018). Ranolazine in High-Risk Patients With Implanted Cardioverter-Defibrillators: The RAID Trial. *J. Am. Coll. Cardiol.* 72 (6), 636–645. doi: 10.1016/j.jacc.2018.04.086

Zaza, A., and Rocchetti, M. (2013). The Late Na+ Current - Origin and Pathophysiological Relevance. *Cardiovasc. Drugs Ther.* 27 (1), 61–68. doi: 10.1007/s10557-012-6430-0

Zhang, T., and Brown, J. H. (2004). Role of Ca2+/calmodulin-dependent protein kinase II in cardiac hypertrophy and heart failure. *Cardiovasc. Res.* 63 (3), 476–486. doi: 10.1016/j.cardiores.2004.04.026

Zhang, Y., Hartmann, H. A., and Satin, J. (1999). Glycosylation Influences Voltage-Dependent Gating of Cardiac and Skeletal Muscle Sodium Channels. *J. Membr. Biol.* 171 (3), 195–207. doi: 10.1007/s002329900571

Zhou, A., Shi, G., Kang, G. J., Xie, A., Liu, H., Jiang, N., et al. (2018). RNA Binding Protein, HuR, Regulates SCN5A Expression Through Stabilizing MEF2C transcription factor mRNA. *J. Am. Heart Assoc.* 7 (9), e007802. doi: 10.1161/JAHA.117.007802

Zygmunt, A. C., Nesterenko, V. V., Rajamani, S., Hu, D., Barajas-Martinez, H., Belardinelli, L., et al. (2011). Mechanisms of atrial-selective block of Na(+) channels by ranolazine: I. Experimental analysis of the use-dependent block. *Am. J. Physiol. Heart Circ. Physiol.* 301 (4), H1606–H1614. doi: 10.1152/ajpheart.00242.2011

5

Challenges and Opportunities for Therapeutic Targeting of Calmodulin Kinase II in Heart

Drew Nassal[1], *Daniel Gratz*[1,2] *and Thomas J. Hund*[1,2,3*]

[1] *The Frick Center for Heart Failure and Arrhythmia and Dorothy M. Davis Heart and Lung Research Institute, The Ohio State University Wexner Medical Center, Columbus, OH, United States,* [2] *Department of Biomedical Engineering, College of Engineering, The Ohio State University, Columbus, OH, United States,* [3] *Department of Internal Medicine, The Ohio State University Wexner Medical Center, Columbus, OH, United States*

Correspondence:
Thomas J. Hund
Thomas.Hund@osumc.edu

Heart failure remains a major health burden around the world. Despite great progress in delineation of molecular mechanisms underlying development of disease, standard therapy has not advanced at the same pace. The multifunctional signaling molecule Ca^{2+}/calmodulin-dependent protein kinase II (CaMKII) has received considerable attention over recent years for its central role in maladaptive remodeling and arrhythmias in the setting of chronic disease. However, these basic science discoveries have yet to translate into new therapies for human patients. This review addresses both the promise and barriers to developing translational therapies that target CaMKII signaling to abrogate pathologic remodeling in the setting of chronic disease. Efforts in small molecule design are discussed, as well as alternative targeting approaches that exploit novel avenues for compound delivery and/or genetic approaches to affect cardiac CaMKII signaling. These alternative strategies provide hope for overcoming some of the challenges that have limited the development of new therapies.

Keywords: calmodulin kinase II, arrhythmias, heart failure, cardiovascular pharmacology, cardiac remodeling

INTRODUCTION

For the past 50 years, therapy based on antagonism of beta adrenergic receptors, angiotensin converting enzyme (ACE), and/or AT2 receptors has been the staple for heart failure (HF) treatment (Bers, 2005). However, the incidence of HF and associated mortality rates continue to grow at an alarming pace, highlighting the need for novel therapies to target pathways that drive HF progression. While the field has shown tremendous strides in understanding mechanisms associated with pathologic remodeling leading to HF, translation of this information into new and effective therapies has been less successful. This review discusses the multifunctional signaling molecule Ca^{2+}/calmodulin-dependent protein kinase II (CaMKII) as an example of both the promise and challenges of developing translational therapies based on our evolving understanding of pathologic remodeling in the setting of chronic disease. Despite the wealth of basic research supporting CaMKII as a master regulator of pathways important for cardiac remodeling and arrhythmia, the field has yet to witness translation of these findings to the clinic. The gap between advances at the bench and new treatments in human patients has not gone unnoticed, and efforts are underway that will hopefully fix the pipeline for development of effective therapy. In this review, we address a brief history of progress in small molecule drug design, followed by consideration of alternative approaches that take advantage of recent advances in novel delivery mechanisms as well as genetic approaches for manipulating CaMKII signaling in the heart. These alternative strategies address the ability to circumvent the challenges and limitations of small molecule drug design while highlighting next-generation therapeutic paradigms.

CAMKII EXPRESSION, STRUCTURE, AND FUNCTION IN HEART

CaMKII is a serine/threonine kinase important for translating changes in the levels of intracellular Ca^{2+}/calmodulin (and other critical second messengers) into adaptations in cell function through direct phosphorylation of a large number of target proteins (Swaminathan et al., 2012; Westenbrink et al., 2013). Diversity in metazoan CaMKII expression arises from existence of four isoforms, α, β, γ, and δ, each encoded by a distinct gene. While α and β isoforms are primarily expressed in the brain where they regulate indispensable mechanisms of long-term potentiation/depression necessary for learning and memory (Silva et al., 1992a; Silva et al., 1992b; Stevens et al., 1994; Coultrap et al., 2014), the δ and γ isoforms are broadly expressed in multiple tissues, including the heart (Bennett et al., 1983; Tobimatsu and Fujisawa, 1989). Notably, CaMKIIδ, the predominant cardiac isoform, undergoes alternative splicing to give rise to CaMKIIδ_b and CaMKIIδ_c variants (Edman and Schulman, 1994). This splicing event confers CaMKIIδ_b with a nuclear localization signal not expressed in CaMKIIδ_c leading to differential subcellular distribution (Srinivasan et al., 1994; Ramirez et al., 1997). Despite important differences, there is high degree of homology across CaMKII isoforms, posing significant challenges for therapy around CaMKII inhibition. Given the ubiquitous nature of CaMKII with expression throughout the body, it is no small task to effectively target isoforms/splice variants involved in cardiac pathophysiology while avoiding those important for normal physiology in heart and other organ systems (e.g., brain) (Little et al., 2009; Peng et al., 2010; Lu et al., 2011b; Beckendorf et al., 2018).

Before considering strategies for targeting CaMKII, it is important to briefly discuss the kinase structure/function relationship. A single molecule of CaMKII is composed of three domains: (1) the N-terminal catalytic domain responsible for ATP binding and kinase function; (2) the regulatory domain responsible for binding Ca^{2+}/calmodulin and subsequent kinase activation; and (3) the C-terminal association domain responsible for the oligomerization of individual CaMKII molecules to create a mature dodecameric-holoenzyme (**Figure 1A**). As will be discussed, the N-terminal catalytic domain has received the most attention for translatable drug design. Inactive CaMKII is folded in a closed conformation where the regulatory domain of each CaMKII monomer acts as a substrate binding the catalytic domain. Additionally, adjacent regulatory domains within the dodecameric structure block the binding of target substrates and ATP, maintaining a self-inhibited state. Activation of CaMKII occurs when Ca^{2+}/calmodulin binds to a defined region in the regulatory domain resulting in a conformation shift that releases the catalytic domain, exposing the kinase substrate and ATP binding sites. Importantly, the regulatory domains of neighboring CaMKII monomers within the holoenzyme are themselves substrates for active CaMKII kinase activity, specifically at Thr287. Phosphorylation of this residue dramatically increases affinity for Ca^{2+}/calmodulin and also prevents reassociation of the regulatory and catalytic domains, creating sustained CaMKII activity through beat-to-beat fluctuations in Ca^{2+} cycling.

In addition to the autophosphorylation at Thr287 maintaining the active conformation, other posttranslational modifications have been identified on the regulatory domain, which maintain an active state and have been associated with cardiac disease states. These include the oxidation of Met281/282 in response to elevated reactive oxygen species (Erickson et al., 2008; He et al., 2011; Purohit et al., 2013; Anderson, 2015), O-linked N-acetylglucosamine (GlcNAcylation) targeting Ser279 as a result of elevated glucose levels (Erickson et al., 2008; Erickson et al., 2013), and reports of S-nitrosylation predicted on Cys290 as a result of increased NO production upon β-AR stimulation (Gutierrez et al., 2013; Erickson et al., 2015). Together, these posttranslational modifications establish a diverse set of pathways that contribute to sustained activation of CaMKII, reinforcing the strong association between CaMKII activity and the development of cardiac disease.

The physiologic targets and consequences of cardiac CaMKII signaling have been thoroughly addressed in previous review articles (Anderson et al., 2011; Westenbrink et al., 2013; Mattiazzi et al., 2015; Mustroph et al., 2017). Therefore, we will only briefly discuss CaMKII targets in the context of cardiac remodeling and disease to lay the foundation for more detailed treatment of efforts to inhibit CaMKII. Ample experimental evidence causally links chronic CaMKII activity to development of cardiac disease and arrhythmias (Maier and Bers, 2002; Swaminathan et al., 2012; Westenbrink et al., 2013). Animal models have shown proof-of-concept studies that transgenic overexpression of CaMKII is sufficient to induce structural and electrical remodeling in the heart, leading to compromised contractility and increased risk for sudden cardiac death (Zhang et al., 2002; Zhang et al., 2003; Wagner et al., 2011). Likewise, genetic and chemical inhibition of CaMKII has been shown to confer protection from the development of dilated cardiomyopathy and sustained contractile performance, following both pressure overload and ischemic stress (Zhang et al., 2005; Backs et al., 2009; Ling et al., 2009). Important when considering translation, human HF has also been associated with an increased expression/activity of CaMKII (Hoch et al., 1999; Kirchhefer et al., 1999). The central role for CaMKII in development of disease stems from its regulation of proteins involved in critical cell functions from Ca^{2+} cycling to mitochondrial function. CaMKII has been implicated in pathologic phosphorylation of a number of Ca^{2+} handling proteins including phospholamban, leading to activation of the sarcoplasmic reticulum (SR) ATP-driven Ca^{2+} pump SERCA2a (Mattiazzi and Kranias, 2014); the ryanodine receptor SR Ca^{2+} release channel (RyR2) (Witcher et al., 1991; Lokuta et al., 1995; Wehrens, 2011), promoting increased

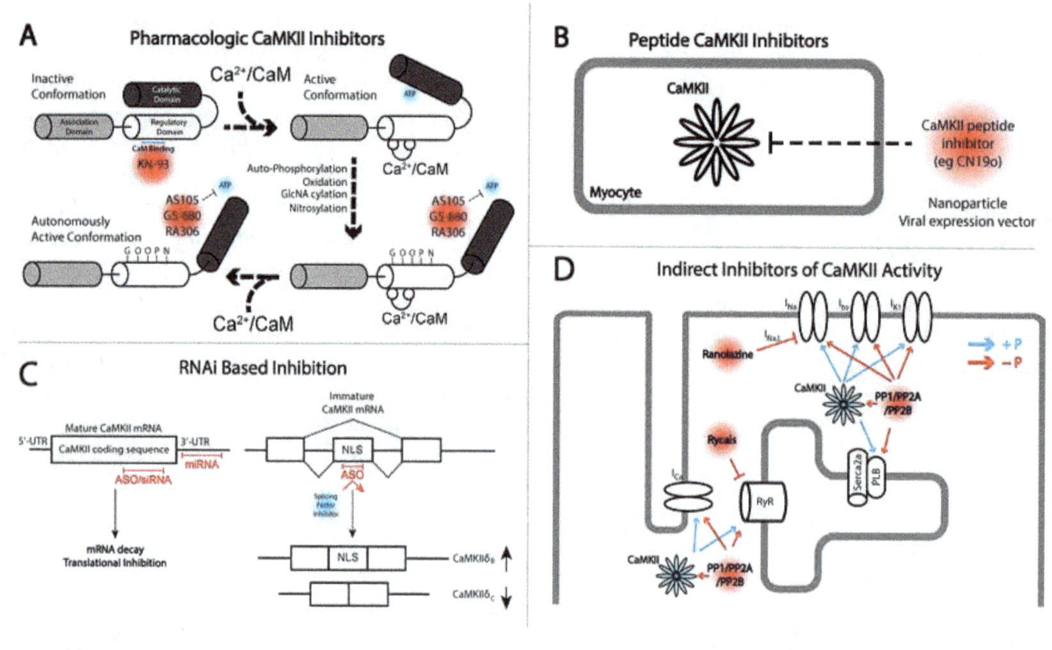

FIGURE 1 | Different approaches for targeting Ca^{2+}/calmodulin-dependent protein kinase II (CaMKII) signaling. **(A)** Depiction of inactive and active monomers of CaMKII showing the association, regulatory, and catalytic domains. The association domain is responsible for interaction with other CaMKII monomers and is necessary for forming the holoenzyme structure, consisting of 12 monomers. In its inactive state, the catalytic domain is obscured by interaction with the regulatory domain. This interaction is disrupted upon the binding of Ca^{2+}/CaM leading to autophosphorylation by neighboring CaMKII monomers, in addition to other posttranslational modifications including oxidation, GlcNAcylation, and nitrosylation, maintaining CaMKII activation even upon release of Ca^{2+}/CaM. KN-93 is a known allosteric inhibitor of CaM binding and therefore preferentially targets CaMKII in the inactive state. CaMKII inhibitors AS105, GS-680, and RA306 are novel pyrimidine-based, ATP-competitive inhibitors that inhibit the activated catalytic domain of CaMKII and represent potential therapeutic agents for translational CaMKII inhibition. **(B)** Peptide inhibitors of CaMKII (e.g., CN19o, refined from CaMKIItide) show favorable selectivity and potency for CaMKII inhibition but face challenges in delivery and bioavailability. Both viral gene delivery and novel advances in nanoparticles offer opportunities for delivery of these agents to the heart. **(C)** RNA interference (RNAi) is a novel approach for inhibiting CaMKII activity at the transcript level. Antisense oligonucleotides (ASOs), small interfering RNA (siRNA), and miRNAs provide opportunity for degrading CaMKII transcripts and/or inhibiting protein translation. ASOs can also be used to interfere with recruitment of splicing factors to enhance concentrations of CaMKIIδ_B which has been shown to have cardioprotective effects. **(D)** Indirect inhibition of CaMKII can be achieved by regulating downstream targets of CaMKII kinase activity. An example comes from the late Na^+ current ($I_{Na,L}$) inhibitor ranolazine, or the RyR stabilizing agents, rycals. Alternatively, protein phosphatases may be targeted to antagonize kinase activity in cardiomyocytes. The development of phosphatase activators for cancer therapeutics may offer opportunity for drug applications in cardiovascular disease.

channel open probability and SR Ca^{2+} leak; and the L-type Ca^{2+} channel $Ca_v1.2$ and associated β-subunits, potentiating current amplitude and slowing inactivation (Hudmon et al., 2005; Grueter et al., 2006). Collectively, these events not only promote activation of hypertrophic remodeling cascades but also heighten the risk for inappropriate membrane potential depolarizations (afterdepolarizations) that serve as arrhythmia triggers (Wu et al., 2002). CaMKII-dependent phosphorylation of other ion channels like the primary cardiac voltage-gated Na^+ channel $Na_v1.5$ enhances late depolarizing current, leading to prolonged action potentials, further disrupting Ca^{2+} handling and providing additional substrates for the formation of arrhythmogenic afterdepolarizations (Koval et al., 2012; Glynn et al., 2015; Howard et al., 2018). Mitochondrial Ca^{2+} entry has also been identified as a target for CaMKII with consequences for mitochondrial function and apoptosis (Joiner et al., 2012; Erickson et al., 2013).

Beyond ion channels, CaMKII has been found to target chromatin remodeling protein class 2 histone deacetylases 4 and 5 (HDAC4/5). The phosphorylation of these proteins induces their nuclear export, freeing the transcription factor MEF2 from its repressed state, contributing to hypertrophic remodeling (Backs et al., 2006; Wu et al., 2006; Backs et al., 2008). Relevant to pathology, CaMKII signaling is notable for the presence of unique dynamical properties including 1) feedback where CaMKII affects downstream targets that in turn alter an input signal for CaMKII activation (Yao et al., 2011; Morotti et al., 2014; Onal et al., 2017); and 2) bistability where CaMKII is capable of toggling between resting and activated equilibrium states (Michalski, 2013). Together, these findings point to CaMKII as a prime candidate for next-generation therapies in managing heart disease in human patients. Despite our thorough understanding of CaMKII structure and function, the development of therapeutics based on this knowledge is in its infancy. Our goal for the remainder of the review will be to provide a comprehensive look at the progressing therapeutic opportunities for inhibiting CaMKII for HF management. Recent reviews have excellently covered the history and progress of CaMKII inhibition (Pellicena and Schulman, 2014;

Mustroph et al., 2017). Here, we will provide an update of recent efforts toward the development of translational pharmacologic agents while considering more novel and unconsidered opportunities in drug delivery and genetic approaches (summarized in **Table 1**).

PHARMACOLOGIC INHIBITORS OF CAMKII

The approach of using pharmacologic inhibitors to target CaMKII activity has been used extensively in basic research with less progress in translational medicine, which is somewhat surprising given the widespread use of protein kinase inhibitors in cancer therapeutics for targeting tumor proliferation and cell survival (Bhullar et al., 2018). In fact, protein kinases are the second most targeted group of proteins, currently with 37 kinase inhibitors having received Food and Drug Administration (FDA) approval for cancer treatment, with another 150 in clinical trials (Bhullar et al., 2018). However, similar compounds have not been successfully developed for therapeutic purposes in the cardiac field due in part to a higher threshold for safety requirements, historical investment being more directed at ion channel blockers for anti-arrhythmics, and a larger burden of clinical trial costs and more uncertain return on investment compared to other therapeutics (Fordyce et al., 2015). Given the growing awareness of the slowdown in cardiovascular drug development (Fordyce et al., 2015) and the dominant academic literature on the contribution of CaMKII in pathologic cardiac remodeling, it seems the community is open and motivated for new pharmacologic drugs for CaMKII inhibition (**Figure 1A**).

Among the first small molecule inhibitors developed for CaMKII was KN-93 (Sumi et al., 1991), which has become one of the most widely used inhibitors in basic research. While its design was not intended for translational use, its prolific use over the years and unique mode of CaMKII inhibition make it important to discuss. While most kinase inhibitors target the ATP-binding domain, KN-93 is unique in that it allosterically disrupts CaM binding and stabilizes the interaction between the enzymatic and regulatory domains as evidenced by measured

TABLE 1 | Properties and limitations of Ca^{2+}/calmodulin-dependent protein kinase II (CaMKII) inhibitory agents.

Inhibitor	Class	Mode of action	Properties and limitations
AS105	Pharmacologic	ATP competitive	Half maximal inhibitory concentration IC50 in the low nM range; shown to improve Ca^{2+} handling in isolated mouse and human cardiomyocytes. Limitations: Activity against CaMKIIα/β/γ, other off-targets, and bioavailability for *in vivo* delivery unknown.
GS-680	Pharmacologic	ATP competitive	IC50 of 2.3 nM for CaMKIIδ with weaker selectivity against CaMKIIα/β/γ and weak interaction with human ether-a-go-go-related gene (hERG). Shown to restore contractility and Ca^{2+} handling in human trabeculae from failing hearts. Limitations: Bioavailability and *in vivo* testing unknown and evidence of potential negative ionotropic effect reversed by isoproterenol treatment.
RA306	Pharmacologic	ATP competitive	IC50 in the 10 nM range for CaMKIIδ/γ with weaker potency against CaMKIIα/β and relatively weak inhibition against hERG, $K_v4.3$, $Na_v1.5$, and $Ca_v1.2$. *In vivo* oral delivery restored contractility in genetic mouse model of dilated cardiomyopathy with minimal drug delivery to the brain. Limitations: Potential inhibition of other kinases associated with cardiac remodeling. Effects on electrical remodeling are not defined. Additional detail needed on acquired disease states like pressure overload.
AC3I/AIP	Peptide	Substrate competitor	IC50 of ~3 μM (AC3I) and 40 nM (AIP). Cardiac specific transgenic models shown to effectively attenuate hypertrophic remodeling, heart failure (HF), and arrhythmias. Limitations: Comprehensive screening of off-targets would be necessary for translational approaches. Existing screens show specificity for CaMKII; however, all isoforms are targeted with equal potency, mandating cardiac specific expression. Bioavailability and cell permeation nonexistent without use of viral vector delivery or potential use of novel nanoparticle delivery.
CaMKIIN	Peptide	Substrate/ regulatory domain competitor	IC50 of 50 nM; however, refinement of the core peptide sequence to the most recent generation (CN19o) has enhanced specificity to CaMKII and improved the IC50 to 0.4 nM. Membrane and mitochondrial associated transgenic expression in mice reduced inflammatory signaling and mitochondrial stress following ischemic injury. Limitations: May impair CaMKII interaction with scaffolding proteins leading to disruption of kinase signaling domains. Lack of bioavailability and cell permeation, requiring viral vector or novel nanoparticle delivery.
Small interfering RNA (siRNA)/ antisense oligonucleotide (ASO)/miRNA	RNAi	Degradation of mRNA, translational inhibition, or alternative splicing	Genetic knockout (KO) of CaMKII in mouse lines has led to improved cardiac performance in multiple disease models. Limitations: *in vivo* therapeutic delivery of RNAi-based agents has not been tested for translational application. Additional limitations include CaMKII targeting in unintended tissues from system delivery.
Ranolazine	Indirect inhibitor of CaMKII signaling	Inhibits late I_{Na}	Shown to reduce late I_{Na} and prevent hypertrophy, HF, and arrhythmias in animal models. Limitations: Clinical trials show uncertain impact preventing atrial fibrillation recurrence, ventricular tachycardia (VT)/ ventricular fibrillation (VF), or improving functional cardiac output in hypertrophic cardiomyopathy.
Rycals (JTV519, S107)	Indirect inhibitor of CaMKII signaling	Stabilizes RyR2	Shown to improve Ca^{2+} handling and ventricular function while protecting against arrhythmias and HF development in both rodents and large animal studies. Clinical investigations performed with S107 to target RyR1 expressed in skeletal muscle for muscular dystrophy treatment
Phosphatase activators	Indirect inhibitor of CaMKII signaling	Dephosphorylation of CaMKII substrates	PP2A activator FTY720 has shown protective capability. Current trend toward phosphatase activators in cancer therapeutics may provide opportunity to examine cardiac effects. Limitations: Transgenic overexpression of phosphatase subunits has been associated with cardiac disease.

FRET signals associated with inactive versus activated structures of CaMKII (Erickson et al., 2011; Erickson et al., 2013). However, this mode of inhibition is thought to be less effective at inhibiting already active CaMKII, including autonomously activated CaMKII as a result of Thr287 autophosphorylation (Vest et al., 2010), which could also extend to additional autonomous modifications of oxidation and GlcNacylation. Another important limitation of KN-93 is that it is not particularly specific or potent against CaMKIIδ, with a half maximal inhibitory concentration (IC50) in a range of 1–4 μM. While KN-93 is reasonably selective for CaMKII over other protein kinases (Gao et al., 2013), it has been found to have a range of off-target effects, including voltage-gated potassium channels (Ledoux et al., 1999; Rezazadeh et al., 2006; Hegyi et al., 2015), L-type Ca^{2+} channels (Anderson et al., 1998), inositol triphosphate receptor Ca^{2+} release (Smyth et al., 2002), and even calmodulin (Johnson et al., 2019).

While KN-93 has proven a valuable research tool, it has not been until recently that concerted efforts have been made to move pharmacological CaMKII inhibition to the clinic. An early effort from the now defunct Scios sought to characterize CaMKII/activity relationships to identify new strategies for inhibiting CaMKII (Mavunkel et al., 2008). From this work, they developed the compound Scios 15b, a cell-permeable, ATP-competitive, pyridimine-based molecule that inhibits CaMKII with an IC50 of 9 nM *in vitro* and 320 nM *in situ*. These initial cell-based assays evaluated CaMKII inhibition by the extent to which it impaired CaMKII-dependent phosphorylation of vimentin. While the compound was not directly investigated with respect to its impact on pathological cardiac remodeling, this work laid the groundwork for the next generation of CaMKII pharmacologics that are being developed, particularly the pyrimidine, ATP-competitive compounds.

Indeed, a more recent novel CaMKII inhibitor, AS105, was also designed as a pyrimidine-based, ATP-competitive molecule by Allosteros Therapeutics following computational optimization of pyrimidine-based CaMKIIδ inhibitors (Neef et al., 2018). Achieving an IC50 in the low nanomolar range for *in vitro* binding, this drug was shown to therapeutically inhibit CaMKII in isolated cardiomyocytes from CaMKIIδ$_C$-overexpressing mice with HF by reducing SR Ca^{2+} leak, improving SR Ca^{2+} loading and Ca^{2+} transient amplitude, and restoring myocyte fractional shortening. Importantly, it was shown to not negatively impact basal excitation–contraction coupling in cardiomyocytes. Moreover, it was able to reduce SR Ca^{2+} leak within isolated human atrial myocytes and suppress arrhythmogenic Ca^{2+} release events. These studies provide promise for the development of a novel CaMKII inhibitor; however, it remains to be seen how specific this drug is for CaMKIIδ compared to CaMKIIα/β/γ and other potential off-targets, as well as its bioavailability.

Another pyrimidine-based, ATP-competitive molecule, GS-680, has been developed by Gilead Sciences (Lebek et al., 2018). GS-680 has a reported CaMKIIδ biochemical IC50 of 2.3 nM, with values 3.1-, 8.7-, and 22.5-fold less potent for CaMKIIγ, α, and β, suggesting a selective potency of CaMKII inhibition for isotypes expressed within the myocardium, minimizing the risk of neuronal side effects. Measurement of phosphorylation levels of phospholamban in neonatal rat ventricular myocytes and neurons treated with GS-680 yielded estimates of EC50 of 98.9 nM and 9,005 nM, respectively, for CaMKII inhibition, consistent with selectivity of the compound for cardiac CaMKII. Moreover, assessment of additional safety factors found the drug to have an EC50 of 3,000 nM for human ether-a-go-go-related gene (hERG) channel inhibition, minimizing the risk of QT prolongation. GS-680 was shown to effectively inhibit premature atrial contractions (PACs) in human atrial trabeculae by exposure to increased external Ca^{2+} (3.5 mM) and isoproterenol (100 nM) and did so in a dose-dependent manner, completely eliminating PACs at 100 and 300 nM concentrations, which occurred in 50% of nontreated samples. In parallel, GS-680 was found to reduce Ca^{2+} sparks and SR Ca^{2+} leak and attenuated triggered activity, as well as increased action potential amplitude and maximal upstroke velocity within isolated human atrial myocytes. However, the drug was found to impair systolic atrial contractions, which was negated after pretreating the tissue with isoproterenol, suggesting that CaMKII inhibition at baseline had a negative ionotropic impact that could be compensated by PKA stimulation. Consistent with this idea, human HF ventricular trabeculae preparations, which are characterized by increased PKA activity and negative force–frequency relationships, experienced improved contractility and increased Ca^{2+} transients at higher pacing frequencies when treated with GS-680, showing that this compound holds promise for the potential treatment of both atrial arrhythmias and HF ventricular remodeling.

Like the compounds just discussed, the most recently designed compound named RA306 developed by Sanofi R&D was derived from a chemical optimization program based on the pyrimidine ATP-competitive class of CaMKII inhibitors (Beauverger et al., 2019). The drug was found to be a potent inhibitor of human CaMKIIδ and γ, the two main cardiac isoforms, having an IC50 of 15 and 25 nM, respectively, in enzymatic caliper assays and below 3 nM for each isoform in a more sensitive P33 assay. CaMKIIβ was also inhibited with an IC50 of 61 nM, and CaMKIIα was weakly inhibited with an IC50 of 420 nM (assessed using caliper assays). There were a limited number of other protein kinases found to be inhibited by the drug including MLK1, SIK, and Pyk2, which have also been associated with adverse cardiac remodeling. RA306 also displayed a favorable ion channel selectivity profile, showing IC50 values for hERG, $K_v4.3$, and $Na_v1.5$ over 30 and 14 μM for $Ca_v1.2$. The therapeutic potential of this compound was tested in a transgenic mouse model of dilated cardiomyopathy, but unique to these studies was the delivery of the drug as an orally bioavailable agent, giving it significant advantage for potential clinical investigation. The drug was found to improve ejection fraction in a genetic mouse model of dilated cardiomyopathy, which associated with reduced levels of phosphorylated phospholamban (Thr17), a direct target of CaMKIIδ. Critically, a five-fold lower exposure for the drug was found in the brain compared to the heart, limiting the potential for off-target impacts of CaMKII inhibition in the brain.

The last several years has seen a strong push in the development of translational pharmacologic agents to inhibit CaMKII for the treatment of pathologic heart conditions. While only one compound (RA306) has been shown to be orally bioavailable, several new agents are available with favorable selectivity and potency profiles. Therefore, based on these efforts, it seems reasonable to remain optimistic about the development of a translationally relevant and novel HF pharmacologic.

PEPTIDE INHIBITORS OF CAMKII

Peptide inhibitors (**Figure 1B**) represent some of the most effective agents to modulate CaMKII for research purposes. The identification of the auto-inhibitory state of the regulatory domain fueled the development of a long inhibitory peptide lacking both the CaM binding domain (Payne et al., 1988; Malinow et al., 1989) and the autophosphorylation residue Thr287 (mutated to be nonphosphorylatable). The result was the generation of the peptide inhibitors autocamtide-2-related inhibitory peptide (AIP) (Ishida et al., 1995) and autocamtide-3 derived inhibitory peptide (AC3-I) (Braun and Schulman, 1995), able to bind the CaMKII catalytic domain but unable to be displaced by canonical CaMKII activation mechanisms. As such, these inhibitors have been delivered through pharmacologic and genetic means to robustly inhibit CaMKII pathologic signaling *in vitro* and *in vivo*, mitigating HF, increasing cardiac function, and preventing lethal cardiac arrhythmias (Zhang et al., 2005; Khoo et al., 2006; Luo et al., 2013; Purohit et al., 2013). Subsequent to the design of these inhibitor peptides, natively expressed inhibitory proteins known as CaMKIINs were discovered. These small proteins were identified through a yeast two-hybrid screen where the CaMKII catalytic domain was used as bait (Chang et al., 1998; Chang et al., 2001), and while they have only been natively detected in the brain, they have been used effectively to target CaMKII activity. Notably, this peptide inhibitor binds with the kinase domain in the active conformation. Indeed, the CaMKIIN inhibitor has been used to limit myocyte death in response to MI, catecholamine stress, and ischemia–reperfusion (Swaminathan et al., 2011; Joiner and Koval, 2014) and reduce the occurrence of arrhythmogenic substrates (Koval et al., 2010) and in particular has utilized localization motifs to inhibit CaMKII within mitochondria or near plasma membrane domains (Joiner et al., 2012). Analysis of the peptide led to refinement and development of a 28-amino acid peptide inhibitor called CaMKIItide (Chang et al., 2001), while further refinement has led to the development of a shortened version only 19 amino acids long called CN19o (Coultrap and Bayer, 2011), with an IC50 of 0.4 nM. This was a >100-fold improvement in the IC50 than the native CaMKIIN, which also led to a stark improvement in the selectivity for CaMKII over other kinases (Coultrap and Bayer, 2011).

While the development and characterization of these highly selective peptide inhibitors has advanced cardiac research, there remains the rather significant challenge of delivery for therapeutic use. The greatest of these challenges is perhaps the limited bioavailability of short peptide sequences *in vivo*. Oral administration would provide limited enteral resorption and intravenous injection for the treatment of a chronic condition would offer challenges with continued compliance, let alone the quick half-life of a short peptide sequence in circulation (Otvos and Wade, 2014). Alternatively, gene therapy could be used to deliver a viral vector which expresses the short peptide. In the last 30 years, there have been four randomized clinical trials employing viral gene delivery for the treatment of HF with reduced ejection fraction (CUPID, CUPID-2, STOP-HF, and AC6) (Penny and Hammond, 2017). While the viral delivery was well tolerated in patients, the greatest burden they faced was insufficient gene transduction, where the patient with the lowest ejection fraction or those receiving the highest viral dosage were the only to experience improved endpoints. While these results do not preclude the future use of gene therapy, they do establish a more rigorous hurdle to overcome to pursue CaMKII inhibition.

A more novel and potentially robust opportunity, however, may reside in recent advances in nanotechnology. A recent report showed the successful delivery of peptide cargo to the heart through the use of biocompatible and biodegradable calcium phosphate nanoparticles introduced by inhalation (Miragoli et al., 2018). This strategy took advantage of the principle that oxygenated blood from the lungs moves from the pulmonary circulation to the heart first. This principle was supported by observations that nanoparticles and particulates from air pollution have been implicated in cardiac dysfunction and arrhythmia (Mills et al., 2009). Not only does the design of these particles allow for delivery to the heart and cell permeation but also protects peptides from enzymatic digestion. This approach has been used for successful delivery of a peptide impacting L-type Ca^{2+} channel expression, resulting in restored cardiac function in a mouse model of diabetic cardiomyopathy (Miragoli et al., 2018). Moreover, peptides have been delivered in a porcine model as well, with minimal delivery to tissues other than the heart. This mode of delivery not only represents a noninvasive and practical means of delivering novel cardiac peptide therapeutics but can take advantage of an already customized potency and precision of CaMKII peptide inhibitors like CaMKIItide or its derivative CN19o.

USE OF RNA INTERFERENCE (RNAI) TO TARGET CAMKII

When it comes to therapeutic treatment of human disease, including cardiac disease, therapeutic intervention falls within two major classes of FDA-approved drugs, small molecules and proteins (Verdine and Walensky, 2007). As has already been discussed, small molecules typically must overcome the burden of target specificity and efficacy and require significant investments of time and resources to make them available for use. Alternatively, protein-based drugs, which frequently take the form of antibodies, display higher specificity, but limitations on size, stability, and deliverability to the right cellular compartments are frequent barriers to their application (Verdine and Walensky, 2007). An alternative approach to the targeting of specific genes implicated in disease may be found in RNA therapeutics (**Figure 1C**). For close to 30 years, RNA drugs [short hairpin RNAs (shRNAs), small-interfering RNAs (siRNAs), microRNAs (miRNAs)] have been used at the bench to target protein expression to identify critical gene targets in disease and signaling pathways. However, their use in clinical settings has been a non-factor given that short single- and double-stranded RNA is extremely susceptible to nuclease digestion, may lead to immune system activation, and is too large and negatively charged to cross cell membranes (Crooke, 1999; Laina et al., 2018). However, significant advances in the design of RNA therapeutics have been able to overcome these challenges to the point that numerous clinical trials are currently underway employing RNAi-based drugs for both cardiac and noncardiac targets (Kaczmarek et al., 2017; Laina et al., 2018).

RNAi therapeutics fall into several different categories, including single-stranded antisense oligonucleotides (ASOs), double-stranded siRNAs, and miRNAs (Laina et al., 2018). ASOs are short (typically 20 base pairs in length) single-stranded synthetic molecules that take advantage of Watson–Crick base-pairing to bind a target mRNA to induce its degradation through endogenous RNAse activity (Crooke, 1999). Depending on the design of the ASO, it can also block ribosomal attachment to reduce target protein expression or even redirect splicing factors to lead to the inclusion or exclusion of targeted exons (Dominski and Kole, 1993; Havens and Hastings, 2016). The latter mode is the mechanism of action of the FDA-approved RNA therapeutic eteplirsen (Exondys 51, Sarepta Therapeutics) for treating Duchenne muscular dystrophy, which induces the skipping of exon 51 of the mutant dystrophin gene and restoring the proper translational reading frame for dystrophin expression (Dystrophy et al., 2013). Therapeutic siRNAs are also synthetic molecules used to silence target genes but are instead double-stranded molecules ranging in length from 19 to 25 base pairs (Siomi and Siomi, 2009). These molecules are recognized by Argonaute 2 and the RNA-induced silencing complex (RISC) and unwound into single-stranded components. The sense strand is degraded and the antisense binds to a target mRNA sequence to induce cleavage by Argonaute 2 and degradation by exonucleases (Sledz et al., 2003; Liu et al., 2004; Rand et al., 2005; Meister, 2013; Ozcan et al., 2015). Finally, miRNAs are endogenous small noncoding RNAs that target multiple mRNAs, silencing target gene expression either by mRNA degradation or translational inhibition. Typically, miRNAs target the 3'-untranslated region (UTR) of the target mRNA through a primary seed sequence eight nucleotides long, with the degree of repression being modulated by the complementarity and nucleotide composition of flanking sequences. These molecules are natively expressed within the cell either under regulation of their own discrete promoter or found within intronic sequences of coding genes. Therefore, therapeutic treatments have focused both on their inhibition through the delivery of antisense sequences acting as complementary decoys to the miRNA as well as direct overexpression of miRNA mimics.

In effect, each of these RNAi-based platforms could theoretically be applied to the inhibition of CaMKII in the heart. While an ASO could be designed with a particular target sequence in mind, there is also precedence for physiologic regulation of CaMKIIδ by a number of native miRNAs to abrogate cardiac remodeling (Wang et al., 2010; Aurora et al., 2012; Cha et al., 2013; He et al., 2013). A multitude of preclinical and clinical trials have employed the use of chemically modified RNAi backbones and encapsulation in nanoparticles to improve pharmacokinetics, escape nuclease activity, enhance target mRNA binding, and minimize toxicity (Lucas and Dimmeler, 2016). Importantly, a major potential advantage in using RNA technology is that it offers the potential for increased precision. Small molecule drugs frequently suffer from impacting unintended secondary targets due to either conservation of enzymatic binding sites (like ATP-competitive sites) or impacting unintended pathways. However, all protein expression is derived from coding mRNA containing nucleic acid sequences significantly more unique to each individual gene, thereby providing a layer of intended target specificity difficult to match through pharmacologic drug design. Even more notably, this precision can even extend to specific isoform targeting of CaMKII. Not only could an siRNA molecule be designed that would specifically target transcripts encoding the CaMKIIδ isoform, circumventing the burden of CaMKII inhibition in the brain where CaMKIIα and β predominate, but may even offer the advantage of specific splice variant targeting of CaMKIIδ by focusing on specific exon–exon junctions unique to each variant. As previous literature has been able to identify, there are splice variant-specific effects of CaMKIIδ in cardiac disease and remodeling, revealing a potential protective role of CaMKIIδ_B, in comparison to the other cardiac variant CaMKIIδ_C (Little et al., 2009; Peng et al., 2010; Lu et al., 2011a).

Moreover, as mentioned, ASO-based therapeutics are also capable of influencing the access of splicing factors to induce the inclusion or skipping of certain exons based on their design. Through such a process, it would be possible to induce a state of increased exon inclusion that favors the variant CaMKIIδ_B, leading to its increased expression relative to CaMKIIδ_C. The consequence of this shift in relative abundances can alter the stoichiometry within the holoenzyme structure, imparting the localization pattern of the isoform that dominates within the complex. Such manipulation of the relative composition has led to the increased nuclear localization of the CaMKIIδ_C isoform when the holoenzyme is composed of more CaMKIIδ_B (Srinivasan et al., 1994). Given that nuclear activity of CaMKIIδ_C has been shown to lead to prosurvival mechanisms within cardiomyocytes and reduced pathologic remodeling (Little et al., 2009; Peng et al., 2010; Lu et al., 2011b), the manipulation of CaMKIIδ at the splicing level through RNA-based mechanisms offers a theoretically plausible mechanism for improving HF treatment that might not even require targeting CaMKII inhibition.

One of the remaining challenges for applying RNA-based CaMKII therapy is selective targeting of heart. Current application of these RNA agents is typically through intravenous or subcutaneous injection, exposing the drugs to systemic circulation. While chemical modification to these drugs can prevent crossing of the blood–brain barrier, this is likely insufficient to prevent undesired consequences for the ubiquitously expressed CaMKIIδ. While this barrier is not unique to RNA therapeutics (also a consideration for small molecule inhibition), there are options that are unique to RNA therapeutics for potentially overcoming this limitation, including gene therapy which could utilize cardiac specific promoters (limited to miRNAs for polymerase compatibility) or local delivery/injection directly into cardiac tissue. There is also exciting opportunity to combine emerging nanoparticle therapy (discussed in previous section) to carry RNA-based drugs instead of peptide cargos through the same inhalation delivery to deliver directly to the heart.

THERAPEUTIC TARGETING OF THE CAMKII SIGNALING PATHWAY

When considering CaMKII as a therapeutic target, it is important to acknowledge opportunities for manipulating the CaMKII signaling pathway without directly targeting the kinase itself. As discussed previously, CaMKII regulates a large number of intracellular substrates (ion channels, transcription factors, Ca^{2+} handling proteins) that may serve as attractive targets for electrical and hypertrophic remodeling. Perhaps the best known example of therapy aimed at a downstream target in the CaMKII pathway comes from ranolazine, an approved antianginal agent that inhibits late Na^+ current among other actions (Rayner-Hartley and Sedlak, 2015). Late Na^+ current, through the actions of the sodium Ca^{2+} exchanger, may impact intracellular Ca^{2+}, contributing to further activation of CaMKII as well as driving the incidence of arrhythmogenic DADs. Ranolazine has been used successfully in rodents and large animals to block these changes and prevent the development of hypertrophy, HF, and arrhythmias (Rastogi et al., 2008; Figueredo et al., 2011; Glynn et al., 2015; Liang et al., 2016; Ellermann et al., 2018; Nie et al., 2019). However, results from clinical trials have been mixed with data supporting that ranolazine is safe with questionable efficacy in preventing AF recurrence (RAFAELLO trial), ventricular tachycardia (VT) or ventricular fibrillation (VF) following implantation of cardioverter defibrillator (RAID trial), or improving functional capacity in hypertrophic cardiomyopathy (RESTYLE-HCM trial) (De Ferrari et al., 2015; Bengel et al., 2017; Olivotto et al., 2018; Zareba et al., 2018).

RyR2 is another potential therapeutic target downstream of CaMKII signaling (Wehrens et al., 2004; Guo et al., 2006; Yang et al., 2007; Wehrens, 2011). Compounds referred to as rycals are small molecules that aim to stabilize RyR2 in its closed conformation through enhanced association with its binding partner calstabin, without blocking the channel or impairing normal Ca^{2+} signaling. JTV519 (K201) is one such compound that has been shown to improve Ca^{2+} leak and left ventricular function in a canine model of HF (Yano et al., 2003). However, translatability of JTV519 is somewhat limited by several off-target effects on other cardiac channels (Kaneko et al., 2009). S107 is another more selective rycal (Bellinger et al., 2008) with demonstrated ability to protect against ventricular arrhythmias in a mouse model with a RyR2 gain-of-function mutation (Lehnart et al., 2008) in addition to reversing the development of HF in a mouse model of constitutively phosphorylated RyR2 (Shan et al., 2010). Molecules such as these are being prepared for clinical testing and represent promising avenues for attenuating the impact of CaMKII activation.

Besides searching downstream of CaMKII for druggable targets, it is important to consider that the functional consequences of any kinase is determined by a delicate balance between the kinase and antagonism by a phosphatase. The majority of phosphatase activity in the heart is due to type-1 phosphatases (PP1) and type-2 phosphatases [PP2A, PP2B (calcineurin)] (El-Armouche and Eschenhagen, 2009), which collectively have been implicated in either dephosphorylating proteins targeted by CaMKII kinase activity or targeting CaMKII directly, removing its autonomous activation (Chiang et al., 2016; Lubbers and Mohler, 2016) (**Figure 1D**). Therefore, it may be possible to balance increased CaMKII activity in disease by simultaneously activating associated phosphatases. For example, the PP2A activator FTY720 has been shown to attenuate hypertrophic remodeling and protect hearts from ischemic injury in the mouse (Egom et al., 2010; Liu et al., 2011; Liu et al., 2013). However, one possible complication with this approach is that increased phosphatase activity has been linked to development of HF (Parra and Rothermel, 2017). Transgenic activation of CaMKII has itself been shown to increase phosphatase activity (Zhang et al., 2002), but it is unclear if this is a compensatory change or a cofactor in driving disease. While maximally activated phosphatase activity is likely to amplify adverse remodeling as the transgenic models have shown, it may be possible to implement a more nuanced approach with the goal of maintaining proper balance between kinase and phosphatase activity. Given that the majority of phosphatase activity is supplied by just three genes, unlike kinases which have numerous members with highly specific functions, phosphatase targeting is regulated by a multitude of binding partners and anchoring proteins (Shi, 2009). $Ca_v1.2$ dephosphorylation for example is dependent on PP2A and its interaction with regulatory subunits B56α and PR59 (Hall et al., 2006; Xu et al., 2010), while spinophilin and regulatory subunit PR130 target PP1 and PP2A to RyR2 (Bers, 2002; Lanner et al., 2010). Future studies may reveal critical subunits which direct phosphatases to relevant CaMKII targets, or to CaMKII itself, through which drug targeting or gene regulation would provide opportunity to influence the extent of that precise interaction. This may provide opportunity to limit adverse outcomes observed in global and unchecked phosphatase induction (Gergs et al., 2004; Hoehn et al., 2015), but clearly a great deal of work is still required to even establish proof of principle.

A unique opportunity for further discerning the potential impact of phosphatase activation may lie in the field of cancer therapeutics. Currently, cancer treatment strategies are beginning to consider phosphatase activators in earnest for tumor disruption (McClinch et al., 2018; Allen-Petersen and Sears, 2019; Remmerie and Janssens, 2019). It is well established that cardiac toxicity is a significant side effect following the use of the common cancer drug, doxorubicin, which has even been associated with CaMKII signaling (Yeh and Bickford, 2009; Sag et al., 2011). Therefore, it would be interesting to observe potential differences in the development of cardiomyopathy with the inclusion of these phosphatase activators when used in conjunction with doxorubicin to provide therapeutic insight and predictive data to the prospect of similar phosphatase activators being utilized for cardioprotective therapies.

Finally, when searching for alternative targets in the CaMKII pathway, it is worth considering scaffolding, cytoskeletal and other interacting proteins important for subcellular localization of CaMKII to specific signaling nanodomains. For example, a role for the cytoskeletal protein β_{IV}-spectrin has been identified in targeting CaMKII to the cardiomyocyte intercalated disc to facilitate regulation of $Na_v1.5$ (Hund et al., 2010). Genetic disruption of β_{IV}-spectrin/CaMKII interaction selectively disrupted the subpopulation of CaMKII at the intercalated disc and prevented stress-induced phosphorylation of $Na_v1.5$. Subsequent studies found that disruption of β_{IV}-spectrin/CaMKII interaction abrogated maladaptive cardiac remodeling in a mouse model of pressure overload (Unudurthi et al., 2018). Thus, it may prove beneficial to develop pharmacological or genetic ways to interfere with spectrin/CaMKII interaction allowing for selective inhibition of a pathological CaMKII subpopulation while leaving the rest of the signaling pathway intact.

CONCLUSION

Given the effectiveness of CaMKII inhibition in improving cardiac function and reducing arrhythmia burden in animal models of disease, it is reasonable to remain optimistic that targeting of CaMKII signaling has a future in cardiac translational therapy. While conventional delivery routes and strategies merit further investigation, it will be important going forward to be aggressive in the search for new delivery routes and targets that may accelerate translation of basic science discoveries to human patients. Recent advances in genetic techniques and/or particle deliveries provide entirely new paradigms for not just treating familial diseases but acquired forms as well. Therefore, the development of CaMKII therapeutics might not only represent a breakthrough for cardiac treatment but, depending on the routes taken, may open up an entirely new branch in the models we use to treat a broader range of disease.

AUTHOR CONTRIBUTIONS

DN, DG, and TH drafted and revised the manuscript.

FUNDING

This work was supported by the National Institutes of Health (grant numbers R01-HL135096 and R01-HL134824 to TH) and the American Heart Association (postdoctoral fellowship to DN).

REFERENCES

Allen-Petersen, B. L., and Sears, R. C. (2019). The use of protein phosphatase 2A activators in combination therapies for pancreas cancer. *Oncotarget* 10, 2008–2009. doi: 10.18632/oncotarget.26772

Anderson, M. E., Braun, A. P., Wu, Y., Lu, T., Wu, Y., Schulman, H., et al. (1998). KN-93, an inhibitor of multifunctional Ca++/calmodulin-dependent protein kinase, decreases early afterdepolarizations in rabbit heart. *J. Pharmacol. Exp. Ther.* 287, 996–1006.

Anderson, M. E., Brown, J. H., and Bers, D. M. (2011). CaMKII in myocardial hypertrophy and heart failure. *J. Mol. Cell. Cardiol.* 51, 468–473. doi: 10.1016/j.yjmcc.2011.01.012

Anderson, M. E. (2015). Oxidant stress promotes disease by activating CaMKII. *J. Mol. Cell. Cardiol.* 89, 160–167. doi: 10.1016/j.yjmcc.2015.10.014

Aurora, A. B., Mahmoud, A. I., Luo, X., Johnson, B. A., van Rooij, E., Matsuzaki, S., et al. (2012). MicroRNA-214 protects the mouse heart from ischemic injury by controlling Ca2+ overload and cell death. *J. Clin. Invest.* 122, 1222–1232. doi: 10.1172/JCI59327

Backs, J., Song, K., Bezprozvannaya, S., Chang, S., and Olson, E. N. (2006). CaM kinase II selectively signals to histone deacetylase 4 during cardiomyocyte hypertrophy. *J. Clin. Invest.* 116, 1853–1864. doi: 10.1172/JCI27438

Backs, J., Backs, T., Bezprozvannaya, S., McKinsey, T. A., and Olson, E. N. (2008). Histone deacetylase 5 acquires calcium/calmodulin-dependent kinase II responsiveness by oligomerization with histone deacetylase 4. *Mol. Cell. Biol.* 28, 3437–3445. doi: 10.1128/MCB.01611-07

Backs, J., Backs, T., Neef, S., Kreusser, M. M., Lehmann, L. H., Patrick, D. M., et al. (2009). The delta isoform of CaM kinase II is required for pathological cardiac hypertrophy and remodeling after pressure overload. *Proc. Natl. Acad. Sci. U. S. A.* 106, 2342–2347. doi: 10.1073/pnas.0813013106

Beauverger, P., Ozoux, M.-L., Bégis, G., Glénat, V., Briand, V., Philippo, M.-C., et al. (2019). Reversion of cardiac dysfunction by a novel orally available calcium/calmodulin-dependent protein kinase II inhibitor, RA306, in a genetic model of dilated cardiomyopathy. *Cardiovasc. Res.* doi: 10.1093/cvr/cvz097

Beckendorf, J., van den Hoogenhof, M. M. G., and Backs, J. (2018). Physiological and unappreciated roles of CaMKII in the heart. *Basic Res. Cardiol.* 113, 29. doi: 10.1007/s00395-018-0688-8

Bellinger, A. M., Reiken, S., Dura, M., Murphy, P. W., Deng, S.-X., Landry, D. W., et al. (2008). Remodeling of ryanodine receptor complex causes "leaky" channels: a molecular mechanism for decreased exercise capacity. *Proc. Natl. Acad. Sci. U. S. A.* 105, 2198–2202. doi: 10.1073/pnas.0711074105

Bengel, P., Ahmad, S., and Sossalla, S. (2017). Inhibition of Late Sodium Current as an Innovative Antiarrhythmic Strategy. *Curr. Heart Fail. Rep.* 14, 179–186. doi: 10.1007/s11897-017-0333-0

Bennett, M. K., Erondu, N. E., and Kennedy, M. B. (1983). Purification and characterization of a calmodulin-dependent protein kinase that is highly concentrated in brain. *J. Biol. Chem.* 258, 12735–12744.

Bers, D. M. (2002). Cardiac excitation-contraction coupling. *Nature* 415, 198–205. doi: 10.1038/415198a

Bers, D. M. (2005). Beyond beta blockers. *Nat. Med.* 11, 379–380. doi: 10.1038/nm0405-379

Bhullar, K. S., Lagarón, N. O., McGowan, E. M., Parmar, I., Jha, A., Hubbard, B. P., et al. (2018). Kinase-targeted cancer therapies: progress, challenges and future directions. *Mol. Cancer* 17, 48. doi: 10.1186/s12943-018-0804-2

Braun, A. P., and Schulman, H. (1995). A non-selective cation current activated via the multifunctional Ca(2+)-calmodulin-dependent protein kinase in human epithelial cells. *J. Physiol.* 488, 37–55. doi: 10.1113/jphysiol.1995.sp020944

Cha, M.-J., Jang, J.-K., Ham, O., Song, B.-W., Lee, S.-Y., Lee, C. Y., et al. (2013). MicroRNA-145 suppresses ROS-induced Ca2+ overload of cardiomyocytes by targeting CaMKIIδ. *Biochem. Biophys. Res. Commun.* 435, 720–726. doi: 10.1016/j.bbrc.2013.05.050

Chang, B. H., Mukherji, S., and Soderling, T. R. (1998). Characterization of a calmodulin kinase II inhibitor protein in brain. *Proc. Natl. Acad. Sci. U. S. A.* 95, 10890–10895. doi: 10.1073/pnas.95.18.10890

Chang, B. H., Mukherji, S., and Soderling, T. R. (2001). Calcium/calmodulin-dependent protein kinase II inhibitor protein: Localization of isoforms in rat brain. *Neuroscience* 102, 767–777. doi: 10.1016/S0306-4522(00)00520-0

Chiang, D. Y., Heck, A. J. R., Dobrev, D., and Wehrens, X. H. T. (2016). Regulating the regulator: insights into the cardiac protein phosphatase 1 interactome. *J. Mol. Cell. Cardiol.* 101, 165–172. doi: 10.1016/j.yjmcc.2016.09.009

Coultrap, S. J., and Bayer, K. U. (2011). Improving a natural CaMKII inhibitor by random and rational design. *PloS One* 6, e25245. doi: 10.1371/journal.pone.0025245

Coultrap, S. J., Freund, R. K., O'Leary, H., Sanderson, J. L., Roche, K. W., Dell'Acqua, M. L., et al. (2014). Autonomous CaMKII mediates both LTP and LTD using a mechanism for differential substrate site selection. *Cell Rep.* 6, 431–437. doi: 10.1016/j.celrep.2014.01.005

Crooke, S. T. (1999). Molecular mechanisms of action of antisense drugs. *Biochim. Biophys. Acta - Gene Struct. Expr.* 1489, 31–43. doi: 10.1016/S0167-4781(99)00148-7

De Ferrari, G. M., Maier, L. S., Mont, L., Schwartz, P. J., Simonis, G., Leschke, M., et al. (2015). Ranolazine in the treatment of atrial fibrillation: results of the dose-ranging RAFFAELLO (ranolazine in atrial fibrillation following an electrical cardioversion) study. *Heart Rhythm.* 12, 872–878. doi: 10.1016/j.hrthm.2015.01.021

Dominski, Z., and Kole, R. (1993). Restoration of correct splicing in thalassemic pre-mRNA by antisense oligonucleotides. *Proc. Natl. Acad. Sci. U. S. A.* 90, 8673–8677. doi: 10.1073/pnas.90.18.8673

Dystrophy, M., Mendell, J. R., and Rodino-klapac, L. R. (2013). Eteplirsen for the treatment of duchenne eteplirsen for the treatment of duchenne muscular dystrophy. *Ann. Neurol.* 74, 637–647. doi: 10.1002/ana.23982

Edman, C. F., and Schulman, H. (1994). Identification and characterization of delta B-CaM kinase and delta C-CaM kinase from rat heart, two new multifunctional Ca2+/calmodulin-dependent protein kinase isoforms. *Biochim. Biophys. Acta* 1221, 89–101. doi: 10.1016/0167-4889(94)90221-6

Egom, E. E. A., Ke, Y., Musa, H., Mohamed, T. M. A., Wang, T., Cartwright, E., et al. (2010). FTY720 prevents ischemia/reperfusion injury-associated arrhythmias in an ex vivo rat heart model via activation of Pak1/Akt signaling. *J. Mol. Cell. Cardiol.* 48, 406–414. doi: 10.1016/j.yjmcc.2009.10.009

El-Armouche, A., and Eschenhagen, T. (2009). Beta-adrenergic stimulation and myocardial function in the failing heart. *Heart Fail. Rev.* 14, 225–241. doi: 10.1007/s10741-008-9132-8

Ellermann, C., Kohnke, A., Dechering, D. G., Kochhäuser, S., Reinke, F., Fehr, M., et al. (2018). Ranolazine prevents levosimendan-induced atrial fibrillation. *Pharmacology.* 102, 3–4. doi: 10.1159/000490572

Erickson, J. R., Joiner, M. A., Guan, X., Kutschke, W., Yang, J., Oddis, C. V., et al. (2008). A dynamic pathway for calcium-independent activation of CaMKII by methionine oxidation. *Cell* 133, 462–474. doi: 10.1016/j.cell.2008.02.048

Erickson, J. R., Patel, R., Ferguson, A., Bossuyt, J., and Bers, D. M. (2011). Fluorescence resonance energy transfer-based sensor camui provides new insight into mechanisms of calcium/calmodulin-dependent protein kinase II activation in intact cardiomyocytes. *Circ. Res.* 109, 729–738. doi: 10.1161/CIRCRESAHA.111.247148

Erickson, J. R., Pereira, L., Wang, L., Han, G., Ferguson, A., Dao, K., et al. (2013). Diabetic hyperglycaemia activates CaMKII and arrhythmias by O-linked glycosylation. *Nature* 502, 372–376. doi: 10.1038/nature12537

Erickson, J. R., Nichols, C. B., Uchinoumi, H., Stein, M. L., Bossuyt, J., and Bers, D. M. (2015). S-nitrosylation induces both autonomous activation and inhibition of calcium/calmodulin-dependent protein Kinase II δ. *J. Biol. Chem.* 290, 25646–25656. doi: 10.1074/jbc.M115.650234

Figueredo, V. M., Pressman, G. S., Romero-Corral, A., Murdock, E., Holderbach, P., and Morris, D. L. (2011). Improvement in left ventricular systolic and diastolic performance during ranolazine treatment in patients with stable angina. *J. Cardiovasc. Pharmacol. Ther.* 16, 168–172. doi: 10.1177/1074248410382105

Fordyce, C. B., Roe, M. T., Ahmad, T., Libby, P., Borer, J. S., Hiatt, W. R., et al. (2015). Cardiovascular drug development: is it dead or just hibernating? *J. Am. Coll. Cardiol.* 65, 1567–1582. doi: 10.1016/j.jacc.2015.03.016

Gao, Y., Davies, S. P., Augustin, M., Woodward, A., Patel, U. A., Kovelman, R., et al. (2013). A broad activity screen in support of a chemogenomic map for kinase signalling research and drug discovery. *Biochem. J.* 451, 313–328. doi: 10.1042/BJ20121418

Gergs, U., Boknik, P., Buchwalow, I., Fabritz, L., Matus, M., Justus, I., et al. (2004). Overexpression of the catalytic subunit of protein phosphatase 2A impairs cardiac function. *J. Biol. Chem.* 279, 40827–40834. doi: 10.1074/jbc.M405770200

Glynn, P., Musa, H., Wu, X., Unudurthi, S. D., Little, S., Qian, L., et al. (2015). Voltageg-gated sodium channel phosphorylation at Ser571 regulates late current, arrhythmia, and cardiac function in vivo. *Circulation.* 132, 567–577. doi: 10.1161/CIRCULATIONAHA.114.015218

Grueter, C. E., Abiria, S. A., Dzhura, I., Wu, Y., Ham, A.-J. L., Mohler, P. J., et al. (2006). L-type Ca2+ channel facilitation mediated by phosphorylation of the beta subunit by CaMKII. *Mol. Cell* 23, 641–650. doi: 10.1016/j.molcel.2006.07.006

Guo, T., Zhang, T., Mestril, R., and Bers, D. M. (2006). Ca2+/Calmodulin-dependent protein kinase II phosphorylation of ryanodine receptor does affect calcium sparks in mouse ventricular myocytes. *Circ. Res.* 99, 398–406. doi: 10.1161/01.RES.0000236756.06252.13

Gutierrez, D. A., Fernandez-Tenorio, M., Ogrodnik, J., and Niggli, E. (2013). NO-dependent Ca MKII activation during β-adrenergic stimulation of cardiac muscle. *Cardiovasc. Res.* 100, 392–401. doi: 10.1093/cvr/cvt201

Hall, D. D., Feekes, J. A., Arachchige Don, A. S., Shi, M., Hamid, J., Chen, L., et al. (2006). Binding of protein phosphatase 2A to the L-type calcium channel Cav1.2 next to Ser1928, its main PKA site, is critical for Ser1928 dephosphorylation. *Biochemistry* 45, 3448–3459. doi: 10.1021/bi051593z

Havens, M. A., and Hastings, M. L. (2016). Splice-switching antisense oligonucleotides as therapeutic drugs. *Nucleic Acids Res.* 44, 6549–6563. doi: 10.1093/nar/gkw533

He, B. J., Joiner, M.-L. A., Singh, M. V., Luczak, E. D., Swaminathan, P. D., Koval, O. M., et al. (2011). Oxidation of CaMKII determines the cardiotoxic effects of aldosterone. *Nat. Med.* 17, 1610–1618. doi: 10.1038/nm.2506

He, J., Jiang, S., Li, F., Zhao, X., Chu, E., Sun, M., et al. (2013). MicroRNA-30b-5p is involved in the regulation of cardiac hypertrophy by targeting CaMKIIδ. *J. Investig. Med.* 61, 604–612. doi: 10.2310/JIM.0b013e3182819ac6

Hegyi, B., Chen-Izu, Y., Jian, Z., Shimkunas, R., Izu, L. T., and Banyasz, T. (2015). KN-93 inhibits IKr in mammalian cardiomyocytes. *J. Mol. Cell. Cardiol.* 89, 173–176. doi: 10.1016/j.yjmcc.2015.10.012

Hoch, B., Meyer, R., Hetzer, R., Krause, E. G., and Karczewski, P. (1999). Identification and expression of delta-isoforms of the multifunctional Ca2 +/calmodulin-dependent protein kinase in failing and nonfailing human myocardium. *Circ. Res.* 84, 713–721. doi: 10.1161/01.RES.84.6.713

Hoehn, M., Zhang, Y., Xu, J., Gergs, U., Boknik, P., Werdan, K., et al. (2015). Overexpression of protein phosphatase 2A in a murine model of chronic myocardial infarction leads to increased adverse remodeling but restores the regulation of β-catenin by glycogen synthase kinase 3β. *Int. J. Cardiol.* 183, 39–46. doi: 10.1016/j.ijcard.2015.01.087

Howard, T., Greer-Short, A., Satroplus, T., Patel, N., Nassal, D., Mohler, P. J., et al. (2018). CaMKII-dependent late Na+ current increases electrical dispersion and arrhythmia in ischemia-reperfusion. *Am. J. Physiol. - Hear. Circ. Physiol.* 315, H794–H801. doi: 10.1152/ajpheart.00197.2018

Hudmon, A., Schulman, H., Kim, J., Maltez, J. M., Tsien, R. W., and Pitt, G. S. (2005). CaMKII tethers to L-type Ca2+ channels, establishing a local and dedicated integrator of Ca2+ signals for facilitation. *J. Cell Biol.* 171, 537–547. doi: 10.1083/jcb.200505155

Hund, T. J., Koval, O. M., Li, J., Wright, P. J., Qian, L., Snyder, J. S., et al. (2010). A βIV-spectrin/CaMKII signaling complex is essential for membrane excitability in mice. *J. Clin. Invest.* 120, 3508–3519. doi: 10.1172/JCI43621

Ishida, A., Kameshita, I., Okuno, S., Kitani, T., and Fujisawa, H. (1995). A novel highly specific and potent inhibitor of calmodulin-dependent protein kinase II. *Biochem. Biophys. Res. Commun.* 212, 806–812. doi: 10.1006/bbrc.1995.2040

Johnson, C. N., Pattanayek, R., Potet, F., Rebbeck, R. T., Blackwell, D. J., Nikolaienko, R., et al. (2019). The CaMKII inhibitor KN93-calmodulin interaction and implications for calmodulin tuning of NaV1.5 and RyR2 function. *Cell Calcium.* 82, 102063. doi: 10.1016/j.ceca.2019.102063

Joiner, M. L. A., and Koval, O. M. (2014). CaMKII and stress mix it up in mitochondria. *Front. Pharmacol.* 5, 67. doi: 10.3389/fphar.2014.00067

Joiner, M.-L. A., Koval, O. M., Li, J., He, B. J., Allamargot, C., Gao, Z., et al. (2012). CaMKII determines mitochondrial stress responses in heart. *Nature* 491, 269–273. doi: 10.1038/nature11444

Kaczmarek, J. C., Kowalski, P. S., and Anderson, D. G. (2017). Advances in the delivery of RNA therapeutics: from concept to clinical reality. *Genome Med.* 9, 60. doi: 10.1186/s13073-017-0450-0

Kaneko, N., Matsuda, R., Hata, Y., and Shimamoto, K. (2009). Pharmacological characteristics and clinical applications of K201. *Curr. Clin. Pharmacol.* 4, 126–131. doi: 10.2174/157488409788184972

Khoo, M. S. C., Li, J., Singh, M. V., Yang, Y., Kannankeril, P., Wu, Y., et al. (2006). Death, cardiac dysfunction, and arrhythmias are increased by calmodulin kinase II in calcineurin cardiomyopathy. *Circulation* 114, 1352–1359. doi: 10.1161/CIRCULATIONAHA.106.644583

Kirchhefer, U., Schmitz, W., Scholz, H., and Neumann, J. (1999). Activity of cAMP-dependent protein kinase and Ca2+/calmodulin-dependent protein kinase in failing and nonfailing human hearts. *Cardiovasc. Res.* 42, 254–261. doi: 10.1016/S0008-6363(98)00296-X

Koval, O. M., Guan, X., Wu, Y., Joiner, M. L., Gao, Z., Chen, B., et al. (2010). Ca V 1.2 β-subunit coordinates CaMKII-triggered cardiomyocyte death and afterdepolarizations. *Proc. Natl. Acad. Sci. U. S. A.* 107, 4996–5000. doi: 10.1073/pnas.0913760107

Koval, O. M., Snyder, J. S., Wolf, R. M., Pavlovicz, R. E., Glynn, P., Curran, J., et al. (2012). Ca2+/calmodulin-dependent protein kinase ii-based regulation of voltage-gated na+ channel in cardiac disease. *Circulation.* 126, 2084–2094. doi: 10.1161/CIRCULATIONAHA.112.105320

Laina, A., Gatsiou, A., Georgiopoulos, G., Stamatelopoulos, K., and Stellos, K. (2018). RNA therapeutics in cardiovascular precision medicine. *Front. Physiol.* 9, 953. doi: 10.3389/fphys.2018.00953

Lanner, J. T., Georgiou, D. K., Joshi, A. D., and Hamilton, S. L. (2010). Ryanodine receptors: structure, expression, molecular details, and function in calcium release. *Cold Spring Harb. Perspect. Biol.* 2, a003996. doi: 10.1101/cshperspect.a003996

Lebek, S., Plößl, A., Baier, M., Mustroph, J., Tarnowski, D., Lücht, C. M., et al. (2018). The novel CaMKII inhibitor GS-680 reduces diastolic SR Ca leak and prevents CaMKII-dependent pro-arrhythmic activity. *J. Mol. Cell. Cardiol.* 118, 159–168. doi: 10.1016/j.yjmcc.2018.03.020

Ledoux, J., Chartier, D., and Leblanc, N. (1999). Inhibitors of calmodulin-dependent protein kinase are nonspecific blockers of voltage-dependent K+ channels in vascular myocytes. *J. Pharmacol. Exp. Ther.* 290, 1165–1174.

Lehnart, S. E., Mongillo, M., Bellinger, A., Lindegger, N., Chen, B.-X., Hsueh, W., et al. (2008). Leaky Ca2+ release channel/ryanodine receptor 2 causes seizures and sudden cardiac death in mice. *J. Clin. Invest.* 118, 2230–2245. doi: 10.1172/JCI35346

Liang, F., Fan, P., Jia, J., Yang, S., Jiang, Z., Karpinski, S., et al. (2016). Inhibitions of late INa and CaMKII act synergistically to prevent ATX-II-induced atrial fibrillation in isolated rat right atria. *J. Mol. Cell. Cardiol.* 94, 122–130. doi: 10.1016/j.yjmcc.2016.04.001

Ling, H., Zhang, T., Pereira, L., Means, C. K., Cheng, H., Gu, Y., et al. (2009). Requirement for Ca2+/calmodulin-dependent kinase II in the transition from pressure overload-induced cardiac hypertrophy to heart failure in mice. *J. Clin. Invest.* 119, 1230–1240. doi: 10.1172/JCI38022

Little, G. H., Saw, A., Bai, Y., Dow, J., Marjoram, P., Simkhovich, B., et al. (2009). Critical role of nuclear calcium/calmodulin-dependent protein kinase IIδB in cardiomyocyte survival in cardiomyopathy. *J. Biol. Chem.* 284, 24857–24868. doi: 10.1074/jbc.M109.003186

Liu, J., Carmell, M. A., Rivas, F. V., Marsden, C. G., Thomson, J. M., Song, J. J., et al. (2004). Argonaute2 is the catalytic engine of mammalian RNAi. *Science* (80-.), 1437–1441. doi: 10.1126/science.1102513

Liu, W., Zi, M., Naumann, R., Ulm, S., Jin, J., Taglieri, D. M., et al. (2011). Pak1 as a novel therapeutic target for antihypertrophic treatment in the heart. *Circulation* 124, 2702–2715. doi: 10.1161/CIRCULATIONAHA.111.048785

Liu, W., Zi, M., Tsui, H., Chowdhury, S. K., Zeef, L., Meng, Q.-J., et al. (2013). A novel immunomodulator, FTY-720 reverses existing cardiac hypertrophy and fibrosis from pressure overload by targeting NFAT (nuclear factor of activated T-cells) signaling and periostin. *Circ. Heart Fail.* 6, 833–844. doi: 10.1161/CIRCHEARTFAILURE.112.000123

Lokuta, A. J., Rogers, T. B., Lederer, W. J., and Valdivia, H. H. (1995). Modulation of cardiac ryanodine receptors of swine and rabbit by a phosphorylation-dephosphorylation mechanism. *J. Physiol.* 487, 609–622. doi: 10.1113/jphysiol.1995.sp020904

Lu, Y.-M., Huang, J., Shioda, N., Fukunaga, K., Shirasaki, Y., Li, X.-M., et al. (2011a). CaMKIIδB mediates aberrant NCX1 expression and the imbalance of NCX1/SERCA in transverse aortic constriction-induced failing heart. *PloS One* 6, e24724. doi: 10.1371/journal.pone.0024724

Lu, Y. M., Huang, J., Shioda, N., Fukunaga, K., Shirasaki, Y., Li, ,. X. M., et al. (2011b). Camkiiδb mediates aberrant NCX1 expression and the imbalance of NCX1/SERCA in transverse aortic Constriction-Induced failing heart. *PloS One* 6, e24724. doi: 10.1371/journal.pone.0024724

Lubbers, E. R., and Mohler, P. J. (2016). Roles and regulation of protein phosphatase 2A (PP2A) in the heart. *J. Mol. Cell. Cardiol.* 101, 127–133. doi: 10.1016/j.yjmcc.2016.11.003

Lucas, T., and Dimmeler, S. (2016). RNA therapeutics for treatment of cardiovascular diseases. *Circ. Res.* 119, 794–797. doi: 10.1161/CIRCRESAHA.116.308730

Luo, M., Guan, X., Luczak, E. D., Lang, D., Kutschke, W., Gao, Z., et al. (2013). Diabetes increases mortality after myocardial infarction by oxidizing CaMKII. *J. Clin. Invest.* 123, 1262–1274. doi: 10.1172/JCI65268

Maier, L. S., and Bers, D. M. (2002). Calcium, calmodulin, and calcium-calmodulin kinase II: heartbeat to heartbeat and beyond. *J. Mol. Cell. Cardiol.* 34, 919–939. doi: 10.1006/jmcc.2002.2038

Malinow, R., Schulman, H., and Tsien, R. W. (1989). Inhibition of postsynaptic PKC or CaMKII blocks induction but not expression of LTP. *Science* (80-.), 862–866. doi: 10.1126/science.2549638

Mattiazzi, A., and Kranias, E. G. (2014). The role of CaMKII regulation of phospholamban activity in heart disease. *Front. Pharmacol.* 5, 5. doi: 10.3389/fphar.2014.00005

Mattiazzi, A., Bassani, R. A., Escobar, A. L., Palomeque, J., Valverde, C. A., Vila Petroff, M., et al. (2015). Chasing cardiac physiology and pathology down the caMKII cascade. *Am. J. Physiol. - Hear. Circ. Physiol.* 308, H1177–H1191. doi: 10.1152/ajpheart.00007.2015

Mavunkel, B., Xu, ,. Y. J., Goyal, B., Lim, D., Lu, Q., Chen, Z., et al. (2008). Pyrimidine-based inhibitors of CaMKIIδ. *Bioorganic Med. Chem. Lett.* 18, 2404–2408. doi: 10.1016/j.bmcl.2008.02.056

McClinch, K., Avelar, R. A., Callejas, D., Izadmehr, S., Wiredja, D., Perl, A., et al. (2018). Small-molecule activators of protein phosphatas 2A for the treatment of castration-resistant prostate cancer. *Cancer Res.* 78, 2065–2080. doi: 10.1158/0008-5472.CAN-17-0123

Meister, G. (2013). Argonaute proteins: functional insights and emerging roles. *Nat. Rev. Genet.* 14, 447–459. doi: 10.1038/nrg3462

Michalski, P. J. (2013). The delicate bistability of CaMKII. *Biophys. J.* 105, 794–806. doi: 10.1016/j.bpj.2013.06.038

Mills, N. L., Donaldson, K., Hadoke, P. W., Boon, N. A., MacNee, W., Cassee, F. R., et al. (2009). Adverse cardiovascular effects of air pollution. *Nat. Clin. Pract. Cardiovasc. Med.* 6, 36–44. doi: 10.1038/ncpcardio1399

Miragoli, M., Ceriotti, P., Iafisco, M., Vacchiano, M., Salvarani, N., Alogna, A., et al. (2018). Inhalation of peptide-loaded nanoparticles improves heart failure. *Sci. Transl. Med.* 10, eaan6205. doi: 10.1126/scitranslmed.aan6205

Morotti, S., Edwards, A. G., Mcculloch, A. D., Bers, D. M., and Grandi, E. (2014). A novel computational model of mouse myocyte electrophysiology to assess the synergy between Na+loading and CaMKII. *J. Physiol.* 592, 1181–1197. doi: 10.1113/jphysiol.2013.266676

Mustroph, J., Neef, S., and Maier, L. S. (2017). CaMKII as a target for arrhythmia suppression. *Pharmacol. Ther.* 176, 22–31. doi: 10.1016/j.pharmthera.2016.10.006

Neef, S., Steffens, A., Pellicena, P., Mustroph, J., Lebek, S., Ort, K. R., et al. (2018). Improvement of cardiomyocyte function by a novel pyrimidine-based CaMKII-inhibitor. *J. Mol. Cell. Cardiol.* 115, 73–81. doi: 10.1016/j.yjmcc.2017.12.015

Nie, J., Duan, Q., He, M., Li, X., Wang, B., Zhou, C., et al. (2019). Ranolazine prevents pressure overload-induced cardiac hypertrophy and heart failure by restoring aberrant Na + and Ca 2+ handling. *J. Cell. Physiol.* 234, 11587–11601. doi: 10.1002/jcp.27791

Olivotto, I., Camici, P. G., Merlini, P. A., Rapezzi, C., Patten, M., Climent, V., et al. (2018). Efficacy of ranolazine in patients with symptomatic hypertrophic cardiomyopathy. *Circ. Hear. Fail.* 11, e004124. doi: 10.1161/CIRCHEARTFAILURE.117.004124

Onal, B., Gratz, D., and Hund, T. J. (2017). Ca2+/calmodulin-dependent kinase II-dependent regulation of atrial myocyte late Na+ current, Ca2+ cycling, and excitability: a mathematical modeling study. *Am. J. Physiol. Heart Circ. Physiol.* 313, H1227–H1239. doi: 10.1152/ajpheart.00185.2017

Otvos, L., and Wade, J. D. (2014). Current challenges in peptide-based drug discovery. *Front. Chem.* 2, 62. doi: 10.3389/fchem.2014.00062

Ozcan, G., Ozpolat, B., Coleman, R. L., Sood, A. K., and Lopez-Berestein, G. (2015). Preclinical and clinical development of siRNA-based therapeutics. *Adv. Drug Deliv. Rev.* 87, 108–119. doi: 10.1016/j.addr.2015.01.007

Parra, V., and Rothermel, B. A. (2017). Calcineurin signaling in the heart: The importance of time and place. *J. Mol. Cell. Cardiol.* 103, 121–136. doi: 10.1016/j.yjmcc.2016.12.006

Payne, M. E., Fong, Y. L., Ono, T., Colbran, R. J., Kemp, B. E., Soderling, T. R., et al. (1988). Calcium/calmodulin-dependent protein kinase II. Characterization of distinct calmodulin binding and inhibitory domains. *J. Biol. Chem.* 263, 7190–7195.

Pellicena, P., and Schulman, H. (2014). CaMKII inhibitors: from research tools to therapeutic agents. *Front. Pharmacol.* 5, 21. doi: 10.3389/fphar.2014.00021

Peng, W., Zhang, Y., Zheng, M., Cheng, H., Zhu, W., Cao, C. M., et al. (2010). Cardioprotection by CaMKII-δB is mediated by phosphorylation of heat shock factor 1 and subsequent expression of inducible heat shock protein 70. *Circ. Res.* 106, 102–110. doi: 10.1161/CIRCRESAHA.109.210914

Penny, W. F., and Hammond, H. K. (2017). Randomized clinical trials of gene transfer for heart failure with reduced ejection fraction. *Hum. Gene Ther.* 28, 378–384. doi: 10.1089/hum.2016.166

Purohit, A., Rokita, A. G., Guan, X., Chen, B., Koval, O. M., Voigt, N., et al. (2013). Oxidized Ca(2+)/calmodulin-dependent protein kinase II triggers atrial fibrillation. *Circulation* 128, 1748–1757. doi: 10.1161/CIRCULATIONAHA.113.003313

Ramirez, M. T., Zhao, X. L., Schulman, H., and Brown, J. H. (1997). The nuclear deltaB isoform of Ca2+/calmodulin-dependent protein kinase II regulates atrial natriuretic factor gene expression in ventricular myocytes. *J. Biol. Chem.* 272, 31203–31208. doi: 10.1074/jbc.272.49.31203

Rand, T. A., Petersen, S., Du, F., and Wang, X. (2005). Argonaute2 cleaves the anti-guide strand of siRNA during RISC activation. *Cell* 123, 621–629. doi: 10.1016/j.cell.2005.10.020

Rastogi, S., Sharov, V. G., Mishra, S., Gupta, R. C., Blackburn, B., Belardinelli, L., et al. (2008). Ranolazine combined with enalapril or metoprolol prevents progressive LV dysfunction and remodeling in dogs with moderate heart failure. *Am. J. Physiol. - Hear. Circ. Physiol.* 295, H2149–H2155. doi: 10.1152/ajpheart.00728.2008

Rayner-Hartley, E., and Sedlak, T. (2015). Ranolazine: a contemporary review. *J. Am. Heart Assoc.* 5, e003196. doi: 10.1161/JAHA.116.003196

Remmerie, M., and Janssens, V. (2019). PP2A: a promising biomarker and therapeutic target in endometrial cancer. *Front. Oncol.* 9, 462. doi: 10.3389/fonc.2019.00462

Rezazadeh, S., Claydon, T. W., and Fedida, D. (2006). KN-93 (2-[N-(2-hydroxyethyl)]-N-(4-methoxybenzenesulfonyl)]amino-N-(4-chlorocinnamyl)-N-methylbenzylamine), a calcium/calmodulin-dependent protein kinase II inhibitor, is a direct extracellular blocker of voltage-gated potassium channels. *J. Pharmacol. Exp. Ther.* 317, 292–299. doi: 10.1124/jpet.105.097618

Sag, C. M., Köhler, A. C., Anderson, M. E., Backs, J., and Maier, L. S. (2011). CaMKII-dependent SR Ca leak contributes to doxorubicin-induced impaired Ca handling in isolated cardiac myocytes. *J. Mol. Cell. Cardiol.* 51, 749–759. doi: 10.1016/j.yjmcc.2011.07.016

Shan, J., Betzenhauser, M. J., Kushnir, A., Reiken, S., Meli, A. C., Wronska, A., et al. (2010). Role of chronic ryanodine receptor phosphorylation in heart failure and β-adrenergic receptor blockade in mice. *J. Clin. Invest.* 120, 4375–4387. doi: 10.1172/JCI37649

Shi, Y. (2009). Serine/threonine phosphatases: mechanism through structure. *Cell* 139, 468–484. doi: 10.1016/j.cell.2009.10.006

Silva, A. J., Paylor, R., Wehner, J. M., and Tonegawa, S. (1992a). Impaired spatial learning in alpha-calcium-calmodulin kinase II mutant mice. *Science* 257, 206–211. doi: 10.1126/science.1321493

Silva, A. J., Stevens, C. F., Tonegawa, S., and Wang, Y. (1992b). Deficient hippocampal long-term potentiation in alpha-calcium-calmodulin kinase II mutant mice. *Science* 257, 201–206. doi: 10.1126/science.1378648

Siomi, H., and Siomi, M. C. (2009). On the road to reading the RNA-interference code. *Nature* 457, 396–404. doi: 10.1038/nature07754

Sledz, C. A., Holko, M., De Veer, M. J., Silverman, R. H., and Williams, B. R. G. (2003). Activation of the interferon system by short-interfering RNAs. *Nat. Cell Biol.* 5, 834–839. doi: 10.1038/ncb1038

Smyth, J. T., Abbott, A. L., Lee, B., Sienaert, I., Kasri, N. N., De Smedt, H., et al. (2002). Inhibition of the inositol trisphosphate receptor of mouse eggs and A7r5 cells by KN-93 via a mechanism unrelated to Ca 2+/calmodulin-dependent protein kinase II antagonism. *J. Biol. Chem.* 277, 35061–35070. doi: 10.1074/jbc.M202928200

Srinivasan, M., Edman, C. F., and Schulman, H. (1994). Alternative splicing introduces a nuclear localization signal that targets multifunctional CaM kinase to the nucleus. *J. Cell Biol.* 126, 839–852. doi: 10.1083/jcb.126.4.839

Stevens, C. F., Tonegawa, S., and Wang, Y. (1994). The role of calcium-calmodulin kinase II in three forms of synaptic plasticity. *Curr. Biol.* 4, 687–693. doi: 10.1016/S0960-9822(00)00153-6

Sumi, M., Kiuchi, K., Ishikawa, T., Ishii, A., Hagiwara, M., Nagatsu, T., et al. (1991). The newly synthesized selective Ca2+/calmodulin dependent protein kinase II inhibitor KN-93 reduces dopamine contents in PC12h cells. *Biochem. Biophys. Res. Commun.* 181, 968–975. doi: 10.1016/0006-291X(91)92031-E

Swaminathan, P. D., Purohit, A., Soni, S., Voigt, N., Singh, M. V., Glukhov, A. V., et al. (2011). Oxidized CaMKII causes cardiac sinus node dysfunction in mice. *J. Clin. Invest.* 121, 3277–3288. doi: 10.1172/JCI57833

Swaminathan, P. D., Purohit, A., Hund, T. J., and Anderson, M. E. (2012). Calmodulin-dependent protein kinase II: linking heart failure and arrhythmias. *Circ. Res.* 110, 1661–1677. doi: 10.1161/CIRCRESAHA.111.243956

Tobimatsu, T., and Fujisawa, H. (1989). Tissue-specific expression of four types of rat calmodulin-dependent protein kinase II mRNAs. *J. Biol. Chem.* 264, 17907–17912. doi: 10.1016/0921-8696(89)90769-X

Unudurthi, S. D., Nassal, D., Greer-Short, A., Patel, N., Howard, T., Xu, X., et al. (2018). βIV-Spectrin regulates STAT3 targeting to tune cardiac response to pressure overload. *J. Clin. Invest.* 128, 5561–5572. doi: 10.1172/JCI99245

Verdine, G. L., and Walensky, L. D. (2007). The challenge of drugging undruggable targets in cancer: lessons learned from targeting BCL-2 family members. *Clin. Cancer Res.* 13, 7264–7270. doi: 10.1158/1078-0432.CCR-07-2184

Vest, R. S., O'Leary, H., Coultrap, S. J., Kindy, M. S., and Bayer, K. U. (2010). Effective post-insult neuroprotection by a novel Ca2+/calmodulin-dependent protein kinase II (CaMKII) inhibitor. *J. Biol. Chem.* 285, 20675–20682. doi: 10.1074/jbc.M109.088617

Wagner, S., Ruff, H. M., Weber, S. L., Bellmann, S., Sowa, T., Schulte, T., et al. (2011). Reactive oxygen species-activated Ca/calmodulin kinase IIδ is required for late I(Na) augmentation leading to cellular Na and Ca overload. *Circ. Res.* 108, 555–565. doi: 10.1161/CIRCRESAHA.110.221911

Wang, X., Zhang, X., Ren, X.-P., Chen, J., Liu, H., Yang, J., et al. (2010). MicroRNA-494 targeting both proapoptotic and antiapoptotic proteins protects against ischemia/reperfusion-induced cardiac injury. *Circulation* 122, 1308–1318. doi: 10.1161/CIRCULATIONAHA.110.964684

Wehrens, X. H. T., Lehnart, S. E., Reiken, S. R., and Marks, A. R. (2004). Ca2+/calmodulin-dependent protein kinase II phosphorylation regulates the cardiac ryanodine receptor. *Circ. Res.* 94, e61–e70. doi: 10.1161/01.RES.0000125626.33738.E2

Wehrens, X. H. T. (2011). CaMKII regulation of the cardiac ryanodine receptor and sarcoplasmic reticulum calcium release. *Hear. Rhythm.* 8, 323–325. doi: 10.1016/j.hrthm.2010.09.079

Westenbrink, B. D., Edwards, A. G., McCulloch, A. D., and Brown, J. H. (2013). The promise of CaMKII inhibition for heart disease: preventing heart failure and arrhythmias. *Expert Opin. Ther. Targets* 17, 889–903. doi: 10.1517/14728222.2013.809064

Witcher, D. R., Kovacs, R. J., Schulman, H., Cefali, D. C., and Jones, L. R. (1991). Unique phosphorylation site on the cardiac ryanodine receptor regulates calcium channel activity. *J. Biol. Chem.* 266, 11144–11152.

Wu, Y., Temple, J., Zhang, R., Dzhura, I., Zhang, W., Trimble, R., et al. (2002). Calmodulin kinase II and arrhythmias in a mouse model of cardiac hypertrophy. *Circulation* 106, 1288–1293. doi: 10.1161/01.CIR.0000027583.73268.E7

Wu, X., Zhang, T., Bossuyt, J., Li, X., McKinsey, T. A., Dedman, J. R., et al. (2006). Local InsP3-dependent perinuclear Ca2+ signaling in cardiac myocyte excitation-transcription coupling. *J. Clin. Invest.* 116, 675–682. doi: 10.1172/JCI27374

Xu, H., Ginsburg, K. S., Hall, D. D., Zimmermann, M., Stein, I. S., Zhang, M., et al. (2010). Targeting of protein phosphatases PP2A and PP2B to the C-terminus of the L-type calcium channel Ca v1.2. *Biochemistry* 49, 10298–10307. doi: 10.1021/bi101018c

Yang, D., Zhu, W.-Z., Xiao, B., Brochet, D. X. P., Chen, S. R. W., Lakatta, E. G., et al. (2007). Ca2+/calmodulin kinase II-dependent phosphorylation of ryanodine receptors suppresses Ca2+ sparks and Ca2+ waves in cardiac myocytes. *Circ. Res.* 100, 399–407. doi: 10.1161/01.RES.0000258022.13090.55

Yano, M., Kobayashi, S., Kohno, M., Doi, M., Tokuhisa, T., Okuda, S., et al. (2003). FKBP12.6-Mediated stabilization of calcium-release channel (ryanodine receptor) as a novel therapeutic strategy against heart failure. *Circulation* 107, 477–484. doi: 10.1161/01.CIR.0000044917.74408.BE

Yao, L., Fan, P., Jiang, Z., Viatchenko-Karpinski, S., Wu, Y., Kornyeyev, D., et al. (2011). Na v 1.5-dependent persistent Na + influx activates CaMKII in rat ventricular myocytes and N 1325 S mice. *Am. J. Physiol. - Cell Physiol.* 301, C577–C586. doi: 10.1152/ajpcell.00125.2011

Yeh, E. T. H., and Bickford, C. L. (2009). Cardiovascular complications of cancer therapy: incidence, pathogenesis, diagnosis, and management. *J. Am. Coll. Cardiol.* 53, 2231–2247. doi: 10.1016/j.jacc.2009.02.050

Zareba, W., Daubert, J. P., Beck, C. A., Huang, D. T., Alexis, J. D., Brown, M. W., et al. (2018). Ranolazine in high-risk patients with implanted cardioverter-defibrillators: The RAID trial. *J. Am. Coll. Cardiol.* 72, 636–645. doi: 10.1016/j.jacc.2018.04.086

Zhang, T., Johnson, E. N., Gu, Y., Morissette, M. R., Sah, V. P., Gigena, M. S., et al. (2002). The cardiac-specific nuclear δ B isoform of Ca 2+/Calmodulin-dependent protein kinase II induces hypertrophy and dilated cardiomyopathy associated with increased protein phosphatase 2A activity. *J. Biol. Chem.* 277, 1261–1267. doi: 10.1074/jbc.M108525200

Zhang, T., Maier, L. S., Dalton, N. D., Miyamoto, S., Ross, J., Bers, D. M., et al. (2003). The δc isoform of CaMKII is activated in cardiac hypertrophy and induces dilated cardiomyopathy and heart failure. *Circ. Res.* 92, 912–919. doi: 10.1161/01.RES.0000069686.31472.C5

Zhang, R., Khoo, M. S. C., Wu, Y., Yang, Y., Grueter, C. E., Ni, G., et al. (2005). Calmodulin kinase II inhibition protects against structural heart disease. *Nat. Med.* 11, 409–417. doi: 10.1038/nm1215

6

Calcium Handling Defects and Cardiac Arrhythmia Syndromes

Kornél Kistamás [1,2], Roland Veress [1], Balázs Horváth [1], Tamás Bányász [1], Péter P. Nánási [1,3] and David A. Eisner [2]*

[1] Department of Physiology, Faculty of Medicine, University of Debrecen, Debrecen, Hungary, [2] Division of Cardiovascular Sciences, School of Medical Sciences, University of Manchester, Manchester, United Kingdom, [3] Department of Dental Physiology, Faculty of Dentistry, University of Debrecen, Debrecen, Hungary

***Correspondence:**
Kornél Kistamás
kistamas.kornel@med.unideb.hu

Calcium ions (Ca^{2+}) play a major role in the cardiac excitation-contraction coupling. Intracellular Ca^{2+} concentration increases during systole and falls in diastole thereby determining cardiac contraction and relaxation. Normal cardiac function also requires perfect organization of the ion currents at the cellular level to drive action potentials and to maintain action potential propagation and electrical homogeneity at the tissue level. Any imbalance in Ca^{2+} homeostasis of a cardiac myocyte can lead to electrical disturbances. This review aims to discuss cardiac physiology and pathophysiology from the elementary membrane processes that can cause the electrical instability of the ventricular myocytes through intracellular Ca^{2+} handling maladies to inherited and acquired arrhythmias. Finally, the paper will discuss the current therapeutic approaches targeting cardiac arrhythmias.

Keywords: calcium signalling, cardiac arrhythmias, catecholaminergic polymorphic ventricular tachycardia, long QT syndrome, atrial fibrillation, reentry, early afterdepolarization, delayed afterdepolarization

INTRODUCTION

Excitation-contraction coupling (E-C coupling) of the cardiac myocytes is a well studied phenomenon. We know that the calcium ion (Ca^{2+}) plays a major role in controlling contraction and force, a feature that was originally described by Sidney Ringer more than a century ago (Ringer, 1883). Since this discovery, it has become clear that changes in intracellular Ca^{2+} concentration ($[Ca^{2+}]_i$) have a significant role in virtually all parts of the human body. Of particular importance is the fact, that within cardiac myocytes, $[Ca^{2+}]_i$ changes must be tightly regulated, so that the heart can beat rhythmically. This means that during the cardiac systole, $[Ca^{2+}]_i$ has to increase to certain levels to make contraction occur and must fall

---

Abbreviations: AF, atrial fibrillation; AP, action potential; APD, action potential duration; AV, atrioventricular; BrS, Brugada syndrome; CaM, calmodulin; CaMKII, Ca^{2+}/calmodulin-dependent protein kinase II; CICR, Ca^{2+}-induced Ca^{2+} release; CPVT, catecholaminergic polymorphic ventricular tachycardia; CSQ2, calsequestrin 2; DAD, delayed afterdepolarization; EAD, early afterdepolarization; EC, excitation-contraction coupling; ERS, early repolarization syndrome; HF, heart failure; ICD, implantable cardiac defibrillator; IVF, idiopathic ventricular fibrillation; LQTS, long QT syndrome; NCX, sodium-calcium exchange; NFAT, nuclear factor of activated T-cells; PKA, protein kinase A; PLN, phospholamban; PMCA, plasma membrane Ca^{2+}-ATPase; PVC, premature ventricular contraction; RSV, relative short term beat-to-beat variability of action potential duration; RyR, ryanodine receptor; SA, sinoatrial; SERCA, sarco/endoplasmic reticulum Ca^{2+}-ATPase; SOCE, store overload-induced Ca^{2+} entry; SOICR, store overload-induced Ca^{2+} release; SQTS, short QT syndrome; SR, sarcoplasmic reticulum; SV, short term beat-to-beat variability of action potential duration; VF, ventricular fibrillation; VT, ventricular tachycardia.

in diastole, allowing the muscle to relax and prepare for the next cardiac cycle. E-C coupling has been reviewed in detail (Bers, 2002; Eisner et al., 2017), here we consider the elementary steps and the events that can lead to electrical disturbances (**Figure 1**).

The normal cardiac action potential (AP) originates in the sinoatrial node and propagates through the heart. In the ventricle the initial depolarization opens voltage-gated sodium channels leading to further depolarization which, in turn, opens the L-type Ca^{2+} channels, causing a large Ca^{2+}-influx (**Figure 1A**). Some Ca^{2+} can also enter *via* T-type Ca^{2+} channels and reverse mode Na^{+}/Ca^{2+} exchange (NCX) (Kohomoto et al., 1994; Sipido et al., 1997). This Ca^{2+} entry triggers a process known as calcium-induced calcium release (CICR), in which Ca^{2+} is released from the sarcoplasmic reticulum (SR) into the cytoplasm *via* ryanodine receptors (RyR), allowing Ca^{2+} to bind to the myofilament protein troponin C, activating the contractile machinery. Normal cardiac function also requires relaxation to occur; this results from a decrease of free cytoplasmic Ca^{2+} levels. Several Ca^{2+} transport pathways are involved in this process, as Ca^{2+} reuptake into the SR by the SR Ca^{2+}-ATPase (SERCA), Ca^{2+} extrusion by the sarcolemmal NCX and plasma membrane Ca^{2+}-ATPase (PMCA) (**Figure 1B**) (Bers, 2000). This normal cardiac function requires perfect coordination of the ion currents and intracellular processes, as any imbalance in Ca^{2+} homeostasis of a cardiac myocyte can lead to electrical disturbances (from cellular AP prolongation to complex arrhythmic storms) (Eisner et al., 2017; Eisner, 2018).

Here we review the role of Ca^{2+} in generating and maintaining cardiac arrhythmias from basic arrhythmia mechanisms to recent progresses in pharmacological challenges and possible future therapies.

CALCIUM IN PATHOPHYSIOLOGY, ARRHYTHMIA MECHANISMS

Arrhythmia mechanisms have multiscale dynamics in the heart. The lower end is the molecular scale, originating from the stochastic behavior of ion channels, resulting from thermodynamic fluctuations (Qu and Weiss, 2015). Next is the cellular scale, with differences in the shape of the APs originating from distant parts of the myocardium (**Figure 2A**). Under some diseased conditions, several mechanisms can lead to electrical disturbances at the cellular level, including early or delayed afterdepolarizations (EAD or DAD, respectively) (**Figures 3A–D**). Whole-cell Ca^{2+} oscillations, developing into propagating Ca^{2+} waves arise when the molecular and cellular dynamics merge at the tissue and organ level. The lower and higher scales tend to have a bidirectional information flow. A good example is when EADs arising during an AP due to abnormal ion currents and Ca^{2+} dynamics, can bring an extra amount of Ca^{2+} into the cell due to L-type Ca^{2+} channel reopening and potentiate Ca^{2+} waves. These multiscale dynamics can lead to life threatening complex arrhythmias.

Normal cardiac automaticity originates in the sinoatrial (SA) node. If SA node impulse generation is impaired, atrioventricular node (AV node) and Purkinje fibers can show automatic activity. These secondary pacemakers are also called latent or subsidiary pacemakers (Antzelevitch and Burashnikov, 2011). SA node pacemaker activity depends on interactions of membrane potential and $[Ca^{2+}]_i$. This "coupled-clock" pacemaker system

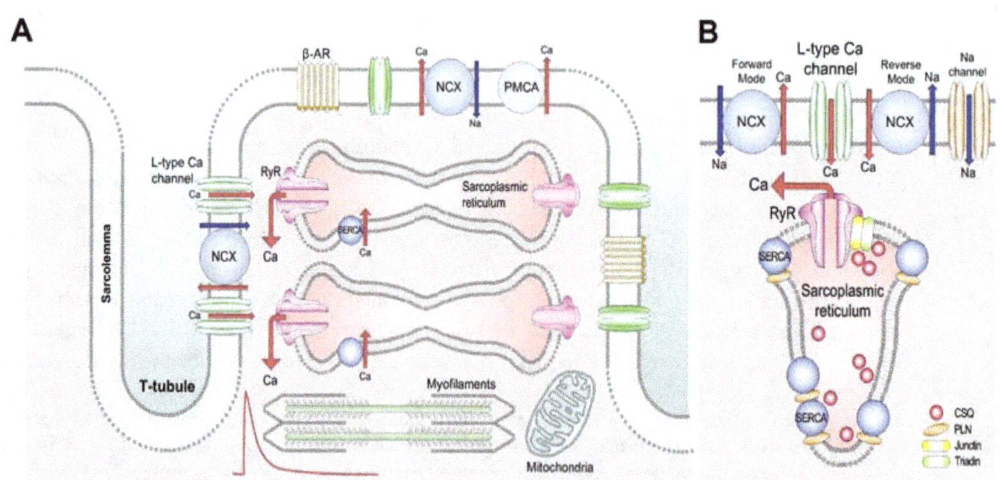

FIGURE 1 | Schematic diagram of the cardiac excitation-contraction coupling. **(A)** Structures involved in Ca^{2+} transport in cardiac mycocytes. Red trace shows a typical systolic Ca^{2+} transient. Briefly, during the Ca^{2+}-induced Ca^{2+} release process, Ca^{2+} entering the cell *via* L-type Ca^{2+} channels releases a larger amount of Ca^{2+} from the sarcoplasmic reticulum to activate the contractile machinery. Ca^{2+} extrusion requires NCX, PMCA, and SERCA. **(B)** Detailed section of the dyad showing the major proteins involved in Ca^{2+} cycling. Reproduced from Eisner et al. used with permission (Eisner et al., 2017). β-AR, β adrenoceptor; NCX, Na^{+}-Ca^{2+} exchange; PMCA, plasma membrane Ca^{2+}-ATPase; RyR, ryanodine receptor; SERCA, sarco/endoplasmic reticulum Ca^{2+}-ATPase; CSQ, calsequestrin; PLN, phospholamban.

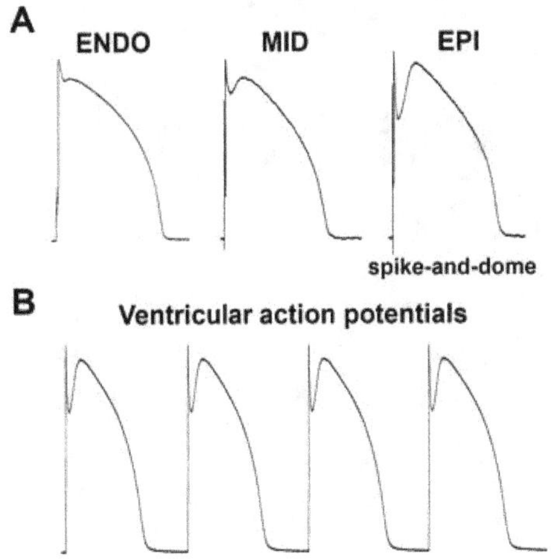

FIGURE 2 | Cellular physiological electrical activities. **(A)** Transmural heterogeneity in the cardiac ventricular action potential, showing (from left to right) recordings from: subendocardium, midmyocardium, and subepicardium. Note the spike-and-dome action potential configuration in the subepicardium. ENDO, subendocardial mycocyte; MID, midmyocardial "M" myocyte; EPI, subepicardial myocyte. **(B)** Series of typical subepicardial ventricular action potentials at normal pacing activity.

is produced by membrane proteins, driving the AP and the intracellular Ca^{2+} cycling molecules (**Figure 4**) (Maltsev et al., 2006; Lakatta, 2010; Joung et al., 2011).

The "membrane clock" implies sarcolemmal proteins, continuously driving the membrane potential to more positive or more negative values. The most important and well-known participant is the hyperpolarization-activated funny current (I_f), working mainly during early diastolic depolarization. The consequent depolarization opens Ca^{2+} channels ($I_{Ca,T}$ and $I_{Ca,L}$) and the pacemaker (slow type) action potential occurs. As in the case of the working myocardium, K^+ currents repolarize the membrane. In the last two decades it has become clear that spontaneous Ca^{2+} release in a cardiac cell is not always pathological. In the "calcium clock" mechanism, spontaneous SR Ca^{2+} release events, the Ca^{2+} sparks activate I_{NCX} and cause late diastolic membrane depolarization. Coupled clock pacemaker system comprises functional interactions between the membrane and calcium clock (**Figure 4**) (Vinogradova et al., 2006; Lakatta and DiFrancesco, 2009; Lakatta et al., 2010).

For physiological contraction and relaxation, not only pacemaker automaticity, but also the impulse conduction system needs to work properly. Spontaneous depolarization from the SA node propagates and depolarizes the distant parts of the cardiac muscle (**Figure 2B**), *via* the SA node, AV node, Bundle of His, Bundle branches, and Purkinje fibers pathway.

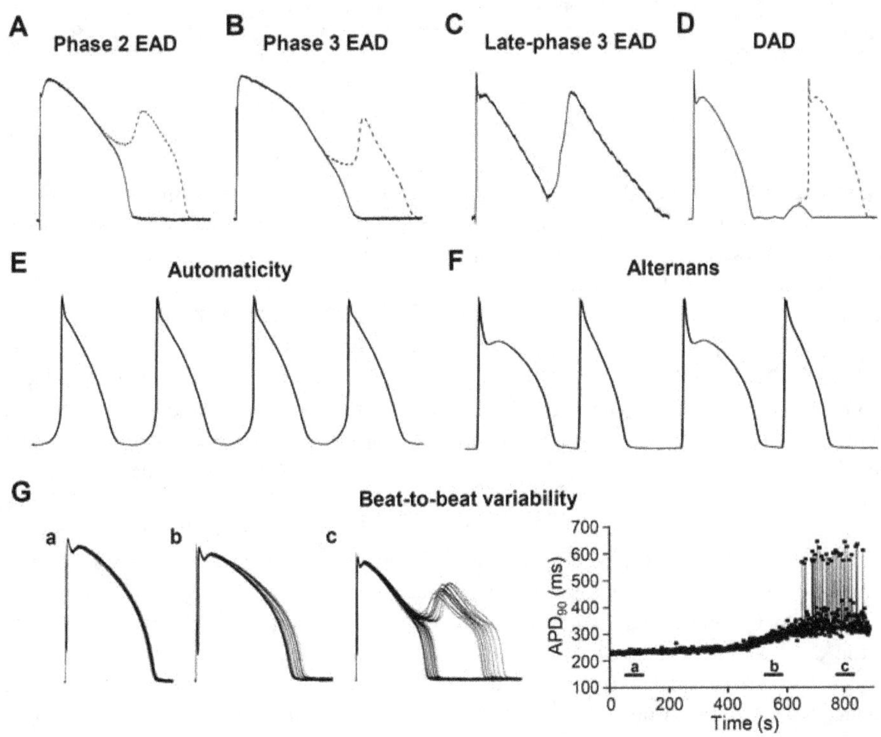

FIGURE 3 | Cellular pathophysiological electrical activities. **(A)** Phase 2 early afterdepolarization (EAD), **(B)** Phase 3 EAD, **(C)** Late-phase 3 EAD, **(D)** Delayed afterdepolarization (DAD) manifesting triggered activity. Ca^{2+} has an important role in generating afterdepolarizations. Underlying mechanisms are described in the relevant sections. **(E)** Automaticity (spontaneous membrane potential oscillations) occurs if the membrane potential of the cells shift to more positive values causing abnormal activity. **(F)** Cardiac voltage alternans, manifesting a long-short-long-short pattern. **(G)** Short term beat-to-beat variability of the action potential duration. **(a)**, **(b)**, and **(c)** show different time points after interventions that increase action potential duration and beat-to-beat variability leading to EAD generation. Right panel of **(G)** shows action potential duration at 90% of the repolarization (APD_{90}) as a function of time.

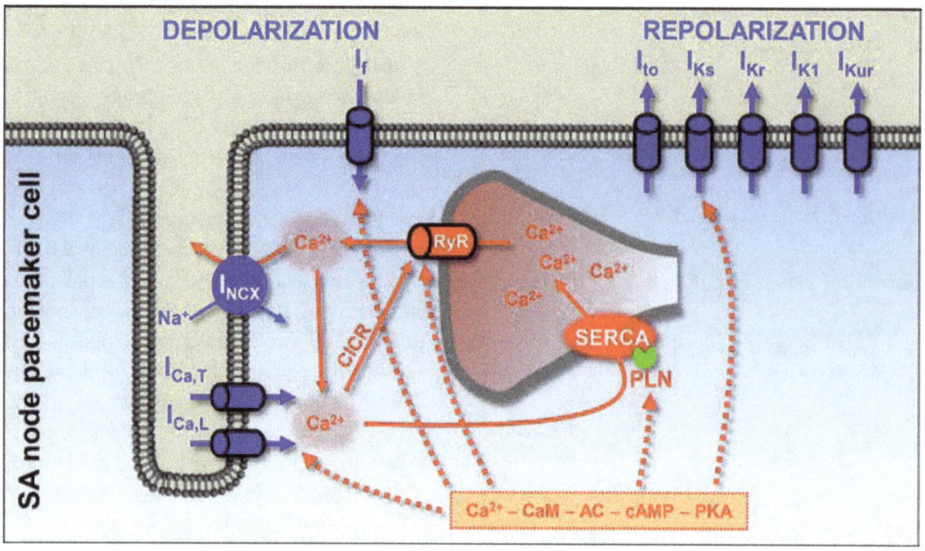

FIGURE 4 | The origin of the heartbeat: coupled-clock pacemaker system in the sinoatrial cells. The pacemaker activity of the SA node originates from the membrane and calcium clock mechanisms. The former is composed of the sarcolemmal channel proteins, and the latter results from sarcoplasmic reticulum and sarcoplasmic Ca^{2+} turnover. At end of the SA action potential the hyperpolarization-activated I_f depolarizes the membrane to a level where Ca^{2+} channels open. In addition, during late diastole, spontaneous SR Ca^{2+} releases further depolarize the membrane by activating I_{NCX}. Ca^{2+} can bind to calmodulin and activate adenylyl cyclase (AC). High constitutive activation of AC leading to high basal level of cAMP (which is needed for protein kinase A-dependent phosphorylation) in SA node cells has been suggested to contribute to the Ca^{2+} overload state. PKA-dependent phosphorylation of phospholamban, $I_{Ca,L}$, and RyR promotes spontaneous Ca^{2+} release. Blue shows the membrane clock and red shows the calcium clock mechanism. Solid arrows show the Ca^{2+}-induced Ca^{2+} release process and spontaneous Ca^{2+} release events *via* RyR; dashed arrows show the phosphorylation targets of the cAMP–PKA pathway. $I_{Ca,L}$, L-type Ca^{2+} current; $I_{Ca,T}$, T-type Ca^{2+} current; I_{NCX}, Na^+-Ca^{2+} exchange; I_f, funny current; I_{to}, transient outward K^+ current; I_{Ks}, slow component of delayed rectifier K^+ current; I_{Kr}, rapid component of delayed rectifier K^+ current; I_{K1}, inward rectifier K^+ current; I_{Kur}, ultra rapid component of delayed rectifier K^+ current; RyR, ryanodine receptor; SERCA, sarcoplasmic reticulum Ca^{2+}-ATPase; PLN, phospholamban; CaM, calmodulin; AC, adenylyl cyclase; PKA, protein kinase A; CICR, Ca^{2+}-induced Ca^{2+} release; SA, sinoatrial.

Cardiac arrhythmia mechanisms can be divided into two main categories: abnormal impulse formation and abnormal impulse conduction. In general, these arrhythmic events occur when the electrical activity of the heart is slower or faster than normal and/or becomes irregular.

Abnormal Impulse Generation

Focal activity (enhanced or abnormal impulse generation) is an important arrhythmogenic mechanism and consists of abnormal automaticity and triggered activity.

Automaticity

In the normal human heart, the SA node generates the propagating APs and determine the heart rate. In the case of parasystole, when the primary pacemaker is bordered by ischemic, infarcted regions the impulse cannot leave the SA node. Under these conditions, parasystolic pacemakers can take over pacemaker activity and fire APs at a lower rate compared to that of the SA node (Gussak et al., 2003). The AV node produces a junctional rhythm of 40 to 60 bpm and Purkinje fibers of about 20 to 40 bpm (Tse, 2016). In diseased hearts (e.g. heart failure, HF) membrane potential of pacemaker cells can shift to more positive values and this depolarization causes abnormal automaticity. Enhanced activity (i.e. tachycardia) increases rate of AP discharge by three mechanisms: threshold potential shifts to more negative, maximum diastolic potential shifts to more positive, and the rate of phase 4 depolarization increases (**Figure 3E**) (Jalife et al., 2009).

Early Afterdepolarization

Aside from the abnormal automaticity, the most common causes of focal activity are the early and delayed afterdepolarizations (EAD and DAD, respectively). EADs occur before the terminal repolarization (phase 2 and phase 3 repolarization) of the AP, while DADs occur after the repolarization when membrane potential reaches the resting levels (**Figure 5**).

EADs usually occur when repolarization reserve is compromised, i.e. reduced outward currents (I_{K1}, I_{Kr}, I_{Ks}) and/or increased inward currents (I_{Na}, window $I_{Ca,L}$, I_{NCX}) (Damiano and Rosen, 1984; Sipido et al., 2007; Benitah et al., 2010; Horvath et al., 2015; Karagueuzian et al., 2017), that is, there is a change in the net membrane current during the plateau (**Figure 5A**). In most of the cases these conditions cause prolongation of the AP, allowing $I_{Ca,L}$ to recover from inactivation (Chiamvimonvat et al., 2017) and as a positive feedback loop, triggering an AP (January and Riddle, 1989) (**Figure 3A**). Alternatively, at membrane potentials negative to the activation threshold for $I_{Ca,L}$, spontaneous Ca^{2+} release from the SR can activate I_{NCX}, driving a depolarizing current by reactivating I_{Na} (**Figure 3B**) (Szabo et al., 1994). In addition, although EADs usually

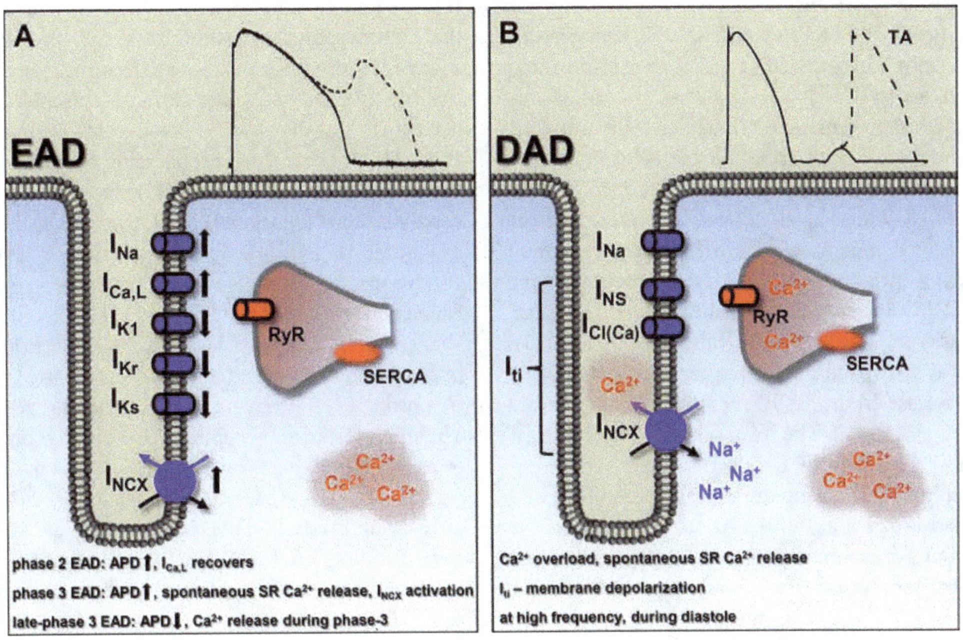

FIGURE 5 | Basic mechanisms of ectopic activity. **(A)** Factors involved in the generation of early afterdepolarizations (EAD). In general, EADs occur when outward currents are reduced (reduced repolarization reserve) and/or the inward currents are enhanced. The currently known types of EADs are consequencies of different etiologies, indicated on **(A)**. Detailed description in the text. Membrane potential recording shows a typical phase 2 EAD. **(B)** Delayed afterdepolarizations (DAD) originate from Ca^{2+} overload and consequently, spontaneous SR Ca^{2+} release which, in turn, generates a depolarizing transient inward (I_{ti}) current. Suprathreshold depolarization can elicit triggered activity. Membrane potential recording shows a typical DAD. EAD, early afterdepolarization; DAD, delayed afterdepolarization; $I_{Ca,L}$, L-type Ca^{2+} current; I_{Na}, Na^+ current; I_{Ks}, slow component of delayed rectifier K^+ current; I_{Kr}, rapid component of delayed rectifier K^+ current; I_{K1}, inward rectifier K^+ current; I_{NCX}, Na^+-Ca^{2+} exchange; I_{NS}, nonselective Ca^{2+}-sensitive cationic currents; $I_{Cl(Ca)}$, Ca^{2+}-activated chloride current; I_{ti}, transient outward current; RyR, ryanodine receptor; SR, sarcoplasmic reticulum; SERCA, sarcoplasmic reticulum Ca^{2+}-ATPase; TA, triggered activity.

occur when the AP duration (APD) is prolonged, some data suggests a novel mechanism, where even shortening of APD can be responsible for generation of EADs (late-phase 3 EAD) (Burashnikov and Antzelevitch, 2003). Late-phase 3 EADs occur particularly under elevated intracellular Ca^{2+} loading (i.e. large Ca^{2+} transient) and are considered as a hybrid between EAD and DAD (**Figure 3C**). At normal APD and at membrane potentials negative to the equilibrium of the I_{NCX} (and $I_{Cl(Ca)}$), these Ca^{2+}-mediated currents are weakly inward. However, if APD is abbreviated, they become strongly inward, allowing an I_{NCX}-driven depolarizing current, when the shorter repolarization allows a stronger (and not spontaneous) Ca^{2+} release from the SR (Burashnikov and Antzelevitch, 2006). The EAD generated under these circumstances interrupts the final phase of the AP. A key difference compared to the previously described EADs (and DADs) is a non-spontaneous Ca^{2+} release in generating late-phase 3 EADs (**Figure 5**). Late-phase 3 EAD also has clinical relevance, as its appearance is immediately following termination of other tachyarrhythmias, such as atrial flutter and fibrillation or ventricular tachycardia and fibrillation (Burashnikov and Antzelevitch, 2006).

The contribution of spontaneous SR Ca^{2+} release and an inward I_{NCX} to the generation of EADs has been described (Priori and Corr, 1990; Volders et al., 1997), furthermore, Volders et al. elegantly demonstrated in isoproterenol induced canine ventricular myocytes that early Ca^{2+} aftertransients and their aftercontractions precede the upstroke of the subsequent EAD so that they are a primary event inducing EADs (Volders et al., 1997). The time course of the EAD generation is characterized by a conditional phase (in other words, an initial delay in repolarization, defined by net membrane current) and the EAD upstroke. In this regard, a significant role of I_{NCX} has been suggested in the initial delay in repolarization, thus in the conditional phase (Volders et al., 2000).

In previous studies, distinct spatial features of afterdepolarization-associated Ca^{2+} transients had been shown; i.e. a heterogenous pattern indicating focal, spontaneous SR Ca^{2+} release in DADs and a homogenous pattern suggesting $I_{Ca,L}$-induced Ca^{2+} release in EADs (Miura et al., 1993; Miura et al., 1995; De Ferrari et al., 1995). However, it must be noted, under certain circumstances (adrenergic stimulation mediated sudden $[Ca^{2+}]_i$ changes), Ca^{2+} release during an EAD is not governed by sarcolemmal Ca^{2+} influx, so that it is spontaneous, which resembles as a heterogenous pattern, just like in the case of DADs (Volders et al., 1997).

In our previous work, EADs were evoked by I_{Kr} blockade (dofetilide), activation of Na+ current ($I_{Na,L}$) (veratridine), and activation of $I_{Ca,L}$ (BAY K8644) at slow pacing rates. Additional application of the Ca^{2+} chelator BAPTA-AM decreased $[Ca^{2+}]_i$ as expected, but either reduced EAD frequency in the presence of dofetilide and veratridine or further increased EAD frequency in the presence of BAY K8644 (direct augmentation of the $I_{Ca,L}$

brings extra Ca^{2+} inflow and is a substrate for increased EAD likelihood). Since BAPTA-AM decreased EAD frequency in the presence of veratridine, but failed to shorten APD, these results contradicts the exclusive role of APD in EAD generation and indicate that an increase in $[Ca^{2+}]_i$ is a significant factor not only for generating DADs, but for evoking EADs as well (Horvath et al., 2015). Moreover, in another set of experiments of Kistamas et al. H_2O_2 significantly increased APD and relative short term beat-to-beat variability (SV) (Kistamas et al., 2015a) and increased the occurrence of EADs on canine ventricular myocytes. Elevation of $[Ca^{2+}]_i$ in H_2O_2 was shown by others which can account for the increased SV and EAD incidence (Goldhaber, 1996; Xie et al., 2009; Szentandrassy et al., 2015; Kistamas et al., 2015). Furthermore, we also showed in guinea pig cardiomyocytes, that spontaneous Ca^{2+} release from the SR mediates ($I_{Na,L}$) induced EADs (Horvath et al., 2013). The two possible mechanisms proposed by Zaza et al. by which $I_{Na,L}$ promotes EAD genesis are (1) the reactivation of $I_{Ca,L}$ during the plateau phase of AP and (2) SR Ca^{2+} overload (Zaza et al., 2008). In our experiments the first EAD occurred at a membrane potential more positive than the window Ca^{2+} current voltage range, meaning that not the reactivation of $I_{Ca,L}$ was responsible for the generation of EADs. In fact, several mechanisms were addressed, showing the SR load was key in formation of the EADs: (a) anemone toxin II (ATX-II) facilitates $I_{Na,L}$ that caused elevated systolic Ca^{2+} transient and SR load, (b) the spontaneous Ca^{2+} wave precedes the first EAD, and (c) Ca^{2+} buffering with BAPTA in the patch pipette abolished EADs (Horvath et al., 2013).

Therefore, our recent knowledge about the factors involved in the development of EADs includes changes in $[Ca^{2+}]_i$ and the amplitude of Ca^{2+} transient, along with the APD and beat-to-beat variability of APD, AP morphology and plateau potential, net membrane current, and the actual availability of L-type Ca^{2+} channels. Regardless of the type of EAD mechanisms, if the depolarizing effect of the EAD on the membrane potential is sufficient to activate I_{Na}, the result will be an abnormal impulse generation, triggered activity (Hoffman and Rosen, 1981).

EADs are more likely to develop in midmyocardial cells and Purkinje fibers than in subepi- or subendocardial cells. There is a difference in ion current composition (less I_{Ks}, more $I_{Na,L}$ in midmyocardial cells), consequently these regions are more prone to AP prolongation (Liu and Antzelevitch, 1995; Zygmunt et al., 2001; Szabo et al., 2005). EADs are generally observed under conditions of ventricular hypertrophy and HF, injured cardiac tissue, or when the myocardium is exposed to catecholamines, hypoxia, acidosis, and pharmacologic agents (Roden, 2004; Roden, 2006). The clinical significance of EADs is clear, as they can either serve as the trigger or as the substrate for initiation and perpetuation of torsade de pointes arrhythmia (Volders et al., 2000). Being as a trigger, as EADs can cause new APs which will be reflected on the ECG as ectopic beats. EADs provide a substrate by causing electrical inhomogeneity in the surrounding tissues.

Delayed Afterdepolarization

DADs are the other common causes of focal activity and were originally described as oscillatory afterpotentials (Ferrier et al., 1973). They occur in diastole, after complete repolarization of the cell (**Figure 5B**). DADs can originate from intracellular Ca^{2+} overload that induces spontaneous SR Ca^{2+} release, resulting in a depolarizing current *via* forward mode I_{NCX} (Mechmann and Pott, 1986). Other nonselective Ca^{2+}-sensitive cationic currents (I_{NS}) and chloride current ($I_{Cl(Ca)}$) may also be involved in DAD generation (Asakura et al., 2014). These three depolarizing currents result in a transient inward current (I_{ti}), which is responsible for the membrane depolarization (**Figure 3D**). Ca^{2+} overload of the cardiac myocytes can occur in several diseases and also in several experimental conditions, e.g. toxic levels of digitalis (Ferrier et al., 1973; Saunders et al., 1973; Rosen et al., 1973), catecholamines (Wit and Cranefield, 1977; Rozanski and Lipsius, 1985; Priori and Corr, 1990), hypokalemia and hypercalcemia (Tse, 2016), hypertrophy, HF (Aronson, 1981; Vermeulen et al., 1994), and rapid heart rates. The amplitude of the generated DAD depends on the size of the Ca^{2+} transient and on the properties of I_{NCX} and the inward rectifier K^+ current (I_{K1}) (Pogwizd et al., 2001; Sung et al., 2006; Maruyama et al., 2010). Subthreshold DADs [appearing as the U wave on the electrocardiogram (ECG)] are small voltage deflections, which although unable to trigger a propagating action potential, may still cause dispersion of excitability, thereby promoting regional conduction block (Rosen et al., 1975; Surawicz, 1998; di Bernardo and Murray, 2002). However, if DADs reach the threshold potential for the opening of Na^+ channels, a spontaneous AP emerges and can result in premature ventricular contraction (PVC). The clinical significance of DAD generation lies in triggered activity that contributes to arrhythmogenesis with catecholaminergic polymorphic ventricular tachycardia (CPVT), atrial fibrillation (AF), and HF. In CPVT and HF, intracellular Ca^{2+} load combines with RyR dysfunction ("leaky" RyR). Under circumstances when the SR becomes loaded (high Ca^{2+} load, fast heart rate, and/or increased adrenergic tone) and/or RyR becomes leaky, spontaneous Ca^{2+} release is favored.

Considering the mechanism of the spontaneous Ca^{2+} release, there are two main patterns. First, focal Ca^{2+} release, when Ca^{2+} signal acts locally (Lipp and Niggli, 1994) and secondly, when the released Ca^{2+} leaves its focus and propagates as a global Ca^{2+} wave through the myocyte (Takamatsu and Wier, 1990; Wier et al., 1987; Cheng et al., 1993).

Unlike the EADs, DADs are always generated at relatively rapid rates (Antzelevitch and Burashnikov, 2011). As mentioned earlier, late-phase 3 EADs are considered as a hybrid between EAD and DAD. A key difference is the time of the SR Ca^{2+} release during the AP (**Figure 5**). Ca^{2+} release occurs during diastole in the case of DAD, while late-phase 3 EAD is generated at the late repolarization of the AP (Fink and Noble, 2010).

Beat-To-Beat Variability of Action Potential Duration

Variations (physiological or pathological) in AP configuration can cause disturbances in Ca^{2+} signaling and the electrical properties of cardiac muscle. In our previous experiments, we determined the beat-to-beat variability of AP duration in isolated canine left ventricular myocytes in several experimental settings (Kistamas et al., 2015a; Kistamas et al., 2015b; Szentandrassy et al., 2015; Magyar et al., 2016), as recent studies suggest the short term beat-to-beat variability (SV) of APD as a novel method for predicting imminent cardiac arrhythmias (Thomsen et al., 2004; Abi-Gerges et al., 2010). Higher variability is considered to be arrhythmic by increasing dispersion of refractoriness (**Figure 3G**). We established the concept of relative short term beat-to-beat variability of APD (RSV) by normalizing the changes of short term variability of APD to the concomitant changes in APD [see (Nanasi et al., 2017] for review). We summarized that RSV was decreased by ion currents involved in the negative feedback regulation of APD ($I_{Ca,L}$, I_{Ks} and I_{Kr}), while it was increased by I_{Na} and I_{to}, and in general, increased if repolarization reserved was compromised. RSV was also increased at faster rates and at increased $[Ca^{2+}]_i$. Transient changes of $[Ca^{2+}]_i$ due to Ca^{2+} released from the SR were the dominant contributor to this process (Kistamas et al., 2015b). High RSV at faster rates can also be explained by the elevated $[Ca^{2+}]_i$, as faster pacing increases $I_{Ca,L}$, ultimately overloading the cell with Ca^{2+} which, in turn, increases RSV.

Cardiac Alternans

A severe form of this beat-to-beat variation is cardiac alternans, where short and long AP duration alternate (**Figure 3F**). Pulse and T-wave alternans can be clinically observed and are considered to be a precursor for cardiac arrhythmias (Rosenbaum et al., 1994; Verrier et al., 2011). Cardiac alternans originates from instabilities of membrane voltage or of Ca^{2+} cycling. At the cellular level, alternans is manifested as beat-to-beat alternations in contraction amplitude (mechanical alternans), APD (electrical or APD alternans), and Ca^{2+} transient amplitude (Ca^{2+} alternans) at constant heart rate. However, because of the bidirectional information flow between membrane voltage and Ca^{2+} cycling, electrical alternans is always influenced by Ca^{2+} alternans, and vice versa (Weiss et al., 2006).

Two mechanisms have been described for Ca^{2+}-driven alternans. One depends on the relationship between SR Ca^{2+} content and the amount of Ca^{2+} released from the SR (Eisner et al., 2000). If this relationship is steep then a small increase of SR Ca^{2+} content will produce a large increase of the amplitude of the Ca^{2+} transient resulting in increased Ca^{2+} efflux *via* I_{NCX} and a decreased influx *via* $I_{Ca,L}$ (Ca^{2+}-dependent inactivation). The net result is a decrease of SR Ca^{2+} content. The next beat therefore arises from a depleted SR resulting in a smaller Ca^{2+} transient and decreased I_{NCX}, so that the cell will gain Ca^{2+} resulting in a larger SR content and Ca^{2+} transient for the third beat (Eisner et al., 2006). Later, it was shown that reduced SERCA pump activity is also needed for an alternating pattern to develop (Shiferaw et al., 2003; Qu et al., 2007; Xie et al., 2008; Li et al., 2009). Another mechanism for Ca^{2+}-driven alternans has been proposed, when on every beat, the SR load is unchanged, however the released amount of Ca^{2+} is alternating beat-to-beat. This kind of alternans results from the refractoriness of the RyRs, without the need for SR Ca^{2+} content alternans (Picht et al., 2006; Shkryl et al., 2012).

Voltage-driven or electrical alternans is determined by APD restitution. Here, the shorter the preceding diastolic interval, the less the APD (Nolasco and Dahlen, 1968). The steeper this relationship, the more likely is alternans to occur. There may be several causes for this APD restitution. The rapid, pacing-induced electrical alternans occurs at fast heart rates (short diastolic intervals, where recovery of $I_{Ca,L}$ is crucial, becoming a key factor in regulating the steepness of APD restitution (Mahajan et al., 2008). Another APD alternating mechanism is driven by I_{to} at slow or normal heart rates and possibly accounts for T-wave alternans in patients with Brugada syndrome (Hopenfeld, 2006). The third type of electrical alternans is mediated by non-inactivating $I_{Ca,L}$ with I_{Ks} at normal or slow rates and possibly cause T-wave alternans in LQTS patients (Wegener et al., 2008). Electrical, restitution-based alternans has been associated with the breakdown of reentry into ventricular fibrillation (VF). At the tissue level, if cellular alternanses in different regions of the ventricle occur in phase with each other (spatially concordant), T-wave alternanses is observed on the ECG. A more malignant form, the spatially discordant APD alternans, manifesting as QRS alternans on the ECG, causes large dispersion of refractoriness, a substrate for reentry. Spatially discordant alternans is a significant cause of wave break, a phenomenon that is essential to VF (Garfinkel, 2007). It has been shown, that interventions that lower the slope of the APD restitution curve can turn multiwave VF to single-wave monomorphic ventricular tachycardia (VT) (Garfinkel et al., 2000; Wu et al., 2002).

Abnormal Impulse Conduction

Abnormal impulse conduction, i.e. reentry, occurs when the AP fails to terminate and has the ability to re-excite tissue regions which have already recovered. This mechanism can be divided into two main types, one with an obstacle (circus type with anatomical or functional barrier) and the other without an obstacle (phase-2 reentry and reflection). The key difference is in refractoriness. Circus movement reentry travels around an anatomic or functional obstacle and all cells are recovered from inactivation, while cells involved in reflection or phase-2 reentry show large differences in recovery from refractoriness with no obstacle in the way of the reentrant wave. In addition, classic nomenclature distinguishes between microreentry and macroreentry, where the reentrant circuit does not or does appear on the surface ECG, respectively.

The myocardium works as a functional syncytium (**Figure 6A**). The elemental components of this system are the gap junctions. Gap junctions form channels (comprised of two neighboring connexons) between adjacent cardiomyocytes and allow the cardiac AP to propagate from cell to cell and thereby initiate contraction. However, gap junction channels are unevenly distributed within the cells, expressing a larger portion of channel proteins at the longitudinal ends of the cells than at the transversal, lateral sides (De Maziere and Scheuermann, 1990; Oosthoek et al., 1993). This anisotropy allows a much larger longitudinal conduction velocity and effective electrical coupling between the adjacent cells (**Figure 6B**). Several conditions are reported to reduce or abolish gap junctional conductance, including increased $[Ca^{2+}]_i$, reduced pH, or lower ATP levels (Dhein, 1998). Uncoupling of the cells may lead to the formation of unidirectional conduction block and reentry type arrhythmias (**Figure 6B**). The hypothesis that Ca^{2+} overload conditions have arrhythmogenic behavior is also supported by experiments in neonatal rat myocytes, where gap junctional conductance was

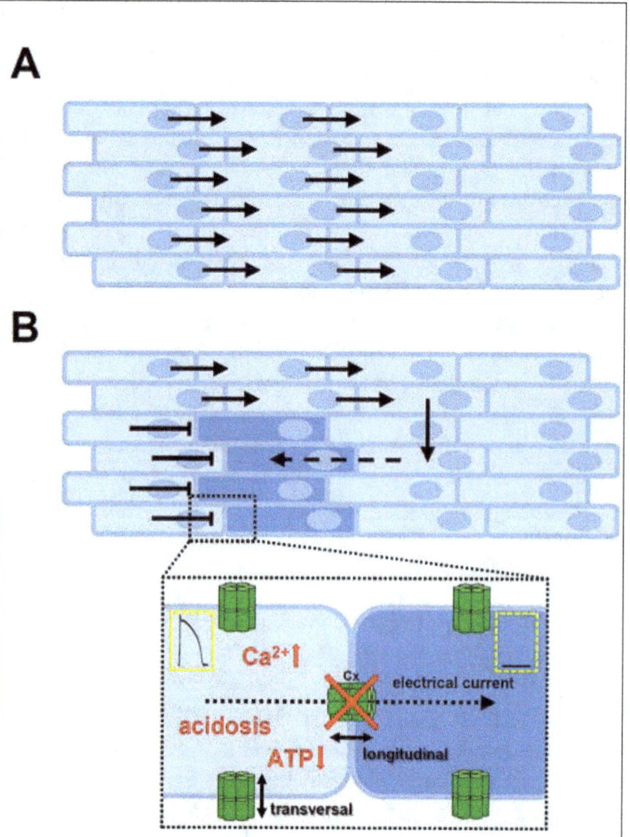

FIGURE 6 | Role of gap junctions in propagating of the cardiac action potential. **(A)** The cardiac tissue is eletrically homogenous if the adjacent cells are coupled by gap junction channels. The anisotropic nature of gap junction channel distribution favors longitudinal over transversal conduction. **(B)** Conditions that decrease or abolish coupling between the cells may cause a unidirectional conduction block and as the electrical impulse propagates around the block it can re-excite those tissue regions due to differences in refractoriness. Insert shows cell-cell connections *via* gap junction channels. The main causes of uncoupling of the cells (showed in red) are elevated intracellular Ca^{2+} concentration, reduction in H^+ concentration, or lower levels of ATP. Cx, connexon; ATP, adenosine triphosphate.

decreased by Ca^{2+} concentrations higher than physiological (Firek and Weingart, 1995), while it was proposed that elevation of $[Ca^{2+}]_i$ by Ca^{2+} entry was more effective in decreasing gap junctional conductance than Ca^{2+} released from internal stores (Lazrak et al., 1994; Chanson et al., 1999). Furthermore, adequate coupling between the cells in the tissue (i.e. low longitudinal resistance) can suppress differences in APD, eliminate EADs, and reduce beat-to-beat variability (Magyar et al., 2015).

In the subsequent sections reentry types are discussed in detail.

Reentry With Anatomical Obstacle (Ring Model)

Reentry was first described in 1906 by Mayer in rings of tissue cut from jellyfish (ring model) (Mayer, 1906). Later work by Mines showed that circus-type reentry can be initiated by electrical stimulation in cardiac muscle and was the first to define the concept of circus movement reentry around an anatomical obstacle (**Figure 7A**) (Mines, 1913; Mines, 1914). The anatomical barrier can be a valve, vessel or scar. The possibility that circus-type reentry can form without an anatomical obstacle was proposed by Garrey (1914).

Initiation of reentry requires a trigger and a substrate. The trigger can be a premature contraction, while tissue substrate is the dispersion of refractoriness. On top of that, fundamental settings are needed for reentry excitation with anatomical obstacle: (1) the impulse initiating the circus movement must propagate in one direction (unidirectional block) and (2) the proportion of absolute and relative refractoriness in the tissue, that is, the reentrant circuit must be long enough to let all areas—within the circuit, distal from the stimulus—recover from refractory (excitable gap), so the circuit can return to its origin and continue as a new cycle (**Figure 7A**). Consequently, (3) the circulating movement would terminate in case of interruption of the reentrant circuit (Mines, 1913). These criteria proposed by Mines are still in use today. The above mentioned excitation is, in fact, a propagating wave. The length of this wave (wavelength) is determined by the distance between the wavefront (phase 0, AP depolarization) and waveback (phase 3, repolarization), that is, creating an arrhythmogenic excitation needs the special properties of refractoriness and conduction velocity (Weiss et al., 2000). If the above three criteria are not met, i.e. in sinus rhythm if the tissue around the anatomical obstacle is homogenous (and the impulse pathway is wide enough), the wavefront can simultaneously propagate in both pathways around the barrier. However, if the tissue is electrically heterogenous, due to dispersion of refractoriness, unidirectional conduction block can form caused by a PVC, i.e. initiating reentry (**Figure 7A**).

Reentry Without Anatomical Obstacle (Functional Block)

In the cases, when there is no anatomical barrier present, functional reentry can still form, maintained only by the electrical properties (dispersion of refractoriness) of the tissue. The best known examples are the leading circle, spiral wave, and figure-of-8 reentry (**Figure 7B**).

The leading circle model was described by Allessie et al., as "the head of the circulating wavefront is continuously biting in its own tail of refractoriness" (Allessie et al., 1977). The main differences compared to the ring model are (1) the length of the circuit is determined by conduction velocity, stimulating efficacy, and refractory period not by an anatomic obstacle, (2) while the length of the circuit is not fixed, it can be altered by changes in electrophysiological properties of the tissue. (3) There is no excitable gap in the leading circle model and (4) a shortcut of the circuit is possible and finally (5) revolution time is proportional to refractory period, while in the ring model, revolution time is inversely related to conduction velocity (**Figure 7B**) (Allessie et al., 1977).

Spiral waves and rotors can be induced in small two-dimensional pieces of cardiac muscle, without an anatomical barrier, and can drift through the tissue (Pertsov et al., 1993). Scroll waves are the three-dimensional forms of spiral waves. Spiral waves can develop both in homogenous and heterogenous tissues and either in stable or in an unstable form (Ikeda et al.,

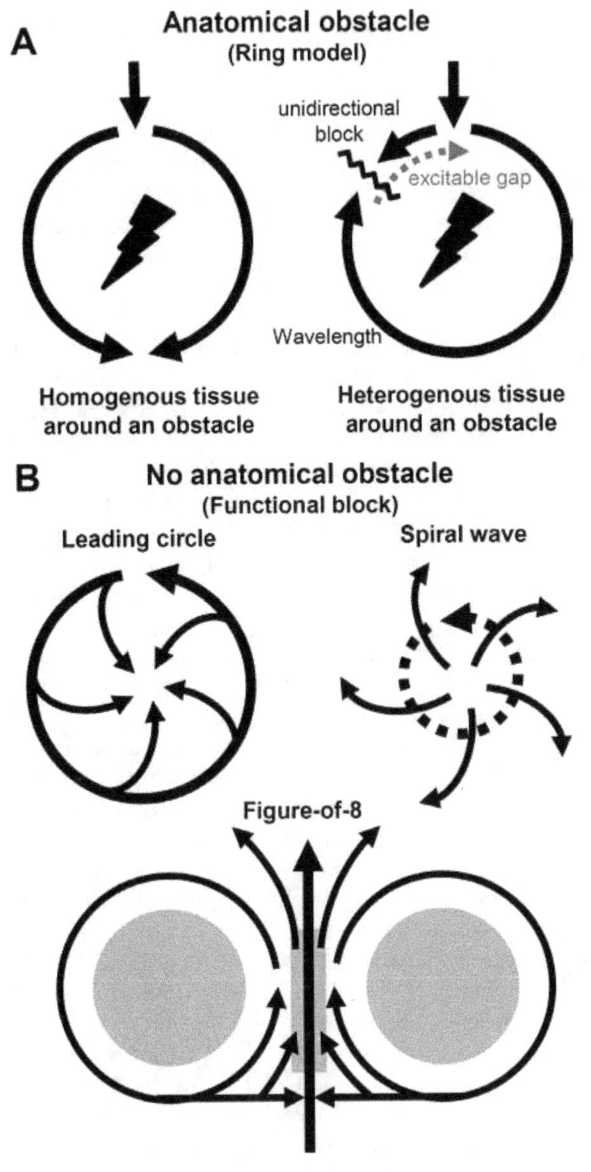

FIGURE 7 | Abnormal impulse conduction. Circus movement reentry types. **(A)** Reentrant wave travels around an anatomical obstacle. If the cardiac tissue around the obstacle is homogenous the impulse conduction is favored in both directions. However, if the tissue is heterogenous (i.e. dispersion of refractoriness), unidirectional block can form initating a reentry circuit. Excitable gap consists of tissue regions that fully and/or partially recovered from refractory period, therefore excitable. **(B)** Circuit movement reentry can form in the absence of an anatomical obstacle (functional block). In the leading circle model the length of the circuit is not determined by the pathway around an obstacle, but rather by conduction velocity, refractory period, and stimulating efficacy where (in the absence of an obstacle) a shortcut of the circuit is possible. Spiral waves reentry (or scroll wave if three-dimensional) drifts through the tissue without an obstacle and the main wave can break up and radiate waves to the neighboring regions. In the model of figure-of-8 the circulating waves appear in pairs and the wavefront can circulate around the functional blocks clockwise and counterclockwise. If the intermediate area (central gray) can be activated by the colliding separated waves, reentry can form.

1996; Davidenko et al., 1992). The former might result in monomorphic VT, while the latter can cause polymorphic VT or torsade de pointes (**Figure 7B**) (Gray et al., 1995).

Figure-of-8 type reentry was first demonstrated by el-Sherif et al. In this case the reentrant wavefront reaches a functional conduction block surrounded by regions of reduced excitability. As conduction is not favored through such tissue, the wavefront drives clockwise and counterclockwise around the two arcs of functional block and beyond the barriers of low excitability the two separated waves can collide. If the conduction is slow enough and the intermediate area can be activated, reentry can form (**Figure 7B**) (el-Sherif et al., 1985; Lazzara, 1988).

Phase-2 Reentry

In the previous reentrant mechanisms, the trigger and the substrate originated from different etiologies, while in the case of phase-2 reentry, trigger and substrate are from the same source. Phase-2 reentry occurs in ischemia (Lukas and Antzelevitch, 1996), Brugada syndrome (Brugada and Brugada, 1992) or under conditions of higher pacing rates and higher extracellular Ca^{2+} concentration (Di Diego and Antzelevitch, 1994). It is caused by severe spatial dispersion of repolarization, that is, spike-and-dome configuration of AP morphology is lost at one site (predominantly at the epicardial region), while preserved at another site and is responsible for the transition to VT and VF. APs without the dome (short APD, early repolarization) can therefore be reexcited and reentry can be initiated (Antzelevitch, 2007). Loss of dome can be explained by a stronger transient outward current (I_{to}) current, and overall by the competitive behavior between I_{Na} and I_{to} (Greenstein et al., 2000; Szabo et al., 2005; Dong et al., 2010). If the actual membrane potential value is more negative than the activation threshold for the $I_{Ca,L}$ then the AP dome vanishes. Cantalapiedra et al. showed in a simplified ionic and in a realistic cardiac model, that the origin of reexcitation is based on the presence of slow Ca^{2+} pulse, produced by the slow inward Ca^{2+} current (I_{si}), so that the slow pulse propagates to the regions of short APs until it triggers a fast pulse (Cantalapiedra et al., 2010). Interestingly, the same research group argued that conditions (e.g. drugs) increasing the $I_{Ca,L}$, to recover the dome or to prevent the loss of dome, decreases dispersion of repolarization, however, also increasing the probability of reexcitation, through the stabilizing effect of the Ca^{2+} conductance ($I_{Ca,L}$) on the slow Ca^{2+} pulse (Cantalapiedra et al., 2009).

Reflection

Reflection is another example of non-circus movement reentry, with a one-dimensional behavior and can be the cause of PVCs or even lethal arrhythmias (Wit et al., 1972; Rosenthal, 1988; Van Hemel et al., 1988). Reflection describes reentry in a linear bundle of a conductive tissue. A stimulus from the proximal region travels through an inexcitable gap and elicits an AP at the distal end. Slow electrotonic currents (inexcitable region can only transmit electrotonic currents) generated by this AP can then propagate in the retrograde direction and reenter and reexcite the proximal elements (Antzelevitch et al., 1980). There must be an adequate conduction delay to let reflection happen (proximal end can recover from refractoriness), depending on the pacing interval and stimulus strength. It was also shown that neither EADs nor automaticity was required for reflection (Cabo and Barr, 1992; Kandel and Roth, 2015).

Biexcitability

A novel wave dynamic, termed biexcitability has been described in recent studies (Chang et al., 2012). In pacemaker regions $I_{Ca,L}$ causes the activation, while in working muscle cells, the upstroke of the AP is driven by I_{Na} and $I_{Ca,L}$. During biexcitability both form of activation can coexist at the same tissue. Under certain conditions, like long QT syndrome, repolarization reserve is compromised, APD prolongs, and EADs can occur. Consequently, there can be a situation where the cells develop two stable membrane potential values (−80 mV and −50 mV) and switches between them (Gadsby and Cranefield, 1977), resulting in a Na^+- and Ca^{2+}-mediated (fast) or a Ca^{2+}-mediated (slow) propagating wavefront. This bi-stable behavior might serve as an explanation for the two different possible outcomes of torsade de pointes. According to Chang et al., in cases where the Ca^{2+}-mediated slow spiral wave is terminated, leads to termination of the torsade de pointes, while if the tissue is sufficiently heterogenous, Na^+ and Ca^{2+}-mediated fast spiral waves degenerate torsade de pointes to VF (Chang et al., 2012; Chang et al., 2013).

DADs can induce focal VT by DAD-mediated triggered activity or initiate reentry. Moreover, unstable Ca^{2+} signaling can dynamically serve as a substrate for reentry, by promoting dispersion of excitability or promoting dispersion of refractoriness (Weiss et al., 2015). In those tissue regions, where subthreshold DADs do not trigger a propagating AP, the resultant small membrane depolarization can still be sufficient to depress excitability by inactivating the fast voltage gated Na^+ channels. This condition can lead to reentry, as the inactivated Na^+ channels form a regional conduction block for impulses generated by suprathreshold DADs (Rosen et al., 1975; Liu et al., 2015). In the latter case, DAD-mediated triggered activity at fast rates can promote Ca^{2+} transient alternans, which in turn causes APD alternans, thereby increasing the dispersion of refractoriness (Sato et al., 2006; Weiss et al., 2006). As previously mentioned, subthreshold EADs can also enhance the dispersion of refractoriness, also creating a reentry substrate.

For more detailed reviews on conduction disorders, see Qu and Weiss (2015) and Antzelevitch and Burashnikov (2011).

The following sections will provide further insights into intracellular Ca^{2+} handling maladies in the most prevalent inherited and acquired arrhythmia syndromes, caused by channelopathies and defects in Ca^{2+} handling genes. Ca^{2+} handling defects also have an arrhythmogenic role in diseases, such as heart failure and cardiomyopathies, however they are beyond the scope of the present review [see recent reviews (Coppini et al., 2018; Johnson and Antoons, 2018; Denham et al., 2018)].

INHERITED SYNDROMES

Catecholaminergic Polymorphic Ventricular Tachycardia

Catecholaminergic Polymorphic Ventricular Tachycardia (CPVT) is a severe arrhythmogenic disorder, manifesting as a bidirectional or polymorphic VT, mainly in young patients with structurally healthy hearts after exercise or acute emotional stress (Reid et al., 1975). As heart rate increases as a result of exercise or emotional stress, the ectopic ventricular trigger increases in complexity, such that VT turns into VF and may lead to syncope or sudden cardiac death (Coumel, 1978; Leenhardt et al., 1995).

The main criteria for CPVT diagnosis are as follows: structurally normal heart (and normal coronary arteries in individuals above 40 years of age), normal QT interval, and adrenergic induced bidirectional or polymorphic VT (Venetucci et al., 2012). CPVT is also diagnosed in patients who carry a pathogenic mutation and in family members of a CPVT index case, fulfilling the above mentioned criteria (Priori et al., 2013). There are also nonspecific features, therefore not diagnostic criteria, including a prominent U wave on the ECG accompanied by sinus bradycardia (Postma et al., 2005).

In CPVT, arrhythmias are induced by Ca^{2+} release from the SR leading to a DAD. The fundamental feature of this process is the Ca^{2+} release unit (Ca^{2+} sparks), where the spontaneous Ca^{2+} release occurs. If sufficient number of release units are activated, a Ca^{2+} wave is born, which depends on the SR Ca^{2+} content and the SR Ca^{2+} threshold (Lukyanenko et al., 1999; Venetucci et al., 2007). Interventions that alter RyR opening will affect SR Ca^{2+} threshold. For example, caffeine increases the open probability of RyR, therefore it is easier to elicit spontaneous Ca^{2+} release (Trafford et al., 2000), on the other hand tetracaine has an opposite effect, by reducing RyR opening, SR Ca^{2+} release threshold is higher (Overend et al., 1997; Venetucci et al., 2006).

In the previous sections we detailed the normal Ca^{2+} cycling and consequences of elevated $[Ca^{2+}]_i$. Briefly, the main arrhythmogenic mechanism in CPVT is due to SR Ca^{2+} release increasing cytoplasmic Ca^{2+} levels, NCX exchanges Ca^{2+} with Na^+, thereby generating I_{ti}. I_{ti} produces DADs and if DADs reach the activation threshold of Na^+ channels, an elicited AP causes triggered activity, which in turn can lead to an extrasystolic heartbeat. Mutations in CPVT have been shown to alter RyR function and increase the occurrence of spontaneous Ca^{2+} release events after sympathetic stimulation (Liu et al., 2006). β-adrenergic activation increases SR Ca^{2+} content, while the same process enhances RyR phosphorylation by Ca^{2+}/calmodulin-dependent protein kinase II (CaMKII) and protein kinase A (PKA) (Kashimura et al., 2010; Liu et al., 2011a; Venetucci et al., 2012). In addition to the phosphorylation by PKA, CaMKII-mediated phosphorylation increases the $I_{Ca,L}$ and SERCA (by removing the inhibitory effect of phospholamban on SERCA) and activates RyR. Simultaneous activation of $I_{Ca,L}$, SERCA (increases SR Ca^{2+} content), and RyR therefore increases the possibility of spontaneous Ca^{2+} release (Maier and Bers, 2007; Hegyi et al., 2019). Experimental data confirmed that higher RyR Ca^{2+} sensitivity alone is not sufficient to elicit spontaneous Ca^{2+} release and that inhibition of CaMKII in a CPVT mouse model prevents arrhythmias (Venetucci et al., 2007; Liu et al., 2011a).

Several CPVT subtypes have been described to date, albeit the two most common types are the CPVT-1 and CPVT-2 (**Table 1**).

CPVT-1 is caused by an autosomal dominant mutation in the RyR2 gene (Swan et al., 1999). This subtype is the most common, accountable for about 60% of all CPVT cases (Laitinen et al., 2001; Priori et al., 2001). RyR exists as a macromolecular complex with many other molecules, such as calsequestrin 2 (CSQ2), FK506 binding protein 1B (FKBP1B or FKBP12.6), FK506 binding protein 1B (FKBP1B or FKBP12.6), PKA, CaMKII, phosphatase 1 (PP1), phosphatase 1 (PP1), phosphatase 2A (PP2A), histidine-rich Ca^{2+} binding protein (HRC), junctin and triadin (Wang et al., 1998; George et al., 2007; Yano et al., 2009; Arvanitis et al., 2011; Szabo et al., 2013). Junctin and triadin mediates interaction between RyR and CSQ2 (Eisner et al., 2017). Most RyR mutations in CPVT are gain-of-function mutations and thereby leading to increased Ca^{2+} sensitivity and RyR channels may open during diastole causing Ca^{2+} leak, particularly during adrenergic stress (Jones et al., 2008). Several hypotheses have been advanced to explain this phenomenon, including the role of FKBP12.6, store overload-induced Ca^{2+} entry (SOCE) and a defective mutation in the RyR 3D conformation (Reiken et al., 2003; Lehnart et al., 2004; Jiang et al., 2005; Yamamoto et al., 2008; Liu et al., 2009; Uchinoumi et al., 2010; Suetomi et al., 2011; Venetucci et al., 2012a).

CPVT-2 is an autosomal recessive gene anomaly in CASQ2-encoded CSQ2 and responsible for about 3–5% of CPVT patients (Lahat et al., 2001). The structure of this intra-SR Ca^{2+} buffer changes Ca^{2+} concentration. At low SR Ca^{2+} concentrations (< 0.6 mmol/L) CSQ2 is a monomer, which is converted to a dimer (0.6–3 mmol/L) or polymer (> 3 mmol/L) at higher Ca^{2+} concentrations (Mitchell et al., 1988; Wang et al., 1998). It has been shown that, in the absence of functional CSQ2, RyR channels open spontaneously, without the need for L-type Ca^{2+} current mediated trigger (Knollmann et al., 2006) and that mutation of CSQ2 destabilizes Ca^{2+} storing capacity of the SR, which in turn alters the Ca^{2+} sensitivity of RyR (Viatchenko-Karpinski et al., 2004). In all CSQ2 mutations (missense, deleterious, nonsense), level of CSQ2 protein is reduced or absent, perhaps because it is more susceptible to degradation (Rizzi et al., 2008; Faggioni et al., 2012). Impaired polymerization (Bal et al., 2010), reduced RyR binding and modulation (Houle et al., 2004; Terentyev et al., 2006) are generally associated with lower SR Ca^{2+} content, higher $[Ca^{2+}]_i$ and Ca^{2+} leak through RyR, these effects

TABLE 1 | Ca^{2+} handling genes associated with inherited arrhythmogenic syndromes.

Syndrome/ Phenotype	Genes	Genetic Locus	Functional effect	Protein	Ref	Syndrome overlap
CPVT-1	RYR2	1q43	GoF	**ryanodine receptor 2**	(Laitinen et al., 2001; Priori et al., 2001)	
CPVT-2	CASQ2	1p13.1	GoF	**calsequestrin 2**	(Lahat et al., 2001)	
CPVT-4	CALM1	14q31–q32	LoF	**calmodulin 1**	(Nyegaard et al., 2012; Sondergaard et al., 2015; Sondergaard et al., 2017)	LQTS-14
CPVT-5	TRDN	6q22.31	LoF	**triadin**	(Chopra et al., 2009)	LQTS-17
LQTS-4	ANK2	4q25–q26	LoF	**ankyrin B**	(Bhuiyan et al., 2013; Mohler et al., 2003)	
LQTS-8 (Timothy syndrome)	CACNA1C	12p13.33	GoF	**$\alpha 1_C$ subunit of LTCC**	(Splawski et al., 2004; Thiel et al., 2008; Boczek et al., 2015; Landstrom et al., 2016)	BrS-3, SQTS-4, ERS/IVF
LQTS-14	CALM1	14q32.11	GoF/LoF	**calmodulin 1**	(Shamgar et al., 2006; Gray and Behr, 2016; Jensen et al., 2018; Wren et al., 2019)	CPVT-4
LQTS-15	CALM2	2p21	LoF	**calmodulin 2**	(Shamgar et al., 2006; Gray and Behr, 2016; Jensen et al., 2018; Wren et al., 2019)	
LQTS-16	CALM3	19q13.32	LoF	**calmodulin 3**	(Shamgar et al., 2006; Gray and Behr, 2016; Jensen et al., 2018; Wren et al., 2019)	
LQTS-17 (Triadin Knockout Syndrome)	TRDN	6q22.31	LoF	**triadin**	(Altmann et al., 2015)	CPVT-5
BrS-3	CACNA1C	12p13.33	LoF	**$\alpha 1_C$ subunit of LTCC**	(Schwartz et al., 1995; Rosero et al., 1997)	SQTS-4, ERS/IVF
BrS-4	CACNB2	10p12.33–p12.31	LoF	**β_2 subunit of LTCC**	(Schwartz et al., 1995; Rosero et al., 1997)	SQTS-5, ERS/IVF
BrS-11	CACNA2D1	7q21.11	LoF	**$\alpha_2\delta_1$ subunit of LTCC**	(Schwartz et al., 1995; Rosero et al., 1997)	SQTS-6, ERS/IVF
BrS-15	TRMP4	19q13.33	GoF/LoF	**transient receptor potential melastatin 4**	(Liu et al., 2013)	
SQTS-4	CACNA1C	12p13.33	LoF	**$\alpha 1_C$ subunit of LTCC**	(Antzelevitch et al., 2007; Bjerregaard et al., 2010)	BrS-3, ERS/IVF
SQTS-5	CACNB2	10p12.33–p12.31	LoF	**β_2 subunit of LTCC**	(Antzelevitch et al., 2007; Bjerregaard et al., 2010)	BrS-4, ERS/IVF
SQTS-6	CACNA2D1	7q21.11	LoF	**$\alpha_2\delta_1$ subunit of LTCC**	(Antzelevitch et al., 2007; Bjerregaard et al., 2010)	BrS-11, ERS/IVF
ERS/IVF	CACNA1C	12p13.33	LoF	**$\alpha 1_C$ subunit of LTCC**	(Priori et al., 2013)	BrS-3, SQTS-4
	CACNB2	10p12.33–p12.31	LoF	**β_2 subunit of LTCC**	(Priori et al., 2013)	BrS-4, SQTS-5
	CACNA2D1	7q21.11	LoF	**$\alpha_2\delta_1$ subunit of LTCC**	(Priori et al., 2013)	BrS-11, SQTS-6

CPVT, catecholaminergic polymorphic ventricular tachycardia; LQTS, long QT syndrome; BrS, Brugada syndrome; SQTS, short QT syndrome; ERS, early repolarization syndrome; IVF, idiopathic ventricular fibrillation; LTCC, L-type Ca^{2+} channel; GoF, gain-of-function; LoF, loss-of-function.

can be augmented by β-stimulation (Song et al., 2007). An interesting feature of CSQ2 protein reduction is a subsequent reduction in triadin and junctin levels. Denegri et al. showed in CSQ2 knock-out animal model that viral gene transfer for *in vivo* replacement of CSQ2 restored normal CSQ2 levels along with triadin and junctin, and ultimately prevented arrhythmias (Denegri et al., 2012).

Other, less frequent gene mutations have also been described, such as autosomal recessive forms of CPVT, the CPVT-3 and CPVT-5, while CPVT-4 is an autosomal dominant form of the inherited syndrome. CPVT-3 subtype is related to the gene encoding trans-2,3-enoyl-CoA reductase-like protein (TECRL) and is first seen at an early age with high likelihood of infant sudden cardiac death (Bhuiyan et al., 2007). When CPVT-3 is studied in induced pluripotent stem cell-derived cardiomyocytes (iPSC-CM) slower Ca^{2+} reuptake, slower Ca^{2+} transient upstroke velocity, and increased APD has been observed, along with norepinephrine-induced DADs, which could be eliminated by flecainide (see below) (Devalla et al., 2016). Mutations in CALM1-encoded calmodulin (CaM) cause the CPVT-4 subtype. *In vitro* experiments showed that this gene anomaly in the C domain compromises Ca^{2+} binding to CaM and impairs interaction between RyR and its CaM-binding domain, leading to an increased open state of RyR (Nyegaard et al., 2012; Sondergaard et al., 2015; Sondergaard et al., 2017). TRDN-encoded triadin mutation results in CPVT-5 subtype, which may cause diastolic Ca^{2+} leak and Ca^{2+} overload. Electron microscopy experiments uncovered fragmentation and reduced contact at the dyadic cleft, thus possibly lacking the negative feedback of SR Ca^{2+} release on the L-type Ca^{2+} channels, so SR Ca^{2+} overload may arise from the uncontrolled Ca^{2+} influx (Chopra et al., 2009).

A possible loss-of-function RyR mutation has also been proposed in a case classified as idiopathic VF, where a reduced SR Ca^{2+} sensitivity was shown (Jiang et al., 2007). Moreover, exercise induced bidirectional VT has been reported in types of long QT syndromes (LQTS-4 and LQTS-7) (**Table 1**) (Mohler et al., 2004; Vega et al., 2009).

Because of the hiding nature of the disease, it is difficult to diagnose CPVT, as patients have normal heart structure and show no symptoms before syncope or sudden cardiac death. However, if diagnosed, there are several therapeutic approaches to CPVT.

Generally speaking, life-long administration of β-blockers is the first choice as treatment. Studies showed that nadolol was clinically effective and a useful prophylactic (Priori et al., 2013). In countries, where nadolol is not available, propranolol was also shown to be effective (Hayashi et al., 2009). Carvedilol has been shown to inhibit store overload-induced Ca^{2+} release (SOICR) and is the only β-blocker to have RyR inhibitory action, albeit it is a less potent β-blocker after all (Zhou et al., 2011). Patients with CPVT are recommended to remove the triggers, in other words to limit or avoid any vigorous physical activities and stressful environments (Priori et al., 2013). In some patients (lacking long-term studies yet) β-blocker and non–dihydropyridine Ca^{2+}-channel blocker (verapamil) combination therapy was shown to be beneficial (Swan et al., 2005; Rosso et al., 2007).

Flecainide administration has been suggested on top of β-blockers to prevent arrhythmias, in CPVT patients refractory to β-blockers alone (Biernacka and Hoffman, 2011; Pott et al., 2011; van der Werf et al., 2011). Flecainide is a Na^{+}-channel blocker drug, specifically a Class Ic antiarrhythmic agent. Several studies, including three retrospective cohorts in human patients with CPVT (Liu et al., 2011; Radwanski et al., 2016; Kannankeril et al., 2017) have shown the effectiveness of flecainide but there is still debate around the mechanism by which it exerts its antiarrhythmic effect. Watanabe et al. concluded that the most important effect of flecainide was blocking the RyR along with the Na^{+}-channel blockade (Watanabe et al., 2009). They hypothesized that blocking RyR reduces the spontaneous Ca^{2+} release events and therefore DADs, while Na^{+}-channel blockade prevents the possibility of triggered activity from any residual DADs (Hilliard et al., 2010). Of the Class Ic antiarrhythmic drugs, only flecainide and propafenone was shown to inhibit RyR activity (Hwang et al., 2011). On the other hand, Liu et al. showed in an animal model of CPVT that although flecainide prevents VT and triggered activity, spontaneous Ca^{2+} release and DADs were still detectable in single myocytes. They concluded that the antiarrhythmic effect of flecainide results from its Na^{+}-channel blocker effect rather than *via* RyR inhibition (Liu et al., 2011b; Bannister et al., 2015). These conflicting results raise the question whether the different effects seen in the previous studies are dependent of a specific genetic mutation. In a recent study, isolated myocytes from Casq2$^{-/-}$ and RyR2R4496C$^{+/-}$ mice were compared (Hwang et al., 2019). It was found that the former produces a stronger proarrhythmic response upon isoproterenol stimulation, but flecainide prevented arrhythmias in both cases. Also independent from the underlying mutation, effect of flecainide decreased at high Ca^{2+} load. An additional drug has also been tested both *in vitro* and *in vivo*. 1,4-benzothiazepine derivative K201 (JTV519) was shown to prevent arrhythmias in mouse models by reducing RyR opening, SERCA activity and $I_{Ca,L}$ (Lehnart et al., 2004; Loughrey et al., 2007).

The latest guidelines recommend implantable cardiac defibrillator (ICD) implantation in patients with diagnosis of CPVT who experience VT, syncope, or cardiac arrest despite the optimal medical treatment (Priori et al., 2013). However, the use of ICDs without concomitant use of β-blockers is dangerous because of the possibility of shock-related electrical storms in these patients (Mohamed et al., 2006; Pflaumer and Davis, 2012). Selective left cardiac sympathetic denervation (LCSD) can be a useful therapeutic method and may be considered in patients with uncontrollable arrhythmias (patients with contraindication to β-blockers; when ICD cannot be implanted; or when recurrent VTs manifest in patients with ICD and β-blockers treatment) (Priori et al., 2013). Pulmonary vein isolation (catheter ablation) was reported to be efficient in some patients with CPVT and AF (Sumitomo et al., 2010), while the possibility of gene therapy was suggested after successful adenoviral vector infection (CASQ2 gene) in R33Q knock-in mutant mouse with dysfunctional CSQ2 (Denegri et al., 2014). Family screening of first degree relatives (clinical evaluation and genetic testing) has been strongly suggested with an optional β-blocker therapy even in the absence of a positive exercise test (Bauce et al., 2002; Hayashi et al., 2009).

Congenital Long QT Syndrome

Congenital long QT syndrome (LQTS) is an inherited cardiac ion channelopathy. LQTS is characterized by a prolonged QT interval on the surface ECG, reflecting the ventricular APD prolongation, which gives rise to risk for syncope, seizures, VT or torsade de pointes and finally VF and sudden cardiac death (Schwartz et al., 2012). Prolongation of APD can happen in an inhomogenous pattern, resulting in an enhanced dispersion of repolarization across the tissue. Delay in repolarization can occur e.g. by genetic defects of key ion currents, namely I_{Ks}, I_{Kr}, or I_{Na}. As mentioned in a previous section, EADs can form if the repolarization reserve is compromised, outward currents are reduced and/or inward currents are increased. In the case of LQTS, inhomogeneity of refractoriness combined with EADs establishes the arrhythmia substrate for VT, torsade de pointes.

The above mentioned conditions are illustrated in the cases of LQTS-1, LQTS-2, and LQTS-3. LQTS-1 is caused by the loss-of-function mutation of KCNQ1 gene ($K_v7.1$) that encodes I_{Ks} (Sanguinetti et al., 1996; Barhanin et al., 1996) while LQTS-2 is also a loss-of-function mutation, but of the KCNH2 channel gene ($K_v11.1$), encoding I_{Kr} (Sanguinetti et al., 1995). LQTS-3 is an inherited gain-of-function mutation of SCN5A Na^+ channel ($Na_v1.5$) encoding I_{Na} (Wang et al., 1995). All three mutations play key role in determining the length of AP and all of them points towards compromised repolarization reserve with decreased outward currents (LQTS1-2) and increased inward current (LQTS-3). LQTS-1–3 account for ~75–85% of the congenital LQTS cases (El-Sherif et al., 2017).

Mutations of several other genes have been described in LQTS patients. Mutations of structural and channel interacting proteins result in: LQTS-4, a loss-of-function mutation of ANK2-encoded ankyrin B and leads to Ca^{2+} overload, QT prolongation, sinus bradycardia, AF, and CPVT (Bhuiyan et al., 2013; Mohler et al., 2003); LQTS-5, a loss-of-function KCNE1-encoded minK mutation, consequential reduction in I_{Ks} (Splawski et al., 1997); LQTS-6, a loss-of-function mutation of KCNE2-encoded MiRP1, causing a faster inactivation time course for I_{Kr}, enhanced $I_{Ca,L}$, and reduced I_f (Lu et al., 2003; Nawathe et al., 2013; Liu et al., 2014); LQTS-9, CAV3-encoded Caveolin 3, causing an enhanced $I_{Na,L}$; and LQTS-11, a mutant A-kinase anchoring protein (AKAP9-Yotiao) results in an abnormal response upon β-stimulation, as mutation reduces interaction between AKAP9 and K_vLQT1 cannel α subunit (KCNQ1, I_{Ks}) leading to dysfunctional response to cAMP and a prolonged APD (QT) (Chen et al., 2007).

LQTS-9 and LQTS-10 (gain-of-function mutation in SCN4B-encoded Na^+ channel $Na_v\beta4$ β-subunit) together resemble the LQTS-3 phenotype as QT prolongation is achieved by increased Na^+ current (Medeiros-Domingo et al., 2007). Mutation of SNTA1-encoded α1-syntrophin is a gain-of-function gene anomaly, causing LQTS-12 by enhancing Na^+ current ($Na_v1.5$) (Wu et al., 2008). LQTS-7 and LQTS-13 are affecting repolarizing K^+ currents and channels. LQTS-7 or Andersen-Tawil type 1 syndrome is caused by the loss-of-function mutation of the KCNJ2-encoded $K_{ir}2.1$ inward rectifier K^+ channel, responsible for I_{K1}, and as I_{K1} is an important player in terminal repolarization, reduction of $K_{ir}2.1$ function prolongs QT interval (Plaster et al., 2001). In LQTS-13, a loss-of-function mutation on KCNJ5-encoded $K_{ir}3.4$ causes loss of acetylcholine activated, G-protein-gated K^+ (I_{KAch}) channel function. I_{KAch} is formed by $K_{ir}3.1$ and $K_{ir}3.4$. Mutation in $K_{ir}3.4$ function disrupts membrane targeting and stability, i.e. reduced membrane expression has been suggested as the cause of LQTS-13 (Yang et al., 2010).

Although most of the LQTS mutant genes are related to K^+ and Na^+ channels (i.e. LQTS-1-3 being ~75–85% of total congenital LQTS), there are several Ca^{2+}-signaling proteins that are linked to the occurrence of long QT intervals, typically causing LQTS-8, LQTS-14, LQTS-15, LQTS-16, and LQTS-17 (**Table 1**).

LQTS-8 is a gain-of-function mutation of the CACNA1C-encoded $\alpha1_C$ subunit of L-type Ca^{2+} channel ($Ca_v1.2$) and is generally associated with Timothy syndrome. Timothy syndrome is a rare (less than 30 patients reported worldwide), but severe multisystem disorder, involving QT prolongation, syndactyly, congenital heart defects, cardiomyopathies, bradycardia (caused by AV block rather than sinus bradycardia), and autism (Splawski et al., 2004). LQTS-8 mutation of the $Ca_v1.2$ leads to (1) a significant reduction in voltage-dependent inactivation of $I_{Ca,L}$, (2) enhanced $I_{Ca,L}$, (3) decreased current density with enhanced window current, and (4) a steeper APD restitution curve (Thiel et al., 2008; Boczek et al., 2015; Landstrom et al., 2016). A lesser inactivation of the steady-state current and/or increased peak current means a higher Ca^{2+} influx, which can in turn prolong APD, therefore QT interval. A steeper APD restitution curve is proarrhythmic, being a substrate for alternans, as detailed in previous chapters. The mutation can also cause T-wave alternans on the ECG by increasing the dispersion of repolarization (Zhu and Clancy, 2007). In iPSC cells of a Timothy syndrome patient, a cyclin-dependent kinase inhibitor, roscovitine was found to shorten APD by partially recovering inactivation of the mutant channel (Yarotskyy et al., 2010; Yazawa et al., 2011). If Timothy syndrome/LQTS-8 is diagnosed, because of the high mortality, ICD implantation is the first choice. ICD is often supplemented with β-blockers, relying on the fact that they are generally effective in LQTS patients. Also, verapamil (Jacobs et al., 2006), mexiletine (Krause et al., 2011), and ranolazine (Shah et al., 2012) have been shown to shorten APD by affecting $I_{Ca,L}$ and reducing the risk of arrhythmias.

LQTS-14–16 are newly described subtypes of LQT syndrome, caused by mutations in the genes coding the ubiquitous Ca^{2+} sensor and binder, calmodulin (CaM). Mutations in CALM1-encoding CaM1, CALM2-encoding CaM2, and CALM3-encoding CaM3 are responsible for producing LQTS-14, LQTS-15, and LQTS-16, respectively. Patients diagnosed with these conditions are usually young and have a high rate of cardiac arrest with severe QT prolongation (Gray and Behr, 2016). CaM is important in the inactivation of Na^+ channels, Ca^{2+}-dependent inactivation of $I_{Ca,L}$ and also important in the trafficking, assembly, and gating of the I_{Ks} channel, KCNQ1 (Shamgar et al., 2006). Gene anomalies, affecting CaM, and therefore, Ca^{2+} binding and/or enhancing $I_{Ca,L}$ can lead to severe APD prolongation. To date, over 20 mutations have been reported in the disease group of calmodulinopathies (Jensen et al., 2018; Wren et al., 2019) associated with LQTS, CPVT, and idiopathic VF. LQTS mutations, e.g. CaM-D130G, CaM-D96V, CaM-N98S, and CaM-F142L are all having impaired Ca^{2+} binding properties at the EF hand domains (Crotti et al., 2013). In CaM-D130G, CaM-D96V, and CaM-N98S mutations impaired CaM-dependent inhibition of RyR was reported, thereby increasing SR Ca^{2+} release due to an increased open state of RyR (Sondergaard et al., 2017; Jensen et al., 2018). Unexpectedly, an LQTS-associated CaM mutation, CaM-F142L did not diminish, but, increased the CaM-dependent RyR gating inhibition and caused faster RyR closing at high $[Ca^{2+}]_i$ (Sondergaard et al., 2017). The authors proposed that the mutation displayed both gain-of-function and loss-of-function properties. In the process of gain-of-function, F142L mutation increases the interactions between the C-domain of CaM and the CaM binding domain of RyR, therefore enhancing RyR inhibition. On the other hand, the loss-of-function effect impairs the ability of the C-domain of CaM to bind free Ca^{2+}, i.e. decreases RyR inhibition. However, at high $[Ca^{2+}]_i$ C-domain of CaM saturates allowing the increased RyR inhibitory effect to be the dominant one (Sondergaard et al., 2017). One might assume an overlap between LQTS and CPVT as diminished inhibitory effect on RyR gating is generally associated with CPVT. In mutant guinea pig cells, it was shown that decreased inhibition of RyR gating with impaired CaM effect on the CaM-dependent inactivation of $I_{Ca,L}$ (i.e. increased $I_{Ca,L}$) may contribute to APD prolongation and that LQTS associated CaM mutations can lead to electrical alternans, a pathological feature of LQTS (Limpitikul et al., 2014).

Recently a novel mutation, LQTS-17 has been proposed, however, the nomenclature is still indistinct. Some reviews refer to LQTS-17 as a mutation in TRDN-encoded triadin, which has also been linked to CPVT-5 (Landstrom et al., 2017). However, Altmann et al., originally identified the autosomal recessive homozygous or compound heterozygous frameshift loss-of-function mutations in TRDN, proposed the term Triadin Knockout Syndrome (TKOS) or TRDN-mediated autosomal-recessive LQTS, rather than LQTS-17 (Altmann et al., 2015). As in the previous case, here is also the possibility of an overlap with CPVT, as QT prolongation and disease appearance at young age is accompanied by arrhythmias that occur during exercise. The possible cellular mechanism includes reduced negative feedback on $I_{Ca,L}$ (i.e. increased $I_{Ca,L}$), increased spontaneous Ca^{2+} release *via* RyR, and promotion of SR Ca^{2+} loading by NCX. It is not clear yet, whether the arrhythmogenic feature is mediated by DAD or EAD, but in a TRDN-null mice model, nifedipine aborted SR Ca^{2+} overload and spontaneous Ca^{2+} release (Chopra et al., 2009).

Although most of the LQTSs are inherited in an autosomal dominant form, there is a relatively rare, autosomal recessive inherited form, causing the Jervell and Lange-Nielsen syndrome (KCNQ1 or KCNE1, leading to reduced I_{Ks}) (Splawski et al., 1997; Duggal et al., 1998). LQTS-related arrhythmias can be triggered by either slow or fast heart rate or by sinus pauses, therefore the relation between the LQTSs and the sinoatrial node is an interesting topic; for details, see the mini-review from Wilders and Verkerk (2018). For a detailed summary chart about LQTSs with the genetic loci, see a recent review of Landstrom et al. (Landstrom et al., 2017).

Pharmacological management of congenital LQTS starts with the administration of β-blockers, irrespective of the genotype (Moss et al., 2000). In one study, propranolol was shown to be the most effective β-blocker (Na^+ channel blockade with limited effects on K^+ channels) (Chockalingam et al., 2012). It should be noted that care is required with the use of β-blockers at low heart rate in LQTS-3 since bradycardia-dependent arrhythmias occur more often in these patients (El-Sherif et al., 2017). It was shown in LQTS-2 patients that besides β-blockers, application of mexiletine may also have positive effects (Kim et al., 2010; Ildarova et al., 2012). As an add-on therapy, in the case of LQTS-3 patients mexiletine (Schwartz et al., 1995), lidocaine, tocainide (Rosero et al., 1997), flecainide (Moss et al., 2005), phenytoin (Vukmir and Stein, 1991), or ranolazine (Moss et al., 2008) can be useful (Priori et al., 2013). In LQTS where mutations cause reduction in K^+ currents, drugs that enhance K^+ currents, nicorandil (Shimizu et al., 1998) or RPR26043 (Kang et al., 2005) were shown to be effective. ICD implantation is recommended for survivors of cardiac arrest or with recurrent syncope while on β-blocker (Priori et al., 2013). Left cardiac sympathetic denervation (LCSD) can also be performed on high-risk patients (arrhythmic events even in the presence of β-blocker/ICD). In addition to drugs or surgical procedures, lifestyle changes, such as avoidance of drugs that lengthen QT interval, identification and correlation of electrolyte abnormalities, avoidance of strenuous exercise (especially swimming in LQTS-1 patients) and abrupt loud noises (LTQS-2) are recommended for patients (Priori et al., 2013).

Brugada Syndrome

Brugada syndrome (BrS) is characterized by ST elevation in V1–V3 ECG leads and is associated with elevated risk of polymorphic VT, VF, and sudden cardiac death (Brugada and Brugada, 1992). Two hypotheses have been proposed to describe the mechanism behind BrS and how ST segment elevation is linked to VT/VF. (Ringer, 1883) In the repolarization hypothesis, the loss of spike-and-dome AP morphology (heterogenous shortening of AP due to predominance of I_{to} over I_{Na} and $I_{Ca,L}$) is suggested in the epicardium of the right ventricular outflow tract, causing an enhanced transmural dispersion of repolarization, i.e. ST elevation (Yan and Antzelevitch, 1999). The arrhythmogenic mechanism is delivered by phase-2 reentry, when the produced extrasystole can occur on the preceding T wave (R-on-T phenomenon), finally initiating VT/VF. (Bers, 2002) The depolarization theory proposes a slowed conduction and delayed activation mechanism in the right ventricular outflow tract as a substrate for reentry (Meregalli et al., 2005).

To date, 23 gene (gain-of-function and also loss-of-function) mutations have been described generating BrS-1–BrS-23 (Gray and Behr, 2016). The most common subtype is BrS-1, mutation affects the SCN5A-encoded α-subunit of the Na^+ channel ($Na_v1.5$) and is accountable for about one third of all BrS (Antzelevitch et al., 2005). Genes, governing Ca^{2+}-signaling molecules are also affected in BrS and causing 10–15% of cases (Burashnikov et al., 2010) (**Table 1**). Loss-of-function mutation of the CACNA1C-encoded α_{1C}-subunit ($Ca_v1.2\alpha1$; BrS-3), the CACNB2-encoded β_2-subunit ($Ca_v\beta2$; BrS-4), and the CACNA2D1-encoded $\alpha_2\delta_1$-subunit ($Ca_v\alpha2\delta1$; BrS-11) of the L-type Ca^{2+} channel (governing $I_{Ca,L}$) have been described with a concomitant reduction of $I_{Ca,L}$ (Antzelevitch et al., 2007). Patients harboring these Ca^{2+} related mutations showed BrS like ECG but with shorter than normal QT intervals. Recently, a new Ca^{2+}-related mutation has been linked to BrS, accounting for about 6% of the cases. Mutation of the TRPM4-encoded Ca^{2+} activated non-selective cation channel transient receptor potential melastatin 4 (TRPM4; BrS-15) can either be gain-of-function or loss-of-function (Liu et al., 2013). TRPM4-mediated current increases APD in atrial muscle and isolated myocytes (Simard et al., 2013), possibly by promoting the plateau (as it is more likely to activate when Ca^{2+} is elevated). Therefore, TRPM4 mutation may change the AP dome and be arrhythmogenic. TRMP4 may also slow down conduction by altering the availability of Na^+ channels (Liu et al., 2013).

There have been pharmacological attempts to manage BrS (isoproterenol, quinidine, procainamide, propafenone, pilsicainide, flecainide), some of them were effective in preventing recurrent episodes of VF or electrical storms, but did not reduce the overall risk of VF (Brugada et al., 2000; Shimizu et al., 2000; Morita et al., 2003; Belhassen et al., 2004; Ohgo et al., 2007). Guidelines are also recommending lifestyle changes (omit drugs that aggravate ST elevation, avoid alcohol and immediate treatment if fevered) and implantation of ICD (Priori et al., 2013).

Short QT Syndrome

Short QT syndrome (SQTS) is a rare inherited syndrome characterized by QT intervals essentially shorter than 360 ms and by an increased incidence of VT/VF mainly in youngsters (Bjerregaard et al., 2010). There are eight different gene mutations, of which three affect $I_{Ca,L}$ (**Table 1**). Loss-of-function mutation of the CACNA1C-encoded α_{1C}-subunit ($Ca_v1.2\alpha1$; SQTS-4), the CACNB2-encoded β_2-subunit ($Ca_v\beta2$; SQTS-5), and the CACNA2D1-encoded $\alpha_2\delta_1$-subunit ($Ca_v\alpha2\delta1$; SQTS-6) of the L-type Ca^{2+} channel, similar to the BrS-3, BrS-4, and BrS-11 phenotype. These mutations decrease $I_{Ca,L}$ (alter current density and activation/inactivation kinetics), cause heterogenous shortening of APD and QT interval, therefore increases dispersion of repolarization (Antzelevitch et al., 2007). Transmural dispersion of repolarization (shortening effect is more pronounced in the epicardium compared to endocardium and midmyocardium) finally serves as a substrate for reentry. These mutations combined with the mutation of SCN5A-encoded α-subunit of the Na^+ channel ($Na_v1.5$) causes an overlapping phenotype of SQTS and BrS.

Early Repolarization Syndrome and Idiopathic Ventricular Fibrillation

Early repolarization syndrome (ERS) is characterized by J-point and ST segment elevation in two or more contiguous leads on ECG (Boineau, 2007). The early repolarization pattern (in the inferior and/or lateral precordial leads) had been considered harmless, but it has recently been associated with idiopathic ventricular fibrillation (IVF) (Rosso et al., 2008). ERS now is diagnosed in IVF survival patients, without other causes of cardiac arrest (channelopathies; structural or non-structural heart diseases, e.g. BrS; metabolic; toxicological; respiratory; and infectious) (Haissaguerre et al., 2008). Seven gene mutations were shown, to date, including loss-of-function mutations of CACNA1C, CACNAB2, and CACNA2D1, as seen in BrS or SQTS (**Table 1**). L-type channel mutations account for 16% of cases (Burashnikov et al., 2010). CaM-F90L mutation was proposed to be linked to IVF phenotype, where the authors speculated that CaM mutations could be arrhythmogenic by altering Ca^{2+} binding and/or binding of target proteins, thus generating a rather insensitive CaM and that the gene anomaly is more pronounced in the Purkinje system (Marsman et al., 2014). Recently, a novel single point mutation in RyR2 (RyR2-H29D) has been linked to IVF phenotype (Cheung et al., 2015). RyR2-H29D mutation was shown to be associated with short-coupled premature ventricular contractions, initiating polymorphic VT. This mutation caused diastolic Ca^{2+} leak at rest by higher open probability and higher frequency of opening of RyR at low diastolic Ca^{2+} levels in a non-PKA phosphorylated state, unlike the typical CPVT-related RyR mutations. Therefore, RyR dysfunction caused by RyR2-H29D mutation may play a role in short-coupled polymorphic VT.

J-point elevation associated malignant arrhythmias have recently been proposed with a new classification, as J-wave syndrome (Antzelevitch and Yan, 2010).

ACQUIRED SYNDROMES

Acquired Long QT Syndrome

In addition to the congenital form, LQTS can also be acquired. The prevalence of acquired LQTS is greater than that of congenital forms (El-Sherif et al., 2019). It is generally caused by adverse, unwanted drug effects and/or electrolyte abnormalities and may predispose to the prolongation of the APD/QT interval, increase in dispersion of refractoriness and to a higher risk for generating EADs, being the substrates for VTs, especially for torsade de pointes VT (El-Sherif and Turitto, 1999).

The above mentioned effects are often seen for the hERG-encoded (human ether-à-go-go-related gene or KCNH2) $K_v11.1$ channel, responsible for I_{Kr} while effects on enhanced $I_{Na,L}$ has also been reported (Yang et al., 2014). The role of dispersion of repolarization in generating tachyarrhythmias (and the role as a preclinical proarrhythmia marker) is further supported by a series of experiments, where DL-sotalol and amiodarone were compared (Milberg et al., 2004). It was shown, that both hERG-blockers increased QT interval, however only DL-sotalol increased transmural dispersion of refractoriness, EADs and torsade de pointes (and caused triangulation of the AP), while amiodarone caused phase-2 prolongation of the AP without triangulation, which is otherwise considered proarrhythmic.

Several other causes of acquired LQTS have been described, including electrolyte disorders (El-Sherif and Turitto, 2011), such as hypokalemia, hypomagnesemia or hypocalcemia, hypothyroidism, hypothermia, but also antidepressant and antipsychotic treatments (Sicouri and Antzelevitch, 2018), female gender, and autoimmune and inflammatory diseases (Lazzerini et al., 2015; Boutjdir et al., 2016). Hypocalcemia causes QT prolongation *via* phase-2 prolongation of AP (Eryol et al., 2003), also longer and late Ca^{2+} influx (due to reduced Ca^{2+}-dependent inactivation of $I_{Ca,L}$) can favor the formation of EADs.

Atrial Fibrillation

The most prevalent cardiac arrhythmia is atrial fibrillation (AF) and this can be classified as paroxysmal (spontaneously self-terminates into sinus rhythm in less than 7 days), persistent (lasts for more than 7 days), long-lasting persistent (AF lasts for more than a year) or permanent AF (without active rhythm control) (Kirchhof et al., 2016). AF is multifactorial. Basic arrhythmogenic mechanisms include Ca^{2+} handling defects such as triggered activity (DAD, late-phase 3 EAD), conduction block (reentry), and Ca^{2+}-driven cardiac alternans and altered Ca^{2+} buffering (Nattel and Dobrev, 2016). DAD-mediated triggered arrhythmias are underlined by Ca^{2+} handling instability in AF, namely RyR dysfunction (increased phosphorylation and open probability), increased SERCA function, increased diastolic SR Ca^{2+} leak and spontaneous SR Ca^{2+} release, increase in Ca^{2+} sparks and waves, enhanced CaMKII function (with subsequent RyR hyperphosphorylation), or reduced $I_{Ca,L}$ (Sood et al., 2008; Neef et al., 2010; Shan et al., 2012; Voigt et al., 2012). Involvement of late-phase 3 EAD has also been shown (Burashnikov and Antzelevitch, 2006). As in most of the AF models APD is abbreviated, this observation can be somewhat surprising, since EADs generally occur at a prolonged APD. However, as we previously described, late-phase 3 EADs occur at shorter APD and at elevated Ca^{2+} loading conditions (such as rapid atrial pacing). These ectopic activities can serve as a trigger for reentry which is considered to be the main arrhythmogenic mechanism in AF. Also, $I_{Ca,L}$ reduction in AF causes APD shortening and promotes reentrant activity (Heijman et al., 2014). Reduction of $I_{Ca,L}$ might be governed by reduction of protein and mRNA levels of the channel (alpha subunit) after rapid pacing. This transcriptional downregulation of Ca^{2+} channel has been proposed to be mediated by activation of calcineurin by Ca^{2+}/CaM, which in turn, regulates nuclear translocation of NFAT (Qi et al., 2008).

A novel, interesting theory has been proposed, namely, Ca^{2+} signaling silencing, as an antiarrhythmic adaptive mechanism in AF (Greiser et al., 2014). The key observation was, that sustained high atrial pacing may not lead to Ca^{2+} instability, suggesting a role of accompanying cardiovascular diseases (e.g. HF) rather than "lone AF" itself in those cases when unstable Ca^{2+} signaling occurs in AF. Ca^{2+} signaling silencing process includes the failure of centripetal intracellular Ca^{2+} signal propagation (also unchanged level of Ca^{2+} sparks and decreased amplitude of the systolic Ca^{2+} transient), remodeling of the RyR complex (reduced protein expression and CaMKII-mediated phosphorylation), and lower Na^+ concentration (consequential reduction in Ca^{2+} load) (Greiser, 2017). The decreased propagation was associated with an increase of cytoplasmic buffer power possibly due to increased Ca^{2+} sensitivity of myofilaments resulting from decreased phosphorylation of troponin I (Greiser et al., 2014). The authors concluded that the Ca^{2+} signaling phenotype in AF patients is a net result offactors that stabilize (i.e. Ca^{2+} signaling silencing) or destabilize it (arrhythmogenic Ca^{2+} instability). Therefore, future therapeutic approaches should identify the substrate (arrhythmia enhancing abnormalities or arrhythmia suppressing Ca^{2+} signaling silencing) and tailor therapies for individual AF patients (Kirchhof et al., 2016; Schotten et al., 2016; Greiser, 2017).

For an excess review about the role of Ca^{2+} in the pathophsiology of AF see the review of Denham et al. (2018).

CONCLUSIONS

In summary, we have reviewed the roles of Ca^{2+} in cardiac E-C-coupling focusing on those defects which lead to cardiac arrhythmias in inherited and acquired syndromes. In the last few decades there have been great advances in the understanding of these arrhythmias, however, there is still a need for more work investigating the physiology and pathophysiology of Ca^{2+} related events. Designing drugs to treat a specific disease type has never been simple; it is enough to think of the early disappointing attempts to block the Na^+ or K^+ channels (CAST and SWORD trials, respectively). Multiple characteristics of novel therapeutic approaches have to be determined and to be considered as a complex, systems problem.

Along with the generally used β-blockers, newly developed selective drugs without proarrhythmic side effects are necessary. While implantable cardiac defibrillators provide longer life expectancy, they cannot prevent the onset of cardiac events. An additional helpful tool would be reliable and effective risk stratification and clinical guidance for all of the syndromes discussed. It should not be overlooked that in the future other genetic mutations may be discovered requiring novel biological therapies. Because of the diversity of inherited and acquired mutations individually tailored therapeutic approaches (gene-specific or mutation-specific pharmacological and/or gene therapy) will be required.

To gain a better understanding of the role of Ca^{2+} in the cardiac arrhythmias data from basic science should meet the clinical practice; translational aspects must be key in all fields of science.

AUTHOR CONTRIBUTIONS

KK conceived the review and drafted the manuscript. KK, RV, BH, TB, PN, and DE revised the manuscript critically for important intellectual content. DE contributed to the critical review of the literature, editing of the manuscript text and review of the figures. All authors approved the final version of the manuscript submitted.

FUNDING

This work was funded by the National Research Development and Innovation Office (NKFIH-K115397). Further support was obtained from GINOP-2.3.2.-15-2016-00040 and EFOP-3.6.2-16-2017-00006 projects, which are co-financed by the European Union and the European Regional Development Fund. The research was financed by the Thematic Excellence Programme of the Ministry for Innovation and Technology in Hungary (ED_18-1-2019-0028), within the framework of the Space Sciences thematic program of the University of Debrecen. This work was supported by the British Heart Foundation Chair Award (grant number: CH/200004/12801).

ACKNOWLEDGMENTS

KK is grateful to his wife Viktoria Csato, PhD who is expecting their twin daughters Zoe Amira and Liza Jazmin, without whom this review would have been completed much earlier. The authors wish to thank Jessica L. Caldwell for the design of **Figure 1**.

REFERENCES

Abi-Gerges, N., Valentin, J. P., and Pollard, C. E. (2010). Dog left ventricular midmyocardial myocytes for assessment of drug-induced delayed repolarization: short-term variability and proarrhythmic potential. *Br. J. Pharmacol.* 159 (1), 77–92. doi: 10.1111/j.1476-5381.2009.00338.x

Allessie, M. A., Bonke, F. I., and Schopman, F. J. (1977). Circus movement in rabbit atrial muscle as a mechanism of tachycardia. III. The "leading circle" concept: a new model of circus movement in cardiac tissue without the involvement of an anatomical obstacle. *Circ. Res.* 41 (1), 9–18. doi: 10.1161/01.res.41.1.9

Altmann, H. M., Tester, D. J., Will, M. L., Middha, S., Evans, J. M., Eckloff, B. W., et al. (2015). Homozygous/compound heterozygous triadin mutations associated with autosomal-recessive long-QT syndrome and pediatric sudden cardiac arrest: elucidation of the triadin knockout syndrome. *Circulation* 131 (23), 2051–2060. doi: 10.1161/CIRCULATIONAHA.115.015397

Antzelevitch, C., and Burashnikov, A. (2011). Overview of basic mechanisms of cardiac arrhythmia. *Cardiac Electrophysiol. Clinics* 3 (1), 23–45. doi: 10.1016/j.ccep.2010.10.012

Antzelevitch, C., and Yan, G. X. (2010). J wave syndromes. *Heart Rhythm* 7 (4), 549–558. doi: 10.1016/j.hrthm.2009.12.006

Antzelevitch, C., Jalife, J., and Moe, G. K. (1980). Characteristics of reflection as a mechanism of reentrant arrhythmias and its relationship to parasystole. *Circulation* 61 (1), 182–191. doi: 10.1161/01.cir.61.1.182

Antzelevitch, C., Brugada, P., Borggrefe, M., Brugada, J., Brugada, R., Corrado, D., et al. (2005). Brugada syndrome: report of the second consensus conference: endorsed by the heart rhythm society and the european heart rhythm association. *Circulation* 111 (5), 659–670. doi: 10.1161/01.CIR.0000152479.54298.51

Antzelevitch, C., Pollevick, G. D., Cordeiro, J. M., Casis, O., Sanguinetti, M. C., Aizawa, Y., et al. (2007). Loss-of-function mutations in the cardiac calcium channel underlie a new clinical entity characterized by ST-segment elevation, short QT intervals, and sudden cardiac death. *Circulation* 115 (4), 442–449. doi: 10.1161/CIRCULATIONAHA.106.668392

Antzelevitch, C. (2007). Heterogeneity and cardiac arrhythmias: an overview. *Heart Rhythm* 4 (7), 964–972. doi: 10.1016/j.hrthm.2007.03.036

Aronson, R. S. (1981). Afterpotentials and triggered activity in hypertrophied myocardium from rats with renal hypertension. *Circ. Res.* 48 (5), 720–727. doi: 10.1161/01.res.48.5.720

Arvanitis, D. A., Vafiadaki, E., Sanoudou, D., and Kranias, E. G. (2011). Histidine-rich calcium binding protein: the new regulator of sarcoplasmic reticulum calcium cycling. *J. Mol. Cell. Cardiol.* 50 (1), 43–49. doi: 10.1016/j.yjmcc.2010.08.021

Asakura, K., Cha, C. Y., Yamaoka, H., Horikawa, Y., Memida, H., Powell, T., et al. (2014). EAD and DAD mechanisms analyzed by developing a new human ventricular cell model. *Prog. Biophys. Mol. Biol.* 116 (1), 11–24. doi: 10.1016/j.pbiomolbio.2014.08.008

Bal, N. C., Sharon, A., Gupta, S. C., Jena, N., Shaikh, S., Gyorke, S., et al. (2010). The catecholaminergic polymorphic ventricular tachycardia mutation R33Q disrupts the N-terminal structural motif that regulates reversible calsequestrin polymerization. *J. Biol. Chem.* 285 (22), 17188–17196. doi: 10.1074/jbc.M109.096354

Bannister, M. L., Thomas, N. L., Sikkel, M. B., Mukherjee, S., Maxwell, C., MacLeod, K. T., et al. (2015). The mechanism of flecainide action in CPVT does not involve a direct effect on RyR2. *Circ. Res.* 116 (8), 1324–1335. doi: 10.1161/CIRCRESAHA.116.305347

Barhanin, J., Lesage, F., Guillemare, E., Fink, M., Lazdunski, M., and Romey, G. (1996). K(V)LQT1 and lsK (minK) proteins associate to form the I(Ks) cardiac potassium current. *Nature* 384 (6604), 78–80. doi: 10.1038/384078a0

Bauce, B., Rampazzo, A., Basso, C., Bagattin, A., Daliento, L., Tiso, N., et al. (2002). Screening for ryanodine receptor type 2 mutations in families with effort-induced polymorphic ventricular arrhythmias and sudden death: early diagnosis of asymptomatic carriers. *J. Am. Coll. Cardiol.* 40 (2), 341–349. doi: 10.1016/s0735-1097(02)01946-0

Belhassen, B., Glick, A., and Viskin, S. (2004). Efficacy of quinidine in high-risk patients with Brugada syndrome. *Circulation* 110 (13), 1731–1737. doi: 10.1161/01.CIR.0000143159.30585.90

Benitah, J. P., Alvarez, J. L., and Gomez, A. M. (2010). L-type Ca(2+) current in ventricular cardiomyocytes. *J. Mol. Cell. Cardiol.* 48 (1), 26–36. doi: 10.1016/j.yjmcc.2009.07.026

Bers, D. M. (2000). Calcium fluxes involved in control of cardiac myocyte contraction. *Circ. Res.* 87 (4), 275–281. doi: 10.1161/01.res.87.4.275

Bers, D. M. (2002). Cardiac excitation-contraction coupling. *Nature* 415 (6868), 198–205. doi: 10.1038/415198a

Bhuiyan, Z. A., Hamdan, M. A., Shamsi, E. T., Postma, A. V., Mannens, M. M., Wilde, A. A., et al. (2007). A novel early onset lethal form of catecholaminergic polymorphic ventricular tachycardia maps to chromosome 7p14-p22. *J. Cardiovasc. Electrophysiol.* 18 (10), 1060–1066. doi: 10.1111/j.1540-8167.2007.00913.x

Bhuiyan, Z. A., Al-Shahrani, S., Al-Aama, J., Wilde, A. A., and Momenah, T. S. (2013). Congenital long QT syndrome: an update and present perspective in Saudi Arabia. *Front. Pediatr.* 1, 39. doi: 10.3389/fped.2013.00039

Biernacka, E. K., and Hoffman, P. (2011). Efficacy of flecainide in a patient with catecholaminergic polymorphic ventricular tachycardia. *Europace* 13 (1), 129–130. doi: 10.1093/europace/euq279

Bjerregaard, P., Nallapaneni, H., and Gussak, I. (2010). Short QT interval in clinical practice. *J. Electrocardiol.* 43 (5), 390–395. doi: 10.1016/j.jelectrocard.2010.06.004

Boczek, N. J., Miller, E. M., Ye, D., Nesterenko, V. V., Tester, D. J., Antzelevitch, C., et al. (2015). Novel Timothy syndrome mutation leading to increase in

CACNA1C window current. *Heart Rhythm.* 12 (1), 211–219. doi: 10.1016/j.hrthm.2014.09.051

Boineau, J. P. (2007). The early repolarization variant-normal or a marker of heart disease in certain subjects. *J. Electrocardiol.* 40 (1), 3.e11–3.e16. doi: 10.1016/j.jelectrocard.2006.04.002

Boutjdir, M., Lazzerini, P. E., Capecchi, P. L., Laghi-Pasini, F., and El-Sherif, N. (2016). Potassium channel block and novel autoimmune-associated long QT syndrome. *Cardiac Electrophysiol. Clinics* 8 (2), 373–384. doi: 10.1016/j.ccep.2016.02.002

Brugada, P., and Brugada, J. (1992). Right bundle branch block, persistent ST segment elevation and sudden cardiac death: a distinct clinical and electrocardiographic syndrome. a multicenter report. *J. Am. Coll. Cardiol.* 20 (6), 1391–1396. doi: 10.1016/0735-1097(92)90253-j

Brugada, R., Brugada, J., Antzelevitch, C., Kirsch, G. E., Potenza, D., Towbin, J. A., et al. (2000). Sodium channel blockers identify risk for sudden death in patients with ST-segment elevation and right bundle branch block but structurally normal hearts. *Circulation* 101 (5), 510–515. doi: 10.1161/01.cir.101.5.510

Burashnikov, A., and Antzelevitch, C. (2003). Reinduction of atrial fibrillation immediately after termination of the arrhythmia is mediated by late phase 3 early afterdepolarization-induced triggered activity. *Circulation* 107 (18), 2355–2360. doi: 10.1161/01.CIR.0000065578.00869.7C

Burashnikov, A., and Antzelevitch, C. (2006). Late-phase 3 EAD. a unique mechanism contributing to initiation of atrial fibrillation. *Pacing Clin. Electrophysiol.* 29 (3), 290–295. doi: 10.1111/j.1540-8159.2006.00336.x

Burashnikov, E., Pfeiffer, R., Barajas-Martinez, H., Delpon, E., Hu, D., Desai, M., et al. (2010). Mutations in the cardiac L-type calcium channel associated with inherited J-wave syndromes and sudden cardiac death. *Heart Rhythm* 7 (12), 1872–1882. doi: 10.1016/j.hrthm.2010.08.026

Cabo, C., and Barr, R. C. (1992). Propagation model using the DiFrancesco-Noble equations. Comparison to reported experimental results. *Med. Biol. Eng. Comput.* 30 (3), 292–302. doi: 10.1007/bf02446967

Cantalapiedra, I. R., Penaranda, A., Mont, L., Brugada, J., and Echebarria, B. (2009). Reexcitation mechanisms in epicardial tissue: role of I(to) density heterogeneities and I(Na) inactivation kinetics. *J. Theor. Biol.* 259 (4), 850–859. doi: 10.1016/j.jtbi.2009.04.021

Cantalapiedra, I. R., Penaranda, A., Echebarria, B., and Bragard, J. (2010). Phase-2 reentry in cardiac tissue: role of the slow calcium pulse. *Phys. Rev. E Stat. Nonlinear Soft Matter Phys.* 82 (1 Pt 1), 011907. doi: 10.1103/PhysRevE.82.011907

Chang, M. G., Sato, D., de Lange, E., Lee, J. H., Karagueuzian, H. S., Garfinkel, A., et al. (2012). Bi-stable wave propagation and early afterdepolarization-mediated cardiac arrhythmias. *Heart Rhythm* 9 (1), 115–122. doi: 10.1016/j.hrthm.2011.08.014

Chang, M. G., de Lange, E., Calmettes, G., Garfinkel, A., Qu, Z., and Weiss, J. N. (2013). Pro- and antiarrhythmic effects of ATP-sensitive potassium current activation on reentry during early afterdepolarization-mediated arrhythmias. *Heart Rhythm* 10 (4), 575–582. doi: 10.1016/j.hrthm.2012.12.017

Chanson, M., Mollard, P., Meda, P., Suter, S., and Jongsma, H. J. (1999). Modulation of pancreatic acinar cell to cell coupling during ACh-evoked changes in cytosolic Ca2+. *J. Biol. Chem.* 274 (1), 282–287. doi: 10.1074/jbc.274.1.282

Chen, L., Marquardt, M. L., Tester, D. J., Sampson, K. J., Ackerman, M. J., and Kass, R. S. (2007). Mutation of an a-kinase-anchoring protein causes long-QT syndrome. *Proc. Natl. Acad. Sci. U. S. A.* 104 (52), 20990–20995. doi: 10.1073/pnas.0710527105

Cheng, H., Lederer, W. J. , and Cannell, M. B. (1993). Calcium sparks: elementary events underlying excitation-contraction coupling in heart muscle. *Science* 262 (5134), 740–744. doi: 10.1126/science.8235594

Cheung, J. W., Meli, A. C., Xie, W., Mittal, S., Reiken, S., Wronska, A., et al. (2015). Short-coupled polymorphic ventricular tachycardia at rest linked to a novel ryanodine receptor (RyR2) mutation: leaky RyR2 channels under non-stress conditions. *Int. J. Cardiol.* 180, 228–236. doi: 10.1016/j.ijcard.2014.11.119

Chiamvimonvat, N., Chen-Izu, Y., Clancy, C. E., Deschenes, I., Dobrev, D., Heijman, J., et al. (2017). Potassium currents in the heart: functional roles in repolarization, arrhythmia and therapeutics. *J. Physiol.* 595 (7), 2229–2252. doi: 10.1113/JP272883

Chockalingam, P., Crotti, L., Girardengo, G., Johnson, J. N., Harris, K. M., van der Heijden, J. F., et al. (2012). Not all beta-blockers are equal in the management of long QT syndrome types 1 and 2: higher recurrence of events under metoprolol. *J. Am. Coll. Cardiol.* 60 (20), 2092–2099. doi: 10.1016/j.jacc.2012.07.046

Chopra, N., Yang, T., Asghari, P., Moore, E. D., Huke, S., Akin, B., et al. (2009). Ablation of triadin causes loss of cardiac Ca2+ release units, impaired excitation-contraction coupling, and cardiac arrhythmias. *Proc. Natl. Acad. Sci. U. S. A.* 106 (18), 7636–7641. doi: 10.1073/pnas.0902919106

Coppini, R., Ferrantini, C., Mugelli, A., Poggesi, C., and Cerbai, E. (2018). Altered Ca(2+) and Na(+) homeostasis in human hypertrophic cardiomyopathy: implications for arrhythmogenesis. *Front. Physiol.* 9, 1391. doi: 10.3389/fphys.2018.01391

Coumel, P. (1978). Catecholaminergic-induced severe ventricular arrhythmias with adams-Stokes syndrome in children: report of four cases. *Br. Heart J.* 40, 28–37.

Crotti, L., Johnson, C. N., Graf, E., De Ferrari, G. M., Cuneo, B. F., Ovadia, M., et al. (2013). Calmodulin mutations associated with recurrent cardiac arrest in infants. *Circulation* 127 (9), 1009–1017. doi: 10.1161/CIRCULATIONAHA.112.001216

Damiano, B. P., and Rosen, M. R. (1984). Effects of pacing on triggered activity induced by early afterdepolarizations. *Circulation* 69 (5), 1013–1025. doi: 10.1161/01.cir.69.5.1013

Davidenko, J. M., Pertsov, A. V., Salomonsz, R., Baxter, W., and Jalife, J. (1992). Stationary and drifting spiral waves of excitation in isolated cardiac muscle. *Nature* 355 (6358), 349–351. doi: 10.1038/355349a0

De Ferrari, G. M., Viola, M. C., D'Amato, E., Antolini, R., and Forti, S. (1995). Distinct patterns of calcium transients during early and delayed afterdepolarizations induced by isoproterenol in ventricular myocytes. *Circulation* 91 (10), 2510–2515. doi: 10.1161/01.cir.91.10.2510

De Maziere, A. M., and Scheuermann, D. W. (1990). Structural changes in cardiac gap junctions after hypoxia and reoxygenation: a quantitative freeze-fracture analysis. *Cell Tissue Res.* 261 (1), 183–194. doi: 10.1007/bf00329451

Denegri, M., Avelino-Cruz, J. E., Boncompagni, S., De Simone, S. A., Auricchio, A., Villani, L., et al. (2012). Viral gene transfer rescues arrhythmogenic phenotype and ultrastructural abnormalities in adult calsequestrin-null mice with inherited arrhythmias. *Circ. Res.* 110 (5), 663–668. doi: 10.1161/CIRCRESAHA.111.263939

Denegri, M., Bongianino, R., Lodola, F., Boncompagni, S., De Giusti, V. C., Avelino-Cruz, J. E., et al. (2014). Single delivery of an adeno-associated viral construct to transfer the CASQ2 gene to knock-in mice affected by catecholaminergic polymorphic ventricular tachycardia is able to cure the disease from birth to advanced age. *Circulation* 129 (25), 2673–2681. doi: 10.1161/CIRCULATIONAHA.113.006901

Denham, N. C., Pearman, C. M., Caldwell, J. L., Madders, G. W. P., Eisner, D. A., Trafford, A. W., et al. (2018). Calcium in the pathophysiology of atrial fibrillation and heart failure. *Front. Physiol.* 9, 1380. doi: 10.3389/fphys.2018.01380

Devalla, H. D., Gelinas, R., Aburawi, E. H., Beqqali, A., Goyette, P., Freund, C., et al. (2016). TECRL, a new life-threatening inherited arrhythmia gene associated with overlapping clinical features of both LQTS and CPVT. *EMBO Mol. Med.* 8 (12), 1390–1408. doi: 10.15252/emmm.201505719

Dhein, S. (1998). Gap junction channels in the cardiovascular system: pharmacological and physiological modulation. *Trends Pharmacol. Sci.* 19 (6), 229–241. doi: 10.1016/s0165-6147(98)01192-4

di Bernardo, D., and Murray, A. (2002). Origin on the electrocardiogram of U-waves and abnormal U-wave inversion. *Cardiovasc. Res.* 53 (1), 202–208. doi: 10.1016/s0008-6363(01)00439-4

Di Diego, J. M., and Antzelevitch, C. (1994). High [Ca2+]o-induced electrical heterogeneity and extrasystolic activity in isolated canine ventricular epicardium. Phase 2 reentry. *Circulation* 89 (4), 1839–1850. doi: 10.1161/01.cir.89.4.1839

Dong, M., Yan, S., Chen, Y., Niklewski, P. J., Sun, X., Chenault, K., et al. (2010). Role of the transient outward current in regulating mechanical properties of canine ventricular myocytes. *J. Cardiovasc. Electrophysiol.* 21 (6), 697–703. doi: 10.1111/j.1540-8167.2009.01708.x

Duggal, P., Vesely, M. R., Wattanasirichaigoon, D., Villafane, J., Kaushik, V., and Beggs, A. H. (1998). Mutation of the gene for IsK associated with both jervell and lange-nielsen and romano-ward forms of long-QT syndrome. *Circulation* 97 (2), 142–146. doi: 10.1161/01.cir.97.2.142

Eisner, D. A., Choi, H. S., Diaz, M. E., O'Neill, S. C., and Trafford, A. W. (2000). Integrative analysis of calcium cycling in cardiac muscle. *Circ. Res.* 87 (12), 1087–1094. doi: 10.1161/01.res.87.12.1087

Eisner, D. A., Li, Y., and O'Neill, S. C. (2006). Alternans of intracellular calcium: mechanism and significance. *Heart Rhythm* 3 (6), 743–745. doi: 10.1016/j.hrthm.2005.12.020

Eisner, D. A., Caldwell, J. L., Kistamas, K., and Trafford, A. W. (2017). Calcium and excitation-contraction coupling in the heart. *Circ. Res.* 121 (2), 181–195. doi: 10.1161/circresaha.117.310230

Eisner, D. A. (2018). Ups and downs of calcium in the heart. *J. Physiol.* 596 (1), 19–30. doi: 10.1113/jp275130

El-Sherif, N., and Turitto, G. (1999). The long QT syndrome and torsade de pointes. *Pacing Clin. Electrophysiol.* 22 (1 Pt 1), 91–110. doi: 10.1111/j.1540-8159.1999.tb00305.x

El-Sherif, N., and Turitto, G. (2011). Electrolyte disorders and arrhythmogenesis. *Cardiol. J.* 18 (3), 233–245.

el-Sherif, N., WB, G., RH, Z., and Hariman, R. (1985). Reentrant ventricular arrhythmias in the late myocardial infarction period. 12. spontaneous versus induced reentry and intramural versus epicardial circuits. *J. Am. Coll. Cardiol.* 6 (1), 124–132. doi: 10.1016/s0735-1097(85)80263-1

El-Sherif, N., Turitto, G., and Boutjdir, M. (2017). Congenital Long QT syndrome and torsade de pointes. *Ann. Noninvasive Electrocardiol.: Off. J. Int. Soc. Holter Noninvasive Electrocardiol. Inc.* 22 (6), e12481. doi: 10.1111/anec.12481

El-Sherif, N., Turitto, G., and Boutjdir, M. (2019). Acquired long QT syndrome and electrophysiology of torsade de pointes. *Arrhythmia Electrophysiol. Rev.* 8 (2), 122–130. doi: 10.15420/aer.2019.8.3

Eryol, N. K., Colak, R., Ozdogru, I., Tanriverdi, F., Unal, S., Topsakal, R., et al. (2003). Effects of calcium treatment on QT interval and QT dispersion in hypocalcemia. *Am. J. Cardiol.* 91 (6), 750–752. doi: 10.1016/s0002-9149(02)03423-9

Faggioni, M., Kryshtal, D. O., and Knollmann, B. C. (2012). Calsequestrin mutations and catecholaminergic polymorphic ventricular tachycardia. *Pediatr. Cardiol.* 33 (6), 959–967. doi: 10.1007/s00246-012-0256-1

Ferrier, G. R., Saunders, J. H., and Mendez, C. (1973). A cellular mechanism for the generation of ventricular arrhythmias by acetylstrophanthidin. *Circ. Res.* 32 (5), 600–609. doi: 10.1161/01.res.32.5.600

Fink, M., and Noble, D. (2010). Pharmacodynamic effects in the cardiovascular system: the modeller's view. *Basic Clin. Pharmacol. Toxicol.* 106 (3), 243–249. doi: 10.1111/j.1742-7843.2009.00534.x

Firek, L., and Weingart, R. (1995). Modification of gap junction conductance by divalent cations and protons in neonatal rat heart cells. *J. Mol. Cell. Cardiol.* 27 (8), 1633–1643. doi: 10.1016/s0022-2828(95)90623-1

Gadsby, D. C., and Cranefield, P. F. (1977). Two levels of resting potential in cardiac Purkinje fibers. *J. Gen. Physiol.* 70 (6), 725–746. doi: 10.1085/jgp.70.6.725

Garfinkel, A., Kim, Y. H., Voroshilovsky, O., Qu, Z., Kil, J. R., Lee, M. H., et al. (2000). Preventing ventricular fibrillation by flattening cardiac restitution. *Proc. Natl. Acad. Sci. U. S. A.* 97 (11), 6061–6066. doi: 10.1073/pnas.090492697

Garfinkel, A. (2007). Eight (or more) kinds of alternans. *J. Electrocardiol.* 40 (6 Suppl), S70–S74. doi: 10.1016/j.jelectrocard.2007.06.011

Garrey, W. E. (1914). The nature of fibrillary contraction of the heart.—its relation to tissue mass and form. *Am. J. Physiology-Legacy Content* 33 (3), 397–414. doi: 10.1152/ajplegacy.1914.33.3.397

George, C. H., Jundi, H., Thomas, N. L., Fry, D. L., and Lai, F. A. (2007). Ryanodine receptors and ventricular arrhythmias: emerging trends in mutations, mechanisms and therapies. *J. Mol. Cell. Cardiol.* 42 (1), 34–50. doi: 10.1016/j.yjmcc.2006.08.115

Goldhaber, J. I. (1996). Free radicals enhance Na+/Ca2+ exchange in ventricular myocytes. *Am. J. Physiol.* 271 (3 Pt 2), H823–H833. doi: 10.1152/ajpheart.1996.271.3.H823

Gray, B., and Behr, E. R. (2016). New insights into the genetic basis of inherited arrhythmia syndromes. *Circ. Cardiovasc. Genet.* 9 (6), 569–577. doi: 10.1161/CIRCGENETICS.116.001571

Gray, R. A., Jalife, J., Panfilov, A. V., Baxter, W. T., Cabo, C., Davidenko, J. M., et al. (1995). Mechanisms of cardiac fibrillation. *Science* 270 (5239), 1222–1223; author reply 4–5. doi: 10.1126/science.270.5239.1222

Greenstein, J. L., Wu, R., Po, S., Tomaselli, G. F., and Winslow, R. L. (2000). Role of the calcium-independent transient outward current I(to1) in shaping action potential morphology and duration. *Circ. Res.* 87 (11), 1026–1033. doi: 10.1161/01.res.87.11.1026

Greiser, M., Kerfant, B. G., Williams, G. S., Voigt, N., Harks, E., Dibb, K. M., et al. (2014). Tachycardia-induced silencing of subcellular Ca2+ signaling in atrial myocytes. *J. Clin. Invest.* 124 (11), 4759–4772. doi: 10.1172/JCI70102

Greiser, M. (2017). Calcium signalling silencing in atrial fibrillation. *J. Physiol.* 595 (12), 4009–4017. doi: 10.1113/JP273045

Gussak, I., Antzelevitch, C., Hammill, S. C., Shen, W. K., and Bjerregaard, P. (2003). *Cardiac Repolarization - Bridging Basic and Clinical Science.* Contemporary Cardiology. (Totowa, New Jersey: Humana Press).

Haissaguerre, M., Derval, N., Sacher, F., Jesel, L., Deisenhofer, I., de Roy, L., et al. (2008). Sudden cardiac arrest associated with early repolarization. *New Engl. J. Med.* 358 (19), 2016–2023. doi: 10.1056/NEJMoa071968

Hayashi, M., Denjoy, I., Extramiana, F., Maltret, A., Buisson, N. R., Lupoglazoff, J. M., et al. (2009). Incidence and risk factors of arrhythmic events in catecholaminergic polymorphic ventricular tachycardia. *Circulation* 119 (18), 2426–2434. doi: 10.1161/CIRCULATIONAHA.108.829267

Hegyi, B., Bers, D. M., and Bossuyt, J. (2019). CaMKII signaling in heart diseases: Emerging role in diabetic cardiomyopathy. *J. Mol. Cell. Cardiol.* 127, 246–259. doi: 10.1016/j.yjmcc.2019.01.001

Heijman, J., Voigt, N., Nattel, S., and Dobrev, D. (2014). Cellular and molecular electrophysiology of atrial fibrillation initiation, maintenance, and progression. *Circ. Res.* 114 (9), 1483–1499. doi: 10.1161/CIRCRESAHA.114.302226

Hilliard, F. A., Steele, D. S., Laver, D., Yang, Z., Le Marchand, S. J., Chopra, N., et al. (2010). Flecainide inhibits arrhythmogenic Ca2+ waves by open state block of ryanodine receptor Ca2+ release channels and reduction of Ca2+ spark mass. *J. Mol. Cell. Cardiol.* 48 (2), 293–301. doi: 10.1016/j.yjmcc.2009.10.005

Hoffman, B. F., and Rosen, M. R. (1981). Cellular mechanisms for cardiac arrhythmias. *Circ. Res.* 49 (1), 1–15. doi: 10.1161/01.res.49.1.1

Hopenfeld, B. (2006). Mechanism for action potential alternans: the interplay between L-type calcium current and transient outward current. *Heart Rhythm* 3 (3), 345–352. doi: 10.1016/j.hrthm.2005.11.016

Horvath, B., Banyasz, T., Jian, Z., Hegyi, B., Kistamas, K., Nanasi, P. P., et al. (2013). Dynamics of the late Na(+) current during cardiac action potential and its contribution to afterdepolarizations. *J. Mol. Cell. Cardiol.* 64, 59–68. doi: 10.1016/j.yjmcc.2013.08.010

Horvath, B., Hegyi, B., Kistamas, K., Vaczi, K., Banyasz, T., Magyar, J., et al. (2015). Cytosolic calcium changes affect the incidence of early afterdepolarizations in canine ventricular myocytes. *Can. J. Physiol. Pharmacol.* 93 (7), 527–534. doi: 10.1139/cjpp-2014-0511

Houle, T. D., Ram, M. L., and Cala, S. E. (2004). Calsequestrin mutant D307H exhibits depressed binding to its protein targets and a depressed response to calcium. *Cardiovasc. Res.* 64 (2), 227–233. doi: 10.1016/j.cardiores.2004.09.009

Hwang, H. S., Hasdemir, C., Laver, D., Mehra, D., Turhan, K., Faggioni, M., et al. (2011). Inhibition of cardiac Ca2+ release channels (RyR2) determines efficacy of class I antiarrhythmic drugs in catecholaminergic polymorphic ventricular tachycardia. *Circ. Arrhythm. Electrophysiol.* 4 (2), 128–135. doi: 10.1161/CIRCEP.110.959916

Hwang, H. S., Baldo, M. P., Rodriguez, J. P., Faggioni, M., and Knollmann, B. C. (2019). Efficacy of flecainide in catecholaminergic polymorphic ventricular tachycardia is mutation-independent but reduced by calcium overload. *Front. Physiol.* 10, 992. doi: 10.3389/fphys.2019.00992

Ikeda, T., Uchida, T., Hough, D., Lee, J. J., Fishbein, M. C., Mandel, W. J., et al. (1996). Mechanism of spontaneous termination of functional reentry in isolated canine right atrium. Evidence for the presence of an excitable but nonexcited core. *Circulation* 94 (8), 1962–1973. doi: 10.1161/01.cir.94.8.1962

Ildarova, R., Shkolnikova, M. A., Kharlap, M., Bereznitskaya, V., and Kalinin, L. (2012). Sodium-channel blockers might contribute to the prevention of ventricular tachycardia in patients with long QT syndrome type 2: a description of 4 cases. *J. Electrocardiol.* 45 (3), 237–243. doi: 10.1016/j.jelectrocard.2012.01.008

Jacobs, A., Knight, B. P., McDonald, K. T., and Burke, M. C. (2006). Verapamil decreases ventricular tachyarrhythmias in a patient with timothy syndrome (LQT8). *Heart Rhythm* 3 (8), 967–970. doi: 10.1016/j.hrthm.2006.04.024

Jalife, J., Delmar, M., Anumonwo, J., Berenfeld, O., and Kalifa, J. (2009). Basic mechanisms of cardiac arrhythmias. *Basic Cardiac Electrophysiol. Clinician* 2.

January, C. T., and Riddle, J. M. (1989). Early afterdepolarizations: mechanism of induction and block. A role for L-type Ca2+ current. *Circ. Res.* 64 (5), 977–990. doi: 10.1161/01.res.64.5.977

Jensen, H. H., Brohus, M., Nyegaard, M., and Overgaard, M. T. (2018). Human calmodulin mutations. *Front. Mol. Neurosci.* 11, 396. doi: 10.3389/fnmol.2018.00396

Jiang, D., Wang, R., Xiao, B., Kong, H., Hunt, D. J., Choi, P., et al. (2005). Enhanced store overload-induced Ca2+ release and channel sensitivity to luminal Ca2+ activation are common defects of RyR2 mutations linked to ventricular tachycardia and sudden death. *Circ. Res.* 97 (11), 1173–1181. doi: 10.1161/01.RES.0000192146.85173.4b

Jiang, D., Chen, W., Wang, R., Zhang, L., and Chen, S. R. (2007). Loss of luminal Ca2+ activation in the cardiac ryanodine receptor is associated with ventricular fibrillation and sudden death. *Proc. Natl. Acad. Sci. U. S. A.* 104 (46), 18309–18314. doi: 10.1073/pnas.0706573104

Johnson, D. M., and Antoons, G. (2018). Arrhythmogenic mechanisms in heart failure: linking beta-adrenergic stimulation, stretch, and calcium. *Front. Physiol.* 9, 1453. doi: 10.3389/fphys.2018.01453

Jones, P. P., Jiang, D., Bolstad, J., Hunt, D. J., Zhang, L., Demaurex, N., et al. (2008). Endoplasmic reticulum Ca2+ measurements reveal that the cardiac ryanodine receptor mutations linked to cardiac arrhythmia and sudden death alter the threshold for store-overload-induced Ca2+ release. *Biochem. J.* 412 (1), 171–178. doi: 10.1042/BJ20071287

Joung, B., Chen, P. S., and Lin, S. F. (2011). The role of the calcium and the voltage clocks in sinoatrial node dysfunction. *Yonsei Med. J.* 52 (2), 211–219. doi: 10.3349/ymj.2011.52.2.211

Kandel, S. M., and Roth, B. J. (2015). The mechanism of reflection type reentry: a simulation study. *J. Cardiovasc. Electrophysiol.* 26 (12), 1370–1375. doi: 10.1111/jce.12815

Kang, J., Chen, X. L., Wang, H., Ji, J., Cheng, H., Incardona, J., et al. (2005). Discovery of a small molecule activator of the human ether-a-go-go-related gene (HERG) cardiac K + channel. *Mol. Pharmacol.* 67 (3), 827–836. doi: 10.1124/mol.104.006577

Kannankeril, P. J., Moore, J. P., Cerrone, M., Priori, S. G., Kertesz, N. J., Ro, P. S., et al. (2017). Efficacy of flecainide in the treatment of catecholaminergic polymorphic ventricular tachycardia: a randomized clinical trial. *JAMA Cardiol.* 2 (7), 759–766. doi: 10.1001/jamacardio.2017.1320

Karagueuzian, H. S., Pezhouman, A., Angelini, M., and Olcese, R. (2017). Enhanced late na and ca currents as effective antiarrhythmic drug targets. *Front. Pharmacol.* 8, 36. doi: 10.3389/fphar.2017.00036

Kashimura, T., Briston, S. J., Trafford, A. W., Napolitano, C., Priori, S. G., Eisner, D. A., et al. (2010). In the RyR2(R4496C) mouse model of CPVT, beta-adrenergic stimulation induces Ca waves by increasing SR Ca content and not by decreasing the threshold for Ca waves. *Circ. Res.* 107 (12), 1483–1489. doi: 10.1161/CIRCRESAHA.110.227744

Kim, J. A., Lopes, C. M., Moss, A. J., McNitt, S., Barsheshet, A., Robinson, J. L., et al. (2010). Trigger-specific risk factors and response to therapy in long QT syndrome type 2. *Heart Rhythm* 7 (12), 1797–1805. doi: 10.1016/j.hrthm.2010.09.011

Kirchhof, P., Benussi, S., Kotecha, D., Ahlsson, A., Atar, D. , Casadei, B., et al. (2016). ESC Guidelines for the management of atrial fibrillation developed in collaboration with EACTS. *Eur. J. Cardiothorac. Surg.* 50 (5), e1–e88. doi: 10.1093/ejcts/ezw313

Kistamas, K., Hegyi, B., Vaczi, K., Horvath, B., Banyasz, T., Magyar, J., et al. (2015a). Oxidative shift in tissue redox potential increases beat-to-beat variability of action potential duration. *Can. J. Physiol. Pharmacol.* 93 (7), 563–568. doi: 10.1139/cjpp-2014-0531

Kistamas, K., Szentandrassy, N., Hegyi, B., Vaczi, K., Ruzsnavszky, F., Horvath, B., et al. (2015b). Changes in intracellular calcium concentration influence beat-to-beat variability of action potential duration in canine ventricular myocytes. *J. Physiol. Pharmacol.* 66 (1), 73–81.

Knollmann, B. C., Chopra, N., Hlaing, T., Akin, B., Yang, T., Ettensohn, K., et al. (2006). Casq2 deletion causes sarcoplasmic reticulum volume increase, premature Ca2+ release, and catecholaminergic polymorphic ventricular tachycardia. *J. Clin. Invest.* 116 (9), 2510–2520. doi: 10.1172/JCI29128

Kohomoto, O., Levi, A. J., and Bridge, J. H. (1994). Relation between reverse sodium-calcium exchange and sarcoplasmic reticulum calcium release in guinea pig ventricular cells. *Circ. Res.* 74 (3), 550–554. doi: 10.1161/01.res.74.3.550

Krause, U., Gravenhorst, V., Kriebel, T., Ruschewski, W., and Paul, T. (2011). A rare association of long QT syndrome and syndactyly: Timothy syndrome (LQT 8). *Clin. Res. Cardiol.* 100 (12), 1123–1127. doi: 10.1007/s00392-011-0358-4

Lahat, H., Pras, E., Olender, T., Avidan, N., Ben-Asher, E., Man, O., et al. (2001). A missense mutation in a highly conserved region of CASQ2 is associated with autosomal recessive catecholamine-induced polymorphic ventricular tachycardia in Bedouin families from Israel. *Am. J. Hum. Genet.* 69 (6), 1378–1384. doi: 10.1086/324565

Laitinen, P. J., Brown, K. M., Piippo, K., Swan, H., Devaney, J. M., Brahmbhatt, B., et al. (2001). Mutations of the cardiac ryanodine receptor (RyR2) gene in familial polymorphic ventricular tachycardia. *Circulation* 103 (4), 485–490. doi: 10.1161/01.cir.103.4.485

Lakatta, E. G., and DiFrancesco, D. (2009). What keeps us ticking: a funny current, a calcium clock, or both? *J. Mol. Cell. Cardiol.* 47 (2), 157–170. doi: 10.1016/j.yjmcc.2009.03.022

Lakatta, E. G., Maltsev, V. A., and Vinogradova, T. M. (2010). A coupled SYSTEM of intracellular Ca2+ clocks and surface membrane voltage clocks controls the timekeeping mechanism of the heart's pacemaker. *Circ. Res.* 106 (4), 659–673. doi: 10.1161/CIRCRESAHA.109.206078

Lakatta, E. G. (2010). A paradigm shift for the heart's pacemaker. *Heart Rhythm* 7 (4), 559–564. doi: 10.1016/j.hrthm.2009.12.013

Landstrom, A. P., Boczek, N. J., Ye, D., Miyake, C. Y., De la Uz, C. M., Allen, H. D., et al. (2016). Novel long QT syndrome-associated missense mutation, L762F, in CACNA1C-encoded L-type calcium channel imparts a slower inactivation tau and increased sustained and window current. *Int. J. Cardiol.* 220, 290–298. doi: 10.1016/j.ijcard.2016.06.081

Landstrom, A. P., Dobrev, D., and Wehrens, X. H. T. (2017). Calcium signaling and cardiac arrhythmias. *Circ. Res.* 120 (12), 1969–1993. doi: 10.1161/CIRCRESAHA.117.310083

Lazrak, A., Peres, A., Giovannardi, S., and Peracchia, C. (1994). Ca-mediated and independent effects of arachidonic acid on gap junctions and Ca-independent effects of oleic acid and halothane. *Biophys. J.* 67 (3), 1052–1059. doi: 10.1016/S0006-3495(94)80570-3

Lazzara, R. (1988). Electrophysiological mechanisms for ventricular arrhythmias. *Clin. Cardiol.* 11 (3 Suppl 2), II1–II4.

Lazzerini, P. E., Capecchi, P. L., and Laghi-Pasini, F. (2015). Long QT syndrome: an emerging role for inflammation and immunity. *Front. Cardiovasc. Med.* 2, 26. doi: 10.3389/fcvm.2015.00026

Leenhardt, A., Lucet, V., Denjoy, I., Grau, F., Ngoc, D. D., and Coumel, P. (1995). Catecholaminergic polymorphic ventricular tachycardia in children. A 7-year follow-up of 21 patients. *Circulation* 91 (5), 1512–1519. doi: 10.1161/01.cir.91.5.1512

Lehnart, S. E., Wehrens, X. H., Laitinen, P. J., Reiken, S. R., Deng, S. X., Cheng, Z., et al. (2004). Sudden death in familial polymorphic ventricular tachycardia associated with calcium release channel (ryanodine receptor) leak. *Circulation* 109 (25), 3208–3214. doi: 10.1161/01.CIR.0000132472.98675.EC

Li, Y., Diaz, M. E., Eisner, D. A., and O'Neill, S. (2009). The effects of membrane potential, SR Ca2+ content and RyR responsiveness on systolic Ca2+ alternans in rat ventricular myocytes. *J. Physiol.* 587 (Pt 6), 1283–1292. doi: 10.1113/jphysiol.2008.164368

Limpitikul, W. B., Dick, I. E., Joshi-Mukherjee, R., Overgaard, M. T., George, A. L.Jr., and Yue, D. T. (2014). Calmodulin mutations associated with long QT syndrome prevent inactivation of cardiac L-type Ca(2+) currents and promote proarrhythmic behavior in ventricular myocytes. *J. Mol. Cell. Cardiol.* 74, 115–124. doi: 10.1016/j.yjmcc.2014.04.022

Lipp, P., and Niggli, E. (1994). Modulation of Ca2+ release in cultured neonatal rat cardiac myocytes. Insight from subcellular release patterns revealed by confocal microscopy. *Circ. Res.* 74 (5), 979–990. doi: 10.1161/01.res.74.5.979

Liu, D. W., and Antzelevitch, C. (1995). Characteristics of the delayed rectifier current (IKr and IKs) in canine ventricular epicardial, midmyocardial, and endocardial myocytes. a weaker IKs contributes to the longer action potential of the M cell. *Circ. Res.* 76 (3), 351–365. doi: 10.1161/01.res.76.3.351

Liu, N., Colombi, B., Memmi, M., Zissimopoulos, S., Rizzi, N., Negri, S., et al. (2006). Arrhythmogenesis in catecholaminergic polymorphic ventricular tachycardia: insights from a RyR2 R4496C knock-in mouse model. *Circ. Res.* 99 (3), 292–298. doi: 10.1161/01.RES.0000235869.50747.e1

Liu, N., Rizzi, N., Boveri, L., and Priori, S. G. (2009). Ryanodine receptor and calsequestrin in arrhythmogenesis: what we have learnt from genetic diseases and transgenic mice. *J. Mol. Cell. Cardiol.* 46 (2), 149–159. doi: 10.1016/j.yjmcc.2008.10.012

Liu, N., Ruan, Y., Denegri, M., Bachetti, T., Li, Y., Colombi, B., et al. (2011a). Calmodulin kinase II inhibition prevents arrhythmias in RyR2(R4496C+/-) mice with catecholaminergic polymorphic ventricular tachycardia. *J. Mol. Cell. Cardiol.* 50 (1), 214–222. doi: 10.1016/j.yjmcc.2010.10.001

Liu, N., Denegri, M., Ruan, Y., Avelino-Cruz, J. E., Perissi, A., Negri, S., et al. (2011b). Short communication: flecainide exerts an antiarrhythmic effect in a mouse model of catecholaminergic polymorphic ventricular tachycardia by increasing the threshold for triggered activity. *Circ. Res.* 109 (3), 291–295. doi: 10.1161/CIRCRESAHA.111.247338

Liu, H., Chatel, S., Simard, C., Syam, N., Salle, L., Probst, V., et al. (2013). Molecular genetics and functional anomalies in a series of 248 Brugada cases with 11 mutations in the TRPM4 channel. *PLoS One* 8 (1), e54131. doi: 10.1371/journal.pone.0054131

Liu, W., Deng, J., Wang, G., Zhang, C., Luo, X., Yan, D., et al. (2014). KCNE2 modulates cardiac L-type Ca(2+) channel. *J. Mol. Cell. Cardiol.* 72, 208–218. doi: 10.1016/j.yjmcc.2014.03.013

Liu, M. B., de Lange, E., Garfinkel, A., Weiss, J. N., and Qu, Z. (2015). Delayed afterdepolarizations generate both triggers and a vulnerable substrate promoting reentry in cardiac tissue. *Heart Rhythm* 12 (10), 2115–2124. doi: 10.1016/j.hrthm.2015.06.019

Loughrey, C. M., Otani, N., Seidler, T., Craig, M. A., Matsuda, R., Kaneko, N., et al. (2007). K201 modulates excitation-contraction coupling and spontaneous Ca2+ release in normal adult rabbit ventricular cardiomyocytes. *Cardiovasc. Res.* 76 (2), 236–246. doi: 10.1016/j.cardiores.2007.06.014

Lu, Y., Mahaut-Smith, M. P., Huang, C. L., and Vandenberg, J. I. (2003). Mutant MiRP1 subunits modulate HERG K+ channel gating: a mechanism for pro-arrhythmia in long QT syndrome type 6. *J. Physiol.* 551 (Pt 1), 253–262. doi: 10.1113/jphysiol.2003.046045

Lukas, A., and Antzelevitch, C. (1996). Phase 2 reentry as a mechanism of initiation of circus movement reentry in canine epicardium exposed to simulated ischemia. *Cardiovasc. Res.* 32 (3), 593–603. doi: 10.1016/S0008-6363(96)00115-0

Lukyanenko, V., Subramanian, S., Gyorke, I., Wiesner, T. F., and Gyorke, S. (1999). The role of luminal Ca2+ in the generation of Ca2+ waves in rat ventricular myocytes. *J. Physiol.* 518 (Pt 1), 173–186. doi: 10.1111/j.1469-7793.1999.0173r.x

Magyar, J., Banyasz, T., Szentandrassy, N., Kistamas, K., Nanasi, P. P., and Satin, J. (2015). Role of gap junction channel in the development of beat-to-beat action potential repolarization variability and arrhythmias. *Curr. Pharma. Des.* 21 (8), 1042–1052. doi: 10.2174/1381612820666141029102443

Magyar, J., Kistamas, K., Vaczi, K., Hegyi, B., Horvath, B., Banyasz, T., et al. (2016). Concept of relative variability of cardiac action potential duration and its test under various experimental conditions. *Gen. Physiol. Biophys.* 35 (1), 55–62. doi: 10.4149/gpb_2015019

Mahajan, A., Shiferaw, Y., Sato, D., Baher, A., Olcese, R., Xie, L. H., et al. (2008). A rabbit ventricular action potential model replicating cardiac dynamics at rapid heart rates. *Biophys. J.* 94 (2), 392–410. doi: 10.1529/biophysj.106.98160

Maier, L. S., and Bers, D. M. (2007). Role of Ca2+/calmodulin-dependent protein kinase (CaMK) in excitation-contraction coupling in the heart. *Cardiovasc. Res.* 73 (4), 631–640. doi: 10.1016/j.cardiores.2006.11.005

Maltsev, V. A., Vinogradova, T. M., and Lakatta, E. G. (2006). The emergence of a general theory of the initiation and strength of the heartbeat. *J. Pharmacol. Sci.* 100 (5), 338–369. doi: 10.1254/jphs.cr0060018

Marsman, R. F., Barc, J., Beekman, L., Alders, M., Dooijes, D., van den Wijngaard, A., et al. (2014). A mutation in CALM1 encoding calmodulin in familial idiopathic ventricular fibrillation in childhood and adolescence. *J. Am. Coll. Cardiol.* 63 (3), 259–266. doi: 10.1016/j.jacc.2013.07.091

Maruyama, M., Joung, B., Tang, L., Shinohara, T., On, Y. K., Han, S., et al. (2010). Diastolic intracellular calcium-membrane voltage coupling gain and postshock arrhythmias: role of purkinje fibers and triggered activity. *Circ. Res.* 106 (2), 399–408. doi: 10.1161/CIRCRESAHA.109.211292

Mayer, A. G. (1906). *Rhythmical Pulsation in Scyphomedusae* (Washington DC: Carnegie Institution of Washington).

Mechmann, S., and Pott, L. (1986). Identification of Na-Ca exchange current in single cardiac myocytes. *Nature* 319 (6054), 597–599. doi: 10.1038/319597a0

Medeiros-Domingo, A., Kaku, T., Tester, D. J., Iturralde-Torres, P., Itty, A., Ye, B., et al. (2007). SCN4B-encoded sodium channel beta4 subunit in congenital long-QT syndrome. *Circulation* 116 (2), 134–142. doi: 10.1161/CIRCULATIONAHA.106.659086

Meregalli, P. G., Wilde, A. A., and Tan, H. L. (2005). Pathophysiological mechanisms of Brugada syndrome: depolarization disorder, repolarization disorder, or more? *Cardiovasc. Res.* 67 (3), 367–378. doi: 10.1016/j.cardiores.2005.03.005

Milberg, P., Ramtin, S., Monnig, G., Osada, N., Wasmer, K., Breithardt, G., et al. (2004). Comparison of the *in vitro* electrophysiologic and proarrhythmic effects of amiodarone and sotalol in a rabbit model of acute atrioventricular block. *J. Cardiovasc. Pharmacol.* 44 (3), 278–286. doi: 10.1097/01.fjc.0000129581.81508.78

Mines, G. R. (1913). On dynamic equilibrium in the heart. *J. Physiol.* 46 (4-5), 349–383. doi: 10.1113/jphysiol.1913.sp001596

Mines, G. R. (1914). On circulating excitations in heart muscle and their possible relation to tachycardia and fibrillation. *Trans. R Soc. Can.* 8, 43–52.

Mitchell, R. D., Simmerman, H. K., and Jones, L. R. (1988). Ca2+ binding effects on protein conformation and protein interactions of canine cardiac calsequestrin. *J. Biol. Chem.* 263 (3), 1376–1381.

Miura, M., Ishide, N., Oda, H., Sakurai, M., Shinozaki, T., and Takishima, T. (1993). Spatial features of calcium transients during early and delayed afterdepolarizations. *Am. J. Physiol.* 265 (2 Pt 2), H439–H444. doi: 10.1152/ajpheart.1993.265.2.H439

Miura, M., Ishide, N., Numaguchi, H., and Takishima, T. (1995). Diversity of early afterdepolarizations in guinea pig myocytes: spatial characteristics of intracellular Ca2+ concentration. *Heart Vessels* 10 (5), 266–274. doi: 10.1007/BF01744906

Mohamed, U., Gollob, M. H., Gow, R. M., and Krahn, A. D. (2006). Sudden cardiac death despite an implantable cardioverter-defibrillator in a young female with catecholaminergic ventricular tachycardia. *Heart Rhythm* 3 (12), 1486–1489. doi: 10.1016/j.hrthm.2006.08.018

Mohler, P. J., Splawski, I., Napolitano, C., Bottelli, G., Sharpe, L., Timothy, K., et al. (2004). A cardiac arrhythmia syndrome caused by loss of ankyrin-B function. *Proc. Natl. Acad. Sci. U. S. A.* 101 (24), 9137–9142. doi: 10.1073/pnas.0402546101

Mohler, P. J., Schott, J. J., Gramolini, A. O., Dilly, K. W., Guatimosim, S., duBell, W. H., et al. (2003). Ankyrin-B mutation causes type 4 long-QT cardiac arrhythmia and sudden cardiac death. *Nature* 421 (6923), 634–639. doi: 10.1038/nature01335

Morita, H., Morita, S. T., Nagase, S., Banba, K., Nishii, N., Tani, Y., et al. (2003). Ventricular arrhythmia induced by sodium channel blocker in patients with Brugada syndrome. *J. Am. Coll. Cardiol.* 42 (9), 1624–1631. doi: 10.1016/j.jacc.2003.06.004

Moss, A. J., Zareba, W., Hall, W. J., Schwartz, P. J., Crampton, R. S., Benhorin, J., et al. (2000). Effectiveness and limitations of beta-blocker therapy in congenital long-QT syndrome. *Circulation* 101 (6), 616–623. doi: 10.1161/01.cir.101.6.616

Moss, A. J., Windle, J. R., Hall, W. J., Zareba, W., Robinson, J. L., McNitt, S., et al. (2005). Safety and efficacy of flecainide in subjects with Long QT-3 syndrome (DeltaKPQ mutation): a randomized, double-blind, placebo-controlled clinical trial. *Ann. Noninvasive Electrocardiol.* 10 (4 Suppl), 59–66. doi: 10.1111/j.1542-474X.2005.00077.x

Moss, A. J., Zareba, W., Schwarz, K. Q., Rosero, S., McNitt, S., and Robinson, J. L. (2008). Ranolazine shortens repolarization in patients with sustained inward sodium current due to type-3 long-QT syndrome. *J. Cardiovasc. Electrophysiol.* 19 (12), 1289–1293. doi: 10.1111/j.1540-8167.2008.01246.x

Nanasi, P. P., Magyar, J., Varro, A., and Ordog, B. (2017). Beat-to-beat variability of cardiac action potential duration: underlying mechanism and clinical implications. *Can. J. Physiol. Pharmacol.* 95 (10), 1230–1235. doi: 10.1139/cjpp-2016-0597

Nattel, S., and Dobrev, D. (2016). Electrophysiological and molecular mechanisms of paroxysmal atrial fibrillation. *Nat. Rev. Cardiol.* 13 (10), 575–590. doi: 10.1038/nrcardio.2016.118

Nawathe, P. A., Kryukova, Y., Oren, R. V., Milanesi, R., Clancy, C. E., Lu, J. T., et al. (2013). An LQTS6 MiRP1 mutation suppresses pacemaker current and is associated with sinus bradycardia. *J. Cardiovasc. Electrophysiol.* 24 (9), 1021–1027. doi: 10.1111/jce.12163

Neef, S., Dybkova, N., Sossalla, S., Ort, K. R., Fluschnik, N., Neumann, K., et al. (2010). CaMKII-dependent diastolic SR Ca2+ leak and elevated diastolic Ca2+ levels in right atrial myocardium of patients with atrial fibrillation. *Circ. Res.* 106 (6), 1134–1144. doi: 10.1161/CIRCRESAHA.109.203836

Nolasco, J. B., and Dahlen, R. W. (1968). A graphic method for the study of alternation in cardiac action potentials. *J. Appl. Physiol.* 25 (2), 191–196. doi: 10.1152/jappl.1968.25.2.191

Nyegaard, M., Overgaard, M. T., Sondergaard, M. T., Vranas, M., Behr, E. R., Hildebrandt, L. L., et al. (2012). Mutations in calmodulin cause ventricular tachycardia and sudden cardiac death. *Am. J. Hum. Genet.* 91 (4), 703–712. doi: 10.1016/j.ajhg.2012.08.015

Ohgo, T., Okamura, H., Noda, T., Satomi, K., Suyama, K., Kurita, T., et al. (2007). Acute and chronic management in patients with Brugada syndrome associated with electrical storm of ventricular fibrillation. *Heart Rhythm* 4 (6), 695–700. doi: 10.1016/j.hrthm.2007.02.014

Oosthoek, P. W., Viragh, S., Lamers, W. H., and Moorman, A. F. (1993). Immunohistochemical delineation of the conduction system. II: The atrioventricular node and Purkinje fibers. *Circ. Res.* 73 (3), 482–491. doi: 10.1161/01.res.73.3.482

Overend, C. L., Eisner, D. A., and O'Neill, S. C. (1997). The effect of tetracaine on spontaneous Ca2+ release and sarcoplasmic reticulum calcium content in rat ventricular myocytes. *J. Physiol.* 502 (Pt 3), 471–479. doi: 10.1111/j.1469-7793.1997.471bj.x

Pertsov, A. M., Davidenko, J. M., Salomonsz, R., Baxter, W. T., and Jalife, J. (1993). Spiral waves of excitation underlie reentrant activity in isolated cardiac muscle. *Circ. Res.* 72 (3), 631–650. doi: 10.1161/01.res.72.3.631

Pflaumer, A., and Davis, A. M. (2012). Guidelines for the diagnosis and management of catecholaminergic polymorphic ventricular tachycardia. *Heart Lung Circ.* 21 (2), 96–100. doi: 10.1016/j.hlc.2011.10.008

Picht, E., DeSantiago, J., Blatter, L. A., and Bers, D. M. (2006). Cardiac alternans do not rely on diastolic sarcoplasmic reticulum calcium content fluctuations. *Circ. Res.* 99 (7), 740–748. doi: 10.1161/01.RES.0000244002.88813.91

Plaster, N. M., Tawil, R., Tristani-Firouzi, M., Canun, S., Bendahhou, S., Tsunoda, A., et al. (2001). Mutations in Kir2.1 cause the developmental and episodic electrical phenotypes of Andersen's syndrome. *Cell* 105 (4), 511–519. doi: 10.1016/s0092-8674(01)00342-7

Pogwizd, S. M., Schlotthauer, K., Li, L., Yuan, W., and Bers, D. M. (2001). Arrhythmogenesis and contractile dysfunction in heart failure: Roles of sodium-calcium exchange, inward rectifier potassium current, and residual beta-adrenergic responsiveness. *Circ. Res.* 88 (11), 1159–1167. doi: 10.1161/hh1101.091193

Postma, A. V., Denjoy, I., Kamblock, J., Alders, M., Lupoglazoff, J. M., Vaksmann, G., et al. (2005). Catecholaminergic polymorphic ventricular tachycardia: RYR2 mutations, bradycardia, and follow up of the patients. *J. Med. Genet.* 42 (11), 863–870. doi: 10.1136/jmg.2004.028993

Pott, C., Dechering, D. G., Reinke, F., Muszynski, A., Zellerhoff, S., Bittner, A., et al. (2011). Successful treatment of catecholaminergic polymorphic ventricular tachycardia with flecainide: a case report and review of the current literature. *Europace* 13 (6), 897–901. doi: 10.1093/europace/euq517

Priori, S. G., and Corr, P. B. (1990). Mechanisms underlying early and delayed afterdepolarizations induced by catecholamines. *Am. J. Physiol.* 258 (6 Pt 2), H1796–H1805. doi: 10.1152/ajpheart.1990.258.6.H1796

Priori, S. G., Napolitano, C., Tiso, N., Memmi, M., Vignati, G., Bloise, R., et al. (2001). Mutations in the cardiac ryanodine receptor gene (hRyR2) underlie catecholaminergic polymorphic ventricular tachycardia. *Circulation* 103 (2), 196–200. doi: 10.1161/01.cir.103.2.196

Priori, S. G., Wilde, A. A., Horie, M., Cho, Y., Behr, E. R., Berul, C., et al. (2013). Executive summary: HRS/EHRA/APHRS expert consensus statement on the diagnosis and management of patients with inherited primary arrhythmia syndromes. *Heart Rhythm* 10 (12), e85–108. doi: 10.1016/j.hrthm.2013.07.021

Qi, X. Y., Yeh, Y. H., Xiao, L., Burstein, B., Maguy, A., Chartier, D., et al. (2008). Cellular signaling underlying atrial tachycardia remodeling of L-type calcium current. *Circ. Res.* 103 (8), 845–854. doi: 10.1161/CIRCRESAHA.108.175463

Qu, Z., and Weiss, J. N. (2015). Mechanisms of ventricular arrhythmias: from molecular fluctuations to electrical turbulence. *Annu. Rev. Physiol.* 77, 29–55. doi: 10.1146/annurev-physiol-021014-071622

Qu, Z., Shiferaw, Y., and Weiss, J. N. (2007). Nonlinear dynamics of cardiac excitation-contraction coupling: an iterated map study. *Phys. Rev. E Stat. Nonlinear Soft Matter Phys.* 75 (1 Pt 1), 011927. doi: 10.1103/PhysRevE.75.011927

Radwanski, P. B., Ho, H. T., Veeraraghavan, R., Brunello, L., Liu, B., Belevych, A. E., et al. (2016). Neuronal Na(+) channels are integral components of pro-arrhythmic Na(+)/Ca(2+) signaling nanodomain that promotes cardiac arrhythmias during beta-adrenergic stimulation. *JACC Basic to Trans. Sci.* 1 (4), 251–266. doi: 10.1016/j.jacbts.2016.04.004

Reid, D. S., Tynan, M., Braidwood, L., and Fitzgerald, G. R. (1975). Bidirectional tachycardia in a child. a study using his bundle electrography. *Br. Heart J.* 37 (3), 339–344. doi: 10.1136/hrt.37.3.339

Reiken, S., Gaburjakova, M., Guatimosim, S., Gomez, A. M., D'Armiento, J., Burkhoff, D., et al. (2003). Protein kinase a phosphorylation of the cardiac calcium release channel (ryanodine receptor) in normal and failing hearts. Role of phosphatases and response to isoproterenol. *J. Biol. Chem.* 278 (1), 444–453. doi: 10.1074/jbc.M207028200

Ringer, S. (1883). A further contribution regarding the influence of the different constituents of the blood on the contraction of the heart. *J. Physiol.* 4 (1), 29–42. doi: 10.1113/jphysiol.1883.sp000120

Rizzi, N., Liu, N., Napolitano, C., Nori, A., Turcato, F., Colombi, B., et al. (2008). Unexpected structural and functional consequences of the R33Q homozygous mutation in cardiac calsequestrin: a complex arrhythmogenic cascade in a knock in mouse model. *Circ. Res.* 103 (3), 298–306. doi: 10.1161/CIRCRESAHA.108.171660

Roden, D. M. (2004). Drug-induced prolongation of the QT interval. *New Engl. J. Med.* 350 (10), 1013–1022. doi: 10.1056/NEJMra032426

Roden, D. M. (2006). Long QT syndrome: reduced repolarization reserve and the genetic link. *J. Internal Med.* 259 (1), 59–69. doi: 10.1111/j.1365-2796.2005.01589.x

Rosen, M. R., Gelband, H., Merker, C., and Hoffman, B. F. (1973). Mechanisms of digitalis toxicity. effects of ouabain on phase four of canine Purkinje fiber transmembrane potentials. *Circulation* 47 (4), 681–689. doi: 10.1161/01.cir.47.4.681

Rosen, M. R., Wit, A. L., and Hoffman, B. F. (1975). Electrophysiology and pharmacology of cardiac arrhythmias. IV. Cardiac antiarrhythmic and toxic effects of digitalis. *Am. Heart J.* 89 (3), 391–399. doi: 10.1016/0002-8703(75)90090-3

Rosenbaum, D. S., Jackson, L. E., Smith, J. M., Garan, H., Ruskin, J. N., and Cohen, R. J. (1994). Electrical alternans and vulnerability to ventricular arrhythmias. *New Engl. J. Med.* 330 (4), 235–241. doi: 10.1056/NEJM199401273300402

Rosenthal, J. E. (1988). Reflected reentry in depolarized foci with variable conduction impairment in 1 day old infarcted canine cardiac tissue. *J. Am. Coll. Cardiol.* 12 (2), 404–411. doi: 10.1016/0735-1097(88)90413-5

Rosero, S. Z., Zareba, W., Robinson, J. L., and Moss, A. J. (1997). Gene-Specific Therapy for Long QT Syndrome. *Ann. Noninvasive Electrocardiol.* 2 (3), 274–278. doi: 10.1111/j.1542-474X.1997.tb00336.x

Rosso, R., Kalman, J. M., Rogowski, O., Diamant, S., Birger, A., Biner, S., et al. (2007). Calcium channel blockers and beta-blockers versus beta-blockers alone for preventing exercise-induced arrhythmias in catecholaminergic polymorphic ventricular tachycardia. *Heart Rhythm* 4 (9), 1149–1154. doi: 10.1016/j.hrthm.2007.05.017

Rosso, R., Kogan, E., Belhassen, B., Rozovski, U., Scheinman, M. M., Zeltser, D., et al. (2008). J-point elevation in survivors of primary ventricular fibrillation and matched control subjects: incidence and clinical significance. *J. Am. Coll. Cardiol.* 52 (15), 1231–1238. doi: 10.1016/j.jacc.2008.07.010

Rozanski, G. J., and Lipsius, S. L. (1985). Electrophysiology of functional subsidiary pacemakers in canine right atrium. *Am. J. Physiol.* 249 (3 Pt 2), H594–H603. doi: 10.1152/ajpheart.1985.249.3.H594

Sanguinetti, M. C., Jiang, C., Curran, M. E., and Keating, M. T. (1995). A mechanistic link between an inherited and an acquired cardiac arrhythmia: HERG encodes the IKr potassium channel. *Cell* 81 (2), 299–307. doi: 10.1016/0092-8674(95)90340-2

Sanguinetti, M. C., Curran, M. E., Zou, A., Shen, J., Spector, P. S., Atkinson, D. L., et al. (1996). Coassembly of K(V)LQT1 and minK (IsK) proteins to form cardiac I(Ks) potassium channel. *Nature* 384 (6604), 80–83. doi: 10.1038/384080a0

Sato, D., Shiferaw, Y., Garfinkel, A., Weiss, J. N., Qu, Z., and Karma, A. (2006). Spatially discordant alternans in cardiac tissue: role of calcium cycling. *Circ. Res.* 99 (5), 520–527. doi: 10.1161/01.RES.0000240542.03986.e7

Saunders, J. H., Ferrier, G. R., and Moe, G. K. (1973). Conduction block associated with transient depolarizations induced by acetylstrophanthidin in isolated canine Purkinje fibers. *Circ. Res.* 32 (5), 610–617. doi: 10.1161/01.res.32.5.610

Schotten, U., Dobrev, D., Platonov, P. G., Kottkamp, H., and Hindricks, G. (2016). Current controversies in determining the main mechanisms of atrial fibrillation. *J. Internal Med.* 279 (5), 428–438. doi: 10.1111/joim.12492

Schwartz, P. J., Priori, S. G., Locati, E. H., Napolitano, C., Cantu, F., Towbin, J. A., et al. (1995). Long QT syndrome patients with mutations of the SCN5A and HERG genes have differential responses to Na+ channel blockade and to increases in heart rate. Implications for gene-specific therapy. *Circulation* 92 (12), 3381–3386. doi: 10.1161/01.cir.92.12.3381

Schwartz, P. J., Crotti, L., and Insolia, R. (2012). Long-QT syndrome: from genetics to management. *Circ. Arrhythmia Electrophysiol.* 5 (4), 868–877. doi: 10.1161/CIRCEP.111.962019

Shah, D. P., Baez-Escudero, J. L., Weisberg, I. L., Beshai, J. F., and Burke, M. C. (2012). Ranolazine safely decreases ventricular and atrial fibrillation in timothy syndrome (LQT8). *Pacing Clin. Electrophysiol.* 35 (3), e62–e64. doi: 10.1111/j.1540-8159.2010.02913.x

Shamgar, L., Ma, L., Schmitt, N., Haitin, Y., Peretz, A., Wiener, R., et al. (2006). Calmodulin is essential for cardiac IKS channel gating and assembly: impaired function in long-QT mutations. *Circ. Res.* 98 (8), 1055–1063. doi: 10.1161/01.RES.0000218979.40770.69

Shan, J., Xie, W., Betzenhauser, M., Reiken, S., Chen, B. X., Wronska, A., et al. (2012). Calcium leak through ryanodine receptors leads to atrial fibrillation in 3 mouse models of catecholaminergic polymorphic ventricular tachycardia. *Circ. Res.* 111 (6), 708–717. doi: 10.1161/CIRCRESAHA.112.273342

Shiferaw, Y., Watanabe, M. A., Garfinkel, A., Weiss, J. N., and Karma, A. (2003). Model of intracellular calcium cycling in ventricular myocytes. *Biophys. J.* 85 (6), 3666–3686. doi: 10.1016/S0006-3495(03)74784-5

Shimizu, W., Kurita, T., Matsuo, K., Suyama, K., Aihara, N., Kamakura, S., et al. (1998). Improvement of repolarization abnormalities by a K+ channel opener in the LQT1 form of congenital long-QT syndrome. *Circulation* 97 (16), 1581–1588. doi: 10.1161/01.cir.97.16.1581

Shimizu, W., Antzelevitch, C., Suyama, K., Kurita, T., Taguchi, A., Aihara, N., et al. (2000). Effect of sodium channel blockers on ST segment, QRS duration, and corrected QT interval in patients with Brugada syndrome. *J. Cardiovasc. Electrophysiol.* 11 (12), 1320–1329. doi: 10.1046/j.1540-8167.2000.01320.x

Shkryl, V., Maxwell, J., Domeier, T., and Blatter, L. (2012). Refractoriness of sarcoplasmic reticulum Ca2+ release determines Ca2+ alternans in atrial myocytes. *Am. J. Physiol. Heart Circ. Physiol.* 302 (11), H2310–H2320. doi: 10.1152/ajpheart.00079.2012

Sicouri, S., and Antzelevitch, C. (2018). Mechanisms underlying the actions of antidepressant and antipsychotic drugs that cause sudden cardiac arrest. *Arrhythmia Electrophysiol. Rev.* 7 (3), 199–209. doi: 10.15420/aer.2018.29.2

Simard, C., Hof, T., Keddache, Z., Launay, P., and Guinamard, R. (2013). The TRPM4 non-selective cation channel contributes to the mammalian atrial action potential. *J. Mol. Cell. Cardiol.* 59, 11–19. doi: 10.1016/j.yjmcc.2013.01.019

Sipido, K. R., Maes, M., and Van de Werf, F. (1997). Low efficiency of Ca2+ entry through the Na(+)-Ca2+ exchanger as trigger for Ca2+ release from the sarcoplasmic reticulum. a comparison between L-type Ca2+ current and reverse-mode Na(+)-Ca2+ exchange. *Circ. Res.* 81 (6), 1034–1044. doi: 10.1161/01.res.81.6.1034

Sipido, K. R., Bito, V., Antoons, G., Volders, P. G., and Vos, M. A. (2007). Na/Ca exchange and cardiac ventricular arrhythmias. *Ann. N. Y. Acad. Sci.* 1099, 339–348. doi: 10.1196/annals.1387.066

Sondergaard, M. T., Tian, X., Liu, Y., Wang, R., Chazin, W. J., Chen, S. R., et al. (2015). Arrhythmogenic calmodulin mutations affect the activation and termination of cardiac ryanodine receptor-mediated Ca2+ release. *J. Biol. Chem.* 290 (43), 26151–26162. doi: 10.1074/jbc.M115.676627

Sondergaard, M. T., Liu, Y., Larsen, K. T., Nani, A., Tian, X., Holt, C., et al. (2017). The Arrhythmogenic Calmodulin p.Phe142Leu mutation impairs c-domain ca2+ binding but not calmodulin-dependent inhibition of the cardiac ryanodine receptor. *J. Biol. Chem.* 292 (4), 1385–1395. doi: 10.1074/jbc.M116.766253

Song, L., Alcalai, R., Arad, M., Wolf, C. M., Toka, O., Conner, D. A., et al. (2007). Calsequestrin 2 (CASQ2) mutations increase expression of calreticulin and ryanodine receptors, causing catecholaminergic polymorphic ventricular tachycardia. *J. Clin. Invest.* 117 (7), 1814–1823. doi: 10.1172/JCI31080

Sood, S., Chelu, M. G., van Oort, R. J., Skapura, D., Santonastasi, M., Dobrev, D., et al. (2008). Intracellular calcium leak due to FKBP12.6 deficiency in mice facilitates the inducibility of atrial fibrillation. *Heart Rhythm* 5 (7), 1047–1054. doi: 10.1016/j.hrthm.2008.03.030

Splawski, I., Tristani-Firouzi, M., Lehmann, M. H., Sanguinetti, M. C., and Keating, M. T. (1997). Mutations in the hminK gene cause long QT syndrome and suppress IKs function. *Nat. Genet.* 17 (3), 338–340. doi: 10.1038/ng1197-338

Splawski, I., Timothy, K. W., Sharpe, L. M., Decher, N., Kumar, P., Bloise, R., et al. (2004). Ca(V)1.2 calcium channel dysfunction causes a multisystem disorder including arrhythmia and autism. *Cell* 119 (1), 19–31. doi: 10.1016/j.cell.2004.09.011

Suetomi, T., Yano, M., Uchinoumi, H., Fukuda, M., Hino, A., Ono, M., et al. (2011). Mutation-linked defective interdomain interactions within ryanodine receptor cause aberrant Ca(2)(+)release leading to catecholaminergic polymorphic ventricular tachycardia. *Circulation* 124 (6), 682–694. doi: 10.1161/CIRCULATIONAHA.111.023259

Sumitomo, N., Nakamura, T., Fukuhara, J., Nakai, T., Watanabe, I., Mugishima, H., et al. (2010). Clinical effectiveness of pulmonary vein isolation for arrhythmic events in a patient with catecholaminergic polymorphic ventricular tachycardia. *Heart Vessels* 25 (5), 448–452. doi: 10.1007/s00380-009-1214-6

Sung, R. J., Wu, S. N., Wu, J. S., Chang, H. D., and Luo, C. H. (2006). Electrophysiological mechanisms of ventricular arrhythmias in relation to Andersen-Tawil syndrome under conditions of reduced IK1: a simulation study. *Am. J. Physiol. Heart Circ. Physiol.* 291 (6), H2597–H2605. doi: 10.1152/ajpheart.00393.2006

Surawicz, B. (1998). U wave: facts, hypotheses, misconceptions, and misnomers. *J. Cardiovasc. Electrophysiol.* 9 (10), 1117–1128. doi: 10.1111/j.1540-8167.1998.tb00890.x

Swan, H., Piippo, K., Viitasalo, M., Heikkila, P., Paavonen, T., Kainulainen, K., et al. (1999). Arrhythmic disorder mapped to chromosome 1q42-q43 causes malignant polymorphic ventricular tachycardia in structurally normal hearts. *J. Am. Coll. Cardiol.* 34 (7), 2035–2042. doi: 10.1016/s0735-1097(99)00461-1

Swan, H., Laitinen, P., Kontula, K., and Toivonen, L. (2005). Calcium channel antagonism reduces exercise-induced ventricular arrhythmias in catecholaminergic polymorphic ventricular tachycardia patients with RyR2 mutations. *J. Cardiovasc. Electrophysiol.* 16 (2), 162–166. doi: 10.1046/j.1540-8167.2005.40516.x

Szabo, B., Sweidan, R., Rajagopalan, C. V., and Lazzara, R. (1994). Role of Na+:Ca2+ exchange current in Cs(+)-induced early afterdepolarizations in Purkinje fibers. *J. Cardiovasc. Electrophysiol.* 5 (11), 933–944. doi: 10.1111/j.1540-8167.1994.tb01133.x

Szabo, G., Szentandrassy, N., Biro, T., Toth, B. I., Czifra, G., Magyar, J., et al. (2005). Asymmetrical distribution of ion channels in canine and human left-ventricular wall: epicardium versus midmyocardium. *Pflugers Archiv.* 450 (5), 307–316. doi: 10.1007/s00424-005-1445-z

Szabo, L., Szentandrassy, N., Kistamas, K., Hegyi, B., Ruzsnavszky, F., Vaczi, K., et al. (2013). Effects of tacrolimus on action potential configuration and transmembrane ion currents in canine ventricular cells. *Naunyn-Schmiedeberg's Arch. Pharmacol.* 386 (3), 239–246. doi: 10.1007/s00210-012-0823-2

Szentandrassy, N., Kistamas, K., Hegyi, B., Horvath, B., Ruzsnavszky, F., Vaczi, K., et al. (2015). Contribution of ion currents to beat-to-beat variability of action potential duration in canine ventricular myocytes. *Pflugers Archiv.* 467 (7), 1431–1443. doi: 10.1007/s00424-014-1581-4

Takamatsu, T., and Wier, W. G. (1990). Calcium waves in mammalian heart: quantification of origin, magnitude, waveform, and velocity. *FASEB J.* 4 (5), 1519–1525. doi: 10.1096/fasebj.4.5.2307330

Terentyev, D., Nori, A., Santoro, M., Viatchenko-Karpinski, S., Kubalova, Z., Gyorke, I., et al. (2006). Abnormal interactions of calsequestrin with the ryanodine receptor calcium release channel complex linked to exercise-induced sudden cardiac death. *Circ. Res.* 98 (9), 1151–1158. doi: 10.1161/01.RES.0000220647.93982.08

Thiel, W. H., Chen, B., Hund, T. J., Koval, O. M., Purohit, A., Song, L. S., et al. (2008). Proarrhythmic defects in Timothy syndrome require calmodulin kinase II. *Circulation* 118 (22), 2225–2234. doi: 10.1161/CIRCULATIONAHA.108.788067

Thomsen, M. B., Verduyn, S. C., Stengl, M., Beekman, J. D., de Pater, G., van Opstal, J., et al. (2004). Increased short-term variability of repolarization predicts d-sotalol-induced torsades de pointes in dogs. *Circulation* 110 (16), 2453–2459. doi: 10.1161/01.CIR.0000145162.64183.C8

Trafford, A. W., Sibbring, G. C., Diaz, M. E., and Eisner, D. A. (2000). The effects of low concentrations of caffeine on spontaneous Ca release in isolated rat ventricular myocytes. *Cell Calcium* 28 (4), 269–276. doi: 10.1054/ceca.2000.0156

Tse, G. (2016). Mechanisms of cardiac arrhythmias. *J. Arrhythmia* 32 (2), 75–81. doi: 10.1016/j.joa.2015.11.003

Uchinoumi, H., Yano, M., Suetomi, T., Ono, M., Xu, X., Tateishi, H., et al. (2010). Catecholaminergic polymorphic ventricular tachycardia is caused by mutation-linked defective conformational regulation of the ryanodine receptor. *Circ. Res.* 106 (8), 1413–1424. doi: 10.1161/CIRCRESAHA.109.209312

van der Werf, C., Kannankeril, P. J., Sacher, F., Krahn, A. D., Viskin, S., Leenhardt, A., et al. (2011). Flecainide therapy reduces exercise-induced ventricular arrhythmias in patients with catecholaminergic polymorphic ventricular tachycardia. *J. Am. Coll. Cardiol.* 57 (22), 2244–2254. doi: 10.1016/j.jacc.2011.01.026

Van Hemel, N. M., Swenne, C. A., De Bakker, J. M., Defauw, J. J., and Guiraudon, G. M. (1988). Epicardial reflection as a cause of incessant ventricular bigeminy. *Pacing Clin. Electrophysiol.* 11 (7), 1036–1044. doi: 10.1111/j.1540-8159.1988.tb03949.x

Vega, A. L., Tester, D. J., Ackerman, M. J., and Makielski, J. C. (2009). Protein kinase A-dependent biophysical phenotype for V227F-KCNJ2 mutation in catecholaminergic polymorphic ventricular tachycardia. *Circ. Arrhythm. Electrophysiol.* 2 (5), 540–547. doi: 10.1161/CIRCEP.109.872309

Venetucci, L. A., Trafford, A. W., Diaz, M. E., O'Neill, S. C., and Eisner, D. A. (2006). Reducing ryanodine receptor open probability as a means to abolish spontaneous Ca2+ release and increase Ca2+ transient amplitude in adult ventricular myocytes. *Circ. Res.* 98 (10), 1299–1305. doi: 10.1161/01.RES.0000222000.35500.65

Venetucci, L. A., Trafford, A. W., and Eisner, D. A. (2007). Increasing ryanodine receptor open probability alone does not produce arrhythmogenic calcium waves: threshold sarcoplasmic reticulum calcium content is required. *Circ. Res.* 100 (1), 105–111. doi: 10.1161/01.RES.0000252828.17939.00

Venetucci, L., Denegri, M., Napolitano, C., and Priori, S. G. (2012). Inherited calcium channelopathies in the pathophysiology of arrhythmias. *Nat. Rev. Cardiol.* 9 (10), 561–575. doi: 10.1038/nrcardio.2012.93

Vermeulen, J. T., McGuire, M. A., Opthof, T., Coronel, R., de Bakker, J. M., Klopping, C., et al. (1994). Triggered activity and automaticity in ventricular trabeculae of failing human and rabbit hearts. *Cardiovasc. Res.* 28 (10), 1547–1554. doi: 10.1093/cvr/28.10.1547

Verrier, R. L., Klingenheben, T., Malik, M., El-Sherif, N., Exner, D. V., Hohnloser, S. H., et al. (2011). Microvolt T-wave alternans physiological basis, methods of measurement, and clinical utility–consensus guideline by international society for holter and noninvasive electrocardiology. *J. Am. Coll. Cardiol.* 58 (13), 1309–1324. doi: 10.1016/j.jacc.2011.06.029

Viatchenko-Karpinski, S., Terentyev, D., Gyorke, I., Terentyeva, R., Volpe, P., Priori, S. G., et al. (2004). Abnormal calcium signaling and sudden cardiac death associated with mutation of calsequestrin. *Circ. Res.* 94 (4), 471–477. doi: 10.1161/01.RES.0000115944.10681.EB

Vinogradova, T. M., Lyashkov, A. E., Zhu, W., Ruknudin, A. M., Sirenko, S., Yang, D., et al. (2006). High basal protein kinase a-dependent phosphorylation drives rhythmic internal Ca2+ store oscillations and spontaneous beating of cardiac pacemaker cells. *Circ. Res.* 98 (4), 505–514. doi: 10.1161/01.RES.0000204575.94040.d1

Voigt, N., Li, N., Wang, Q., Wang, W., Trafford, A. W., Abu-Taha, I., et al. (2012). Enhanced sarcoplasmic reticulum Ca2+ leak and increased Na+-Ca2+ exchanger function underlie delayed afterdepolarizations in patients with chronic atrial fibrillation. *Circulation* 125 (17), 2059–2070. doi: 10.1161/CIRCULATIONAHA.111.067306

Volders, P. G., Kulcsar, A., Vos, M. A., Sipido, K. R., Wellens, H. J., Lazzara, R., et al. (1997). Similarities between early and delayed afterdepolarizations induced by isoproterenol in canine ventricular myocytes. *Cardiovasc. Res.* 34 (2), 348–359. doi: 10.1016/s0008-6363(96)00270-2

Volders, P. G., Vos, M. A., Szabo, B., Sipido, K. R., de Groot, S. H., Gorgels, A. P., et al. (2000). Progress in the understanding of cardiac early afterdepolarizations and torsades de pointes: time to revise current concepts. *Cardiovasc. Res.* 46 (3), 376–392. doi: 10.1016/s0008-6363(00)00022-5

Vukmir, R. B., and Stein, K. L. (1991). Torsades de pointes therapy with phenytoin. *Ann. Emerg. Med.* 20 (2), 198–200. doi: 10.1016/s0196-0644(05)81223-5

Wang, Q., Shen, J., Splawski, I., Atkinson, D., Li, Z., Robinson, J. L., et al. (1995). SCN5A mutations associated with an inherited cardiac arrhythmia, long QT syndrome. *Cell* 80 (5), 805–811. doi: 10.1016/0092-8674(95)90359-3

Wang, S., Trumble, W. R., Liao, H., Wesson, C. R., Dunker, A. K., and Kang, C. H. (1998). Crystal structure of calsequestrin from rabbit skeletal muscle sarcoplasmic reticulum. *Nat. Struct. Biol.* 5 (6), 476–483. doi: 10.1038/nsb0698-476

Watanabe, H., Chopra, N., Laver, D., Hwang, H. S., Davies, S. S., Roach, D. E., et al. (2009). Flecainide prevents catecholaminergic polymorphic ventricular tachycardia in mice and humans. *Nat. Med.* 15 (4), 380–383. doi: 10.1038/nm.1942

Wegener, F. T., Ehrlich, J. R., and Hohnloser, S. H. (2008). Amiodarone-associated macroscopic T-wave alternans and torsade de pointes unmasking the inherited long QT syndrome. *Europace* 10 (1), 112–113. doi: 10.1093/europace/eum252

Weiss, J. N., Chen, P. S., Qu, Z., Karagueuzian, H. S., and Garfinkel, A. (2000). Ventricular fibrillation: how do we stop the waves from breaking? *Circ. Res.* 87 (12), 1103–1107. doi: 10.1161/01.res.87.12.1103

Weiss, J. N., Karma, A., Shiferaw, Y., Chen, P. S., Garfinkel, A., and Qu, Z. (2006). From pulsus to pulseless: the saga of cardiac alternans. *Circ. Res.* 98 (10), 1244–1253. doi: 10.1161/01.RES.0000224540.97431.f0

Weiss, J. N., Garfinkel, A., Karagueuzian, H. S., Nguyen, T. P., Olcese, R., Chen, P. S., et al. (2015). Perspective: a dynamics-based classification of ventricular arrhythmias. *J. Mol. Cell. Cardiol.* 82, 136–152. doi: 10.1016/j.yjmcc.2015.02.017

Wier, W. G., Cannell, M. B., Berlin, J. R., Marban, E., and Lederer, W. J. (1987). Cellular and subcellular heterogeneity of [Ca2+]i in single heart cells revealed by fura-2. *Science* 235 (4786), 325–328. doi: 10.1126/science.3798114

Wilders, R., and Verkerk, A. O. (2018). Long QT syndrome and sinus bradycardia-a mini review. *Front. Cardiovasc. Med.* 5, 106. doi: 10.3389/fcvm.2018.00106

Wit, A. L., and Cranefield, P. F. (1977). Triggered and automatic activity in the canine coronary sinus. *Circ. Res.* 41 (4), 434–445. doi: 10.1161/01.res.41.4.434

Wit, A. L., Hoffman, B. F., and Cranefield, P. F. (1972). Slow conduction and reentry in the ventricular conducting system. I. return extrasystole in canine purkinje fibers. *Circ. Res.* 30 (1), 1–10. doi: 10.1161/01.res.30.1.1

Wren, L. M., Jimenez-Jaimez, J., Al-Ghamdi, S., Al-Aama, J. Y., Bdeir, A., Al-Hassnan, Z. N., et al. (2019). Genetic mosaicism in calmodulinopathy. *Circ. Genom. Precis. Med.* 12 (9), 375–385. doi: 10.1161/CIRCGEN.119.002581

Wu, T. J., Lin, S. F., Weiss, J. N., Ting, C. T., and Chen, P. S. (2002). Two types of ventricular fibrillation in isolated rabbit hearts: importance of excitability and action potential duration restitution. *Circulation* 106 (14), 1859–1866. doi: 10.1161/01.cir.0000031334.49170.fb

Wu, G., Ai, T., Kim, J. J., Mohapatra, B., Xi, Y., Li, Z., et al. (2008). alpha-1-syntrophin mutation and the long-QT syndrome: a disease of sodium channel disruption. *Circ. Arrhythmia Electrophysiol.* 1 (3), 193–201. doi: 10.1161/CIRCEP.108.769224

Xie, L. H., Sato, D., Garfinkel, A., Qu, Z., and Weiss, J. N. (2008). Intracellular Ca alternans: coordinated regulation by sarcoplasmic reticulum release, uptake, and leak. *Biophys. J.* 95 (6), 3100–3110. doi: 10.1529/biophysj.108.130955

Xie, L. H., Chen, F., Karagueuzian, H. S., and Weiss, J. N. (2009). Oxidative-stress-induced afterdepolarizations and calmodulin kinase II signaling. *Circ. Res.* 104 (1), 79–86. doi: 10.1161/CIRCRESAHA.108.183475

Yamamoto, T., Yano, M., Xu, X., Uchinoumi, H., Tateishi, H., Mochizuki, M., et al. (2008). Identification of target domains of the cardiac ryanodine receptor to correct channel disorder in failing hearts. *Circulation* 117 (6), 762–772. doi: 10.1161/CIRCULATIONAHA.107.718957

Yan, G. X., and Antzelevitch, C. (1999). Cellular basis for the Brugada syndrome and other mechanisms of arrhythmogenesis associated with ST-segment elevation. *Circulation* 100 (15), 1660–1666. doi: 10.1161/01.cir.100.15.1660

Yang, Y., Yang, Y., Liang, B., Liu, J., Li, J., Grunnet, M., et al. (2010). Identification of a Kir3.4 mutation in congenital long QT syndrome. *Am. J. Hum. Genet.* 86 (6), 872–880. doi: 10.1016/j.ajhg.2010.04.017

Yang, T., Chun, Y. W., Stroud, D. M., Mosley, J. D., Knollmann, B. C., Hong, C., et al. (2014). Screening for acute IKr block is insufficient to detect torsades de pointes liability: role of late sodium current. *Circulation* 130 (3), 224–234. doi: 10.1161/CIRCULATIONAHA.113.007765

Yano, M., Yamamoto, T., Kobayashi, S., and Matsuzaki, M. (2009). Role of ryanodine receptor as a Ca(2)(+) regulatory center in normal and failing hearts. *J. Cardiol.* 53 (1), 1–7. doi: 10.1016/j.jjcc.2008.10.008

Yarotskyy, V., Gao, G., Du, L., Ganapathi, S. B., Peterson, B. Z., and Elmslie, K. S. (2010). Roscovitine binds to novel L-channel (CaV1.2) sites that separately affect activation and inactivation. *J. Biol. Chem.* 285 (1), 43–53. doi: 10.1074/jbc.M109.076448

Yazawa, M., Hsueh, B., Jia, X., Pasca, A. M., Bernstein, J. A., Hallmayer, J., et al. (2011). using induced pluripotent stem cells to investigate cardiac phenotypes in Timothy syndrome. *Nature* 471 (7337), 230–234. doi: 10.1038/nature09855

Zaza, A., Belardinelli, L., and Shryock, J. C. (2008). Pathophysiology and pharmacology of the cardiac "late sodium current." *Pharmacol. Ther.* 119 (3), 326–339. doi: 10.1016/j.pharmthera.2008.06.001

Zhou, Q., Xiao, J., Jiang, D., Wang, R., Vembaiyan, K., Wang, A., et al. (2011). Carvedilol and its new analogs suppress arrhythmogenic store overload-induced Ca2+ release. *Nat. Med.* 17 (8), 1003–1009. doi: 10.1038/nm.2406

Zhu, Z. I., and Clancy, C. E. (2007). L-type Ca2+ channel mutations and T-wave alternans: a model study. *Am. J. Physiol. Heart Circulatory Physiol.* 293 (6), H3480–H3489. doi: 10.1152/ajpheart.00476.2007

Zygmunt, A. C., Eddlestone, G. T., Thomas, G. P., Nesterenko, V. V., and Antzelevitch, C. (2001). Larger late sodium conductance in M cells contributes to electrical heterogeneity in canine ventricle. *Am. J. Physiol. Heart Circulatory Physiol.* 281 (2), H689–H697. doi: 10.1152/ajpheart.2001.281.2.H689

Sacubitril/Valsartan Improves Left Atrial and Left Atrial Appendage Function in Patients with Atrial Fibrillation and in Pressure Overload-Induced Mice

Ya Suo†, Meng Yuan†, Hongmin Li†, Yue Zhang, Ying Li, Huaying Fu, Fei Han, Changhui Ma, Yuanyuan Wang, Qiankun Bao and Guangping Li**

Tianjin Key Laboratory of Ionic-Molecular Function of Cardiovascular Disease, Department of Cardiology, Tianjin Institute of Cardiology, the Second Hospital of Tianjin Medical University, Tianjin, China

***Correspondence:**
Qiankun Bao,
baoqiankun@tmu.edu.cn
Guangping Li
tic_tjcardiol@126.com

†These authors have contributed equally to this work

LCZ696 (sacubitril/valsartan) is an angiotensin receptor-neprilysin inhibitor and has shown beneficial effects in patients with heart failure. However, whether LCZ696 protects against left atrial (LA) and LA appendage (LAA) dysfunction is still unclear. The present study aimed to assess the efficacy of LCZ696 for improving the function of LA and LAA. We performed both a retrospective study comparing LCZ696 with angiotensin receptor blockers (ARBs) to assess the efficacy of LCZ696 in patients with atrial fibrillation and an animal study in a mouse model with pressure overload. LA peak systolic strain, LAA emptying flow velocity, and LAA ejection fraction (LAAEF) were significantly increased in patients with LCZ696 as compared with ARBs ($p = 0.024$, $p = 0.036$, $p = 0.026$, respectively). Users of LCZ696 had a lower incidence of spontaneous echocardiography contrast ($p = 0.040$). Next, patients were divided into two groups (LAAEF $\leq$ 20% and > 20%). Administration of LCZ696 in patients with LAAEF > 20% was more frequent than LAAEF $\leq$ 20% ($p = 0.032$). Even after controlling for LAA dysfunction-related risk factors (age, atrial fibrillation type, old myocardial infarction, hypertension, congestive heart failure, and prior stroke or transient ischemic attack), use of LCZ696 remained significantly associated with reduced probability of LAAEF $\leq$ 20% [odds ratio = 0.011; 95% confidence interval (0.000–0.533), $p = 0.023$]. To further confirmed effect of LCZ696 in LA function, we constructed a post-transverse aortic constriction model in mice. Mice with LCZ696 treatment showed lower LA dimension and higher left ventricular ejection fraction and LAA emptying flow velocity as compared with mice with vehicle or valsartan treatment. Meanwhile, as compared with vehicle or valsartan, LCZ696 significantly decreased LA fibrosis in mice. In summary, we provide evidence that LCZ696 may be more effective in improving LA and LAA function than ARBs in both humans and mice, which suggests that LCZ696 might be evaluated as a direct therapeutic for atrial remodeling and AF.

Keywords: sacubitril/valsartan, atrial fibrillation, left atrial function, left atrial appendage thrombus, atrial fibrosis

INTRODUCTION

Patients with cardiogenic embolic stroke have a high prevalence of non-valvular atrial fibrillation (AF), which is associated with a five-fold increased risk of stroke and a two-fold increased risk of both dementia and mortality (Fuster et al., 2006). In AF patients, impaired atrial emptying might cause atrial blood stasis and enlargement of left atrial (LA), which could further offer a suitable terrain for thrombus formation. The left atrial appendage (LAA) is an important attachment and reservoir of LA, and its effective contraction can prevent blood stasis. AF confers an increased risk of stroke owing to the formation of atrial thrombus, usually in the LAA (Takada et al., 2001). Therefore, it is necessary to preserve the mechanical function of LAA to prevent LAA thrombosis and cardiogenic stroke in patients with AF (Perez et al., 1997; Verhorst et al., 1997). Several parameters measured by transesophageal echocardiography (TEE) can reflect LAA dysfunction (Zabalgoitia et al., 1998), which can result in LAA thrombus (LAAT) formation. Spontaneous echocardiographic contrast (SEC, caused by blood stasis or low-velocity blood flow), reduced LAA emptying flow velocity (LAAeV), and LAA ejection fraction (LAAEF) can be used as effective markers for stratifying thromboembolic risk in patients with AF (Kamp et al., 1999).

Activation of the renin-angiotensin-aldosterone system (RAAS) in atrial local tissue leads to structural and electrophysiological remodeling of the atrium, which further increases the susceptibility of atrial arrhythmia and promotes the occurrence of AF (Healey et al., 2005). LA and LAA function decline with mechanical remodeling of the left atrium, and thrombus is more likely to form within the LAA (Sparks et al., 1999). With atrial fibrosis, conduction abnormalities result in increased AF vulnerability (Jalife, 2014; Jalife and Kaur, 2015; Miragoli and Glukhov, 2015; Nattel, 2017). Recent studies have implicated that inhibition of RAAS activation can moderate atrial remodeling, thereby improving the occurrence and development of AF (Jibrini et al., 2008). In previous work, we demonstrated that administration of RAAS inhibitors in patients with AF might reduce the risk of LAAT by moderating atrial remodelling (Suo et al., 2018). In addition, natriuretic peptides (NPs) are critical regulators of cardiac structure and electrophysiology, modulating ion channel function in the heart, including the atrium (Moghtadaei et al., 2016). NPs also have anti-fibrotic effects (Rose and Giles, 2008), so they may play a protective role against AF development.

LCZ696 (sacubitril/valsartan) is a representative drug targeting both the RAAS and NP systems, which blocks the angiotensin receptor (AT1), and prevents the degradation of NPs *via* inhibiting neprilysin (Voors et al., 2013). In clinical studies, LCZ696 could improve New York Heart Association classification and cardio-renal function in patients with different types of heart failure, including heart failure with reduced left ventricular ejection fraction (HFrEF) and heart failure with preserved left ventricular ejection fraction (HFpEF) (Solomon et al., 2012; Balmforth et al., 2019). In the PARAMOUNT study, patients with LCZ696 showed a significant decrease in LA diameter than patients with valsartan (Solomon et al., 2012). However, whether the administration of LCZ696 could protect against LA and LAA dysfunction has not been elucidated.

Therefore, we undertook this work including both a retrospective study comparing LCZ696 with AT1 blockers (ARBs) to assess the efficacy of LCZ696 in patients with AF and an animal study in a mouse model with pressure overload. LCZ696 was more effective than ARBs in preserving LA and LAA function. Even when controlling for risk factors associated with LAA dysfunction, use of LCZ696 remained significantly associated with reduced risk of LAAEF ≤ 20%. In addition, we verified that LCZ696 improved LA and LAA function and decreased atrial fibrosis in mice with pressure overload. Thus, LCZ696 might have potential therapeutic value in preventing the incidence of cardiogenic embolic stroke in patients with AF.

MATERIALS AND METHODS

Study Population

We conducted a retrospective study of all consecutive adult AF patients admitted to the Second Hospital of Tianjin Medical University from October 1, 2017, to March 31, 2019, and underwent both TEE and transthoracic echocardiography (TTE) on the same day. The total number of all patients was 468, and 81 patients were eventually included in the analysis on the basis of exclusion criteria (see below). AF and its different types were defined according to ESC guidelines for the management of AF (Kirchhof et al., 2016) The researchers were unaware of the results and recorded the required data, including demographic details, LAAT-related risk factors, and LCZ696 or ARB use. Patients who used LCZ696 or ARBs for more than 12 weeks were assigned to the LCZ696 group and ARB group, respectively. LCZ696 (cat. no. H20170362) and valsartan (cat. no. H20040217) were purchased from Novartis Pharma Schweiz AG. The CHA_2DS_2–VASc [congestive heart failure, hypertension, age ≥75 years (doubled), diabetes mellitus, prior stroke or transient ischemic attack or thromboembolism (doubled), vascular disease, age 65 to 74 years, sex category] point score system was used for stratifying ischemic stroke risk among patients with non-valvular AF. Other clinical data including vascular disease (peripheral arterial disease, carotid disease, venous thromboembolic disease, or renal artery stenosis), hyperlipidemia (hypercholesterolemia,

Abbreviations: AF, atrial fibrillation; ARB, angiotensin receptor blocker; BMI, body mass index; CHD, coronary heart diseases; E:e' ratio, The ratio of the early transmitral flow velocity and the early mitral annular velocity; LA, left atrial; LAA, left atrial appendage; LAAEF, left atrial appendage ejection fraction; LAAeV, left atrial appendage emptying flow velocity; LAAT, left atrial appendage thrombus; LAD, left atrial dimension; LAVmax, maximal left atrial volume; LVDd, left ventricular end-diastolic diameter; LVDs, left ventricular end-systolic diameter; LVEF, left ventricular ejection fraction; LVPWd, left ventricular posterior wall thickness diameter; LVSTd, left ventricular interventricular septum thickness diameter; NPs, natriuretic peptides; OMI, old myocardial infarction; RAAS, renin-angiotensin-aldosterone system; SEC, spontaneous echocardiographic contrast; TAC, transverse aortic constriction; TEE, transesophageal echocardiography; TGF-β1, transforming growth factor-β1; TIA, transient ischemic attack; TTE, transthoracic echocardiography.

hypertriglyceridemia, mixed hyperlipidemia, and low-/high-density lipoproteinemia), smoking history (active smoking history accumulated over 6 months), drinking history (alcohol average >120 g/week), and anti-platelet drug use (aspirin and/or clopidogrel for > 12 weeks) were collected.

Patients who did not receive anti-coagulant therapy were excluded from this study. Other exclusion criteria were acute myocardial infarction, significant valvular disease, congenital heart disease, left ventricular (LV) systolic dysfunction [LV ejection fraction (LVEF) ≤ 40%], severe respiratory disease, pulmonary hypertension, and inadequate quality of echocardiographic images. The dysfunction of LA and LAA was the outcome of this study. The Local Ethics Committee approved the study protocol, with all study subjects providing written informed consent (**Figure 1**).

Echocardiography Measurements

Echocardiography examination involved using a commercial ultrasonography system (IE33, Philips Healthcare, Inc.). TTE involved using a 1–5 MHz phased S5-1 probe, and TEE a 2–7 MHz 3D matrix array X7-2t probe. All images were analyzed by using off-line post-processing with QLAB Software.

The following parameters were evaluated in standard views with standard techniques (Lang et al., 2005): LV end-diastolic diameter (LVDd), LVEF, LA dimension (LAD), maximal LA volume (LAVmax), and ratio of early transmittal flow velocity and early mitral annular velocity (E:e' ratio). Spectral Doppler tissue imaging was used to measure tissue Doppler velocity; the septal annuli was selected in this study. LA was divided into 13 segments, and LA peak systolic strain during ventricular systole was calculated by the mean of all 13 segments.

An echocardiographer reviewed all TEE images to determine whether LAAT, SEC, reduced LAAeV, and LAAEF were present. The echocardiographer was blinded to the clinical data and results of TTE. LAAT was defined as a uniformly and circumscribed echo-dense intra-cavitary mass in multiple imaging planes, distinct from the pectinate muscles, and LAA endocardium (Aschenberg et al., 1986). SEC was defined as dynamic "smoke-like" echoes with the characteristic swirling motion during the entire cardiac cycle (Fatkin et al., 1994). The LAAeV was obtained at a depth of 1/3 from the LAA orifice with pulsed Doppler. Then, a 3D-TEE study was performed to visualize various LAA structures. LAAEF was calculated by using the QLAB 3DQ plug-in. We measured LAA volume from the basal short-axis view in the transverse scan. LAAEF was calculated as [(maximum volume - minimum

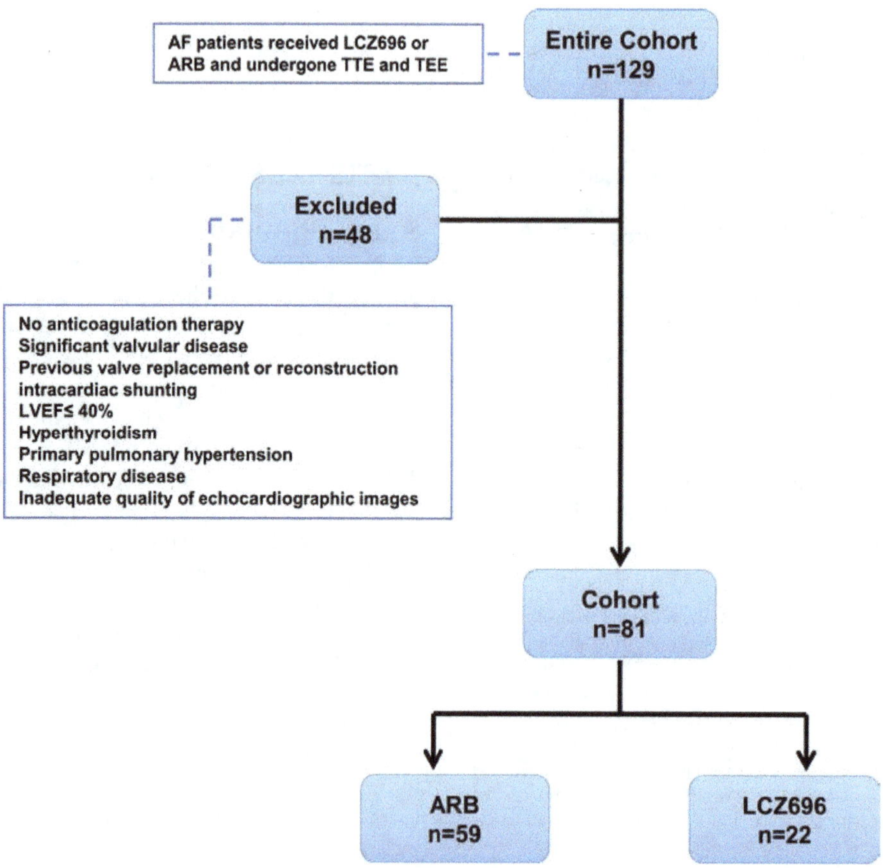

FIGURE 1 | Study design displaying inclusion/exclusion and patient group assignments. AF, atrial fibrillation; ARB, angiotensin receptor blocker; TTE, transthoracic echocardiography; TEE, transesophageal echocardiography; LVEF, left ventricular ejection fraction.

volume)/maximum volume × 100%] (**Figures 2A , B**). The researcher carefully measured the parameters and calculated the mean values from five cardiac cycles.

Animal Study

Animal procedures were approved and conducted in accordance with the Experimental Animal Administration Committee of Tianjin Medical University. Male C57BL/6J mice at 8–10 weeks of age were randomly assigned to transverse aortic constriction (TAC) surgery or sham surgery. All mice were housed in a controlled environment (20 ± 2°C, 12-hr/12-hr light/dark cycle). TAC surgery was performed as described (Wang et al., 2016). Briefly, after mice were anesthetized, the transverse aorta was ligated with a 27-G needle. Mice in the sham surgery group underwent similar surgical procedures without ligation of the transverse aorta. At 8 weeks after surgery, TAC mice were randomized to treatment with LCZ696 (60 mg/kg body weight perorally, n = 6), valsartan (48 mg/kg body weight perorally, n = 6), or no treatment (n = 6) for another 4 weeks. Mice were given valsartan or LCZ696 dissolved in corn oil or only corn oil every day by oral gavage.

Echocardiography Measurements of Mice

TTE was performed on all mice at baseline (8 weeks post-TAC surgery) and 4 weeks post-randomization by using a Vevo 2100 System with an MS400 Linear Array Transducer (VisualSonics, ON, Canada) as described (Gao et al., 2011) After mice were weighed and anesthetized by inhalation of 1.5% isoflurane, they were placed on a heating mat to maintain normothermia (35°C). LAD, LV interventricular septum thickness diameter (IVSTd), LV posterior wall thickness diameter (LVPWd), LVDd, and LVEF were measured. LAAeV was obtained on the parasternal short-axis view (**Figure 3 A**). After final echocardiography examination, mice were immediately sacrificed for heart tissues.

Histology of Heart Tissues

Heart tissues were fixed in 10% neutral-buffered formalin for 24 h at room temperature and embedded in paraffin, then sectioned at 5 μm for staining. Collagen deposition was stained with Masson's trichrome stain (Sigma-Aldrich, MO) and Sirius Red stain (Solarbio Life Sciences, Beijing) according to the manufacturer's instructions. Images of the sections were captured under an Olympus Inverted Microscope (IX53, Tokyo) and fibrotic areas were semi-quantitatively determined by using ImageJ v1.52.

Statistical Analyses

All statistical analyses were performed with SPSS v23.0 (SPSS, Chicago, IL, USA). Results are presented as mean ± standard deviation (SD) or mean±SEM for continuous variables and percentage of the total number of patients for categorical variables. Student *t*-test was used to compare continuous variables. Chi-square and the Fisher exact test were used for nominal variables. Univariate analysis was performed with the chi-square test. Variables significant on univariate logistic regression analysis ($p < 0.05$) were entered into the multiple regression analysis. Logistic regression analysis (with the enter method) was performed to identify independent predictors of depressed LAAEF. The risk was expressed as odd ratios (OR) with 95% confidence intervals (CIs). Statistical analysis involved use of GraphPad Prism 7 (Version 7.04), by one-way ANOVA. The criterion for statistical significance was $P < 0.05$.

RESULTS

Sacubitril/Valsartan Is More Effective Than Angiotensin Receptor Blockers for Improving Left Atrial and Left Atrial Appendage Function in Patients With Atrial Fibrillation

Initially, we identified 129 patients with AF who used LCZ696 or ARBs and received TTE and TEE during hospitalization from 2017 to 2019; 81 were included in the analysis: 22 (27.2%) received LCZ696 and 59 (72.8%) received ARBs (**Figure 1**). The mean age of 81 patients was 62.76 ± 8.19 years; 55.6% were male (**Table 1**). The baseline clinical characteristics were comparable between the two groups (**Table 1**). The two groups did not differ in LVDd, LVEF, LAD, LAVmax, or E:e' ratio (**Table 2**). However, users of LCZ696 had a lower incidence of SEC and higher LAAeV, LAAEF, and LA peak systolic strain as compared with users of ARBs (**Table 2**, **Figure 2**). LAAT occurred in 21% of 81 patients, including 22.0% users of ARBs and 18.2% users of LCZ696 ($p = 0.705$) (**Table 2**).

Next, the 81 patients were divided into two groups according to the cutoff for LAAEF defined as 20% (LAAEF ≤ 20% and > 20%) (Iwama et al., 2012). Demographic, echocardiographic parameters and clinical characteristics of the patients with LAAEF≤ 20% or > 20% are shown in **Table 3**. Patients with LAAEF > 20% were younger than those with LAAEF ≤ 20% (61.4 ± 8.6 *vs.* 65.2 ± 6.9 years) ($p < 0.05$) (**Table 3**). CHA_2DS_2-VASc score was significantly higher for patients with LAAEF ≤ 20% than > 20% ($p < 0.05$). As compared with patients with LAAEF > 20%, those with LAAEF ≤ 20% had a higher prevalence of long-standing persistent AF (continuous AF >12 months duration), persistent AF (continuous AF sustained < 7 days), old myocardial infarction (OMI), prior stroke or transient ischemic attack, congestive heart failure, and hypertension. The proportion of LCZ696 users was higher for patients with LAAEF > 20% than ≤ 20% (35.3 *vs.* 13.3%) ($p < 0.05$). LAAeV, LVEF, and LA peak systolic strain were significantly lower for patients with LAAEF ≤ 20% than > 20%. Patients with LAAEF ≤ 20% had significantly higher E:e' ratio, LAD, LAVmax, LVDd, and incidence of SEC and LAAT than those with LAAEF > 20% ($p < 0.01$) (**Table 3**).

Logistic regression analysis was performed to identify independent clinical predictors of LAAEF ≤ 20% (**Table 4**). Univariate analysis demonstrated prior stroke or transient ischemic attack, congestive heart failure, categories of AF type, OMI, hypertension, and age as significantly positively associated with LAAEF ≤ 20%, except for use of LCZ696, which was significantly negatively associated with LAAEF ≤ 20%. However, only prior stroke or transient ischemic attack, AF type, hypertension, age ≥ 65 years, and use of LCZ696 were associated

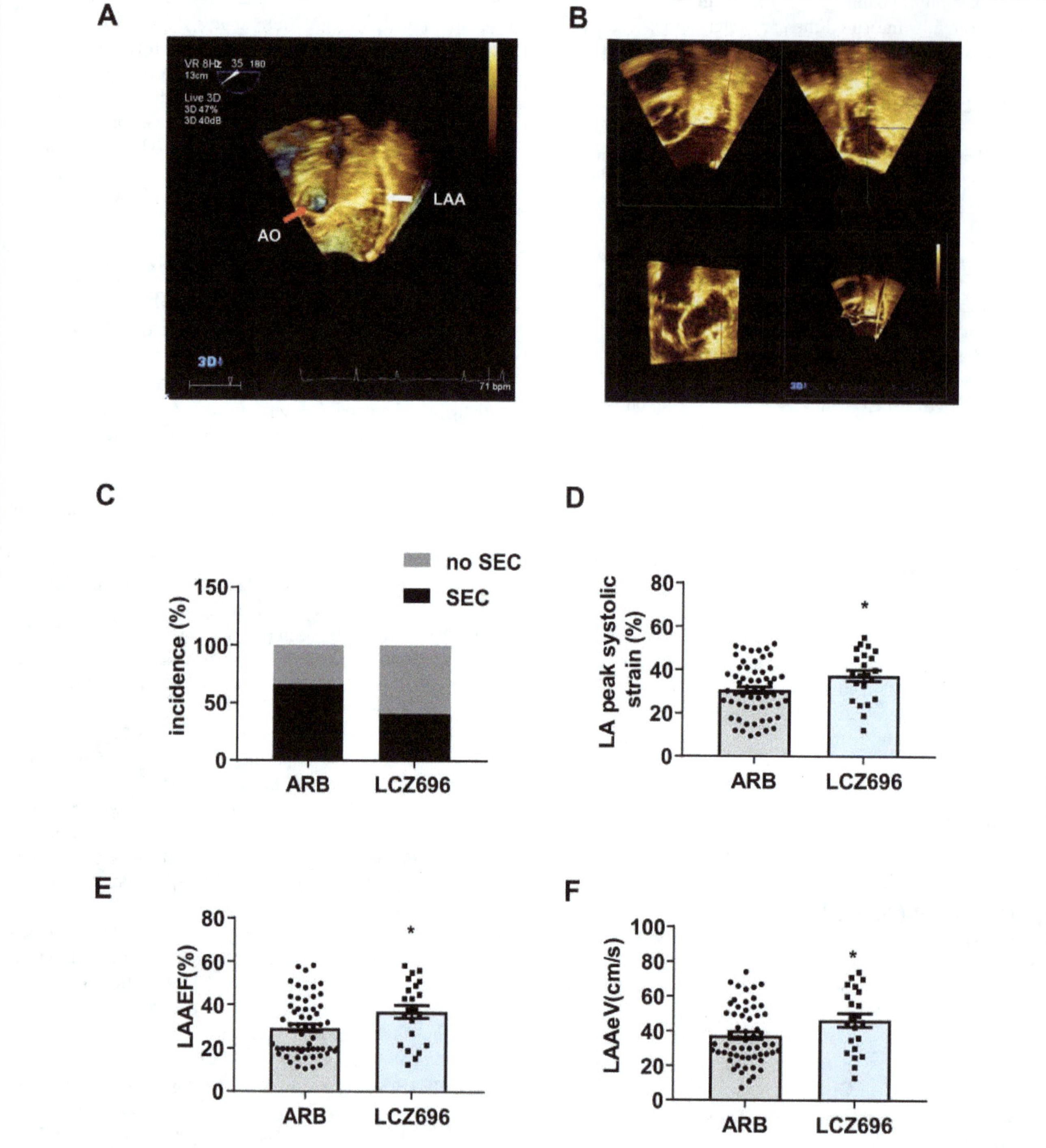

FIGURE 2 | Sacubitril/valsartan is more effective than angiotensin receptor blockers for improving left atrial and left atrial appendage function in patients with atrial fibrillation. **(A)** 3D transesophageal echocardiography (3D-TEE) showing the left atrial appendage (LAA) from the basal short-axis view in the transverse scan. The white arrow indicates the LAA, and the red arrow indicates the aorta (AO). **(B)** QLAB 3DQ plug-in showing LAA. The LAA short axes were aligned by using QLab-3DQ software, allowing visualization of the LAA orifice in the multiplanar reconstruction mode. **(C)** Incidence of spontaneous echocardiographic contrast (SEC), **(D)** LA peak systolic strain, **(E)** LAA ejection fraction (LAAEF), and **(F)** LAA emptying flow velocity (LAAeV). Data are mean ± SD, $^*P < 0.05$, unpaired two-tail *t* test.

with LAAEF ≤ 20% after multivariable adjustments (**Table 4**). Hypertension was associated with a higher risk of LAAEF≤ 20% [OR = 9.797; 95% CI (1.202–79.883); $p = 0.033$]. Congestive heart failure and OMI were not significantly correlated with LAA dysfunction. After controlling for factors related to LAAEF, the use of LCZ696 remained significantly associated with reduced probability of LAAEF ≤ 20% [OR = 0.011; 95% CI (0.000–0.533), $p = 0.023$).

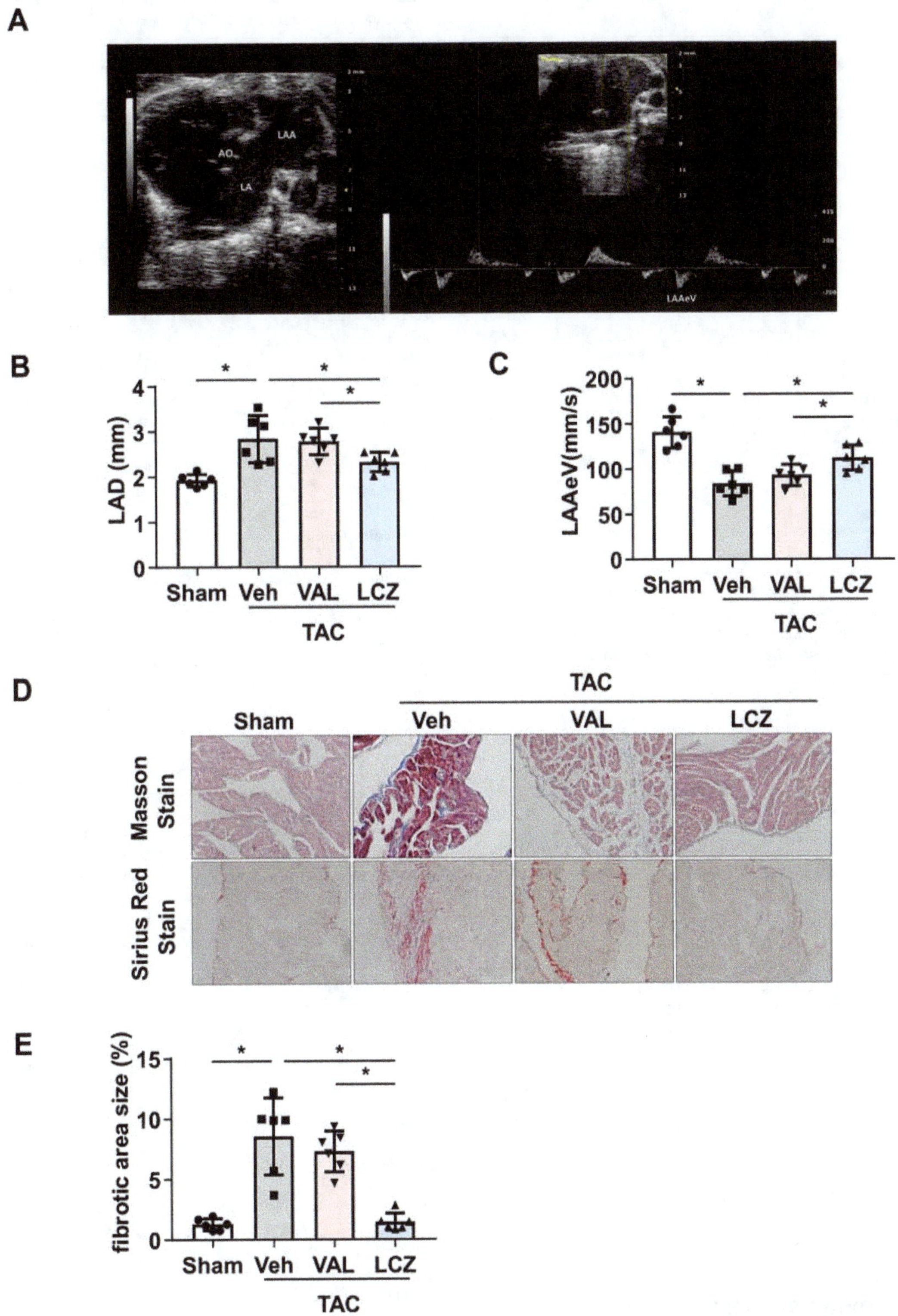

FIGURE 3 | Sacubitril/valsartan is more effective than valsartan for protecting left atrial (LA) and left atrial appendage (LAA) function and decreasing LA fibrosis in mice after pressure overload.**(A)** 2D echocardiography showing LA, LAA, aorta (AO), and LAA emptying flow velocity (LAAeV) from the basal short-axis view. **(B, C)** Left atrial dimension (LAD) and LAAeV quantified by echocardiography. **(D)** Representative images of Masson staining and Sirius Red staining of LA. Scale bar, 100 μm. **(E)** Quantification of the fibrotic area in **(D)**. TAC, transverse aortic constriction; Veh, vehicle; VAL, valsartan; LCZ, LCZ696. Data are mean ± SEM, n = 6 mice per group, *$P < 0.05$, one-way ANOVA.

TABLE 1 | Baseline characteristics of sacubitril/valsartan and angiotensin receptor blocker users.

Variables	LCZ696 n = 22	ARBs n = 59	*P* value
Age, years	60.454 ± 8.410	63.627 ± 8.014	0.135
Age ≥ 65 years, %	31.8%	47.5%	0.206
Male sex, %	63.6%	52.5%	0.371
BMI, kg/m^2	25.865 ± 3.669	26.189 ± 3.785	0.731
AF type, %			0.933
Paroxysmal AF	68.2%	71.2%	
Persistent AF	22.7%	22.0%	
Long-standing persistent	9.1%	6.8%	
OMI, %	27.3%	16.9%	0.351
Vascular disease, %	4.5%	5.1%	1.000
CHD, %	90.9%	71.2%	0.062
Hyperlipidemia, %	68.2%	66.1%	0.860
Hypertension, %	59.1%	71.2%	0.300
Diabetes mellitus, %	36.4%	23.7%	0.255
Congestive heart failure, %	22.7%	13.6%	0.325
Prior stroke or TIA, %	27.3%	20.3%	0.554
CHA_2DS_2–VASc Score, mean±SD	2.454 ± 1.738	2.644 ± 1.471	0.625
Smoking history, %	45.5%	39.0%	0.598
Drinking history, %	27.3%	22.0%	0.621
Antiplatelet drugs, %	68.2%	55.9%	0.318

BMI, body mass index; OMI, old myocardial infarction; CHD, coronary heart diseases; TIA, transient ischemic attack; AF, atrial fibrillation; CHA_2DS_2–VASc Score, congestive heart failure, hypertension, age ≥75 years (doubled), diabetes mellitus, prior stroke or transient ischemic attack or thromboembolism (doubled), vascular disease, age 65 to 74 years, sex category.

TABLE 2 | Echocardiographic parameters for sacubitril/valsartan and angiotensin receptor blocker users.

Variables	LCZ696 n = 22	ARB n = 59	*P* value
LAD, mm	38.814 ± 2.910	40.244 ± 3.960	0.127
LAVmax, ml	48.713 ± 11.652	52.630 ± 13.926	0.244
LA peak systolic strain, %	37.536 ± 11.679	30.727 ± 11.892	0.024
LVDd, mm	50.075 ± 5.460	49.468 ± 5.950	0.677
LVEF, %	53.163 ± 6.456	56.558 ± 7.095	0.053
E:e' ratio	11.040 ± 4.404	12.420 ± 4.327	0.208
LAAeV, cm/s	46.459 ± 18.250	31.481 ± 16.363	0.036
LAAEF, %	37.050 ± 14.289	29.413 ± 13.215	0.026
SEC, %	40.9%	66.1%	0.040
LAAT, %	18.2%	22.0%	0.705

Data are mean ± SD unless indicated. LAD, left atrial dimension; LAVmax, maximal left atrial volume; LVDd, left ventricular end-diastolic diameter; LVEF, left ventricular ejection fraction; E,e' ratio, the ratio of the early transmitral flow velocity and the early mitral annular velocity; LAAeV, left atrial appendage emptying flow velocity; LAAEF, left atrial appendage ejection fraction; SEC, spontaneous echocardiographic contrast; LAAT, left atrial appendage thrombus.

Sacubitril/Valsartan Was More Effective Than Valsartan in Protecting Left Atrial and Left Atrial Appendage Function and Decreasing LA Fibrosis in Mice With Pressure Overload

To detect the efficiency of LCZ696 in protecting LA and LAA function, we used the TAC mouse model, a pressure overload-induced LA and LAA dysfunction model. TAC surgery increased LAD, LVSTd, LVPWd, LVDd, and LVDs as compared with sham mice (**Table 5**). In addition, LAAeV and LVEF were significantly decreased after 8 weeks of TAC surgery.

TABLE 3 | Clinical and echocardiography parameters for patients with left atrial appendage ejection fraction ≤ 20% or LAAEF > 20%.

Variables	LAAEF ≤ 20% n = 30	LAAEF > 20% n = 51	*P* value
Age, years	65.17 ± 6.85	61.35 ± 8.64	0.042
Age≥65 years, %	63.3%	31.4%	0.005
Male sex, %	65.5%	56.3%	0.238
BMI, kg/m^2	26.10 ± 3.5	26.1 ± 3.90	0.996
AF type, %			0.000
Paroxysmal AF	40.0%	88.2%	
Persistent AF	43.3%	9.8%	
Long-standing persistent AF	16.7%	2.0%	
OMI, %	33.3%	11.8%	0.019
Vascular disease, %	6.7%	3.9%	0.624
CHD, %	80.0%	74.5%	0.573
Hyperlipidemia, %	70.0%	64.7%	0.625
Hypertension, %	93.3%	52.9%	0.000
Diabetes mellitus, %	20.0%	31.4%	0.266
Congestive heart failure, %	30.0%	7.8%	0.013
Prior stroke or TIA, %	42.3%	9.8%	0.000
CHA_2DS_2–VASc score	3.57 ± 1.406	2.02 ± 1.32	0.000
Smoking history, %	36.7%	43.1%	0.567
Drinking history, %	20.0%	25.5%	0.573
Antiplatelet drugs, %	66.7%	54.9%	0.298
LCZ696, %	13.3%	35.3%	0.032
LAD, mm	42.55 ± 3.20	38.27 ± 3.08	0.000
LAVmax, ml	59.3 ± 13.8	47.02 ± 10.94	0.000
LA peak systolic strain, %	22.27 ± 8.79	38.64 ± 9.5	0.000
LVDd, mm	51.62 ± 6.67	48.47 ± 4.91	0.017
LVEF, %	52.5 ± 7.5	57.48 ± 6.13	0.002
E:e' ratio	14.01 ± 4.24	10.89 ± 4.04	0.001
LAAeV, cm/s	24.79 ± 8.83	48.82 ± 14.6	0.000
LAAEF, %	17.18 ± 3.09	39.90 ± 10.32	0.000
SEC, %	100%	35.3%	0.000
LAAT, %	50.0%	3.9%	0.000

Data are mean ± SD unless indicated.
LAAT, left atrial appendage thrombus; BMI, body mass index; OMI, old myocardial infarction; CHD, coronary heart diseases; TIA, transient ischemic attack; AF, atrial fibrillation; LAD, left atrial dimension; LAVmax, maximal left atrial volume; LVDd, left ventricular end-diastolic diameter; LVEF, left ventricular ejection fraction; E,e' ratio, the ratio of the early transmitral flow velocity and the early mitral annular velocity; LAAeV, left atrial appendage emptying flow velocity; LAAEF, left atrial appendage ejection fraction; SEC, spontaneous echocardiographic contrast; LAAT, left atrial appendage thrombus.

TABLE 4 | Factors associated with left atrial appendage emptying flow velocity ≤ 20% on multiple regression analyses.

Variables	Odds ratio	95% CI	*P* value
Age ≥ 65 years	7.675	1.183–49.805	0.033
AF type			0.007
OMI	5.465	0.461–64.757	0.178
Hypertension	9.797	1.202–79.883	0.033
CHF	3.095	0.127–75.434	0.488
Prior stroke or TIA	10.474	1.305–76.018	0.027
LCZ696	0.011	0.000–0.533	0.023

LAAEF, left atrial appendage ejection fraction; OMI, old myocardial infarction; CHF, congestive heart failure; TIA, transient ischemic attack; CI, confidence interval.

Next, mice were treated with LCZ696, valsartan, or vehicle for another 4 weeks. LAD was decreased and LAAeV increased in mice with LCZ696 as compared with vehicle and valsartan (**Table 6** and **Figures 3B, C**), which suggests that LCZ696 is more effective than valsartan in protecting LA and LAA function. Consistent with a previous report in rabbits (Torrado et al., 2018), in mice, LVEF was significantly improved with LCZ696 as compared with valsartan (**Table 6**). Moreover, Masson and Sirius red stain demonstrated that LCZ696 reduced fibrosis in the LAA induced by pressure overload as compared with valsartan (**Figures 3D, E**). Together, our data indicate that LCZ696 might be more effective in attenuating LA and LAA dysfunction induced by pressure overload than valsartan in mice.

DISCUSSION

In the present study, we found that the use of LCZ696 was associated with improved LA and LAA function in patients with AF evaluated by echocardiography. In addition, LCZ696 was more effective than valsartan at moderating atrial fibrosis and protecting LA and LAA function in mice with pressure overload. Therefore, our study demonstrated a critical role for LCZ696 in protecting against LA/LAA structural remodeling and dysfunction.

Structural and electrophysiological remodeling of the atrial myocardium increases the susceptibility to arrhythmia and AF development (Burstein and Nattel, 2008). Fibrosis is an important pathophysiological basis of structural and electrophysiological remodelling (Burstein and Nattel, 2008). Atrial fibrosis leads to mechanical dysfunction of the atria and blood stasis in the atria, which leads to thrombosis in the LAA (Kamp et al., 1999; Sparks et al., 1999). The activation of RAAS results in adverse hemodynamic effects, hypertrophy, and especially the stimulation of fibrosis (Burstein and Nattel, 2008). Therefore, RAAS inhibitors containing angiotensin-converting enzyme inhibitors or ARBs are involved in the upstream treatment of AF. Inhibiting RAAS can reduce atrial fibrosis and dilated atrial volume, further delaying AF development (Nakashima and Kumagai, 2007). Our previous retrospective study demonstrated that the incidence of LAAT was reduced and echocardiography indicators related to left atrial remodeling were improved in patients with angiotensin-converting enzyme inhibitor/ARB treatment (Suo et al., 2018).

LCZ696 contains valsartan and the neprilysin inhibitor pro-drug sacubitril (AHU-377, which can be converted by enzymatic cleavage into the active neprilysin inhibiting metabolite LBQ657) in one compound (Gu et al., 2010). Neprilysin degrades biologically active NPs, including atrial NP, B-type natriuretic peptide, and C-type natriuretic peptide,

TABLE 5 | Baseline echocardiography parameters for mice under transverse aortic constriction surgery for 8 weeks.

Variables	Sham	TAC		
		Vehicle	Valsartan	LCZ696
LVSTd, mm	0.611 ± 0.038	0.827 ± 0.064*	0.813 ± 0.040*	0.801 ± 0.051*
LVPWd, mm	0.624 ± 0.036	0.818 ± 0.048*	0.856 ± 0.049*	0.800 ± 0.048*
LVDd, mm	3.330 ± 0.187	3.714 ± 0.195*	3.673 ± 0.362*	3.724 ± 0.312*
LVDs, mm	2.156 ± 0.211	2.907 ± 0.120*	2.882 ± 0.311*	2.895 ± 0.196*
LVEF, %	65.739 ± 6.776	44.477 ± 5.286*	44.339 ± 5.850*	45.315 ± 4.888*
LAD, mm	1.900 ± 0.105	2.236 ± 0.345*	2.222 ± 0.241*	2.221 ± 0.266*
LAAeV, mm/s	155.158 ± 17.184	125.858 ± 9.976*	122.349 ± 15.125*	127.932 ± 24.030*

Data are mean ± SEM.
*LVSTd, left ventricular interventricular septum thickness diameter; LVPWd, left ventricular posterior wall thickness diameter; LVDd, left ventricular end-diastolic diameter; LVDs, left ventricular end-systolic diameter; LVEF, left ventricular ejection fraction; LAD, left atrial dimension; LAAeV, left atrial appendage emptying flow velocity. *P< 0.05 versus sham.*

TABLE 6 | Echocardiography analysis of pressure overload-induced mice after 4-week treatment.

Variables	Sham	TAC		
		Vehicle	Valsartan	LCZ696
IVSTd, mm	0.632 ± 0.025§	1.005 ± 0.106*§	0.911 ± 0.078*#	0.865 ± 0.055*#
LVPWd, mm	0.630 ± 0.062#§	1.021 ± 0.101*§	0.961 ± 0.057*	0.887 ± 0.036*#
LVDd, mm	3.462 ± 0.223#§	4.177 ± 0.213*§	3.981 ± 0.362*	3.821 ± 0.222*#
LVDs, mm	2.360 ± 0.187#§	3.356 ± 0.198*§	3.197 ± 0.282*§	2.922 ± 0.224*#
LVEF, %	60.526 ± 7.265#§	40.508 ± 6.427*§	40.866 ± 3.219*§	47.759 ± 3.904*#
LAD, mm	1.927 ± 0.137#	2.842 ± 0.524*§	2.781 ± 0.293*§	2.318 ± 0.213#
LAAeV, mm/s	140.700 ± 17.257#§	84.079 ± 13.869*§	93.286 ± 11.785*§	112.170 ± 13.688*#

Data are mean ± SEM.
*IVSTd, left ventricular interventricular septum thickness diameter; LVPWd, left ventricular posterior wall thickness diameter; LVDd, left ventricular end-diastolic diameter; LVDs, left ventricular end-systolic diameter; LVEF, left ventricular ejection fraction; LAD, left atrial dimension; LAA eV, LAA emptying flow velocity. *P< 0.05 versus Sham. #P< 0.05 versus TAC + vehicle. §P< 0.05 versus LCZ696.*

which are critical regulators of atrial electrophysiology and structure (Moghtadaei et al., 2016). In contrast to the cardiovascular effects of RAAS, the NP system of hormones protects cardiac structure and function (Nathisuwan, 2002). Atrial deficiency and low levels of atrial natriuretic peptide were found associated with atrial fibrosis and AF recurrence (van den Berg et al., 2004). The effects of the NP system on cardiac remodeling have been implicated as a possible mechanism (van den Berg et al., 2004; Nishikimi et al., 2006). Therefore, NPs might play a protective role in AF development. Angiotensin II, endothelin 1, and transforming growth factor-β1 (TGF-β1) promote hypertrophic and fibrotic actions in cardiomyocytes and fibroblasts, whereas NPs *in vivo* and *in vitro* were shown to antagonize angiotensin II, endothelin 1 and TGF-β1 (Tamura et al., 2000; Nishikimi et al., 2006). However, neprilysin can degrade angiotensin II as well. Thus, a neprilysin inhibitor cannot be used to treat AF in monotherapy because activation of angiotensin II signaling pathways limits its beneficial effect in a feedback increase of NP levels (Richards et al., 1993). Simultaneous addition of ARBs and a neprilysin inhibitor to culture media of rat fibroblasts and cardiomyocytes was more effective than ARBs alone in inhibiting biochemical indicators of cardiac fibrosis and hypertrophy (von Lueder et al., 2013). Therefore, inhibition of both RAAS and neprilysin might have greater potential clinical benefit for neprilysin inhibitors in AF treatment.

LA strain assessed by 2D speckle tracking was inversely correlated with the burden of LA fibrosis analyzed by MRI (Kuppahally et al., 2010). Moreover, LA peak systolic strain can independently predict LA reverse mechanical and structural remodelling (Machino-Ohtsuka et al., 2013). These results suggest that LA peak systolic strain is related to LA function, according to the principle of strain, and useful for evaluating LA reservoir function (Kokubu et al., 2007). LAA acts as an important attachment and reservoir of LA, and its effective contraction can prevent blood stasis and LAAT formation (Tabata et al., 1998; Al-Saady et al., 1999). Moreover, LAA plays an important pathophysiological function when left atrial volume and pressure overload (Nakajima et al., 2010). LAAEF was an independent determinant of LAAT according to previous multivariate logistic regression analysis. And a LAAEF of 20% was the optimal cutoff value for predicting LAAT (Iwama et al., 2012). Compared with 2D imaging, 3D TEE imaging shows the clearer stereoscopic anatomical structure of LAA and more effective evaluation of the LAA function. Lower LAEF and LAAeV in AF patients were associated with increased risk of SEC and LAAT formation (Petersen et al., 2015).

In this study, patients using LCZ696 showed a lower incidence of SEC and greater LA peak systolic strain and LAAeV as compared with ARB users. LAAEF in patients receiving LCZ696 was significantly increased. Multiple regression analysis indicated LCZ696 independently associated with increased LAAEF. These results suggest that LCZ696 can improve LA and LAA function. However, we found no significant differences in incidence of LAAT, LAD, and LAVmax between the two groups. Since atrial dysfunction may occur before atrial structural changes in AF patients, a longer follow-up time is needed to observe atrial structural changes.

We also found hypertension as an independent predictor of LAAEF ≤ 20% [OR = 9.797; 95% CI (1.202–79.883); $p = 0.033$]. Regression models showed no interaction between hypertension and LCZ696 use. This result was consistent to the results of PARAMOUNT study, which demonstrated that the benefit of LCZ696 for reducing LAD and N-terminal pro-brain natriuretic peptide level were independent of the blood pressure-lowering effect. Although LCZ696 showed a better anti-hypertensive effect than valsartan, the two drugs were similar in tolerability (Ruilope et al., 2010; Solomon et al., 2012).

The study contains two limitations. First, we performed a hospital-based retrospective study and could not assess the dosage-related effects. Thus, larger, prospective studies are needed to ascertain the benefit of LCZ696 in AF. Second, the underlying molecular mechanism of the beneficial effect of LCZ696 is still unknown. In summary, this study showed that LCZ696 might be associated with improved LA and LAA function and had potential therapeutic value in preventing the incidence of cardiogenic embolic stroke in patients with AF.

AUTHOR CONTRIBUTIONS

QB and GL contributed conception and design of the study. CM and YW organized the database. YS and HL performed the statistical analysis. YS and MY wrote the first draft of the manuscript. YZ, YL, HF, and FH wrote sections of the manuscript. All authors contributed to manuscript revision, read and approved the submitted version.

FUNDING

This work was supported by grants from the National Natural Science Foundation of China (81800251, 81570304, 81800297).

REFERENCES

Al-Saady, N. M., Obel, O. A., and Camm, A. J. (1999). Left atrial appendage: structure, function, and role in thromboembolism. *Heart.* 82, 547–554. doi: 10.1136/hrt.82.5.547

Aschenberg, W., Schluter, M., Kremer, P., Schroder, E., Siglow, V., and Bleifeld, W. (1986). Transesophageal two-dimensional echocardiography for the detection of left atrial appendage thrombus. *J. Am. Coll Cardiol.* 7, 163–166. doi: 10.1016/S0735-1097(86)80275-3

Balmforth, C., Simpson, J., Shen, L., Jhund, P. S., Lefkowitz, M., Rizkala, A. R., et al. (2019). Outcomes and effect of treatment according to etiology in hfref: an analysis of paradigm-hf. *JACC Heart Fail* 7, 457–465. doi: 10.1016/j.jchf.2019.02.015

Burstein, B., and Nattel, S. (2008). Atrial fibrosis: Mechanisms and clinical relevance in atrial fibrillation. *J. Am. Coll. Cardiol.* 51, 802–809. doi: 10.1016/j.jacc.2007.09.064

Fatkin, D., Herbert, E., and Feneley, M. P. (1994). Hematologic correlates of spontaneous echo contrast in patients with atrial fibrillation and implications for thromboembolic risk. *Am. J. Cardiol.* 73, 672–676. doi: 10.1016/0002-9149(94)90932-6

Fuster, V., Ryden, L. E., Cannom, D. S., Crijns, H. J., Curtis, A. B., Ellenbogen, K. A., et al. (2006). Acc/aha/esc 2006 guidelines for the management of patients with atrial fibrillation–executive summary: a report of the american college of cardiology/american heart association task force on practice guidelines and the european society of cardiology committee for practice guidelines (writing committee to revise the 2001 guidelines for the management of patients with atrial fibrillation). *J. Am. Coll. Cardiol.* 48, 854–906. doi: 10.1016/j.jacc.2006.07.009

Gao, S., Ho, D., Vatner, D. E., and Vatner, S. F. (2011). Echocardiography in mice. *Curr. Protoc. Mouse Biol.* 1, 71–83. doi: 10.1002/9780470942390.mo100130

Gu, J., Noe, A., Chandra, P., Al-Fayoumi, S., Ligueros-Saylan, M., Sarangapani, R., et al. (2010). Pharmacokinetics and pharmacodynamics of lcz696, a novel dual-acting angiotensin receptor-neprilysin inhibitor (arni). *J. Clin. Pharmacol.* 50, 401–414. doi: 10.1177/0091270009343932

Healey, J. S., Baranchuk, A., Crystal, E., Morillo, C. A., Garfinkle, M., Yusuf, S., et al. (2005). Prevention of atrial fibrillation with angiotensin-converting enzyme inhibitors and angiotensin receptor blockers: A meta-analysis. *J. Am. Coll. Cardiol.* 45, 1832–1839. doi: 10.1016/j.jacc.2004.11.070

Iwama, M., Kawasaki, M., Tanaka, R., Ono, K., Watanabe, T., Hirose, T., et al. (2012). Left atrial appendage emptying fraction assessed by a feature-tracking echocardiographic method is a determinant of thrombus in patients with nonvalvular atrial fibrillation. *J. Cardiol.* 59, 329–336. doi: 10.1016/j.jjcc.2012.01.002

Jalife, J. (2014). Mechanisms of persistent atrial fibrillation. *Curr. Opin. Cardiol.* 29, 20–27. doi: 10.1097/HCO.0000000000000027

Jalife, J., and Kaur, K. (2015). Atrial remodeling, fibrosis, and atrial fibrillation. *Trends Cardiovasc. Med.* 25, 475–484. doi: 10.1016/j.tcm.2014.12.015

Jibrini, M. B., Molnar, J., and Arora, R. R. (2008). Prevention of atrial fibrillation by way of abrogation of the renin-angiotensin system: a systematic review and meta-analysis. *Am. J. Ther.* 15 (1), 36–43. doi: 10.1097/MJT.0b013e31804beb59

Kamp, O., Verhorst, P. M., Welling, R. C., and Visser, C. A. (1999). Importance of left atrial appendage flow as a predictor of thromboembolic events in patients with atrial fibrillation. *Eur. Heart J.* 20, 979–985. doi: 10.1053/euhj.1998.1453

Kirchhof, P., Benussi, S., Kotecha, D., Ahlsson, A., Atar, D., Casadei, B., et al. (2016). Esc guidelines for the management of atrial fibrillation developed in collaboration with eacts. *Eur. Heart J.* 37, 2893–2962. doi: 10.1093/eurheartj/ehw210

Kokubu, N., Yuda, S., Tsuchihashi, K., Hashimoto, A., Nakata, T., Miura, T., et al. (2007). Noninvasive assessment of left atrial function by strain rate imaging in patients with hypertension: a possible beneficial effect of renin-angiotensin system inhibition on left atrial function. *Hypertens. Res.* 30, 13–21. doi: 10.1291/hypres.30.13

Kuppahally, S. S., Akoum, N., Burgon, N. S., Badger, T. J., Kholmovski, E. G., Vijayakumar, S., et al. (2010). Left atrial strain and strain rate in patients with paroxysmal and persistent atrial fibrillation: relationship to left atrial structural remodeling detected by delayed-enhancement mri. *Circ. Cardiovasc. Imaging* 3, 231–239. doi: 10.1161/CIRCIMAGING.109.865683

Lang, R. M., Bierig, M., Devereux, R. B., Flachskampf, F. A., Foster, E., Pellikka, P. A., et al. (2005). Recommendations for chamber quantification: a report from the american society of echocardiography's guidelines and standards committee and the chamber quantification writing group, developed in conjunction with the european association of echocardiography, a branch of the european society of cardiology. *J. Am. Soc Echocardiogr.* 18, 1440–1463. doi: 10.1016/j.echo.2005.10.005

Machino-Ohtsuka, T., Seo, Y., Ishizu, T., Yanaka, S., Nakajima, H., Atsumi, A., et al. (2013). Significant improvement of left atrial and left atrial appendage function after catheter ablation for persistent atrial fibrillation. *Circ. J.* 77, 1695–1704. doi: 10.1253/circj.CJ-12-1518

Miragoli, M., and Glukhov, A. V. (2015). Atrial fibrillation and fibrosis: Beyond the cardiomyocyte centric view. *Biomed. Res. Int.* 2015, 798768. doi: 10.1155/2015/798768

Moghtadaei, M., Polina, I., and Rose, R. A. (2016). Electrophysiological effects of natriuretic peptides in the heart are mediated by multiple receptor subtypes. *Prog. Biophys. Mol. Biol.* 120, 37–49. doi: 10.1016/j.pbiomolbio.2015.12.001

Nakajima, H., Seo, Y., Ishizu, T., Yamamoto, M., Machino, T., Harimura, Y., et al. (2010). Analysis of the left atrial appendage by three-dimensional transesophageal echocardiography. *Am. J. Cardiol.* 106, 885–892. doi: 10.1016/j.amjcard.2010.05.014

Nakashima, H., and Kumagai, K. (2007). Reverse-remodeling effects of angiotensin ii type 1 receptor blocker in a canine atrial fibrillation model. *Circ. J.* 71, 1977–1982. doi: 10.1253/circj.71.1977

Nathisuwan, S. (2002). Talbert RL. A review of vasopeptidase inhibitors: a new modality in the treatment of hypertension and chronic heart failure. *Pharmacotherapy* 22, 27–42. doi: 10.1592/phco.22.1.27.33502

Nattel, S. (2017). Molecular and cellular mechanisms of atrial fibrosis in atrial fibrillation. *JACC Clin. Electrophysiol.* 3, 425–435. doi: 10.1016/j.jacep.2017.03.002

Nishikimi, T., Maeda, N., and Matsuoka, H. (2006). The role of natriuretic peptides in cardioprotection. *Cardiovasc. Res.* 69, 318–328. doi: 10.1016/j.cardiores.2005.10.001

Perez, Y., Duval, A. M., Carville, C., Weber, H., Cachin, J. C., Castaigne, A., et al. (1997). Is left atrial appendage flow a predictor for outcome of cardioversion of nonvalvular atrial fibrillation? A transthroacic and transesophageal echocardiographic study. *Am. Heart J.* 134, 745–751. doi: 10.1016/S0002-8703(97)70059-0

Petersen, M., Roehrich, A., Balzer, J., Shin, D. I., Meyer, C., Kelm, M., et al. (2015). Left atrial appendage morphology is closely associated with specific echocardiographic flow pattern in patients with atrial fibrillation. *Europace.* 17, 539–545. doi: 10.1093/europace/euu347

Richards, A. M., Wittert, G. A., Crozier, I. G., Espiner, E. A., Yandle, T. G., Ikram, H., et al. (1993). Chronic inhibition of endopeptidase 24.11 in essential hypertension: evidence for enhanced atrial natriuretic peptide and angiotensin ii. *J. Hypertens.* 11, 407–416. doi: 10.1097/00004872-199304000-00011

Rose, R. A., and Giles, W. R. (2008). Natriuretic peptide c receptor signalling in the heart and vasculature. *J. Physiol.* 586, 353–366. doi: 10.1113/jphysiol.2007.144253

Ruilope, L. M., Dukat, A., Bohm, M., Lacourciere, Y., Gong, J., and Lefkowitz, M. P. (2010). Blood-pressure reduction with lcz696, a novel dual-acting inhibitor of the angiotensin ii receptor and neprilysin: a randomised, double-blind, placebo-controlled, active comparator study. *Lancet* 375, 1255–1266. doi: 10.1016/S0140-6736(09)61966-8

Solomon, S. D., Zile, M., Pieske, B., Voors, A., Shah, A., Kraigher-Krainer, E., et al. (2012). The angiotensin receptor neprilysin inhibitor lcz696 in heart failure with preserved ejection fraction: a phase 2 double-blind randomised controlled trial. *Lancet.* 380, 1387–1395. doi: 10.1016/S0140-6736(12)61227-6

Sparks, P. B., Mond, H. G., Vohra, J. K., Yapanis, A. G., Grigg, L. E., and Kalman, J. M. (1999). Mechanical remodeling of the left atrium after loss of atrioventricular synchrony. A long-term study in humans. *Circulation* 100, 1714–1721. doi: 10.1161/01.CIR.100.16.1714

Suo, Y., Zhang, Y., Wang, Y., Yuan, M., Kariyawasam, S., Tse, G., et al. (2018). Renin-angiotensin system inhibition is associated with reduced risk of left atrial appendage thrombosis formation in patients with atrial fibrillation. *Cardiol. J.* 25, 611–620. doi: 10.5603/CJ.a2017.0112

Tabata, T., Oki, T., Yamada, H., Iuchi, A., Ito, S., Hori, T., et al. (1998). Role of left atrial appendage in left atrial reservoir function as evaluated by left atrial appendage clamping during cardiac surgery. *Am. J. Cardiol.* 81, 327–332. doi: 10.1016/S0002-9149(97)00903-X

Takada, T., Yasaka, M., Nagatsuka, K., Minematsu, K., and Yamaguchi, T. (2001). Blood flow in the left atrial appendage and embolic stroke in nonvalvular atrial fibrillation. *Eur. Neurol.* 46, 148–152. doi: 10.1159/000050788

Tamura, N., Ogawa, Y., Chusho, H., Nakamura, K., Nakao, K., Suda, M., et al. (2000). Cardiac fibrosis in mice lacking brain natriuretic peptide. *Proc. Natl. Acad. Sci. U. S. A.* 97, 4239–4244. doi: 10.1073/pnas.070371497

Torrado, J., Cain, C., Mauro, A. G., Romeo, F., Ockaili, R., Chau, V. Q., et al. (2018). Sacubitril/valsartan averts adverse post-infarction ventricular remodeling and preserves systolic function in rabbits. *J. Am. Coll. Cardiol.* 72, 2342–2356. doi: 10.1016/j.jacc.2018.07.102

van den Berg, M. P., van Gelder, I. C., and van Veldhuisen, D. J. (2004). Depletion of atrial natriuretic peptide during longstanding atrial fibrillation. *Europace* 6, 433–437. doi: 10.1016/j.eupc.2004.04.006

Verhorst, P. M., Kamp, O., Welling, R. C., Van Eenige, M. J., and Visser, C. A. (1997). Transesophageal echocardiographic predictors for maintenance of sinus rhythm after electrical cardioversion of atrial fibrillation. *Am. J. Cardiol.* 79, 1355–1359. doi: 10.1016/S0002-9149(97)00139-2

von Lueder, T. G., Sangaralingham, S. J., Wang, B. H., Kompa, A. R., Atar, D., Burnett, J. C., et al. (2013). Renin-angiotensin blockade combined with natriuretic peptide system augmentation: Novel therapeutic concepts to combat heart failure. *Circ. Heart Fail.* 6, 594–605. doi: 10.1161/CIRCHEARTFAILURE.112.000289

Voors, A. A., Dorhout, B., and van der Meer, P. (2013). The potential role of valsartan + ahu377 (lcz696) in the treatment of heart failure. *Expert Opin. Investig. Drugs* 22, 1041–1047. doi: 10.1517/13543784.2013.797963

Wang, Z., Zhang, X. J., Ji, Y. X., Zhang, P., Deng, K. Q., Gong, J., et al. (2016). The long noncoding rna chaer defines an epigenetic checkpoint in cardiac hypertrophy. *Nat. Med.* 22, 1131–1139. doi: 10.1038/nm.4179

Zabalgoitia, M., Halperin, J. L., Pearce, L. A., Blackshear, J. L., Asinger, R. W., and Hart, R. G. (1998). Transesophageal echocardiographic correlates of clinical risk of thromboembolism in nonvalvular atrial fibrillation. Stroke prevention in atrial fibrillation iii investigators. *J. Am. Coll. Cardiol.* 31, 1622–1626. doi: 10.1016/S0735-1097(98)00146-6

8

Blinded *In Silico* Drug Trial Reveals the Minimum Set of Ion Channels for Torsades de Pointes Risk Assessment

Xin Zhou[1*]*, Yusheng Qu*[2]*, Elisa Passini*[1]*, Alfonso Bueno-Orovio*[1]*, Yang Liu*[3]*, Hugo M. Vargas*[2] *and Blanca Rodriguez*[1*]

[1] Department of Computer Science, British Heart Foundation Centre of Research Excellence, University of Oxford, Oxford, United Kingdom, [2] SPARC, Amgen Research, Amgen Inc., Thousand Oaks, CA, United States, [3] GAU, Amgen Research, Amgen Inc., South San Francisco, CA, United States

***Correspondence:**
Xin Zhou
xin.zhou@cs.ox.ac.uk
Blanca Rodriguez
blanca.rodriguez@cs.ox.ac.uk

Torsades de Pointes (TdP) is a type of ventricular arrhythmia which could be observed as an unwanted drug-induced cardiac side effect, and it is associated with repolarization abnormalities in single cells. The pharmacological evaluations of TdP risk in previous years mainly focused on the hERG channel due to its vital role in the repolarization of cardiomyocytes. However, only considering drug effects on hERG led to false positive predictions since the drug action on other ion channels can also have crucial regulatory effects on repolarization. To address the limitation of only evaluating hERG, the Comprehensive in Vitro Proarrhythmia Assay initiative has proposed to systematically integrate drug effects on multiple ion channels into *in silico* drug trial to improve TdP risk assessment. It is not clear how many ion channels are sufficient for reliable TdP risk predictions, and whether differences in IC_{50} and Hill coefficient values from independent sources can lead to divergent *in silico* prediction outcomes. The rationale of this work is to investigate the above two questions using a computationally efficient population of human ventricular cells optimized to favor repolarization abnormality. Our blinded results based on two independent data sources confirm that simulations with the optimized population of human ventricular cell models enable efficient in silico drug screening, and also provide direct observation and mechanistic analysis of repolarization abnormality. Our results show that 1) the minimum set of ion channels required for reliable TdP risk predictions are Nav1.5 (peak), Cav1.2, and hERG; 2) for drugs with multiple ion channel blockage effects, moderate IC_{50} variations combined with variable Hill coefficients can affect the accuracy of *in silico* predictions.

Keywords: Torsades de Pointes, drug cardiotoxicity, ion channels, *in silico* drug trials, human ventricular action potential

INTRODUCTION

Cardiotoxicity is a major cause of drug withdrawal from the pharmaceutical market, and its earlier detection and assessment could largely speed up the evaluation of target compounds in the drug development process. For instance, drug-induced Torsades de Pointes (TdP) is a type of ventricular arrhythmia linked to sudden cardiac death. It is generally accepted that early afterdepolarizations (EADs) occurring during the repolarization phase of action potentials (APs) can trigger premature events, and then give rise to TdP (Vandersickel et al., 2014: Vandersickel et al., 2015). Drugs that block the hERG current (I_{Kr}) can inhibit the repolarization process, leading to AP duration (APD) prolongation, and facilitating EAD generation (Jurkiewicz and Sanguinetti, 1993; Guo et al., 2011; Pueyo et al., 2011; Dutta et al., 2016). Therefore, prolongation of APD (reflected in the electrocardiogram as QTc interval prolongation) is often used as a surrogate to assess TdP risk. I_{Kr} inhibition and QTc prolongation are sensitive but not very specific for predicting ventricular pro-arrhythmia risk. Inhibition of other cardiac ion channels, especially sodium and calcium channels, may mitigate the effects of hERG blockage and reduce pro-arrhythmic risk and EAD generation (Bril et al., 1996; Martin et al., 2004; Sager et al., 2014; Britton et al., 2017).

Since hERG assays alone can lead to false positives in predicting TdP risk and repolarization abnormalities, Kramer et al. measured concentration-response relationships of hERG, Nav1.5 peak (the fast sodium current, I_{Na}), and Cav1.2 (the L-type calcium current, I_{CaL}) currents for 32 torsadogenic and 23 non-torsadogenic drugs from multiple pharmacological classes (Kramer et al., 2013). A logistic regression analysis showed that risk prediction based on the three channels improved accuracy with respect to using solely hERG block (Kramer et al., 2013).

To overcome the limitation of hERG inhibition as the main evaluation criteria, the Comprehensive in Vitro Proarrhythmia Assay (CiPA) initiative, sponsored by the Food and Drug Administration (FDA) among others, has proposed a new paradigm to integrate drug effects on multiple ion channels into *in silico* modeling to evaluate the propensity for EADs and repolarization instabilities (Sager et al., 2014; Colatsky et al., 2016). Driven by the scheme of CiPA, recent experimental studies have comprehensively analyzed the effects of clinical drugs on up to seven ionic currents (Crumb et al., 2016).

Building on *in vitro* ion channel data, *in silico* TdP risk prediction has shown promising results using several approaches. One strategy for *in silico* TdP risk stratification is to utilize machine learning algorithms to derive TdP risk metrics. Strong performance was achieved using principal component analysis, support vector machine classifications, and logistic regression classifiers, based on ion channel blockage data and features of simulated AP and intracellular calcium transients (Lancaster and Sobie, 2016; Parikh et al., 2017). Another strategy is to use simple classification models to analyze the balance between depolarization and repolarization blockages (Mistry et al., 2015). However, statistical analysis and machine learning classifications do not enable direct observations of pro-arrhythmic repolarization abnormalities (RAs), and make mechanistic interpretations difficult. Alternatively, using RAs as the main metric, simulations using a population of over 1,000 human ventricular cell models with random ionic current variations yielded 89% accuracy in TdP predictions (Passini et al., 2017). The accuracy was higher using RAs in the virtual human cell population than using a single model or APD prolongation, and also higher compared to experimental animal models. The simulation results also revealed mechanistic ion channel properties underlying RAs: for example, weaker I_{NaK} (the sodium potassium pump current) favored RA, which was related to proarrhythmic clinical conditions such as acute myocardial ischemia (Passini et al., 2017).

Normal repolarization involves complex interactions and contributions of multiple ionic currents, which include some redundancy for the robustness of this critical part of the cardiac cycle, namely the so-called repolarization reserve (Roden, 1998; Roden Dan, 2008; Roden and Abraham, 2011). The subclinical change in some currents may not directly lead to RA but the lower repolarization reserve in these scenarios provides vulnerable conditions for RA generation when ion channel blockers are superimposed (Roden, 1998; Roden Dan., 2008; Roden and Abraham, 2011). Inspired by the mechanistic ion channel properties revealed in a previous study (Passini et al., 2017), a population of human ventricular cell models was designed to favor RA by introducing lower repolarization reserve as weaker repolarization currents and stronger depolarization currents (Passini et al., 2019).

In this study, we performed blinded *in silico* drug trials for 85 reference compounds using the optimized virtual human cell population by (Passini et al., 2019), to investigate the following questions: 1) what is the minimum set of ion channels needed for good TdP risk predictions; 2) how different are *in silico* prediction outcomes using IC_{50} and Hill coefficient values from two independent and highly cited sources?

The significance of blinding in this study is twofold: 1) no iterations of model calibration were done to improve predictions, and this enabled a clear and independent validation of the simulations for the use of drug induced TdP risk prediction; 2) blinding also mimicked the preclinical stage of drug development when the side effects were unknown before large clinical trials, and no additional information such as the effects of metabolites can be taken into account, therefore the blinded simulations

Abbreviations: AP, action potential; APD, action potential duration; CiPA, Comprehensive in Vitro Proarrhythmia Assay initiative; EAD, early afterdepolarization; $EFTPC_{max}$, maximal effective free therapeutic concentration; FDA, Food and Drug Administration; IC_{50}, the concentration for 50% ion channel inhibition; I_{CaL}, the L-type calcium current; I_{Na}, the fast sodium current; I_{NaCa}, the sodium-calcium exchanger current; I_{NaK}, the sodium potassium pump current; I_{NaL}, the late sodium current; I_{K1}, the inward rectifier potassium current; I_{Kr}, the hERG current, also known as the rapid delayed rectifier potassium current; I_{Ks}, the slow delayed rectifier potassium current; I_{to}, the transient outward potassium current; ORd model, O'Hara-Rudy dynamic human ventricular action potential model; QTc, Q-T interval on electrocardiogram corrected with heart rate; RA, repolarization abnormality; RF, repolarization failure; TdP, Torsades de Pointes; TP, true positive; TN, true negative; FP, false positive; FN, false negative; PPV, positive predictive value; NPV, negative predictive value.

reflected better the new compound evaluation process. The accuracy of the blinded prediction and its low computational cost demonstrated the potential applicability of this *in silico* approach in cost and animal use reduction for drug development in pharmaceutical industry.

MATERIALS AND METHODS

Optimization of the Population of Human Ventricular Models

The baseline model used in this study is the O'Hara-Rudy dynamic (ORd) human endocardial ventricular AP model (O'Hara et al., 2011), developed using data from over 100 human hearts, with modifications to the fast sodium channel (Passini et al., 2016). It includes detailed representation of the potassium, sodium and calcium sarcolemmal currents, as well as intracellular calcium handling (including SERCA pump and calcium-induced calcium release mechanism). A computationally efficient population of 107 human ventricular AP models constructed in (Passini et al., 2019) was used for the assessment of RAs, as a surrogate for pro-arrhythmic mechanisms under drug action. Based on established knowledge of ionic profiles more likely to develop drug induced RA (Passini et al., 2017), the population of models was constructed by varying nine key ionic conductances to represent electrophysiological variability, then constrained and calibrated using the human data (Britton et al., 2017). Conductances were varied unevenly to allow weaker I_{Kr}, I_{Ks} (the slow delayed rectifier potassium current) and I_{NaK}, and stronger I_{NaL} (the late sodium current), I_{CaL}, and I_{NaCa} (the sodium-calcium exchanger current) (**Supplementary Material Table S1**) (Passini et al., 2019). The low repolarization reserve introduced in the population is also representative of different pathological conditions, such as long QT syndrome (Schwartz Peter. et al., 2012), hypertrophic cardiomyopathy (Coppini et al., 2013), and heart failure (Shamraj et al., 1993; Ambrosi et al., 2013). The full list of parameters for the optimized population is provided in the **Supplementary Material Table S5**.

Datasets

The sources and the names of all the compounds were blinded during the *in silico* test. *In silico* drug trials were performed for two groups of reference compounds at multiple concentrations. Drug/ionic current interactions were simulated using a simple pore-block drug model (Brennan et al., 2009). For each drug, IC_{50} and Hill coefficient were the input parameters used to describe each ionic current block as in previous studies (Mirams et al., 2011; Passini et al., 2017).

Dataset I consisted of 30 compounds, for which IC_{50} and Hill coefficients were available for seven ionic currents: I_{Na}, I_{NaL}, I_{to} (the transient outward potassium current), I_{Kr}, I_{Ks}, I_{K1} (the inward rectifier potassium current), and I_{CaL} (Crumb et al., 2016). Dataset II had 55 compounds, with IC_{50} and Hill coefficients available for only three ion channels: I_{Na}, I_{Kr}, and I_{CaL} (Kramer et al., 2013). The full lists of IC_{50} and Hill coefficient values for both datasets are provided in the **Supplementary Material Table S6**. For each compound, five concentrations were tested: 1, 3, 10, 30, and 100 folds of their maximal effective free therapeutic concentration ($EFTPC_{max}$).

Simulation Environment

Virtual Assay (v.2.4.800 © 2014 Oxford University Innovation Ltd. Oxford, UK), a user-friendly C++ based software package was previously developed for the simulation of drug effects on virtual cardiac AP populations. Virtual Assay uses the ordinary differential equation solver CVODE to implement backward differentiation formula with adaptive time steps (Hindmarsh et al., 2005; Serban and Hindmarsh, 2008), and relative and absolute tolerances equal to 1e-5 and 1e-7, respectively. As shown previously in (Passini et al., 2017), similar simulations of virtual AP traces can be achieved using MATLAB (Mathworks Inc. Natwick, MA, USA) or any other software to solve ordinary differential equations. The effect of a drug at a testing concentration was simulated as conductance reductions which were based on the IC_{50} values and Hill coefficients from the blinded datasets. For each concentration of each compound, the drug assay was conducted on the population of models at a pacing frequency of 1Hz for 150 beats, and the AP traces of the last beat were used for analysis as in (Passini et al., 2017). The choice of the pacing frequency was based on clinical reports that pacing rates slower than 70 beats per minute were more relevant to TdP occurrence while faster pacing can suppress TdP (Viskin et al., 2000; Pinski et al., 2002; Kurisu et al., 2008). For all the simulated traces, APD was calculated as APD_{90} (AP duration at 90% of repolarization), and TdP risk prediction was conducted by analyzing the morphology of simulated AP traces to detect RAs, as described below.

In silico TdP Risk Analysis

TdP risk prediction was calculated based on the occurrence of two types of RAs in the population of human models, encompassing EADs and repolarization failure (RF). The two types of RAs were defined when positive derivatives were found in the membrane voltage (V_m) after 150 ms following the AP peak (for EADs), or the membrane voltage failed to reach resting membrane voltage (V_m >-40 mV) at the end of the last beat (for RF). In order to ensure the accuracy of automated RA detection, simulation traces were also visually examined to check for potential misclassifications caused by the algorithm.

Aggregated results at the population level are presented using a scoring system (TdP risk score) as introduced in (Passini et al., 2017) according to the following formula (where n*RAc* is the number of models showing RA at a tested concentration *c*, W*c* = $EFTPC_{max}$ / *c* is the weight inversely related to the tested concentration *c*, and N is the total number of models in the population).

$$TdP\ \ risk\ \ score = \frac{\sum_c (Wc * nRAc)}{N * \sum_c Wc}$$

The analysis of TdP scores was also performed blindly. The TdP risk score integrated RA occurrence at multiple concentrations, and was computed in MATLAB. Logarithmic scale was considered to maximize the visual separation of TdP score between safe and risky drugs. Zero risk was approximated for visualization with machine precision (10^{-16}). For special cases where access to individual ionic currents and ion channel gating variables was needed, the same drug trials were repeated in MATLAB to obtain more detailed information.

Evaluations of the *In Silico* Prediction Results

After the blinded *in silico* prediction, the TdP risk of each compound was compared against the current clinical reports in the literature. Multiple sources were referenced for classification as in (Kramer et al., 2013), including CredibleMeds® (Woosley et al, 2019), available on www.crediblemeds.org, (Redfern et al., 2003), publications on QT studies, and FDA-generated package inserts. Considering the risk classifications of some drugs are debatable, we also evaluated the prediction accuracy by only applying the CredibleMeds® classification. For this, compounds with any type of TdP risk (known, possible or conditional) were considered to be risky even if the risk may only occur under specific conditions such as overdose or interactions with other drugs (**Supplementary Material Figures S1–S4, Tables S2–S4**).

Prediction results were classified as true positive (TP, both clinical reports and *in silico* predictions were risky), true negative (TN, both clinical reports and *in silico* predictions were safe), false positive (FP, no clinical risk reports but *in silico* predictions were risky), and false negative (FN, *in silico* predicted to be safe but clinically reported to be risky). Sensitivity, specificity, positive predictive value (PPV), and negative predictive value (NPV) were computed separately for Dataset I and II based on the number of TP, TN, FP, and FN predictions. Accuracy was defined as the sum of TPs and TNs divided by the total number of drugs. Each drug is referred to with the name and a roman number to differentiate the two datasets.

Statistical Analysis

The formula for TdP score calculation is a deterministic algorithm using the same models for all drugs, and therefore no statistical algorithm was used for calculating TdP risk for individual drugs. Pairwise linear correlation was performed between TdP scores and drug induced APD prolongations using MATLAB.

RESULTS

In Silico Prediction of TdP Risk Considering All Available Ion Channel Data and All Assessed Concentrations

The TdP risk scores were computed for both groups of compounds, and in both cases risky and safe compounds were identified. In Dataset I, unblinding the compounds revealed a sensitivity of 85% and a specificity of 80% (**Table 1**), and the overall accuracy was 83%, with 3 FN predictions and 2 FP predictions. As illustrated in **Figure 1A** for Dataset I,

TABLE 1 | Accuracy of the *in silico* Torsades de Pointes (TdP) risk predictions using the population of 107 human ventricular cell models with maximum testing concentrations of 100×$EFTPC_{max}$.

	Dataset I		Dataset II	
	Clinical TdP (+)	**Clinical TdP (-)**	**Clinical TdP (+)**	**Clinical TdP (-)**
In silico (+)	17	2	25	7 **4**
In silico (-)	3	8	7	16 **19**
Sensitivity	85%		78%	**78%**
Specificity	80%		70%	**83%**
PPV	89%		78%	**86%**
NPV	73%		70%	**73%**
Accuracy	83%		75%	**80%**

For Dataset II, bold scores indicate the true accuracy of the model predictions after fixing the misclassifications of the automated repolarization abnormality (RA) detection algorithm.

simulations with 11 out of 30 compounds yielded no RAs and thus no TdP risk, whereas 19 compounds induced RA in the population of 107 human ventricular cell models. Among the Dataset I compounds that produced RAs, Quinidine I demonstrated the highest risk, with a TdP score of 0.78, while Azithromycin I showed a mild risk with a TdP score of 10^{-3}.

In Dataset II, 23 out of 55 compounds did not induce RAs, while the remaining 22 compounds produced RAs according to the automated RA detection algorithm (**Figure 1B**). Ibutilide II had the highest TdP score of 1, and Solifenacin II had a very mild TdP score of $6{\cdot}10^{-5}$. Unblinding the compounds revealed a sensitivity of 78% and a specificity of 70% (**Table 1**), with 7 FN predictions and 7 FP predictions from the automated RA detection.

Further visual examination of the raw AP traces revealed that 3 of the risky compounds detected by the automated algorithm (highlighted in black squares in **Figure 1B**) did not induce RAs, and the misclassification was caused by delayed AP peaks (**Supplementary Material, Figures S5A–C**). The misclassifications only happened for traces produced under 100×$EFTPC_{max}$. Fixing the misclassification caused by the automated RA detection algorithm revealed simulations had a true sensitivity of 78%, a specificity of 83%, and an overall accuracy of 80% (**Table 1**, highlighted in bold).

The overall prediction accuracy against the CredibleMeds® drug classifications was similar (**Supplementary Material Figure S1, Table S2**). There were however some differences. Our classifications of Saquinavir, Ranolazine, Dasatinib, Donepezil, Metronidazole, Piperacillin were non-risky based on multiple sources such as CredibleMeds®, publications on QT studies, and package labels, but the latest CredibleMeds® database (accessed 2018-11-28) classify them as risky. The simulation results showed Ranolazine, Metronidazole, and Piperacillin induced RA, while Saquinavir, Dasatinib, and Donepezil did not induce RA.

After unblinding the compounds, we explored whether different pacing rates can affect the predictive accuracy of the simulations by applying a faster pacing rate of 2Hz and a slower pacing rate of 0.5 Hz at 10x $EFTPC_{max}$ for the compounds in Dataset I. The simulation results showed that slower pacing tended to induce more EADs (**Supplementary Figure S7**), but

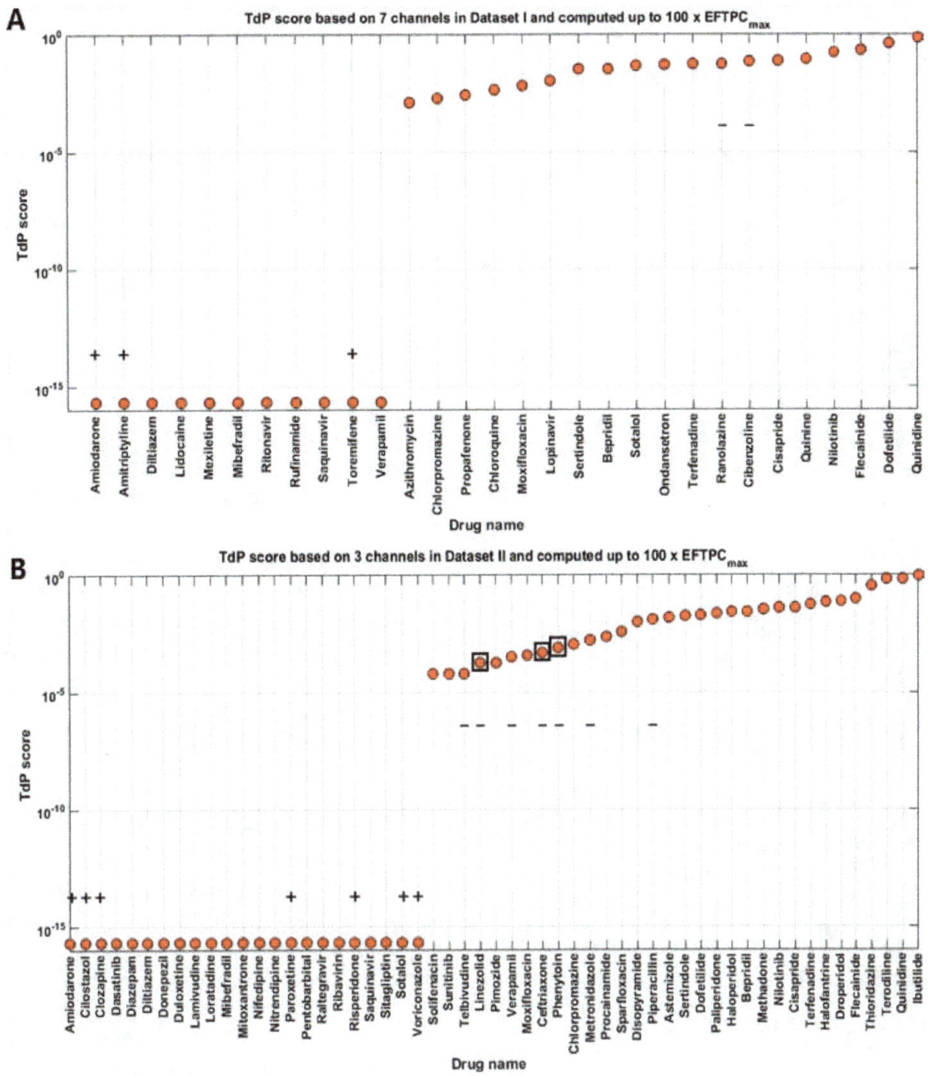

FIGURE 1 | Torsades de Pointes (TdP) risk assessment based on all the available ion channel inputs and up to 100×EFTPC$_{max}$. **(A)** Dataset I TdP risk assessment based on all data from 7 ion channels (Crumb et al., 2016). **(B)** Dataset II TdP risk assessment based on all information from 3 ion channels (Kramer et al., 2013). Classifications inconsistent with current clinical reports are labeled with black "+" and "–": "+" implies the true classification should be risky, while "–" means the true classification should be safe. Black squares in panel **(B)** highlight the compounds whose TdP risk was generated by the misclassification of the automated algorithm, and visual examinations of the simulated AP traces revealed they did not produce repolarization abnormalities (RAs).

no qualitative differences were observed for the FN (Amiodarone I, Amitriptyline I and Toremifene I) and FP compounds in terms of RA generation (Cibenzoline I and Ranolazine I) (**Supplementary Figures S8** and **S9**).

Action Potential Prolongation and TdP Risk

Since many compounds can block hERG and cause prolongation of APD, and excessive APD prolongation can also be a TdP risk factor, the relationship between TdP risk and APD prolongation at low doses was also evaluated. A good linear correlation was found between the overall TdP risk score and the APD prolongation at 1 × EFTPC$_{max}$ (r^2 = 0.96) (**Figure 2**, upper panel). Ibutilide II, which had the biggest TdP score of 1 and yielded the biggest APD prolongation, induced RFs in the population even at the lowest tested dose. Quinidine I (TdP score = 0.78), Quinidine II (TdP score = 0.70), Terodiline II (TdP score = 0.67), Dofetilide I (TdP score = 0.43), and Thioridazine II (TdP score = 0.36) induced significant APD prolongation and EADs at the lowest testing dose (**Figure 3**). Flecainide I (TdP score = 0.22), Nilotinib I (TdP score = 0.17), Quinine I (TdP score = 0.09), Terfenadine I (TdP score = 0.05), and Flecainide II (TdP score = 0.10) did not induce RAs at 1×EFTPC$_{max}$. However, they can lead to APD prolongation of more than 100 ms, and four of these compounds led to EADs when the testing concentration was increased to 3×EFTPC$_{max}$ (**Figure 4**).

Although a good linear correlation was found between very high risk TdP scores and APD prolongation at 1×EFTPC$_{max}$,

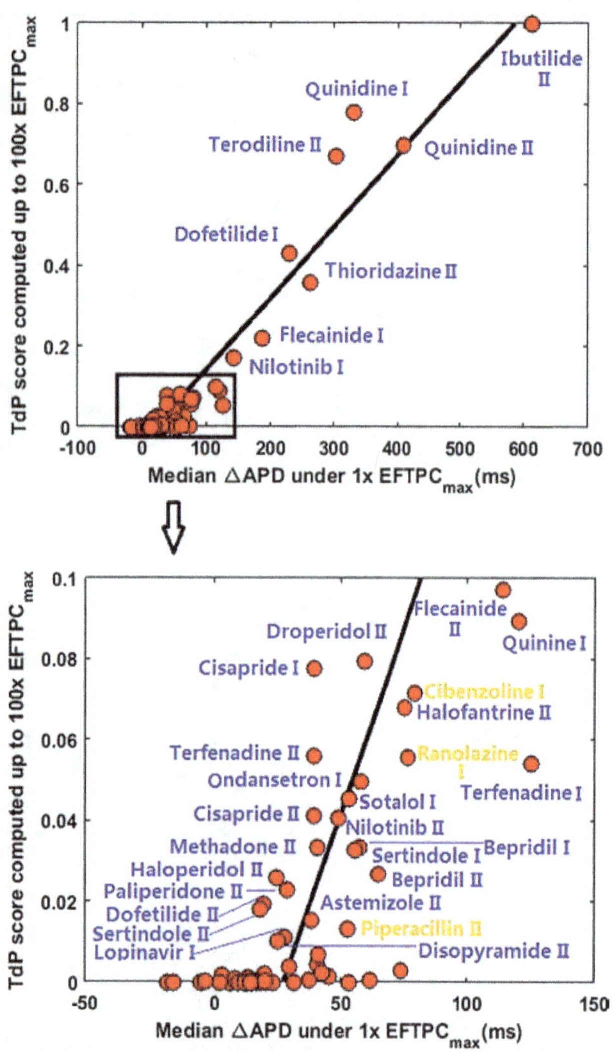

FIGURE 2 | Correlation between action potential duration (APD) prolongation and Torsades de Pointes (TdP) risk score at 1×EFTPCmax for all 85 compounds. ΔAPD=APDdrug-APDcontrol. Blue labels indicate true positive predictions, and yellow labels indicate false positive results. If CredibleMeds® classification was used, Ranolazine I and Piperacillin II would be true positive (blue) instead of false positive.

APD prolongation was less well correlated with low TdP risk scores. As shown in the lower panel of **Figure 2**, with similar low TdP scores close to 0, some compounds showed APD prolongations of up to 70 ms, while others showed very small APD prolongations of less than 20 ms.

Reducing Maximum Testing Concentration Does Not Improve the RA-Based TdP Risk Stratification

In the clinical situation, the maximally-achieved plasma exposure is determined by drug absorption, distribution, metabolism and excretion in an individual whose genetic background and physical condition have significant effects on pharmacokinetics (Tamargo et al., 2017). Therefore, we considered high concentrations of up to 100×EFTPC$_{max}$ in the formerly discussed evaluation of TdP risk. Some compounds with intermediate TdP risk scores elicited RAs only at the highest tested concentration. In order to assess the effects of maximum tested concentrations, we also compared the TdP score calculated with maximum concentrations up to 30×EFTPC$_{max}$. As shown in **Figure 5A** (Dataset I) and **Figure 5B** (Dataset II), predictions were not significantly affected for drugs with either the highest or lowest TdP scores. However, in a few cases, the risk classification can be qualitatively different. For Dataset I, decreasing the maximum testing concentration to 30×EFTPC$_{max}$ led to 2 extra FNs: Azithromycin and Chlorpromazine. Even when classified as risky at 100×EFTPC$_{max}$, these two compounds had the lowest TdP scores among the risky category. For Dataset II, decreasing maximum concentration converted several FPs predictions to TNs but also generated 5 extra FNs.

For both groups, FN predictions cannot be improved under lower concentrations. Therefore decreasing the maximum testing concentrations reduced the sensitivity in the predictions for both datasets, while the specificity was not affected for Dataset I but was improved for Dataset II. Similar results were obtained using the latest CredibleMeds® TdP risk classifications **Supplementary Material** (**Supplementary Material Figure S2, Table S3**). Therefore, based on the overall accuracy, changing maximum testing concentration to 30×EFTPC$_{max}$ does not improve the quality of predictions (**Table 2**).

Using Only hERG Decreases the Specificity of Predictions

For Dataset I compounds, IC$_{50}$/Hill coefficient values are available for seven ion channels, while for Dataset II the information is available for three ion channels. In order to understand how many ion channels are necessary to achieve sufficient prediction accuracy, we also compared the effect of varying the number of affected ion channels. **Figure 6A** compares prediction results for 7, 4 (I_{Na}+I_{NaL}+I_{Kr}+I_{CaL}), 3 (I_{Na}+I_{Kr}+I_{CaL}), and 1 (I_{Kr}) channel only for Dataset I. For these compounds, there was no qualitative difference between the predictions based on information from 7, 4, and 3 channels (1 exception for Saquinavir I). However, if only hERG block (I_{Kr}) was considered, TdP scores were frequently higher, and five safe compounds were misclassified to FP, leading to a significant loss of specificity and overall lower accuracy (**Table 3**).

For Dataset II, the results from 3 channels and only hERG were also compared. Similarly, only considering I_{Kr} block increased the TdP scores in a number of cases (altering the magnitude of predicted TdP risks), and the classification of seven compounds was changed to risky (4 FP and 3 TPs, **Figure 6B**). It was noted that the three compounds misclassified by the automated algorithm when using 3 channels (Ceftriazone II, Linezolid II and Phenytoin II) did induce RAs when only considering hERG block (**Supplementary Material**, **Figures S5D–F**). Therefore, the specificity for Dataset II was also compromised as in Dataset I by using hERG only, leading to lower overall accuracy. Similar effects were observed using CredibleMeds® classifications (**Supplementary Material Figure S3,**

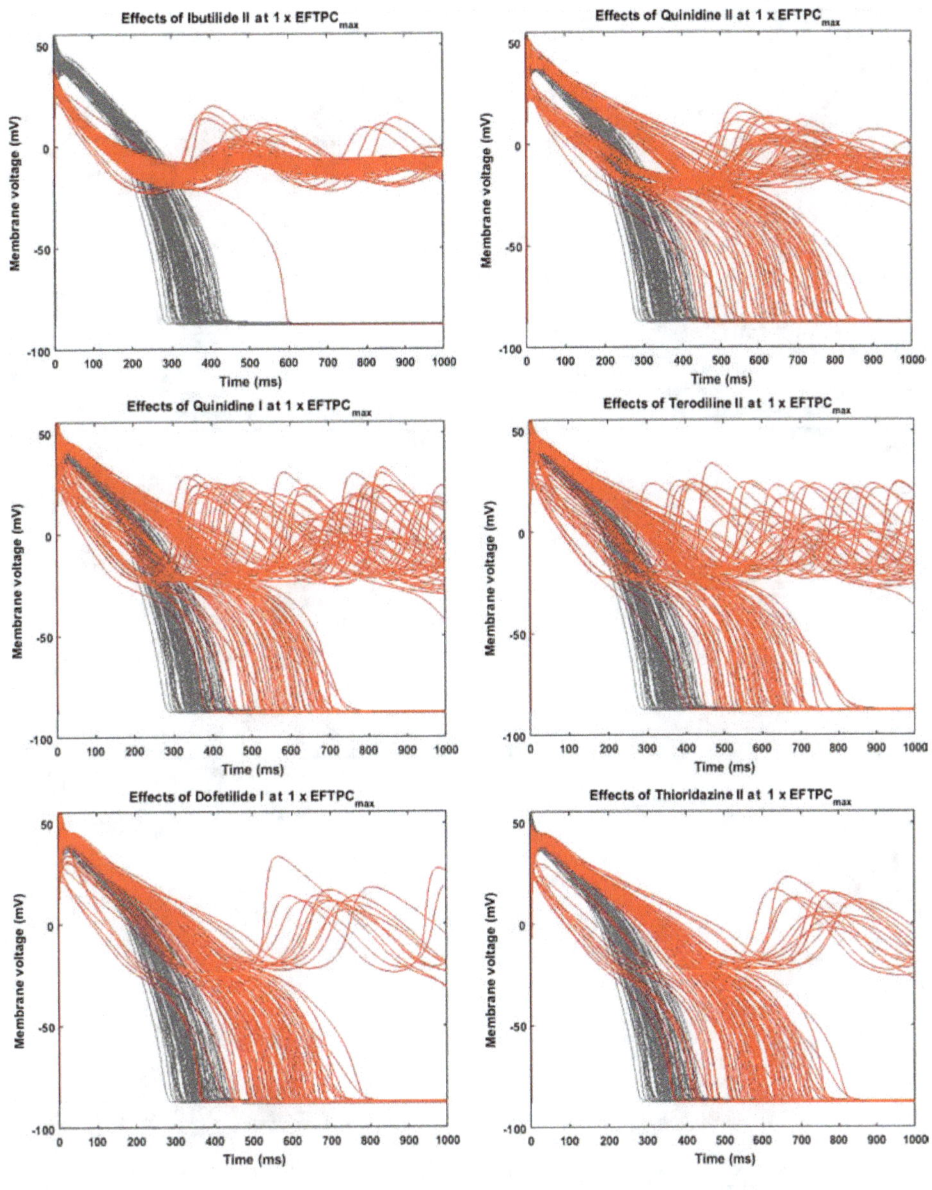

FIGURE 3 | Representative compounds that induce repolarization abnormalities at $1\times EFTPC_{max}$. Grey, control condition; red, drug action.

Table S4). Overall, considering hERG alone decreases the specificity of the predictions for both datasets (**Table 3**).

The higher RA inducibility when considering hERG alone was mainly due to I_{CaL} re-activation under lower repolarization reserve. For example, when only hERG block was applied to Linezolid II, RFs were observed at $100\times EFTPC_{max}$, with re-opening of the I_{CaL} activation gate (gate *d* in the ORd model) leading to oscillations in I_{CaL} and membrane potential (**Figure 7**, red traces). When hERG block alone was applied but the re-activation of I_{CaL} was inhibited (post upstroke inhibition of gate *d*), RFs were successfully suppressed (**Figure 7**, black traces). Since Linezolid II has a strong blockage effect on the L-type calcium channel, the consideration of all three channels yielded a much lower AP plateau. This further inhibited I_{CaL}, preventing the occurrence of a positive feedback loop of I_{CaL} re-activation to trigger RAs (**Figure 7**, blue traces).

Moderate Changes in IC_{50}s Combined With Variable Hill Coefficients Are Relevant to Divergent Prediction Outcomes

The ion channel information for Datasets I and II used in this *in silico* study came from different experimental groups, but they both contain information for the 16 compounds listed in **Figure 8**. In **Figure 8**, we listed the IC_{50} and Hill coefficient values of the three common ion channels between both datasets: hERG, Cav1.2 and Nav1.5-peak. For most compounds, the

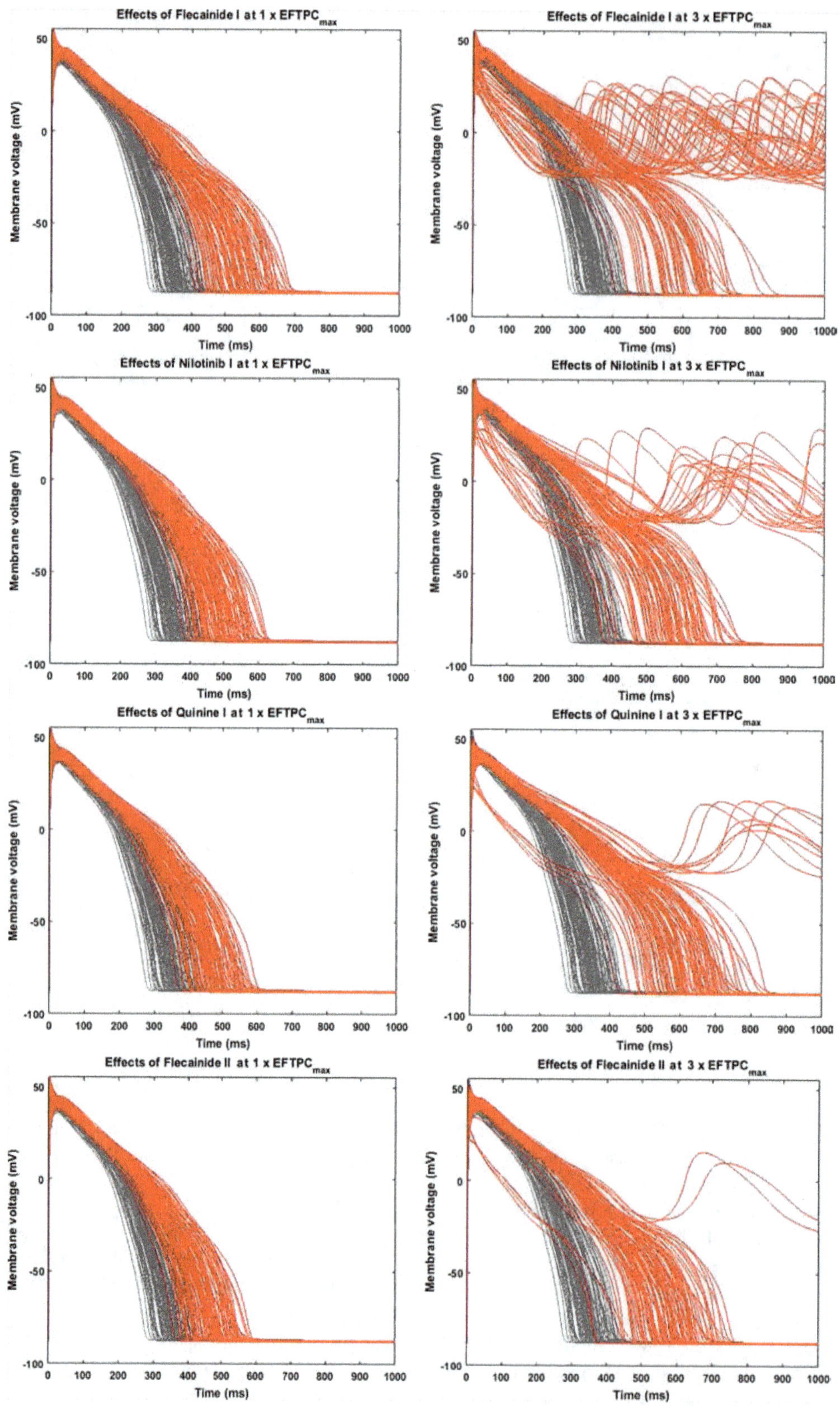

FIGURE 4 | Representative compounds that prolong action potential duration (APD) at $1{\times}EFTPC_{max}$ and induce repolarization abnormalities at $3{\times}EFTPC_{max}$. Grey, control condition; red, drug action.

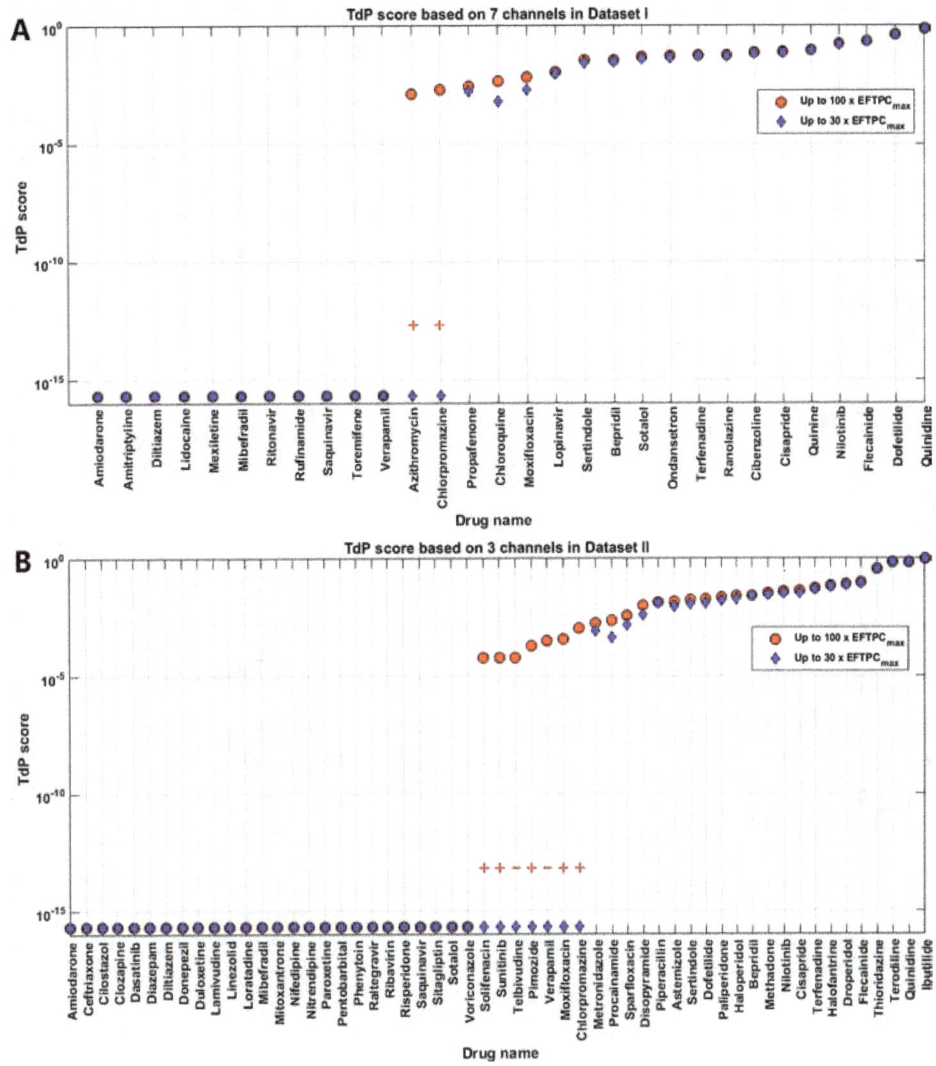

FIGURE 5 | Comparison of Torsades de Pointes (TdP) risk between up to 30×EFTPC$_{max}$ and 100×EFTPC$_{max}$ for Dataset I **(A)** and Dataset II **(B)**. Red "+" and "–" show the classification changes caused by lower testing concentrations: "+" implies the true classification should be risky, while "–" means the true classification should be safe. The three Dataset II compounds whose TdP risk was misclassified by the automated algorithm were corrected in this figure.

TABLE 2 | Comparisons of the *in silico* Torsades de Pointes (TdP) risk predictions between maximum testing concentrations of 30× and 100×EFTPC$_{max}$.

	Dataset I		Dataset II		
	100×EFTPC$_{max}$	**30×EFTPC$_{max}$**	**100×EFTPC$_{max}$**		**30×EFTPC$_{max}$**
Sensitivity	85%	75%	78%	**78%**	63%
Specificity	80%	80%	70%	**83%**	91%
PPV	89%	88%	78%	**86%**	91%
NPV	73%	62%	70%	**73%**	64%
Accuracy	83%	77%	75%	**80%**	75%

For Dataset II, bold scores indicate the true accuracy of the model predictions after fixing the misclassifications of the automated repolarization abnormality (RA) detection algorithm.

differences in ion channel IC_{50} datasets were moderate (<3-fold), while variations of Hill coefficient values were more significant between the two datasets. Despite the differences in IC_{50}s, Hill coefficients and the number of affected ion channels, for 14 out of the 16 compounds, *in silico* predictions based on the two independent datasets are consistent: almost all correct, except for Amiodarone (**Figure 8**).

For Sotalol and Verapamil, *in silico* predictions based on the seven currents from Dataset I produced the correct outcome, while the predictions based on Dataset II lead to FP for Verapamil and FN for Sotalol. Applying only the blockages of hERG, Cav1.2 and Nav1.5-peak in Dataset I for Sotalol and Verapamil still produced correct classification results for both

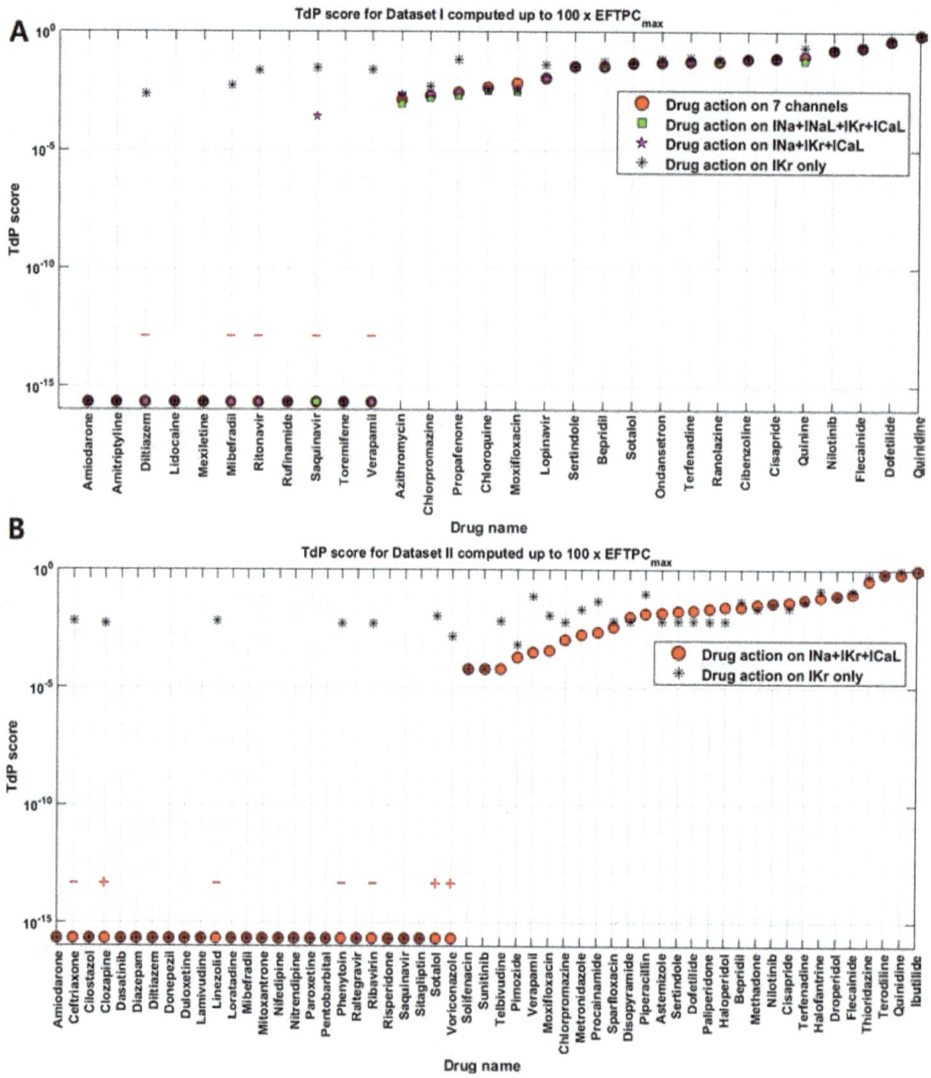

FIGURE 6 | Comparison of Torsades de Pointes (TdP) risk for different subsets of ion channel information for Dataset I **(A)** and Dataset II **(B)**. Red "+" and "–" show the classification changes caused by different ion channel profiles: "+" implies the true classification should be risky, while "–" means the true classification should be safe. The three Dataset II compounds whose TdP risk was misclassified by the automated algorithm were corrected in this figure, and they did induce repolarization abnormalities (RAs) under hERG only simulations.

compounds (**Figure 6A**). This evidenced that it was not the number of ion channels but the different input values between the two datasets what led to the divergent prediction outcomes for these two drugs.

For Sotalol, the Cav1.2 IC_{50} value was much smaller with a steeper concentration-response curve (bigger Hill coefficient) in Dataset II. This corresponded to a more potent calcium channel blockage (100% blockage in Dataset II versus 20% blockage in Dataset I at 100x $EFTPC_{max}$), providing the explanation for the FN prediction of Sotalol II. Verapamil II displayed very slow repolarization under $100 \times EFTPC_{max}$, with several models failing to reach resting membrane potential at the end of the simulation time (**Supplementary Figure S6A**). The difference in the prediction outcome of Verapamil between the two groups was

TABLE 3 | Comparisons of the *in silico* Torsades de Pointes (TdP) risk predictions between different sets of ion channel profiles.

	Dataset I				Dataset II	
	7 channels	4 channels	3 channels	1 channel (hERG)	3 channels	1 channel (hERG)
Sensitivity	85%	85%	85%	85%	78% **78%**	88%
Specificity	80%	80%	70%	30%	70% **83%**	65%
PPV	89%	89%	85%	71%	78% **86%**	78%
NPV	73%	73%	70%	50%	70% **73%**	79%
Accuracy	83%	83%	80%	67%	75% **80%**	78%

For Dataset II, bold scores indicate the true accuracy of the model predictions of 3 channels after fixing the misclassifications of the automated repolarization abnormality (RA) detection algorithm.

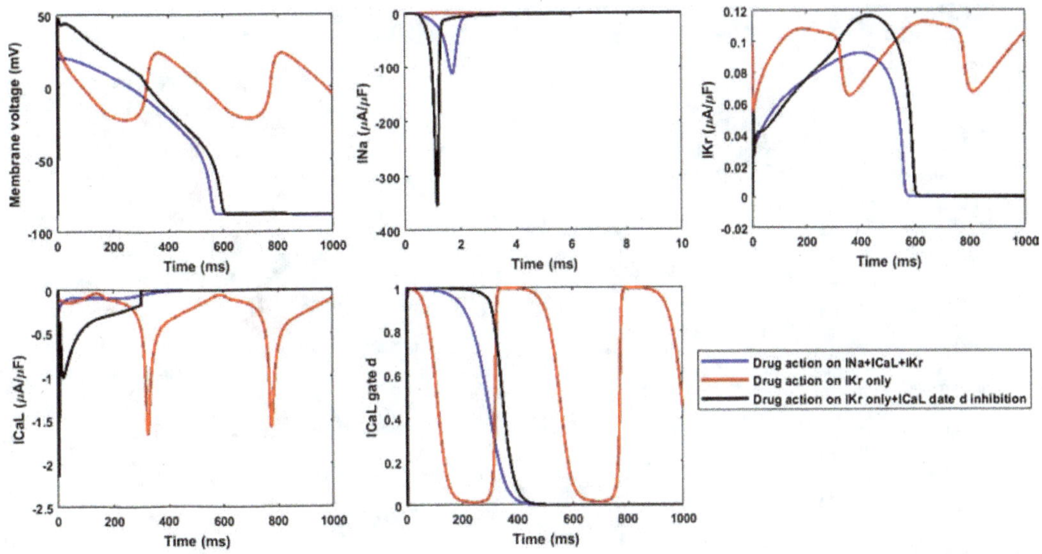

FIGURE 7 | The lack of inhibition to I_{CaL} re-activation by only considering hERG block leads to higher inducibility of repolarization abnormalities for 100×EFTPC$_{max}$ Linezolid II. Gate *d* is the activation gate of I_{CaL}.

due to the distinct input values in the two datasets: in Dataset II, Verapamil's IC_{50} for hERG was about half the value that in Dataset I. In addition, the EFTPC$_{max}$ concentration in Dataset II was almost doubled (**Figure 8**).

If the lower EFTPC$_{max}$ in Dataset I (0.045 μM) was applied to the ionic profile of Verapamil II, RFs still occurred at 100×EFTPC$_{max}$ (**Supplementary Figure S6B**), which proved the role of IC_{50}s and Hill coefficients underlying the FP prediction. Therefore, for drugs with a multi-channel effect, moderate IC_{50} variations (<3-fold) combined with variable Hill coefficients can affect the accuracy of prediction outcomes.

DISCUSSION

In this study, we blindly performed 85 *in silico* drug trials for a total of 69 compounds based on two independent ion channel datasets with 16 overlapping drugs, using a computationally efficient population of human ventricular cell models. The main findings are the following:

1) For both datasets, the overall performance of the prediction was strong, with respective maximum accuracies of 83% and 80% for Dataset I and Dataset II.

2) When considering RAs for TdP prediction, decreasing the maximum testing concentration led to lower sensitivity without significant improvement of specificity, resulting in an optimal testing concentration of 100×EFTPC$_{max}$.

3) I_{CaL} re-activation under reduced repolarization reserve caused by hERG block was the key mechanism underlying RAs. Calcium channel block decreased the propensity to RA. Therefore, only using hERG data decreased the specificity of predictions, and the optimal number of ion channels to achieve sufficient prediction accuracy was three: Nav1.5 (peak only), Cav1.2, and hERG.

4) For compounds with multiple ion channel potencies, moderate variations (<3-fold) in IC_{50} input values combined with variable Hill coefficients can lead to divergent prediction results.

An Optimized Population of Human ORd-Based Models as an Efficient Tool for *In Silico* Risk Prediction and Mechanism Analysis

In this study, we used an optimized population of 107 models for blinded *in silico* drug trials, and we achieved accuracies of 83% for Dataset I and 80% for Dataset II if visual examination of the AP traces was performed. We showed that by using a small population of models that is more susceptible for RAs with uneven variations of the ionic currents, similar prediction accuracy can be achieved as a large population with even ionic current variations. Our results showed that this optimized population of models achieved a slightly lower accuracy than the previous population of 1,213 human ventricular models (Passini et al., 2017), but the computing efficiency was improved by 90% due to much smaller population size. Therefore, designing the optimized population of models is proved to be an efficient strategy to perform TdP risk prediction and physiological analysis (Passini et al., 2019).

We used the simple pore block model in this study, because it only required conventional measurements such as IC_{50} values and Hill coefficients. Other modeling studies have used more complex representations of ion channel kinetics under drug actions, such as Markov representations of the sodium (Morotti et al., 2014; Yang et al., 2016) or the hERG channels (Romero et al., 2015; Li et al., 2017) to incorporate the drug binding states. However, in order to gain sufficient experimental data to achieve accurate representations for these more detailed

Drug	hERG IC50 (Hill coefficient)		Cav1.2 IC50 (Hill coefficient)		Nav1.5-peak IC50 (Hill coefficient)		EFTPCmax		TdP Risk	In Silico	In Silico
	I	II	I	II	I	II	I	II		I	II
Amiodarone	0.941 (0.6)	0.86 (0.12)	1.281 (0.6)	1.9 (0.2)	4.577 (0.7)	15.9 (2.1)	0.0007	0.0008	+	-	-
Bepridil	0.149 (0.9)	0.16 (0.02)	2.808 (0.6)	1 (0.2)	2.929 (1.2)	2.3 (0.3)	0.0315	0.035	+	+	+
Chlorpromazine	1.118 (0.9)	1.5 (0.1)	8.192 (0.8)	3.4 (0.3)	4.536 (2.0)	3 (0.4)	0.0345	0.038	+	+	+
Cisapride	0.012 (1.3)	0.02 (0.003)	∞	11.8 (1.3)	∞	337 (94.6)	0.0026	0.003	+	+	+
Diltiazem	6.569 (0.8)	13.2 (0.7)	0.112 (0.7)	0.76 (0.08)	∞	22.4 (2.2)	0.1275	0.122	-	-	-
Dofetilide	0.001 (0.6)	0.03 (0.004)	∞	26.7 (4.3)	∞	162.1 (23.6)	0.0021	0.002	+	+	+
Flecainide	0.692 (0.8)	1.5 (0.07)	25.599 (1.4)	27.1 (3.2)	6.677 (1.9)	6.2 (0.6)	0.7529	0.753	+	+	+
Mibefradil	0.307 (0.9)	1.7 (0.1)	0.652 (1.1)	0.51 (0.04)	5.866 (1.0)	5.6 (0.5)	0.0106	0.012	-	-	-
Moxifloxacin	93.041 (0.6)	86.2 (10.5)	∞	173 (26.3)	922.727 (1.0) *	1112 (383.9)	3.5625	10.96	+	+	+
Nilotinib	0.091 (0.8)	1 (0.1)	∞	17.5 (2.7)	∞	13.3 (2.3)	0.0604	0.172	+	+	+
Quinidine	0.343 (1.0)	0.72 (0.08)	∞	6.4 (0.7)	18.8152 (1.0) *	14.6 (1.0)	0.8429	3.237	+	+	+
Saquinavir	3.477 (1.0)	16.9 (0.8)	3.161 (1.4)	1.9 (0.3)	15.568 (1.2)	12.1 (1.0)	0.4172	0.13	-	-	-
Sertindole	0.011 (0.8)	0.033 (0.001)	∞	6.3 (0.5)	∞	6.9 (1.2)	0.0016	0.002	+	+	+
Sotalol	86.369 (0.9)	111.4 (14.6)	5976.92 (1.0) *	193.3 (37.8)	∞	7013.9 (2955.8)	14.6864	14.69	+	+	-
Terfenadine	0.019 (0.6)	0.05 (0.004)	0.7 (0.7)	0.93 (0.07)	∞	2 (0.2)	0.009	0.009	+	+	+
Verapamil	0.499 (1.1)	0.25 (0.03)	0.202 (1.1)	0.2 (0.02)	∞	32.5 (4.2)	0.045	0.088	-	-	+

FIGURE 8 | Comparison of the input ion channel IC_{50} values (µM), Hill coefficients, $EFTPC_{max}$ (µM), and *in silico* prediction results for the 16 common compounds between the two datasets. * indicate the cases where IC_{50s} were estimated based on the percentage of ion channel blockage at the maximum tested concentration, with h equal to 1.

drug binding models, more specialized experimental protocols and settings are normally needed, which can be a speed limiting step for efficient screening of new compounds. The simple pore block model, on the other hand, enables a more efficient experimental data collection and potentially a faster application in new drug screening.

Another advantage of using populations of models with electrophysiological variability is that it enables direct observations of RAs after applying drug actions, which can be used to provide physiological insights. Although logistic regression models or machine learning algorithms can also achieve good performances in TdP risk classifications based on the ratios of IC_{50} and EFTPC (Kramer et al., 2013), or features of AP and intracellular calcium transients (Lancaster and Sobie, 2016), some of these algorithms do not enable direct observations of RAs, which compromises the mechanistic explorations for TdP risk. Combining machine learning algorithms and modeling could also be a useful new strategy (Parikh et al., 2017).

Factors Affecting the Accuracy of Blinded *In Silico* TdP Risk Predictions

Although this blinded drug analysis using a small population of models achieved good accuracy for both groups of compounds, examination of some wrong predictions showed that additional information can be crucial for prediction outcome. For example, the predictions for Amiodarone were FN for both datasets in this study. However, if considering the possible lower plasma protein binding reported in literature (Lalloz et al., 1984; Latini et al., 1984), then testing at higher concentrations led to RAs occurrence with Amiodarone (Passini et al., 2017). Similarly, when taking into account the effect of Paliperidone, which is the major active metabolite of Risperidone, Passini et al. produced correct TdP risk classifications for Risperidone (Passini et al., 2017), since Paliperidone plays a more important role in QT prolongation (Suzuki et al., 2012). The information on drug metabolism was not optimized in this study because all compounds were blinded during the simulation process. A recent analysis by (Leishman, 2019) highlights the critical need to address contributions from clinically relevant metabolites in the qualification process to assure that the predictive performance of a new in silico model can address the pro-arrhythmic risk of exposure to both the parent drug and metabolites.

Another factor that affected the prediction accuracy was the definition of RAs. Based on our current definition, three compounds in Dataset II (Ceftriazone II, Linezolid II and Phenytoin II) were misclassified as RAs by the automated algorithm due to their very weak upstrokes and late peaks at the highest testing concentration (**Supplementary Material Figure S5**).

Correcting such misclassifications led to a higher accuracy of 80% for Dataset II. This change in prediction revealed that, on one hand, standardized criteria should be proposed for the definition of RAs, especially if models are to be used for high-throughput drug screening; on the other hand, there are exceptional AP morphologies produced by high dose drugs that may require manual inspections and alternative explanations.

In addition, the accurate classifications of TdP-positive or TdP-negative drugs are benchmarks that are crucial in assessing the performance of *in-silico* modeling. Due to the controversial classification of TdP risk for some drugs, the performance of *in-silico* modeling would be affected. Finally, the inputs, i.e., ion channel potencies determined experimentally, and $EFTPC_{max}$ obtained clinically, determine the accuracy of TdP prediction.

TdP Scores Computed Up to 30 Folds of $EFTPC_{max}$ Are Not Sufficient for the *In Silico* Predictions of Conditional TdP Risk

In order to incorporate the effects of inter-subject variability in drug binding and metabolism rates, as well as the uneven intra-subject drug distributions in the body, drug overdose is often used in both *in vitro* animal experimental tests and *in silico* simulations. In rabbit isolated Langendorff hearts, $30\times EFTPC_{max}$ was shown to be sufficient without incurring TdP risk of potentially beneficial drugs (Lawrence et al., 2006). In this study, we also explored the effect of maximum testing concentration on the accuracy of predictions. We found that decreasing the testing concentration to $30\times EFTPC_{max}$ can only improve specificity of predictions for Dataset II, but at the same time, the lower maximum testing concentration led to more FN predictions. For both datasets, the overall accuracy was lower under $30\times EFTPC_{max}$. Similarly, the previous study using 1213 models also showed that the optimal maximum testing concentration is $100\times EFTPC_{max}$ for the best accuracy (Passini et al., 2017).

We also noted that some FN predictions in this study (Clozapine II, Paroxetine II, Voriconazole II, and also Saquinavir II, Dasatinib II if considering CredibleMeds® classifications), were also FN in the previous 1,213 population of models. Interestingly, although classified as risky, these FN compounds were considered to have possible or conditional TdP risk under the latest classification of CredibleMeds®. Cilostazol II (and Donepezil II by CredibleMeds® classification) only induced EAD in one model under $100\times EFTPC_{max}$ in the previous population, corresponding to the lowest TdP scores in the risky category (Passini et al., 2017). Therefore, for compounds with possible or conditional TdP risk, more detailed investigations need to be performed to take into account other factors in addition to the overdose, such as existing disease conditions, drug interaction, and metabolites. In our recently published paper, we reported the electromechanical window as a sensitive biomarker to improve the prediction of TdP risk for 40 reference compounds under lower tested concentrations (Passini et al., 2019), and future studies can test the prediction accuracy of combining electromechanical window for compounds with conditional TdP risk.

In Silico Drug Trials Based on Nav1.5, Cav1.2, and hERG Generate Robust Prediction Results Without Compromising Efficiency

Previous experiments conducted in isolated ventricular myocytes or Langendorff-perfused animal hearts showed compounds with sodium or calcium blockage effects such as Lidocaine, Ranolazine, Nifedipine and Verapamil, can suppress EAD and prevent hERG blocker-induced TdP (Abrahamsson et al., 1996; Milberg et al., 2005; Yamada et al., 2008; Farkas et al., 2009; Milberg et al., 2012; Parikh et al., 2012). Therefore, it is essential to extend the TdP risk prediction from hERG-based analysis to a multiple-channel assay, which is the principle underlying this study and the CiPA initiative (Sager et al., 2014; Colatsky et al., 2016). In this study, we compared the effects of simulating only hERG blockage against simulating multiple ion channel blockages. For Dataset I, where the analysis was based on seven ion channel data from (Crumb et al., 2016), peak Nav1.5, Cav1.2, and hERG were the minimum set of ion channels with best efficiency for predictions, while for specific drugs, which have strong potency on other ion channels, predictions could improve by including these additional effects in simulations. As for the Dataset II prediction, based on data from (Kramer et al., 2013), only considering hERG significantly decreased specificity, and although sensitivity was slightly improved, the overall accuracy was also compromised. This is consistent with the previous hypothesis underlying CiPA, i.e., that simulating multiple channel blockages achieve more accurate predictions than only considering hERG (Gintant, 2011).

By using human ventricular cell models of electrophysiology, we were able to provide mechanistic explanations of the increased inducibility of RAs under hERG block. Our results showed that I_{CaL} re-activation was the key mechanism of RAs under hERG block, which was consistent with the mechanism revealed by sheep Purkinje fiber experiments (January et al., 1988; January and Riddle, 1989) and previous modeling investigations (Zeng and Rudy, 1995; Passini et al., 2016). Therefore, if calcium block effect is not considered, the TdP risk of a compound may be overestimated.

Moderate Variations in IC_{50}s Combined With Variable Hill Coefficients Affect *In Silico* Prediction Accuracy

IC_{50}s as well as the steepness of the concentration-response curve of a same drug can vary across experiments and datasets (Kirsch et al., 2004; Yao et al., 2005; Milnes et al., 2010; Fermini et al., 2016; Passini et al., 2017). In this study, we also aimed to explore the effect of IC_{50} and Hill coefficient inputs on the stability of *in silico* predictions. By comparing the simulation results of 16 common drugs, 14 drugs showed consistent results across datasets. Considering the same ion channels (Nav1.5-peak,

Cav1.2, and hERG), the overall accuracy for the 16 common drugs was slightly higher using the Crumb's input values (14 correct) than the Kramer's values (13 correct). This difference could originate from the experimental measurements: 1) the patch clamp experiments in the Crumb's dataset was performed manually and mostly at physiological temperature, while in Kramer's dataset, the experiments were conducted using automated patch clamp at ambient temperature; 2) for hERG and Cav1.2, Crumb's dataset used AP waveform voltage protocols, while Kramer's data were generated using step protocols (Kramer et al., 2013; Crumb et al., 2016). These differences in experimental settings may have contributed to the variability in IC_{50} and Hill coefficient measurements, and some variations in key ionic currents may lead to divergent simulation outcomes. For instance, the low IC_{50} value and steep concentration-response curve of Cav1.2 explained the FN prediction of Sotalol II.

From EADs to Clinical TdP Risk

In clinical settings, patients with structural heart disease and electrophysiological remodeling are at highest risk for drug induced arrhythmia. Experimental work showed that cardiomyocytes isolated from structural heart disease patients with a history of ventricular tachycardia were significantly more prone to the development of EADs (Coppini et al., 2013), and EADs were frequently observed in whole heart experimental recordings of aged or diseased animals, as well as in human whole ventricle simulations (Morita et al., 2009; Milberg et al., 2012; Dutta et al., 2016; Van Nieuwenhuyse et al., 2017). In this study we considered an optimized population of models with low repolarization reserve, including weak I_{Kr}, I_{Ks}, and I_{NaK}, together with strong I_{NaL}, I_{CaL}, and I_{NaCa}, which are observed in multiple diseases, such as long QT syndrome (Schwartz Peter et al., 2012), hypertrophic cardiomyopathy (Coppini et al., 2013), and heart failure (Shamraj et al., 1993; Ambrosi et al., 2013). Therefore, the optimized population of models was designed to favor the generation of EAD and RF, but also to include possible electrophysiological remodeling occurring in patients at higher risk of developing drug-induced arrhythmias.

EADs have been frequently observed in single cells as well as in whole-heart and tissue experimental recordings and simulations in human and animal hearts (Sato et al., 1993; Morita et al., 2009; Sato et al., 2009; Milberg et al., 2012; Coppini et al., 2013; Dutta et al., 2016; Van Nieuwenhuyse et al., 2017). Additional pro-arrhythmic mechanisms such as increased dispersion of repolarization can also provide the substrate for the development of reentrant arrhythmia, and drugs with hERG blockage effects can amplify the intrinsic spatial dispersion of repolarization (Antzelevitch, 2005; Dutta et al., 2016). For instance, low therapeutic concentrations of quinidine preferentially prolonged APD in the midmyocardial cells (Antzelevitch et al., 1999), creating a vulnerable condition across the ventricular wall. In addition, cellular coupling has important roles in modulating EAD generations at tissue level (Pueyo et al., 2011). Although electrotonic coupling can smooth the chaotic EAD behavior (Weiss et al., 2010), regional EADs can propagate into the heterogeneous substrates, resulting in reentry and TdP patterns (Dutta et al., 2016; Vandersickel et al., 2016).

One effective approach to include the tissue effects in TdP risk predictions is whole ventricle simulations (Sato et al., 2009; Moreno et al., 2011; Trayanova, 2011; Dutta et al., 2016; Vandersickel et al., 2016; Martinez-Navarro et al., 2019), however they are computationally much more expensive than the current cell model population which has already shown strong performance. In this study we did not aim to equate EADs and TdP, but rather to use EADs as a pro-arrhythmic risk marker that is mechanistically linked to TdP. Given that the predictive accuracy of populations of models is high, computationally expensive simulations are not necessary. However, whole-ventricular simulations are very valuable for investigating mechanisms of arrhythmia as shown by (Sato et al., 2009; Moreno et al., 2011; Trayanova, 2011; Dutta et al., 2016; Vandersickel et al., 2016; Martinez-Navarro et al., 2019). Whole heart electrophysiology is also complicated by heart rate changes, which are regulated by the autonomic nervous system and hormones. For example Isoproterenol, a β-adrenergic receptor agonist, was used to terminate TdP by increasing heart rate and decreasing the dispersion of repolarization (Surawicz, 1989). Future studies could be performed by evaluating an agent's TdP risk under β-adrenergic stimulations (Heijman et al., 2011; Tomek et al., 2017; Tomek et al., 2019).

CONCLUSION

Through this blinded *in silico* drug trial, we demonstrated that computer simulations utilizing optimized population of human ventricular cell models are useful tools for high-throughput TdP risk predictions, and the minimum set of ion channels required for reliable predictions with highest computational efficiency are Nav1.5 (peak), Cav1.2, and hERG. For drugs with a multi-channel effect, moderate IC_{50} variations (<3-fold) combined with variable Hill coefficients could affect the accuracy of *in silico* predictions.

AUTHOR CONTRIBUTIONS

All the authors conceived and designed the study. XZ performed the in silico drug assays, analyzed simulation results, and drafted the manuscript. YQ provided blinded drug potency datasets and performed drug classifications. XZ and YQ prepared the figures. YL tested the software. XZ, YQ, EP, AB-O, YL, HV and BR interpreted the results. All the authors edited and revised the manuscript.

FUNDING

This study was funded by Amgen Inc. This work was supported by a Wellcome Trust Fellowship in Basic Biomedical Sciences to BR (100246/Z/12/Z and 214290/Z/18/Z) and a British Heart Foundation (BHF) Intermediate Basic Science Fellowship to AB-O (FS/17/22/32644). The authors also acknowledge additional support from the CompBioMed Centre of Excellence in Computational Biomedicine (European Commission Horizon 2020 research and innovation programme, grant agreement No. 675451), an NC3Rs Infrastructure for Impart Award (NC/P001076/1), and the Oxford BHF Centre of Research Excellence (RE/13/1/30181) and the TransQST project (Innovative Medicines Initiative 2 Joint Undertaking under grant agreement No 116030, receiving support from the European Union's Horizon 2020 research and innovation programme and EFPIA). This work made use of the facilities of the UK National Supercomputing Service (Archer Leadership Award e462, Archer RAP Award 00180) and a PRACE project (2017174226).

REFERENCES

Abrahamsson, C., Carlsson, L., and Duker, G. (1996). Lidocaine and nisoldipine attenuate almokalant-induced dispersion of repolarization and early afterdepolarizations *in vitro*. *J. Cardiovasc. Electrophysiol.* 7, 1074–1081. doi: 10.1111/j.1540-8167.1996.tb00483.x

Ambrosi, C. M., Yamada, K. A., Nerbonne, J. M., and Efimov, I. R. (2013). Gender differences in electrophysiological gene expression in failing and non-failing human hearts. *PloS One* 8, e54635. doi: 10.1371/journal.pone.0054635

Antzelevitch, C., Shimizu, W., Yan, G. X., Sicouri, S., Weissenburger, J., Nesterenko, V. V., et al. (1999). The M cell: its contribution to the ECG and to normal and abnormal electrical function of the heart. *J. Cardiovasc. Electrophysiol.* 10, 1124–1152. doi: 10.1111/j.1540-8167.1999.tb00287.x

Antzelevitch, C. (2005). Role of transmural dispersion of repolarization in the genesis of drug-induced torsades de pointes. *Heart Rhythm* 2, S9–S15. doi: 10.1016/j.hrthm.2004.09.011

Brennan, T., Fink, M., and Rodriguez, B. (2009). Multiscale modelling of drug-induced effects on cardiac electrophysiological activity. *Eur. J. Pharm. Sci.* 36, 62–77. doi: 10.1016/j.ejps.2008.09.013

Bril, A., Gout, B., Bonhomme, M., Landais, L., Faivre, J. F., Linee, P., et al. (1996). Combined potassium and calcium channel blocking activities as a basis for antiarrhythmic efficacy with low proarrhythmic risk: experimental profile of BRL-32872. *J. Pharmacol. Exp. Ther.* 276, 637–646.

Britton, O. J., Bueno-Orovio, A., Virág, L., Varró, A., and Rodriguez, B. (2017). The electrogenic Na(+)/K(+) pump is a key determinant of repolarization abnormality susceptibility in human ventricular cardiomyocytes: a population-based simulation study. *Front. Physiol.* 8, 278. doi: 10.3389/fphys.2017.00278

Colatsky, T., Fermini, B., Gintant, G., Pierson, J. B., Sager, P., Sekino, Y., et al. (2016). The comprehensive in vitro proarrhythmia assay (CiPA) initiative - update on progress. *J. Pharmacol. Toxicol. Methods* 81, 15–20. doi: 10.1016/j.vascn.2016.06.002

Coppini, R., Ferrantini, C., Yao, L., Fan, P., Del Lungo, M., Stillitano, F., et al. (2013). Late sodium current inhibition reverses electromechanical dysfunction in human hypertrophic cardiomyopathy. *Circulation* 127, 575–584. doi: 10.1161/CIRCULATIONAHA.112.134932

Crumb, W. J., Vicente, J., Johannesen, L., and Strauss, D. G. (2016). An evaluation of 30 clinical drugs against the comprehensive in vitro proarrhythmia assay (CiPA) proposed ion channel panel. *J. Pharmacol. Toxicol. Methods* 81, 251–262. doi: 10.1016/j.vascn.2016.03.009

Dutta, S., Mincholé, A., Zacur, E., Quinn, T. A., Taggart, P., and Rodriguez, B. (2016). Early afterdepolarizations promote transmural reentry in ischemic human ventricles with reduced repolarization reserve. *Prog. Biophys. Mol. Biol.* 120, 236–248. doi: 10.1016/j.pbiomolbio.2016.01.008

Farkas, A. S., Makra, P., Csík, N., Orosz, S., Shattock, M. J., Fülöp, F., et al. (2009). The role of the Na+/Ca2+ exchanger, I(Na) and I(CaL) in the genesis of dofetilide-induced torsades de pointes in isolated, AV-blocked rabbit hearts. *Br. J. Pharmacol.* 156, 920–932. doi: 10.1111/j.1476-5381.2008.00096.x

Fermini, B., Hancox, J. C., Abi-Gerges, N., Bridgland-Taylor, M., Chaudhary, K. W., Colatsky, T., et al. (2016). A new perspective in the field of cardiac safety testing through the comprehensive *in vitro* proarrhythmia assay paradigm. *J. Biomol. Screen* 21, 1–11. doi: 10.1177/1087057115594589

Gintant, G. (2011). An evaluation of hERG current assay performance: translating preclinical safety studies to clinical QT prolongation. *Pharmacol. Ther.* 129, 109–119. doi: 10.1016/j.pharmthera.2010.08.008

Guo, D., Liu, Q., Liu, T., Elliott, G., Gingras, M., Kowey, P. R., et al. (2011). Electrophysiological properties of HBI-3000: a new antiarrhythmic agent with multiple-channel blocking properties in human ventricular myocytes. *J. Cardiovasc. Pharmacol.* 57, 79–85. doi: 10.1097/FJC.0b013e3181ffe8b3

Heijman, J., Volders, P. G. A., Westra, R. L., and Rudy, Y. (2011). Local control of β-adrenergic stimulation: effects on ventricular myocyte electrophysiology and Ca2+-transient. *J. Mol. Cell. Cardiol.* 50, 863–871. doi: 10.1016/j.yjmcc.2011.02.007

Hindmarsh, A. C., Brown, P. N., Grant, K. E., Lee, S. L., Serban, R., Shumaker, D. E., et al. (2005). SUNDIALS: suite of nonlinear and differential/algebraic equation solvers. *ACM Trans. Math. Software* 31, 363–396. doi: 10.1145/1089014.1089020

January, C. T., and Riddle, J. M. (1989). Early afterdepolarizations: mechanism of induction and block. a role for L-type Ca2+ current. *Circ. Res.* 64, 977–990. doi: 10.1161/01.res.64.5.977

January, C. T., Riddle, J. M., and Salata, J. J. (1988). A model for early afterdepolarizations: induction with the Ca2+ channel agonist Bay K 8644. *Circ. Res.* 62, 563–571. doi: 10.1161/01.res.62.3.563

Jurkiewicz, N. K., and Sanguinetti, M. C. (1993). Rate-dependent prolongation of cardiac action potentials by a methanesulfonanilide class III antiarrhythmic agent. specific block of rapidly activating delayed rectifier K+ current by dofetilide. *Circ. Res.* 72, 75–83. doi: 10.1161/01.res.72.1.75

Kirsch, G. E., Trepakova, E. S., Brimecombe, J. C., Sidach, S. S., Erickson, H. D., Kochan, M. C., et al. (2004). Variability in the measurement of hERG potassium channel inhibition: effects of temperature and stimulus pattern. *J. Pharmacol. Toxicological Methods* 50, 93–101. doi: 10.1016/j.vascn.2004.06.003

Kramer, J., Obejero-Paz, C. A., Myatt, G., Kuryshev, Y. A., Bruening-Wright, A., Verducci, J. S., et al. (2013). MICE models: superior to the HERG model in predicting Torsade de Pointes. *Sci. Rep.* 3, 2100. doi: 10.1038/srep02100

Kurisu, S., Inoue, I., Kawagoe, T., Ishihara, M., Shimatani, Y., Nakama, Y., et al. (2008). Torsade de pointes associated with bradycardia and takotsubo cardiomyopathy. *Can. J. Cardiol.* 24, 640–642. doi: 10.1016/s0828-282x(08)70653-6

Lalloz, M. R., Byfield, P. G., Greenwood, R. M., and Himsworth, R. L. (1984). Binding of amiodarone by serum proteins and the effects of drugs, hormones and other interacting ligands. *J. Pharm. Pharmacol.* 36, 366–372. doi: 10.1111/j.2042-7158.1984.tb04400.x

Lancaster, M. C., and Sobie, E. A. (2016). Improved prediction of drug-induced torsades de pointes through simulations of dynamics and machine learning algorithms. *Clin. Pharmacol. Ther.* 100, 371–379. doi: 10.1002/cpt.367

Latini, R., Tognoni, G., and Kates, R. E. (1984). Clinical pharmacokinetics of amiodarone. *Clin. Pharmacokinet.* 9, 136–156. doi: 10.2165/00003088-198409020-00002

Lawrence, C. L., Bridgland-Taylor, M. H., Pollard, C. E., Hammond, T. G., and Valentin, J.-P. (2006). A rabbit langendorff heart proarrhythmia model:

predictive value for clinical identification of Torsades de Pointes. *Br. J. Pharmacol.* 149, 845–860. doi: 10.1038/sj.bjp.0706894

Leishman, D. J. (2019). Improving prediction of torsadogenic risk in the CiPA in silico model by appropriately accounting for clinical exposure. *J. Pharmacol. Toxicol. Methods* 101, 106654. doi: 10.1016/j.vascn.2019.106654

Li, Z., Dutta, S., Sheng, J., Tran, P. N., Wu, W., Chang, K., et al. (2017). Improving the *In Silico* assessment of Proarrhythmia risk by combining hERG (Human Ether-à-go-go-Related Gene) channel-drug binding kinetics and multichannel pharmacology. *Circ. Arrhythm Electrophysiol.* 10, e004628. doi: 10.1161/CIRCEP.116.004628

Martin, R. L., McDermott, J. S., Salmen, H. J., Palmatier, J., Cox, B. F., and Gintant, G. A. (2004). The utility of hERG and repolarization assays in evaluating delayed cardiac repolarization: influence of multi-channel block. *J. Cardiovasc. Pharmacol.* 43, 369–379. doi: 10.1097/00005344-200403000-00007

Martinez-Navarro, H., Mincholé, A., Bueno-Orovio, A., and Rodriguez, B. (2019). High arrhythmic risk in antero-septal acute myocardial ischemia is explained by increased transmural reentry occurrence. *Sci. Rep.* 9, 16803. doi: 10.1038/s41598-019-53221-2

Milberg, P., Reinsch, N., Osada, N., Wasmer, K., Mönnig, G., Stypmann, J., et al. (2005). Verapamil prevents torsade de pointes by reduction of transmural dispersion of repolarization and suppression of early afterdepolarizations in an intact heart model of LQT3. *Basic Res. Cardiol.* 100, 365–371. doi: 10.1007/s00395-005-0533-8

Milberg, P., Fink, M., Pott, C., Frommeyer, G., Biertz, J., Osada, N., et al. (2012). Blockade of I(Ca) suppresses early afterdepolarizations and reduces transmural dispersion of repolarization in a whole heart model of chronic heart failure. *Br. J. Pharmacol.* 166, 557–568. doi: 10.1111/j.1476-5381.2011.01721.x

Milnes, J. T., Witchel, H. J., Leaney, J. L., Leishman, D. J., and Hancox, J. C. (2010). Investigating dynamic protocol-dependence of hERG potassium channel inhibition at 37°C: Cisapride versus dofetilide. *J. Pharmacol. Toxicological Methods* 61, 178–191. doi: 10.1016/j.vascn.2010.02.007

Mirams, G. R., Cui, Y., Sher, A., Fink, M., Cooper, J., Heath, B. M., et al. (2011). Simulation of multiple ion channel block provides improved early prediction of compounds' clinical torsadogenic risk. *Cardiovasc. Res.* 91, 53–61. doi: 10.1093/cvr/cvr044

Mistry, H. B., Davies, M. R., and Di Veroli, G. Y. (2015). A new classifier-based strategy for *in-silico* ion-channel cardiac drug safety assessment. *Front. Pharmacol.* 6, 59. doi: 10.3389/fphar.2015.00059

Moreno, J. D., Zhu, Z. I., Yang, P.-C., Bankston, J. R., Jeng, M.-T., Kang, C., et al. (2011). A computational model to predict the effects of class I anti-arrhythmic drugs on ventricular rhythms. *Sci. Transl. Med.* 3, 98ra83. doi: 10.1126/scitranslmed.3002588

Morita, N., Sovari, A. A., Xie, Y., Fishbein, M. C., Mandel, W. J., Garfinkel, A., et al. (2009). Increased susceptibility of aged hearts to ventricular fibrillation during oxidative stress. *Am. J. Physiol. Heart Circ. Physiol.* 297, H1594–H1605. doi: 10.1152/ajpheart.00579.2009

Morotti, S., Edwards, A. G., McCulloch, A. D., Bers, D. M., and Grandi, E. (2014). A novel computational model of mouse myocyte electrophysiology to assess the synergy between Na+ loading and CaMKII. *J. Physiol.* 592, 1181–1197. doi: 10.1113/jphysiol.2013.266676

O'Hara, T., Virág, L., Varró, A., and Rudy, Y. (2011). Simulation of the undiseased human cardiac ventricular action potential: model formulation and experimental validation. *PloS Comput. Biol.* 7, e1002061. doi: 10.1371/journal.pcbi.1002061

Parikh, A., Mantravadi, R., Kozhevnikov, D., Roche, M. A., Ye, Y., Owen, L. J., et al. (2012). Ranolazine stabilizes cardiac ryanodine receptors: a novel mechanism for the suppression of early afterdepolarization and torsades de pointes in long QT type 2. *Heart Rhythm* 9, 953–960. doi: 10.1016/j.hrthm.2012.01.010

Parikh, J., Gurev, V., and Rice, J. J. (2017). Novel two-step classifier for Torsades de Pointes risk stratification from direct features. *Front. Pharmacol.* 8, 816. doi: 10.3389/fphar.2017.00816

Passini, E., Mincholé, A., Coppini, R., Cerbai, E., Rodriguez, B., Severi, S., et al. (2016). Mechanisms of pro-arrhythmic abnormalities in ventricular repolarisation and anti-arrhythmic therapies in human hypertrophic cardiomyopathy. *J. Mol. Cell. Cardiol.* 96, 72–81. doi: 10.1016/j.yjmcc.2015.09.003

Passini, E., Britton, O. J., Lu, H. R., Rohrbacher, J., Hermans, A. N., Gallacher, D. J., et al. (2017). Human *in silico* drug trials demonstrate higher accuracy than animal models in predicting clinical pro-arrhythmic cardiotoxicity. *Front. Physiol.* 8, 668. doi: 10.3389/fphys.2017.00668

Passini, E., Trovato, C., Morissette, P., Sannajust, F., Bueno-Orovio, A., and Rodriguez, B. (2019). Drug-induced shortening of the electromechanical window is an effective biomarker for *in silico* prediction of clinical risk of Arrhythmias. *Br. J. Pharmacol.* 176, 3819–3833 doi: 10.1111/bph.14786

Pinski, S. L., Eguía, L. E., and Trohman, R. G. (2002). What is the minimal pacing rate that prevents torsades de pointes? Insights from patients with permanent pacemakers. *Pacing Clin. Electrophysiol.* 25, 1612–1615. doi: 10.1046/j.1460-9592.2002.01612.x

Pueyo, E., Corrias, A., Virág, L., Jost, N., Szél, T., Varró, A., et al. (2011). A multiscale investigation of repolarization variability and its role in cardiac arrhythmogenesis. *Biophys. J.* 101, 2892–2902. doi: 10.1016/j.bpj.2011.09.060

Redfern, W. S., Carlsson, L., Davis, A. S., Lynch, W. G., MacKenzie, I., Palethorpe, S., et al. (2003). Relationships between preclinical cardiac electrophysiology, clinical QT interval prolongation and torsade de pointes for a broad range of drugs: evidence for a provisional safety margin in drug development. *Cardiovasc. Res.* 58, 32–45. doi: 10.1016/S0008-6363(02)00846-5

Roden, D. M., and Abraham, R. L. (2011). Refining repolarization reserve. *Heart Rhythm* 8, 1756–1757. doi: 10.1016/j.hrthm.2011.06.024

Roden Dan, M. (2008). Repolarization Reserve. *Circulation* 118, 981–982. doi: 10.1161/CIRCULATIONAHA.108.798918

Roden, D. M. (1998). Taking the "idio" out of "idiosyncratic": predicting torsades de pointes. *Pacing Clin. Electrophysiol.* 21, 1029–1034. doi: 10.1111/j.1540-8159.1998.tb00148.x

Romero, L., Trenor, B., Yang, P.-C., Saiz, J., and Clancy, C. E. (2015). *In silico* screening of the impact of hERG channel kinetic abnormalities on channel block and susceptibility to acquired long QT syndrome. *J. Mol. Cell. Cardiol.* 87, 271–282. doi: 10.1016/j.yjmcc.2015.08.015

Sager, P. T., Gintant, G., Turner, J. R., Pettit, S., and Stockbridge, N. (2014). Rechanneling the cardiac proarrhythmia safety paradigm: a meeting report from the cardiac safety research consortium. *Am. Heart J.* 167, 292–300. doi: 10.1016/j.ahj.2013.11.004

Sato, T., Hirao, K., and Hiejima, K. (1993). The relationship between early afterdepolarization and the occurrence of torsades de pointes–an in vivo canine model study. *Jpn. Circ. J.* 57, 543–552. doi: 10.1253/jcj.57.543

Sato, D., Xie, L.-H., Sovari, A. A., Tran, D. X., Morita, N., Xie, F., et al. (2009). Synchronization of chaotic early afterdepolarizations in the genesis of cardiac arrhythmias. *Proc. Natl. Acad. Sci. U.S.A.* 106, 2983–2988. doi: 10.1073/pnas.0809148106

Schwartz Peter, J., Lia, Crotti, and Insolia, R. (2012). Long-QT Syndrome. *Circulation: Arrhythmia Electrophysiology* 5, 868–877. doi: 10.1161/CIRCEP.111.962019

Serban, R., and Hindmarsh, A. C. (2008). CVODES: The Sensitivity-Enabled ODE Solver in SUNDIALS. *ASME 2005 International Design Engineering Technical Conferences and Computers and Information in Engineering Conference* in (American Society of Mechanical Engineers Digital Collection), 257–269. doi: 10.1115/DETC2005-85597

Shamraj, O. I., Grupp, I. L., Grupp, G., Melvin, D., Gradoux, N., Kremers, W., et al. (1993). Characterisation of Na/K-ATPase, its isoforms, and the inotropic response to ouabain in isolated failing human hearts. *Cardiovasc. Res.* 27, 2229–2237. doi: 10.1093/cvr/27.12.2229

Surawicz, B. (1989). Electrophysiologic substrate of torsade de pointes: dispersion of repolarization or early afterdepolarizations? *J. Am. Coll. Cardiol.* 14, 172–184. doi: 10.1016/0735-1097(89)90069-7

Suzuki, Y., Fukui, N., Watanabe, J., Ono, S., Sugai, T., Tsuneyama, N., et al. (2012). QT prolongation of the antipsychotic risperidone is predominantly related to its 9-hydroxy metabolite paliperidone. *Hum. Psychopharmacol.* 27, 39–42. doi: 10.1002/hup.1258

Tamargo, J., Rosano, G., Walther, T., Duarte, J., Niessner, A., Kaski, J. C., et al. (2017). Gender differences in the effects of cardiovascular drugs. *Eur. Heart J. Cardiovasc. Pharmacother.* 3, 163–182. doi: 10.1093/ehjcvp/pvw042

Tomek, J., Rodriguez, B., Bub, G., and Heijman, J. (2017). β-Adrenergic receptor stimulation inhibits proarrhythmic alternans in postinfarction border zone cardiomyocytes: a computational analysis. *Am. J. Physiol. Heart Circ. Physiol.* 313, H338–H353. doi: 10.1152/ajpheart.00094.2017

Tomek, J., Hao, G., Tomková, M., Lewis, A., Carr, C., Paterson, D. J., et al. (2019). β-adrenergic receptor stimulation and alternans in the border zone of a healed infarct: an ex vivo study and computational investigation of arrhythmogenesis. *Front. Physiol.* 10. doi: 10.3389/fphys.2019.00350

Trayanova, N. A. (2011). Whole-heart modeling: applications to cardiac electrophysiology and electromechanics. *Circ. Res.* 108, 113–128. doi: 10.1161/CIRCRESAHA.110.223610

Van Nieuwenhuyse, E., Seemann, G., Panfilov, A. V., and Vandersickel, N. (2017). Effects of early afterdepolarizations on excitation patterns in an accurate model of the human ventricles. *PloS One* 12, e0188867. doi: 10.1371/journal.pone.0188867

Vandersickel, N., Kazbanov, I. V., Nuitermans, A., Weise, L. D., Pandit, R., and Panfilov, A. V. (2014). A study of early afterdepolarizations in a model for human ventricular tissue. *PloS One* 9, e84595. doi: 10.1371/journal.pone.0084595

Vandersickel, N., Kazbanov, I. V., Defauw, A., Pijnappels, D. A., and Panfilov, A. V. (2015). Decreased repolarization reserve increases defibrillation threshold by favoring early afterdepolarizations in an in silico model of human ventricular tissue. *Heart Rhythm* 12, 1088–1096. doi: 10.1016/j.hrthm.2015.01.033

Vandersickel, N., Boer, T. P., de, Vos, M. A., and Panfilov, A. V. (2016). Perpetuation of torsade de pointes in heterogeneous hearts: competing foci or re-entry? *J. Physiol.* 594, 6865–6878. doi: 10.1113/JP271728

Viskin, S., Glikson, M., Fish, R., Glick, A., Copperman, Y., and Saxon, L. A. (2000). Rate smoothing with cardiac pacing for preventing torsade de pointes. *Am. J. Cardiol.* 86, K111–K115. doi: 10.1016/S0002-9149(00)01228-5

Weiss, J. N., Garfinkel, A., Karagueuzian, H. S., Chen, P.-S., and Qu, Z. (2010). Early afterdepolarizations and cardiac arrhythmias. *Heart Rhythm* 7, 1891–1899. doi: 10.1016/j.hrthm.2010.09.017

Woosley, R., Heise, C., and Romero, K. (2019). CredibleMeds :: Home. *QTdrugs List.* Available at: https://crediblemeds.org/ [Accessed November 28, 2018].

Yamada, M., Ohta, K., Niwa, A., Tsujino, N., Nakada, T., and Hirose, M. (2008). Contribution of L-type Ca2+ channels to early afterdepolarizations induced by I Kr and I Ks channel suppression in guinea pig ventricular myocytes. *J. Membr. Biol.* 222, 151–166. doi: 10.1007/s00232-008-9113-9

Yang, P.-C., El-Bizri, N., Romero, L., Giles, W. R., Rajamani, S., Belardinelli, L., et al. (2016). A computational model predicts adjunctive pharmacotherapy for cardiac safety via selective inhibition of the late cardiac Na current. *J. Mol. Cell. Cardiol.* 99, 151–161. doi: 10.1016/j.yjmcc.2016.08.011

Yao, J.-A., Du, X., Lu, D., Baker, R. L., Daharsh, E., and Atterson, P. (2005). Estimation of potency of HERG channel blockers: impact of voltage protocol and temperature. *J. Pharmacol. Toxicological Methods* 52, 146–153. doi: 10.1016/j.vascn.2005.04.008

Zeng, J., and Rudy, Y. (1995). Early afterdepolarizations in cardiac myocytes: mechanism and rate dependence. *Biophys. J.* 68, 949–964. doi: 10.1016/S0006-3495(95)80271-7

9

Antiarrhythmic Properties of Ranolazine: Inhibition of Atrial Fibrillation Associated TASK-1 Potassium Channels

*Antonius Ratte[1,2,3], Felix Wiedmann[1,2,3], Manuel Kraft[1,2,3], Hugo A. Katus[1,2,3] and Constanze Schmidt[1,2,3]**

[1] Department of Cardiology, University of Heidelberg, Heidelberg, Germany, [2] DZHK (German Centre for Cardiovascular Research), partner site Heidelberg/Mannheim, University of Heidelberg, Heidelberg, Germany, [3] HCR, Heidelberg Centre for Heart Rhythm Disorders, University of Heidelberg, Heidelberg, Germany

***Correspondence:**
Constanze Schmidt
Constanze.Schmidt@med.uni-heidelberg.de

Background: Atrial fibrillation (AF) is the most common sustained cardiac arrhythmia and one of the major causes of cardiovascular morbidity and mortality. Despite good progress within the past years, safe and effective treatment of AF remains an unmet clinical need. The anti-anginal agent ranolazine has been shown to exhibit antiarrhythmic properties *via* mainly late I_{Na} and I_{Kr} blockade. This results in prolongation of the atrial action potential duration (APD) and effective refractory period (ERP) with lower effect on ventricular electrophysiology. Furthermore, ranolazine has been shown to be effective in the treatment of AF. TASK-1 is a two-pore domain potassium (K_{2P}) channel that shows nearly atrial specific expression within the human heart and has been found to be upregulated in AF, resulting in shortening the atrial APD in patients suffering from AF. We hypothesized that inhibition TASK-1 contributes to the observed electrophysiological and clinical effects of ranolazine.

Methods: We used *Xenopus laevis* oocytes and CHO-cells as heterologous expression systems for the study of TASK-1 inhibition by ranolazine and molecular drug docking simulations to investigate the ranolazine binding site and binding characteristics.

Results: Ranolazine acts as an inhibitor of TASK-1 potassium channels that inhibits TASK-1 currents with an IC_{50} of 30.6 ± 3.7 μM in mammalian cells and 198.4 ± 1.1 μM in *X. laevis* oocytes. TASK-1 inhibition by ranolazine is not frequency dependent but shows voltage dependency with a higher inhibitory potency at more depolarized membrane potentials. Ranolazine binds within the central cavity of the TASK-1 inner pore, at the bottom of the selectivity filter.

Conclusions: In this study, we show that ranolazine inhibits TASK-1 channels. We suggest that inhibition of TASK-1 may contribute to the observed antiarrhythmic effects of Ranolazine. This puts forward ranolazine as a prototype drug for the treatment of atrial arrhythmia because of its combined efficacy on atrial electrophysiology and lower risk for ventricular side effects.

Keywords: atrial fibrillation, ranolazine, antiarrhythmic drugs, TASK-1, K_{2P}3.1, KCNK3

INTRODUCTION

Atrial fibrillation (AF) is a common cardiac rhythm disorder and one of the major causes of stroke, acute heart failure, sudden death, and cardiovascular morbidity (January et al., 2014). Despite good progress within the last years, safe and effective management of patients suffering from AF remains a major health issue, as current pharmacological, interventional or surgical therapeutic strategies are restricted by insufficient efficacy and often severe adverse effects (Kirchhof et al., 2016). Annual recurrence rates of AF after pharmacological cardioversion, for instance, range from 40 to 70% (Guerra et al., 2017). Furthermore, drug treatment with antiarrhythmic drugs (AADs) is often discontinued because of poor tolerability or adverse effects (Lafuente-Lafuente et al., 2015). For this reason, the development of safe and effective AADs for the treatment of AF is crucial (Dobrev and Nattel 2010).

Ranolazine is a drug originally introduced as an anti-anginal agent (Nash and Nash 2008) that has later been shown to exhibit antiarrhythmic properties *via* inhibition of different ion currents, especially the late phase of the inward sodium current (late I_{Na}) and the rapidly activating delayed rectifier potassium current (I_{Kr}) (Gupta et al., 2015). Because ranolazine predominantly prolongs atrial rather than ventricular action potential duration (APD) and effective refractory period (ERP) (Burashnikov et al., 2007; Antzelevitch and Burashnikov 2009), it appears to be particularly effective in AF (Guerra et al., 2017), thus far attributed to an atrial-selective sodium channel block (Sossalla et al., 2010; Antzelevitch et al., 2011).

TASK-1 (tandem of P domains in a weak inward rectifying K^+ channel (TWIK)-related acid sensitive K^+ channel 1; $K_{2P}3.1$) is a member of the two-pore-domain potassium channel (K_{2P}) family. This heterologous group comprises 15 members that share a unique structure of four transmembrane domains and two pore-forming loops per subunit which assemble as dimers (Goldstein et al., 2001). Regulated by a variety of physiological stimuli (extracellular pH, G-protein-mediated pathways, polyunsaturated fatty acids, temperature and mechanical stress) they provide a background "leak" potassium conductance modulating the cell's resting membrane potential and cellular excitability (Feliciangeli et al., 2015). Their role in controlling cellular excitability predestines K_{2P} channels as potential players in diverse biological functions.

TASK-1 channels are widely expressed in various tissues, including the cerebral cortex (Vu et al., 2015), the brainstem retrotrapezoid (Mulkey et al., 2007) and pre-Botzinger regions (Koizumi et al., 2010), the carotid bodies (Buckler et al., 2000), hypoglossal and spinal cord motor neurons (Lazarenko et al., 2010), pulmonary artery smooth muscle (Olschewski et al., 2006), and the adrenal cortex (Czirjak and Enyedi 2002). They contribute in the regulation of oxygen sensing (Koizumi et al., 2010), endocrine secretion (Davies et al., 2008), auto-immune inflammation (Bittner et al., 2009), apoptosis (Lauritzen et al., 2003), and pulmonary blood pressure (Olschewski et al., 2006).

In the heart, TASK-1 is reported to modulate cardiac conduction, repolarization, and heart rate (Decher et al., 2011; Donner et al., 2011). Knockout or pharmacological inhibition of TASK-1 results in prolonged atrial APD and atrial ERP (Wirth et al., 2003; Putzke et al., 2007; Wirth et al., 2007; Decher et al., 2011; Skarsfeldt et al., 2016). Please note that some of the mentioned studies used inhibitors that are referred to as $K_V1.5$ blockers (AVE0118 and AVE1231 (A293), developed by Sanofi, Paris, France). These inhibitors, however, later turned out to be much more potent TASK-1 blockers (Kiper et al., 2015). Wirth et al. (2007) demonstrated that TASK-1 blockade induced a prolongation of only atrial but not ventricular refractoriness and an associated inhibition of atrial vulnerability to arrhythmia. The prolongation of atrial refractoriness was even more pronounced in tachypacing induced AF and there were no effects on ECG intervals and ventricular repolarization. Within the human heart, TASK-1 has recently been shown to be predominantly expressed in the atrium as well, and TASK-1 inhibition results in prolonged APD on isolated human atrial cardiomyocytes (Schmidt et al., 2015). Because of enhanced TASK-1 currents under the condition of AF, the effect is even more pronounced and thus similar to the results obtained from large animal models. APD prolongation *via* TASK-1 blockade is expected to suppress AF and the 'atrial selectivity' of TASK-1 blockade by limiting the mode of action to atrial tissue, thereby reducing the risk of pro-arrhythmogenic effects in the ventricles, highlights the potential clinical significance of TASK-1 blockade for the treatment of AF in patients (Schmidt et al., 2017).

We hypothesized that ranolazine inhibits TASK-1 currents and that TASK-1 inhibition contributes to the observed antiarrhythmic effects of ranolazine. We chose *Xenopus laevis* oocytes and Chinese Hamster Ovary (CHO) cells as heterologous expression systems for detailed study of the biophysical characteristics of TASK-1 blockade by ranolazine. We further used *in silico* docking simulations and mutagenesis screen to explore structural determinants of TASK-1 blockade.

MATERIALS AND METHODS

Molecular Biology

Complementary DNAs encoding human TWIK-1 (KCNK1; GenBank accession number NM_002245), TREK-1 (KCNK2; EF165334), TASK-1 (KCNK3; NM_002246), and TASK-3 (KCNK9; NM_016601) were kindly provided by Steve Goldstein (Chicago, IL, USA). Human TRESK cDNA (KCNK18; NM_181840) was obtained from C. Spencer Yost (San Francisco, CA, USA). Amplification of human TRAAK (KCNK4; EU978935), TASK-2 (KCNK5; EU978936), TWIK-2 (KCNK6; EU978937), TREK-2 (KCNK10; EU978939), THIK-1 (KCNK13; EU978942), TALK-1 (KCNK16; EU978943), and TALK-2 (KCNK17; EU978944) was previously described (Gierten et al., 2008). For *in vitro* transcription, cDNAs were subcloned into pRAT, a dual-purpose expression vector containing a cytomegalovirus promotor for mammalian expression and a T7 promotor for copy (c)RNA synthesis. All TASK-1 mutants reported in this study were generated using the QuikChange II Site-Directed Mutagenesis Kit (Agilent, Santa Clara, CA, USA) and synthetic mutant oligonucleotide primers. Sequences of all plasmid constructs were verified by DNA sequencing (GATC Biotech, Konstanz, Germany). After vector linearization with XbaI (New England Biolabs, Ipswich, MA, USA), plasmids were transcribed using the T7 mMessage mMachine kit (Thermo Fisher Scientific Inc., Waltham, MA, USA). Integrity of cRNA transcripts was assessed by agarose gel electrophoresis and cRNA concentrations were determined using Nanodrop spectrophotometry (ND-1000, peqLab Biotechnology GmbH, Erlangen, Germany).

Cell Culture

Chinese hamster ovary (CHO) cells (CLS Cat# 603479/p746_CHO, RRID : CVCL_0213) were cultured in Dulbecco's modified Eagle's medium (DMEM, Thermo Fisher Scientific Inc., Waltham, MA, USA) supplemented with 10% fetal bovine serum (FBS, Thermo Fisher Scientific Inc., Waltham, MA, USA), 100 U/ml penicillin G sodium and 100 μg/ml streptomycin sulphate in an atmosphere of 95% humidified air and 5% CO_2 at 37 °C. Cells were passaged regularly and seeded on glass cover slips prior to treatment. Transient transfections of CHO cells (passage 10–20) were performed using FuGENE HD transfection reagent (Promega, Madison, WI, USA) according to the manufacturer's instructions. Cells were co-transfected with 2.2 μg pRAT-hTASK-1 plasmid DNA and 1.1 μg green fluorescent protein (GFP) plasmid DNA (pEGFP-N1; Clontech Laboratories, Mountain View, CA, USA) per 35 mm petri dish. Patch Clamp recordings were performed 24–36 h after transfection only on green fluorescent cells.

X. Laevis Oocyte Preparation

This study was carried out in accordance with the directive 2010/63/EU of the European Parliament, and the current version of the German Law on the Protection of Animals. Approval for experiments involving *X. laevis* was granted by Regierungspräsidium Karlsruhe (institutional approval numbers A-38/11 and G-221/12). For detailed information on oocyte preparation please refer to the supplementary methods.

Electrophysiology

Two-electrode voltage clamp (TEVC) recordings from *X. laevis* oocytes were performed one to three days after cRNA injection using an OC-725C Oocyte Clamp amplifier (Warner Instruments, Hamden, CT, USA), a Digidata 1322A Series (Axon Instruments, Foster City, CA, USA) and pClamp 10 software (Molecular Devices, San José, CA, USA). Current recordings from CHO cells were carried out using the whole-cell patch clamp technique with an Axopatch 200B amplifier (Axon Instruments, Foster City, CA, USA), an Axon Digidata 1550B series (Axon Instruments, Foster City, CA, USA), and pClamp 10 software (Molecular Devices, San José, CA, USA). For detailed information about solutions and test protocols please refer to the supplementary methods.

Molecular Modelling and *In Silico* Drug Docking

Because the crystal structure of the human TASK-1 channel was not revealed yet, we built homology models using the SWISS-MODEL platform (Benkert et al., 2011; Bertoni et al., 2017; Waterhouse et al., 2018). Four models were generated based on the structures of TWIK-1 (protein data bank (PDB) ID: 3UMK) (Miller and Long 2012), TREK-1 (PDB ID: 6CQ6) (Lolicato et al., 2017), TREK-2 (PDB ID: 4XDL) (Dong et al., 2015) and TRAAK (PDB ID: 4RUE) (Lolicato et al., 2014). Quality assessment of the newly generated TASK-1 homology models was performed using MolProbidity (Davis et al., 2007).

Molecular docking calculations were performed using AutoDock Vina (Trott and Olson 2010). Analysis of protein–ligand interactions was performed using PLIP (Salentin et al., 2015). Three-dimensional visualizations of *in silico* simulations and dockings were generated with PyMOL 1.8 (PyMOL Molecular Graphics System, Schrödinger, LLC, New York, NY, USA).

Data Analysis and Statistics

PCLAMP (Molecular Devices, San José, CA, USA), GraphPad Prism 6 (GraphPad Software Inc., La Jolla, CA, USA) and Microsoft Excel (Microsoft, Redmond, WA, USA) software was used for data acquisition and analysis. The concentration required for 50% block of current (half-maximal inhibitory concentration (IC_{50})) was calculated from Hill plots using Prism 6 (GraphPad). Data are expressed as the mean ± standard error of the mean (SEM) unless stated otherwise. Paired and unpaired t-tests (two-tailed tests) were applied to compare the statistical significance of the results. $P < 0.05$ was considered statistically significant. Multiple comparisons were performed using one-way analysis of variance (ANOVA). If the hypothesis of equal means could be rejected, post-hoc comparisons of groups were made and the probability values were adjusted for multiple comparisons using the Bonferroni correction.

Materials

Ranolazine-dihydrochloride was obtained from Selleck Chemicals (Munich, Germany) and dissolved in water to a 100 mM stock solution. Aliquots of the stock solution were stored at −20 °C and diluted to the desired concentration with the bath solution on the day of experiments. The dilution of Ranolazine did not affect the pH of the bath solution.

RESULTS

Ranolazine Inhibits Human Task-1 Channels

To probe the inhibitory effects of ranolazine on human TASK-1 channels, TASK-1 was expressed in *X. laevis* oocytes. After a stabilization period with no significant current amplitude changes (15 min) ranolazine was administered for 30 min. Application of 100 μM ranolazine inhibited TASK-1 currents by 17.4 ± 2% (**Figure 1A**, n = 6, p = 0.018). Inhibitory effects were completely reversible. Current levels reached 100 ± 30% (n = 6) after 15 min washout period. TASK-1 channels were blocked with an IC_{50} of 30.6 ± 3.7 μM in CHO cells, and 198.4 ± 1.1 μM in oocytes, analyzed at +20 mV (**Figures 1C, D**). This 6.5-fold difference is consistent with previous findings that IC_{50} values determined in oocytes are mostly higher than those determined in mammalian cells (Streit et al., 2011; Schmidt et al., 2013). The maximum inhibition of 67.3 ± 4.5% in oocytes and 58.5 ± 6.9% in CHO cells was achieved with ranolazine concentrations of 1 mM and 100 μM,

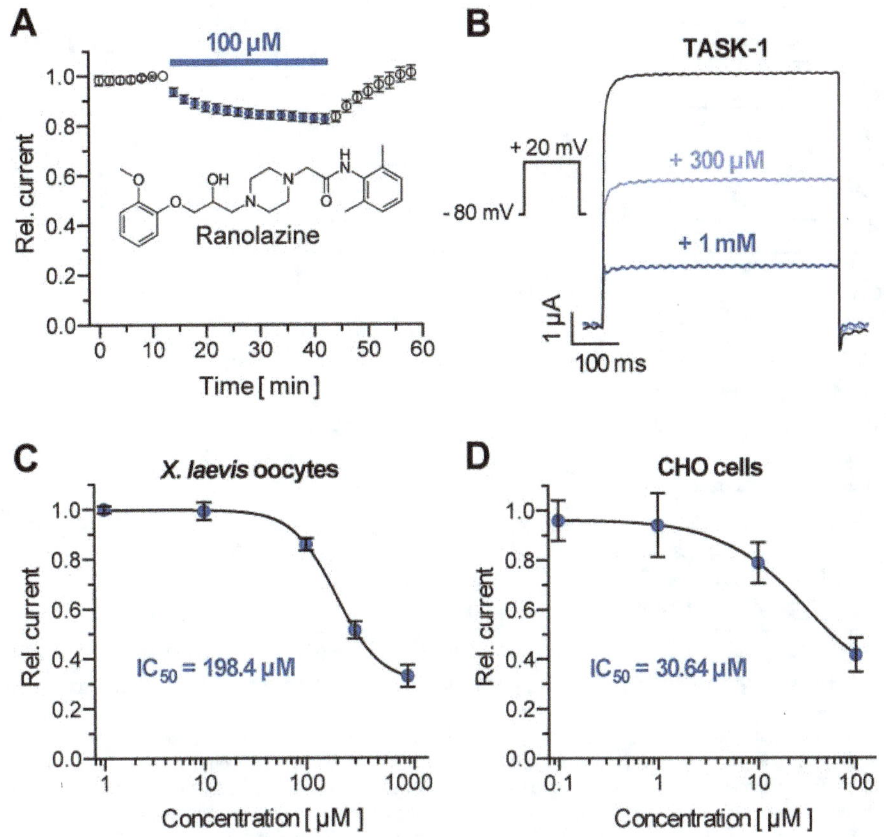

FIGURE 1 | Effect of ranolazine on TASK-1 current. **(A)** Time course of TASK-1 current reduction during ranolazine application (n = 6); currents are normalized to their respective value before ranolazine application after a stabilization period with no significant amplitude changes. **(B)** Representative TASK-1 current recordings evoked by applying a test pulse from −80 mV to +20 mV under control conditions and after 30 min incubation with 300 µM and 1 mM ranolazine. **(C)** Dose–response curve of TASK-1 inhibition by ranolazine in *X. laevis* oocytes. Currents are normalized to their respective values under control conditions (n = 5 – 10). **(D)** Dose–response curve of TASK-1 inhibition by ranolazine in CHO cells. Currents are normalized to their respective values under control conditions (n = 5). Data are given as mean ± SEM.

respectively. Administration of higher concentrations (3 mM in oocytes, 300 µM in CHO cells) led to cell instability and death. We used a concentration of 300 µM ranolazine for further experiments in *X. laevis* oocytes in order to achieve 50% current inhibition.

Biophysical Characteristics of TASK-1 Channel Blockade by Ranolazine

TASK-1 channels show electrophysiologic characteristics that are typical for most K_{2P} channels. They exhibit strong outward rectification with minimal inward current (0.69 ± 0.07 µA at −140 mV, n = 10) and a higher open probability at more depolarized membrane potentials (**Figures 2A, C, D**). **Figure 2A** illustrates representative current recordings of TASK-1 under control conditions and after application of 300 µM ranolazine for 30 min. Ranolazine (300 µM) inhibited TASK-1 currents by 48.79 ± 3.52% (analyzed at the end of the +20 mV test pulse, n = 10, p = 0.0004). Ranolazine also altered the resting membrane potential (RMP) from −66.57 ± 2.62 mV (control conditions, n = 10) to −63.55 ± 2.89 mV (300 µM ranolazine, n = 10, p = 0.0012, **Figure 2B**). Inhibitory effects of ranolazine showed voltage dependency, with less inhibition of inward currents (6.57 ± 2.55% to 11.07 ± 4.51% inhibition at voltages between −140 and −100 mV, n = 10) as compared to outward currents (44.56 ± 3.42% to 55.3 ± 3.87% inhibition at voltages between −40 and +60 mV, n = 10, **Figure 2E**). This resulted in an altered current-voltage (I-V) relationship under ranolazine treatment (**Figure 2D**).

Macroscopic TASK-1 currents in heterologous expression systems activate in two phases. Currents activate quickly to approximately 85% of their respective maximum amplitude within the first 50 ms, followed by a markedly slower additional activation time course. Thus, TASK-1 currents may be divided into an instantaneous and a sustained current component. **Figures 3A, B** illustrate the inhibition of TASK-1 currents by ranolazine during a 7.5 s test pulse from −80 mV to +20 mV (n = 6). The maximum inhibition of 48.67 ± 4.45% was reached after 10 ms and remained unchanged over the 7.5 s test pulse. Additionally, TASK-1 inhibition by ranolazine did not show frequency dependency (**Figure 3C**). The slight difference between 0.1 Hz and 1 Hz may be attributed to higher cell instability at higher stimulation frequencies, as this difference was also observed under control conditions in absence of ranolazine.

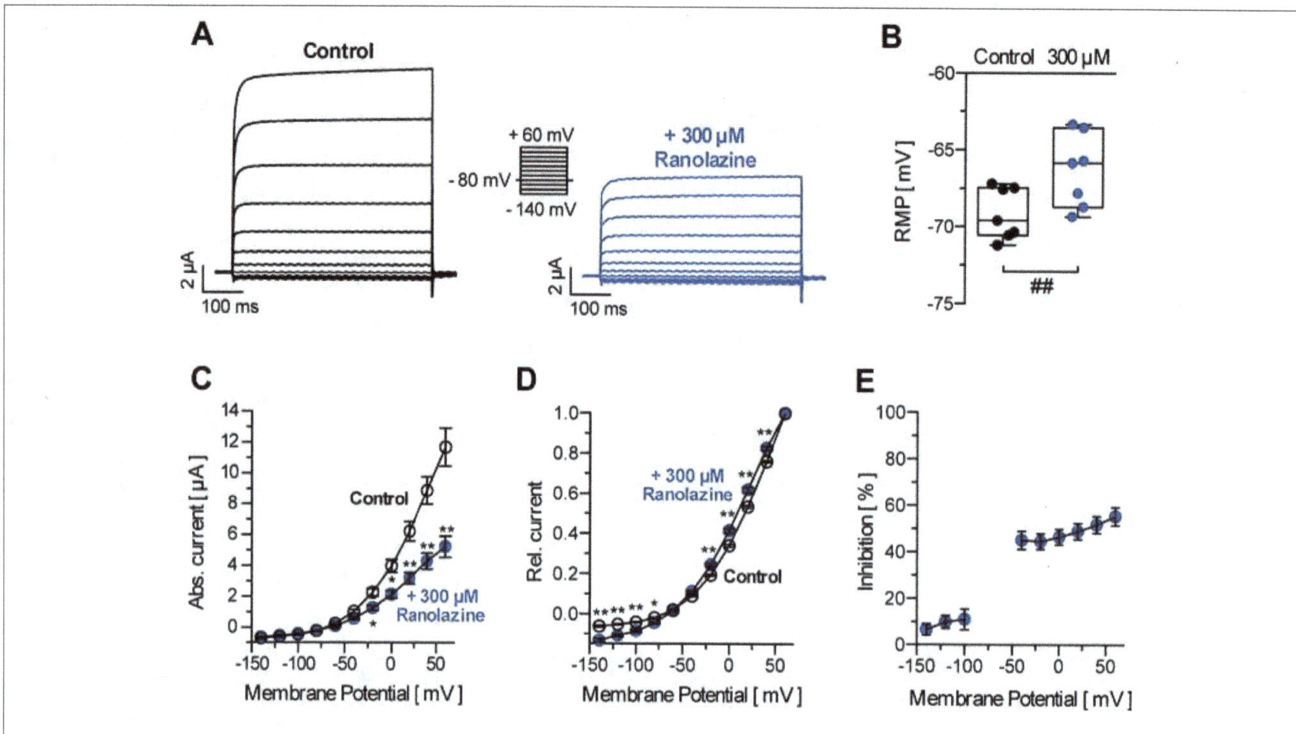

FIGURE 2 | (A) Representative TASK-1 current recordings evoked by applying the displayed pulse protocol under control conditions and after 30 min incubation with ranolazine (300 µM). **(B)** Resting membrane potentials (RMP) in *X. laevis* oocytes before and after 30 min incubation with 300 µM ranolazine (n = 7). Boxes indicate the first and third quartile, whiskers indicate the minimum and maximum, and bands inside the boxes indicate the median; ##p < 0.01, paired t-test. **(C)** Activation curve of TASK-1 current; amplitudes are plotted against the respective test potential under control conditions and after 30 min incubation with ranolazine (n = 10); *p < 0.05, **p < 0.01, unpaired t-test vs. control conditions. **(D)** Amplitudes are normalized to the maximum current amplitude at +60 mV (n = 10); *p < 0.05, **p < 0.01, unpaired t-test vs. control conditions. **(E)** Dependency of TASK-1 current inhibition by ranolazine on membrane potential (n = 10). Data are given as mean ± SEM.

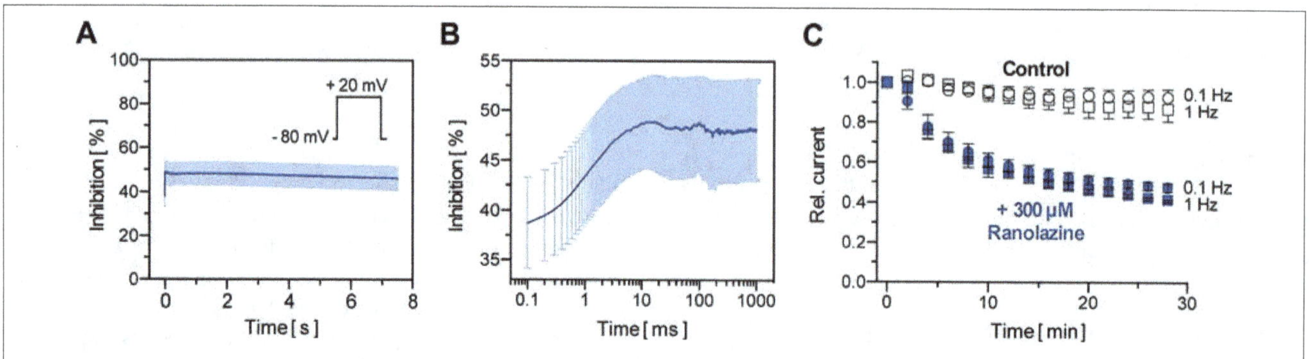

FIGURE 3 | Biophysical properties of TASK-1 blockade by ranolazine. **(A)** The inhibition of TASK-1 current is displayed over a 7.5 s test pulse from –80 mV to +20 mV (n = 6). **(B)** Representation of the first 1000 ms of (A) on a logarithmic time scale (n = 6). **(C)** Frequency dependency of TASK-1 blockade by ranolazine; current amplitudes obtained during 30 min stimulation from –80 mV to +20 mV at stimulation rates of 0.1 Hz and 1 Hz are displayed under control conditions and during administration of 300 µM Ranolazine (n = 5–6). Currents are normalized to their respective values after a stabilization period. Data are given as mean ± SEM.

Effects of Ranolazine on Other Human Two-Pore Domain Potassium (K_{2P}) Channels

We further tested inhibitory effects of ranolazine on other channels within the K_{2P} channel family using a similar approach as reported in **Figure 1A**. Ranolazine (300 µM) was administered after a stabilization period with no significant current amplitude changes (15–20 min). Inhibition of ion currents was quantified after 30 min of ranolazine administration (**Figure 4**). Ranolazine showed small inhibitory effects on TREK-1 (7.35 ± 1.66%, n = 5, p = 0.026) and TRAAK (3.32 ± 1.29%, n = 5, p = 0.045), and more pronounced inhibition of TASK-2 (30.02 ± 6.42%, n = 5, p = 0.037), TALK-1 (23.04 ± 3.06%, n = 5, p = 0.0003), TALK-2 (34.88 ± 2.47%, n = 5, p = 0.024) and TASK-3 currents (28.28 ± 2.1%, n = 5, p = 0.028). Effects on TREK-2 and TRESK were not significant. Ranolazine treatment of THIK-1 lead to slightly enhanced currents (+4.98 ± 0.66%, n = 5, p = 0.002). Taken together, ranolazine favorably inhibits K_{2P} channels that are acid sensitive (TASK-1, TASK-2, TASK-3) or alkaline sensitive (TALK-1, TALK-2).

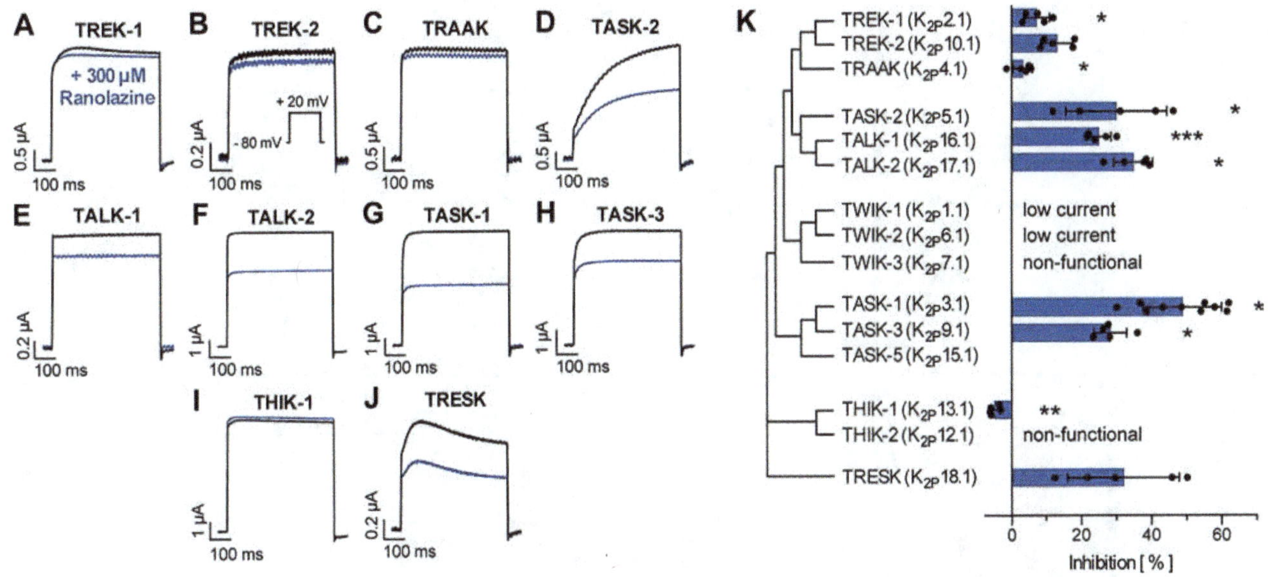

FIGURE 4 | Effect of ranolazine on different members of the K_{2P} channel family. **(A–J)** Representative current recordings evoked by a test pulse from −80 mV to +20 mV under control conditions and after 30 min incubation ranolazine. **(K)** Current inhibition by 300 µM ranolazine is displayed for the different K_{2P} channel family members. Data are given as mean ± SEM. *$p < 0.05$, **$p < 0.01$, ***$p < 0.001$, paired t-test vs. control measurements.

Protein–Ligand Interaction Profile of Ranolazine in the TASK-1 Inner Pore

TASK-1 potassium channels contain four ion binding positions (S1–S4) within the selectivity filter. For *in silico* docking calculations potassium ions were either positioned at S1 and S3 or at S2 and S4 (**Figures 5A, B**). Ten ranked docking poses were calculated for each configuration. The amount and character of the protein–ligand interactions of all docking poses is summarized in **Figure 5C** and displayed separately for the different ion binding configurations. Ranolazine is suggested to form hydrogen bonds with the threonine residues on position T93 and T199 and additional hydrophobic interactions with other pore lining residues. Different ion occupations within the selectivity filter only resulted in a slightly altered interaction profile with fewer hydrogen bonds formed by ranolazine and the threonine residues T93 and T199, and more hydrophobic interactions at position L232.

Ranolazine Inhibition Depends on Amino Acid Residues Located at the Inner Pore of TASK-1

We further investigated the binding site of ranolazine within the TASK-1 inner pore, by individually mutating amino acids that were either predicted to contribute to ranolazine binding in molecular docking simulations, or have been identified as binding site for the high affinity blockers S20951 (A1899) and AVE1231 (A293) (Streit et al., 2011; Wiedmann et al., 2019). Variants T93A, I118A and T199A produced very low current amplitudes that did not allow reasonable pharmacology testing. Inhibitory effects of ranolazine on the functionally active TASK-1 mutants were quantified after 30 min ranolazine incubation at the end of a 500 ms test pulse from −80 mV to +20 mV. **Figure 6 A-H** indicates representative current recordings evoked by a test pulse from -80 mV to +20 mV under control conditions and after 30 min incubation with ranolazine. **Figure 6I** summarizes the current inhibition by 300 µM ranolazine on the different TASK-1 pore mutants. Inhibition of TASK-1 by 300 µM ranolazine was significantly reduced in channel variants L122A (from 48.79 ± 3.52% in wild type (WT) channels to 8.1 ± 3.94% in the mutant variant, n = 5, $p < 0.0001$), L239A (reduced to 22.69 ± 6.73%, n = 5, $p = 0.0007$), and N240A (reduced to 24.29 ± 1.92%, n = 5, $p = 0.0016$). The inhibitory potency of ranolazine remained unchanged in channel variants F125A, Q126A, L232A, and I235A. Note that the amino acids that were included in our mutagenesis screen all line the central cavity of the TASK-1 inner pore (**Figure 6 J-N**).

We further performed *in silico* docking simulations on TASK-1 alanine mutants at positions T93, L122, F125, T199, L232, and I235 that had been identified as the most relevant residues for ranolazine binding in the initial WT docking simulation. The results (summarized in **Figure 7**) suggest, that in channel variants F125A, L232A and I235A, ranolazine was still able to bind and form protein-ligand interactions at the altered binding site. In channel variant L122A the ability to form protein-ligand interactions was impaired; especially the number of relatively stable hydrogen bonds was significantly reduced compared to WT. More detailed information on the individual interaction profiles of ranolazine and the different TASK-1 mutant variants can be found in the supplementary material (**Supplementary Figure S3**).

Figure 8 illustrates the best ranked ranolazine docking pose for WT TASK-1 calculated by AutoDock Vina. Ranolazine is suggested to build a flat layer that binds within the central cavity of the TASK-1 inner pore at the bottom of the selectivity filter occluding the lumen. Ranolazine is located in close proximity (< 4 Å) to amino acid residues L122 and L239 that have also been shown to be relevant for drug binding in the mutagenesis screen. However, N240 is not predicted to contribute to direct drug binding, although the mutant N240A showed reduced ranolazine inhibition.

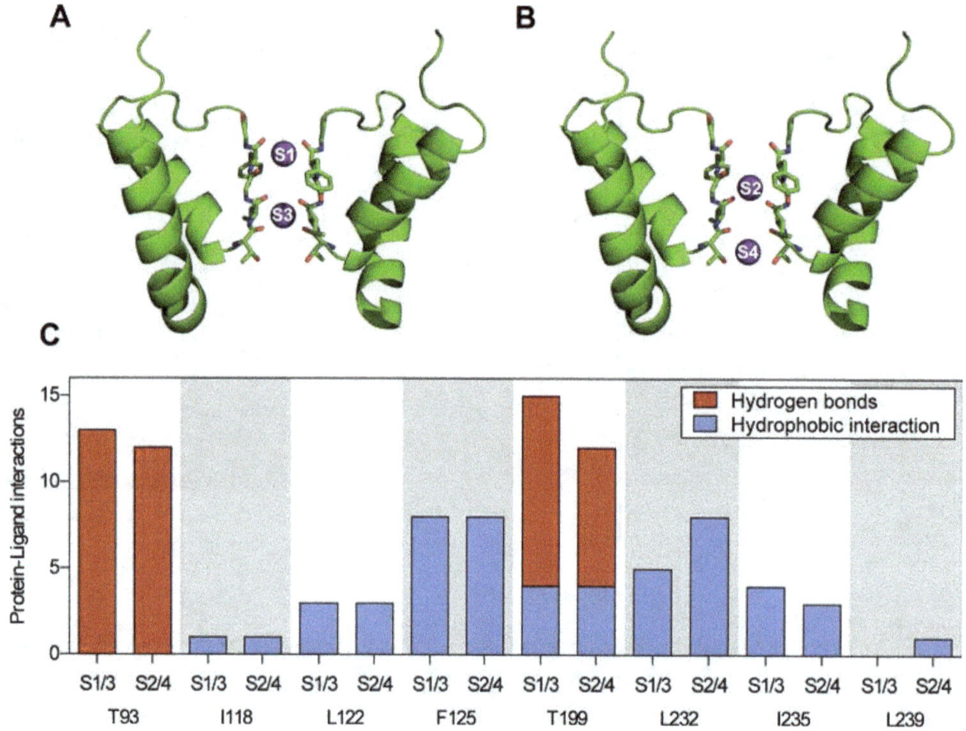

FIGURE 5 | Summary of protein–ligand interactions of all calculated docking poses of ranolazine at the inner pore of the wild type (WT) TASK-1 model (T16cq6). **(A, B)** Docking calculations have been performed with potassium ions either at positions S1 and S3, or at positions S2 and S4. **(C)** Each calculation yielded 10 ranked docking poses, resulting in a total of 20 poses. Protein–ligand interactions have been analyzed using PLIP (Salentin et al., 2015). The amount and character of the interactions is displayed for the individual amino acid residues that interact with ranolazine.

In the illustrated docking pose ranolazine is also predicted to interact with residues F125 and L232, that showed no alteration of inhibition in the experimental data. Ranolazine is further predicted to form hydrogen bonds with residues T93 and T199. The relevance of T93 and T199 could not be validated experimentally due to too small current amplitudes of channel variants T93A and T199A.

DISCUSSION

The development of safe and effective AADs for the treatment of AF is a major clinical challenge (Dobrev and Nattel 2010). Within the past years ranolazine has been identified to deploy potent antiarrhythmic properties and to be effective in the treatment of AF (Guerra et al., 2017). Here we show that ranolazine acts as an inhibitor of the atrial selective TASK-1 potassium channel.

For the prevention of post-operative atrial fibrillation (POAF), ranolazine has been shown to be even more effective than amiodarone (Miles et al., 2011). In this retrospective trial there was no difference in the incidence of adverse events. Ranolazine, however, is considered to be substantially safer in use than amiodarone or other AADs, because it has less proarrhythmic effects on the ventricles (Gupta et al., 2015). This seems to be due to a differential impact on atrial and ventricular cardiomyocytes (Antzelevitch et al., 2011). Burashnikov et al. (2007) noticed that ranolazine was able to prolong the atrial APD and ERP in canine cardiomyocytes with only little effect on the ventricular action potential (AP). They attributed this effect to the inhibition of peak I_{Na} only in atrial but not ventricular cardiomyocytes and therefore proposed atrial-selective sodium channel blockade by ranolazine as a strategy for the treatment of atrial fibrillation (Burashnikov et al., 2007). The mechanism of the atrial-selective block of Na^+ channels has been explained primarily by the rapid dissociation kinetics of ranolazine, a more negative half-inactivation voltage ($V_{0.5}$) in atrial cells than in ventricular cells and a more depolarized RMP in atrial cells. Unblocking of sodium channels is commonly associated with the resting state of the sodium channel (Carmeliet and Mubagwa 1998). Because of a more negative half-inactivation voltage ($V_{0.5}$) in atrial cells than in ventricular cells, a greater fraction of atrial sodium channels would remain in the inactivated state. Therefore the proportion of time that channels are in the resting state would be reduced and hence the dissociation of ranolazine would be slower. Additionally, the availability of sodium channels and the number of channels in the resting state would be further reduced by a more depolarized RMP in atrial cells and the recovery of sodium channels from the inactivated to the resting state is reported to be slower in atrial cells (Antzelevitch and Burashnikov 2009; Nesterenko et al., 2011). Literature regarding a different $V_{0.5}$ in atrial vs. ventricular cardiomyocytes, however, is inconsistent (Sakakibara et al., 1992; Sakakibara et al., 1993; Hiroe et al., 1997; Li et al., 2002). Caves et al. (2017) could recently reproduce atrial selectivity of I_{Na} block by ranolazine in rabbit, providing further evidence that this might be a key element in the atrial-ventricular differences in the action of ranolazine (Caves et al., 2017).

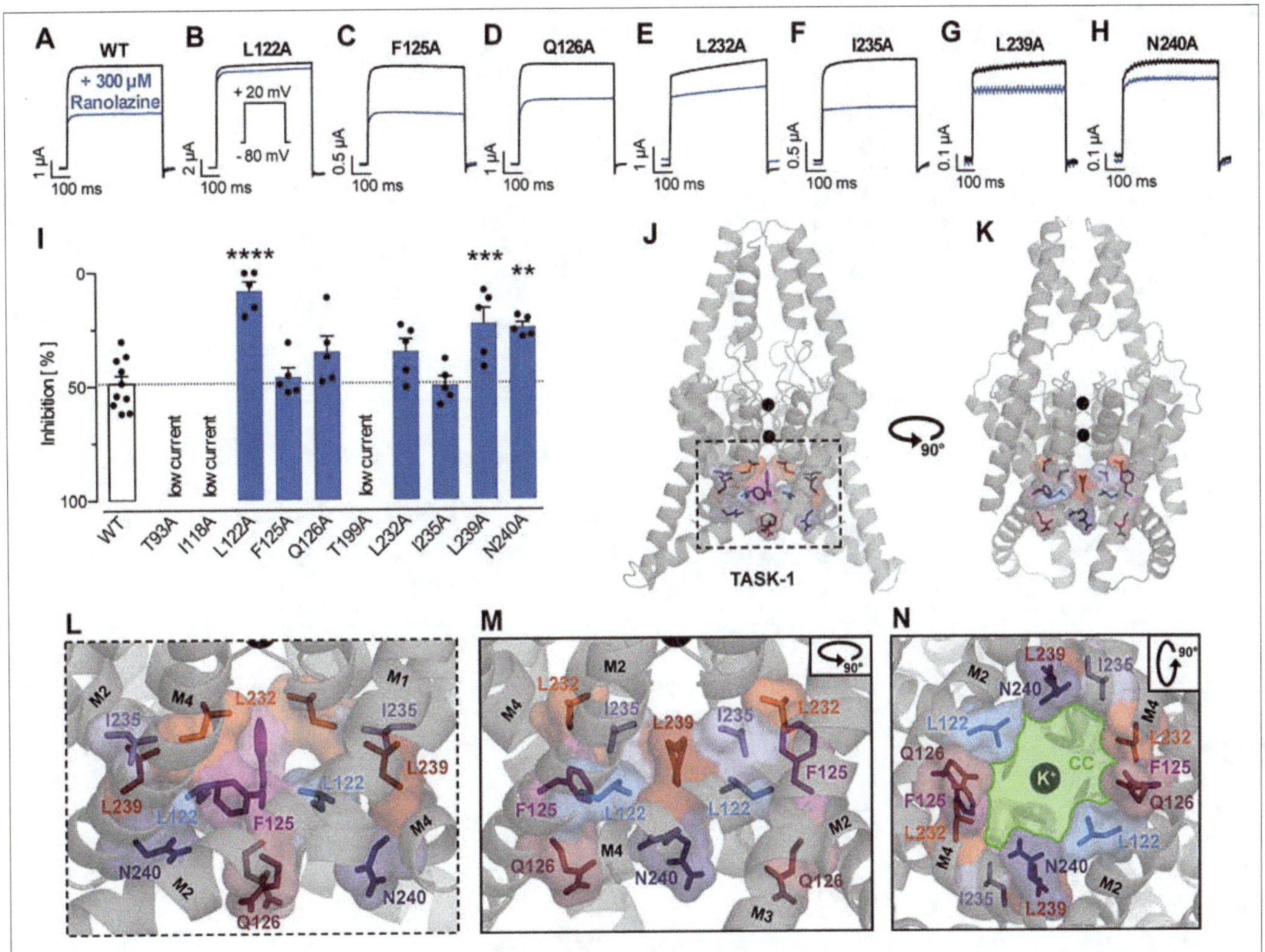

FIGURE 6 | Effect of ranolazine on TASK-1 pore mutants. **(A–H)** Representative current recordings evoked by a test pulse from −80 mV to +20 mV under control conditions and after 30 min incubation with ranolazine. **(I)** Current inhibition by 300 µM ranolazine on the different TASK-1 pore mutants, $^{**}p < 0.01$, $^{***}p < 0.001$, $^{****}p < 0.0001$, one-way ANOVA and post-hoc Bonferroni's multiple comparisons test of WT vs. the respective mutant. **(J, K)** TASK-1 homology model based on TREK-1 illustrating the location of amino acid residues included in the mutagenesis screen. **(L)** Zoom into the inner pore region. **(M)** Lateral view as in panel **(L)** but from a different angle [as in panel **(K)**]. **(N)** View from inside the cell into the central cavity (CC) of the inner pore. Note how the displayed residues line the central cavity (illustrated in green) of the TASK-1 inner pore.

Another explanation for the differential impact on APD prolongation in atrial and ventricular cardiomyocytes lies in the differences of AP configuration between the two cell types that have direct influence on the net effect of simultaneous late I_{Na} and I_{Kr} blockade. Ventricular APs have a more prominent plateau phase than atrial APs. This suggest that there is a smaller late I_{Na} in atrial cells that may result in a shift towards a greater AP prolonging effect of I_{Kr} blockade in atrial cells, whereas in ventricular cells the inhibition of a larger late I_{Na} may offset the I_{Kr} blockade (Du et al., 2014).

We propose that inhibition of TASK-1 potassium channels may contribute to the observed electrophysiological effects of ranolazine. Inhibition of TASK-1 by specific inhibitors has been described to prolong atrial APD and ERP before (Wirth et al., 2003; Wirth et al., 2007; Decher et al., 2011; Donner et al., 2011; Skarsfeldt et al., 2016). Furthermore, the nearly atrial specific expression of TASK-1 could, at least in part, explain the differential behavior of ranolazine between atrial and ventricular tissue (Limberg et al., 2011; Schmidt et al., 2015; Schmidt et al., 2017). The IC_{50} of TASK-1 inhibition by ranolazine is determined at 30.64 µM in mammalian cells which is slightly beyond therapeutic free plasma levels of 2–13.35 µM (Jerling 2006; Undrovinas et al., 2006; EMA 2009; Antzelevitch et al., 2011). Considering that ranolazine has its highest antiarrhythmic potency when administered in high doses, inhibition of TASK-1 current would still be expected *in vivo*. At plasma levels of 10 µM an inhibition of 20% of TASK-1 current is expected. It has to be noticed, however, that TASK-1 blockade by ranolazine is always likely to be less extensive than late I_{Na} (IC_{50} 5.9–15 µM) (Fredj et al., 2006; Antzelevitch et al., 2011) or I_{Kr} blockade (IC_{50} 8–12 µM) (Rajamani et al., 2008; Du et al., 2014). Therefore, the clinical relevance of TASK-1 blockade by ranolazine remains speculative.

We identified the TASK-1 central cavity of the inner pore as the binding site of ranolazine. This binding site overlaps with that of other both high and low affinity blockers of TASK-1 (Streit et al., 2011; Kiper et al., 2015; Schmidt et al., 2018; Wiedmann et al., 2019). The binding configuration of ranolazine within the TASK-1 inner pore is also similar to results published by Du et al. (2014)

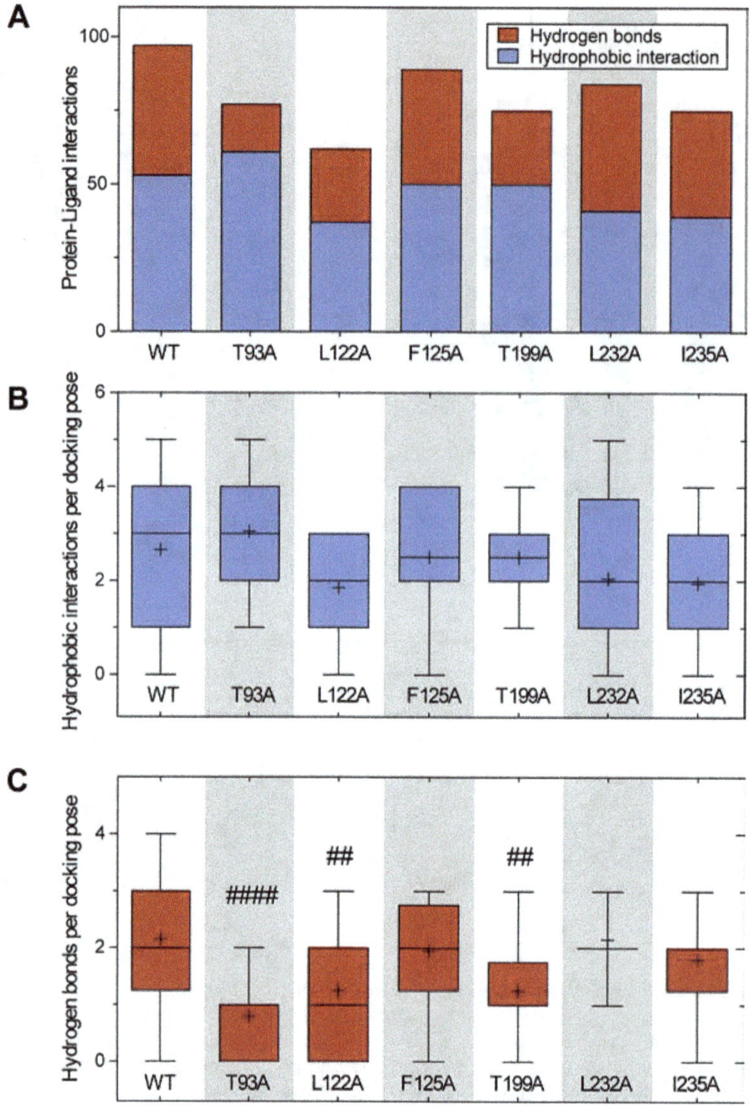

FIGURE 7 | Comparison of the amount of protein–ligand interactions for the docking poses of WT and mutant channels. **(A)** Total amount and character of protein–ligand interactions of all 20 docking poses for the respective channel variant. **(B, C)** Boxplots indicating the amount of hydrophobic interactions **(B)** and hydrogen bonds **(C)** per docking pose. Boxes indicate the first and third quartile, whiskers indicate the minimum and maximum, bands inside the boxes indicate the median, and + indicates the mean. ##p < 0.01, ####p < 0.0001vs. WT. Note that variant L122A that has been identified as being most relevant for ranolazine binding in the experimental data, also forms the fewest interactions in the *in silico* simulations. More detailed information on the interaction profiles of ranolazine and the individual mutant variants can be found in **Supplementary Figure S3**.

for the human Ether à go go Related Gene (hERG) channel, the recombinant equivalent of I_{Kr}. In both TASK-1 and hERG, ranolazine lies high within the inner pore in a horizontal orientation below the selectivity filter where it may form hydrogen bonds with serine or threonine residues (Du et al., 2014). In both channels ranolazine can make additional hydrophobic interactions with pore lining residues (**Figures 5** and **8**). The structural basis for the higher inhibitory potency of ranolazine in hERG may result from a more optimal orientation of the pore lining side chains in hERG, especially in the inactivated state (Chen et al., 2002; Du et al., 2014). Evidence for this hypothesis comes from the observation that mutations of hERG outside the binding site that attenuate channel inactivation and influence configuration of the pore lining side chains to non-optimal arrangements, largely reduce the inhibitory potency of ranolazine without changing the binding site itself (Du et al., 2014).

The binding site is also similar to that in sodium channels, where ranolazine has been shown to interact over a larger surface area that spans from the inner pore to the side fenestration region (Fredj et al., 2006; Nguyen et al., 2019). In sodium channels, access to this binding site is most likely through the cytosolic mouth to the pore and therefore requires opening of the activation gate (Fredj et al., 2006; Wang et al., 2008; Caves et al., 2017). This mechanism provides the structural basis of the use-dependent block of sodium channels (Catterall 2012). In TASK-1, however, the inner pore region is constitutively open and therefore accessible for inhibitors. This may explain why we do not observe use-dependent block of

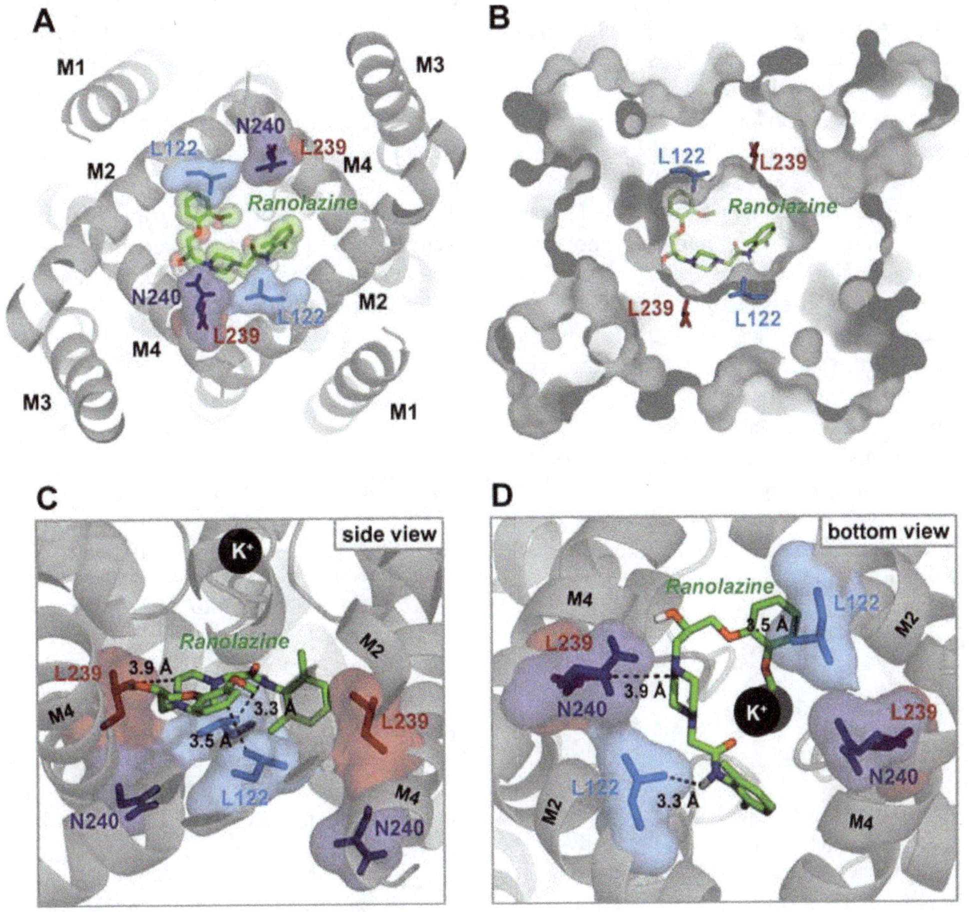

FIGURE 8 | Ranolazine binds to the central cavity of the inner pore. **(A)** View from inside the cell into the central cavity. Ranolazine binds in close proximity to L122 and L239 occluding the lumen of the inner pore. **(B)** Same view as in **(A)** but with TASK-1 surface representation illustrating how ranolazine embeds within the inner pore. **(C)** Zoom into the central cavity illustrating the binding mode and the distance to the residues identified as binding site in the mutagenesis screen. Note that ranolazine does not directly interact with N240. **(D)** Similar zoom as in panel **(C)** but from inside the cell. Note that ranolazine interacts with L122 residues from both monomers.

TASK-1 by ranolazine. Another consequence of the TASK-1 drug binding site being constitutively accessible is that drug dissociation can occur at all time, whereas in sodium channels it requires the channel to be in the resting state (Antzelevitch et al., 2011). This may partly explain the higher inhibitory potency of ranolazine in sodium channels than in the constitutively open TASK-1 channel.

The side fenestrations mentioned earlier as being part of the drug binding site have recently been suggested to play an important role in K_{2P} channel pharmacology by providing an "anchor" for stable binding of inhibitors (Ramirez et al., 2017). In our T16cq6 model (where the model template is TREK-2) the side fenestrations are closed. Therefore, ranolazine is binding solely within the inner pore of TASK-1. When docking ranolazine to the T13ukm model (model template TWIK-1), where the side fenestrations are open, we observe similar binding modes as in the T16cq6 model (**Supplementary Figure S4**). However, with the side fenestrations open, the binding site indeed spans from the inner pore to the entrance of the side fenestrations, because the side chains of L122 and L239 are partly facing towards the fenestrations. Nevertheless, the significance of the side fenestrations in TASK-1 remains speculative, because the structure of TASK-1 has not been revealed yet, and the fenestration state of TASK-1 homology models is ultimately depending on the template used for homology modelling (open fenestrations in TWIK-1, closed fenestrations in TREK-2).

Single mutants F125A, Q126A, L232A and I235A showed no difference in ranolazine blockade, although being predicted to be relevant for ranolazine binding in the *in silico* docking calculations or being identified as binding site for the high affinity blockers S20951 (A1899) and AVE1231 (A293). The reason could be the relatively small size of the ranolazine molecule compared to S20951 and AVE1231. Ranolazine appears to be able to fold into different conformations and hence bind at different sites within the inner pore. The molecular interactions between ranolazine and its binding site are mostly hydrophobic interactions. Only with residues T93 and T199 it forms more stable hydrogen bonds. The ability to form hydrogen bonds appears to be impaired in channel variant L122A, possibly explaining the fact that inhibition by ranolazine is almost abolished in this single mutant.

Study Limitations

Of note, channel variant N240A impedes ranolazine binding without being proposed to be part of the binding site in the *in silico* simulations. It remains unclear whether this is due to methodological limitations of homology modelling and docking simulations or results from interferences of the large asparagine side chain with structural domain morphology, therefore impeding the accessibility to the TASK-1 inner pore for inhibitors. The latter would be supported by the observation that movements or alterations of the M4 transmembrane domain (where N240 is located) affect channel gaiting in other K_{2P} channels (Bagriantsev et al., 2011; Lolicato et al., 2014). However, results obtained by homology modelling are naturally largely influenced by the template that is chosen for modelling. We therefore tried to assess the models quality to our best possibilities. To assess possible influences of the fenestration state of our model, we performed additional docking simulations on the T1ukm model. Of course, deeper insights in this regard would require the solvation of the TASK-1 crystal structure.

Another limitation of this study is that a direct effect of the TASK-1 mutants on channel gating and therefore possible allosteric effects on TASK-1 pharmacology cannot be ruled out. Nevertheless, measurements of an inhibitor's potency on different central pore mutants and comparisons with *in silico* docking simulations on homology models has been a widely accepted strategy in the field thus far.

CONCLUSIONS

This study adds to the action profile of ranolazine. We demonstrate that ranolazine is a TASK-1 inhibitor and suggest that TASK-1 inhibition may contribute to the antiarrhythmic effects of ranolazine. We propose that TASK-1 inhibition could, at least in part, explain the atrial selectivity of APD-prolongation by ranolazine. Even though the efficacy of ranolazine in AF might not yet be optimal, our findings put forward ranolazine as a prototype drug for the treatment of atrial arrhythmia because of its combined efficacy on atrial electrophysiology and lower risk for ventricular side effects.

AUTHOR CONTRIBUTIONS

AR, CS, and HK conceived and designed the experiments. AR, FW, and MK carried out the experiments. AR, FW, MK, and CS contributed to the interpretation of the results. AR and CS visualized the data and wrote the manuscript. HK and CS supervised the project. All authors provided critical feedback and helped shape the research, analysis and manuscript by providing important intellectual content. Further, all persons designated as authors qualify for authorship, and all those who qualify for authorship are listed. All authors agree to be accountable for all aspects of the work in ensuring that questions related to the accuracy or integrity of any part of the work are appropriately investigated and resolved. All authors approved the final version of the manuscript.

FUNDING

This study was supported in part by research grants from the University of Heidelberg Faculty of Medicine [Rahel Goitein-Straus Scholarship and Olympia-Morata Scholarship (to CS)], the German Center for Cardiovascular Research [Excellence Grant (to CS)], the German Heart Foundation/ German Foundation of Heart Research [Grant F/41/15 (to CS), Grant F/35/18 (to FW and CS) and a Kaltenbach Scholarship (to AR and FW)], and the German Research Foundation [Grant SCHM 3358/1-1 (to CS)]. FW was supported by a German Cardiac Society Otto-Hess Scholarship and Research Scholarship. We acknowledge financial support by Deutsche Forschungsgemeinschaft within the funding programme Open Access Publishing, by the Baden-Württemberg Ministry of Science, Research and the Arts and by Ruprecht-Karls-Universität Heidelberg.

ACKNOWLEDGMENTS

We thank Katrin Kupser and Sabine Höllriegel for the excellent technical support.

REFERENCES

Antzelevitch, C., and Burashnikov, A. (2009). A trial-selective sodium channel block as a novel strategy for the management of atrial fibrillation. *J. Electrocardiol.* 42 (6), 543–548. doi: 10.1016/j.jelectrocard.2009.07.007

Antzelevitch, C., Burashnikov, A., Sicouri, S., and Belardinelli, L. (2011). Electrophysiologic basis for the antiarrhythmic actions of ranolazine. *Heart Rhythm* 8 (8), 1281–1290. doi: 10.1016/j.hrthm.2011.03.045

Bagriantsev, S. N., Peyronnet, R., Clark, K. A., Honore, E., and Minor, D. L. Jr. (2011). Multiple modalities converge on a common gate to control K2P channel function. *Embo J.* 30 (17), 3594–3606. doi: 10.1038/emboj.2011.230

Benkert, P., Biasini, M., and Schwede, T. (2011). Toward the estimation of the absolute quality of individual protein structure models. *Bioinformatics* 27 (3), 343–350. doi: 10.1093/bioinformatics/btq662

Bertoni, M., Kiefer, F., Biasini, M., Bordoli, L., and Schwede, T. (2017). Modeling protein quaternary structure of homo- and hetero-oligomers beyond binary interactions by homology. *Sci. Rep.* 7 (1), 10480. doi: 10.1038/s41598-017-09654-8

Bittner, S., Meuth, S. G., Gobel, K., Melzer, N., Herrmann, A. M., and Simon, O. J. (2009). TASK1 modulates inflammation and neurodegeneration in autoimmune inflammation of the central nervous system. *Brain* 132 (Pt 9), 2501–2516. doi: 10.1093/brain/awp163

Buckler, K. J., Williams, B. A., and Honore, E. (2000). An oxygen-, acid- and anaesthetic-sensitive TASK-like background potassium channel in rat arterial chemoreceptor cells. *J. Physiol.* 525 Pt 1, 135–142. doi: 10.1111/j.1469-7793.2000.00135.x

Burashnikov, A., Di Diego, J. M., Zygmunt, A. C., Belardinelli, L., and Antzelevitch, C. (2007). Atrium-selective sodium channel block as a strategy for suppression of atrial fibrillation: differences in sodium channel inactivation between atria and ventricles and the role of ranolazine. *Circulation* 116 (13), 1449–1457. doi: 10.1161/CIRCULATIONAHA.107.704890

Carmeliet, E., and Mubagwa, K. (1998). Antiarrhythmic drugs and cardiac ion channels: mechanisms of action. *Prog. Biophys. Mol. Biol.* 70 (1), 1–72. doi: 10.1016/S0079-6107(98)00002-9

Catterall, W. A. (2012). Voltage-gated sodium channels at 60: structure, function and pathophysiology. *J. Physiol.* 590 (11), 2577–2589. doi: 10.1113/jphysiol.2011.224204

Caves, R. E., Cheng, H., Choisy, S. C., Gadeberg, H. C., Bryant, S. M., and Hancox, J. C. (2017). Atrial-ventricular differences in rabbit cardiac voltage-gated Na^+ currents: basis for atrial-selective block by ranolazine. *Heart Rhythm* 14 (11), 1657–1664. doi: 10.1016/j.hrthm.2017.06.012

Chen, J., Seebohm, G., and Sanguinetti, M. C. (2002). Position of aromatic residues in the S6 domain, not inactivation, dictates cisapride sensitivity of HERG and eag potassium channels. *Proc. Natl. Acad. Sci. U. S. A.* 99 (19), 12461–12466. doi: 10.1073/pnas.192367299

Czirjak, G., and Enyedi, P. (2002). TASK-3 dominates the background potassium conductance in rat adrenal glomerulosa cells. *Mol. Endocrinol.* 16 (3), 621–629. doi: 10.1210/mend.16.3.0788

Davies, L. A., Hu, C., Guagliardo, N. A., Sen, N., Chen, X., and Talley, E. M. (2008). TASK channel deletion in mice causes primary hyperaldosteronism. *Proc. Natl. Acad. Sci. U. S. A.* 105 (6), 2203–2208. doi: 10.1073/pnas.0712000105

Davis, I. W., Leaver-Fay, A., Chen, V. B., Block, J. N., Kapral, G. J., and Wang, X. (2007). MolProbity: all-atom contacts and structure validation for proteins and nucleic acids. *Nucleic Acids Res.* 35 (Web Server issue), W375–W383. doi: 10.1093/nar/gkm216

Decher, N., Wemhoner, K., Rinne, S., Netter, M. F., Zuzarte, M., and Aller, M. I. (2011). Knock-out of the potassium channel TASK-1 leads to a prolonged QT interval and a disturbed QRS complex. *Cell Physiol. Biochem.* 28 (1), 77–86. doi: 10.1159/000331715

Dobrev, D., and Nattel, S. (2010). New antiarrhythmic drugs for treatment of atrial fibrillation. *Lancet* 375 (9721), 1212–1223. doi: 10.1016/S0140-6736(10)60096-7

Dong, Y. Y., Pike, A. C., Mackenzie, A., McClenaghan, C., Aryal, P., and Dong, L. (2015). K2P channel gating mechanisms revealed by structures of TREK-2 and a complex with Prozac. *Science* 347 (6227), 1256–1259. doi: 10.1126/science.1261512

Donner, B. C., Schullenberg, M., Geduldig, N., Huning, A., Mersmann, J., and Zacharowski, K. (2011). Functional role of TASK-1 in the heart: studies in TASK-1-deficient mice show prolonged cardiac repolarization and reduced heart rate variability. *Basic Res. Cardiol.* 106 (1), 75–87. doi: 10.1007/s00395-010-0128-x

Du, C., Zhang, Y., El Harchi, A., Dempsey, C. E., and Hancox, J. C. (2014). Ranolazine inhibition of hERG potassium channels: drug-pore interactions and reduced potency against inactivation mutants. *J. Mol. Cell Cardiol.* 74, 220–230. doi: 10.1016/j.yjmcc.2014.05.013

EMA (2009, 20/05/2019). Ranexa: EPAR - Product Information. *Eur. Med. Agency*. https://www.ema.europa.eu/en/documents/product-information/ranexa-epar-product-information_en.pdf.

Feliciangeli, S., Chatelain, F. C., Bichet, D., and Lesage, F. (2015). The family of K2P channels: salient structural and functional properties. *J. Physiol.* 593 (12), 2587–2603. doi: 10.1113/jphysiol.2014.287268

Fredj, S., Sampson, K. J., Liu, H., and Kass, R. S. (2006). Molecular basis of ranolazine block of LQT-3 mutant sodium channels: evidence for site of action. *Br. J. Pharmacol.* 148 (1), 16–24. doi: 10.1038/sj.bjp.0706709

Gierten, J., Ficker, E., Bloehs, R., Schlomer, K., Kathofer, S., and Scholz, E. (2008). Regulation of two-pore-domain (K2P) potassium leak channels by the tyrosine kinase inhibitor genistein. *Br. J. Pharmacol.* 154 (8), 1680–1690. doi: 10.1038/bjp.2008.213

Goldstein, S. A., Bockenhauer, D., O'Kelly, I., and Zilberberg, N. (2001). Potassium leak channels and the KCNK family of two-P-domain subunits. *Nat. Rev. Neurosci.* 2 (3), 175–184. doi: 10.1038/35058574

Guerra, F., Romandini, A., Barbarossa, A., Belardinelli, L., and Capucci, A. (2017). "Ranolazine for rhythm control in atrial fibrillation: a systematic review and meta-analysis.". *Int. J. Cardiol.* 227, 284–291. doi: 10.1016/j.ijcard.2016.11.103

Gupta, T., Khera, S., Kolte, D., Aronow, W. S., and Iwai, S. (2015). Antiarrhythmic properties of ranolazine: a review of the current evidence. *Int. J. Cardiol.* 187, 66–74. doi: 10.1016/j.ijcard.2015.03.324

Hiroe, K., Hisatome, I., Tanaka, Y., Ahmmed, G. U., Sasaki, N., and Shimoyama, M. (1997). Tonic block of the Na+ current in single atrial and ventricular guinea-pig myocytes, by a new antiarrhythmic drug, Ro 22-9194. *Fundam. Clin. Pharmacol.* 11 (5), 402–407. doi: 10.1111/j.1472-8206.1997.tb00202.x

January, C. T., Wann, L. S., Alpert, J. S., Calkins, H., Cigarroa, J. E., and Cleveland, J. C. Jr. (2014). 2014 AHA/ACC/HRS guideline for the management of patients with atrial fibrillation: a report of the American College of Cardiology/American Heart Association Task Force on Practice Guidelines and the Heart Rhythm Society. *J. Am. Coll. Cardiol.* 64 (21), e1–76. doi: 10.1016/j.jacc.2014.03.022

Jerling, M. (2006). Clinical pharmacokinetics of ranolazine. *Clin. Pharmacokinet.* 45 (5), 469–491. doi: 10.2165/00003088-200645050-00003

Kiper, A. K., Rinne, S., Rolfes, C., Ramirez, D., Seebohm, G., and Netter, M. F. (2015). Kv1.5 blockers preferentially inhibit TASK-1 channels: TASK-1 as a target against atrial fibrillation and obstructive sleep apnea? *Pflugers Arch.* 467 (5), 1081–1090. doi: 10.1007/s00424-014-1665-1

Kirchhof, P., Benussi, S., Kotecha, D., Ahlsson, A., Atar, D., and Casadei, B. (2016). 2016 ESC Guidelines for the management of atrial fibrillation developed in collaboration with EACTS. *Eur. Heart J.* 37 (38), 2893–2962. doi: 10.1093/eurheartj/ehw210

Koizumi, H., Smerin, S. E., Yamanishi, T., Moorjani, B. R., Zhang, R., and Smith, J. C. (2010). TASK channels contribute to the K+-dominated leak current regulating respiratory rhythm generation *in vitro*. *J. Neurosci.* 30 (12), 4273–4284. doi: 10.1523/JNEUROSCI.4017-09.2010

Lafuente-Lafuente, C., Valembois, L., Bergmann, J. F., and Belmin, J. (2015). Antiarrhythmics for maintaining sinus rhythm after cardioversion of atrial fibrillation. *Cochrane Database Syst. Rev.* (3), Cd005049. doi: 10.1002/14651858.CD005049.pub4

Lauritzen, I., Zanzouri, M., Honore, E., Duprat, F., Ehrengruber, M. U., and Lazdunski, M. (2003). K+-dependent cerebellar granule neuron apoptosis. Role of task leak K+ channels. *J. Biol. Chem.* 278 (34), 32068–32076. doi: 10.1074/jbc.M302631200

Lazarenko, R. M., Willcox, S. C., Shu, S., Berg, A. P., Jevtovic-Todorovic, V., and Talley, E. M. (2010). Motoneuronal TASK channels contribute to immobilizing effects of inhalational general anesthetics. *J. Neurosci.* 30 (22), 7691–7704. doi: 10.1523/JNEUROSCI.1655-10.2010

Li, G. R., Lau, C. P., and Shrier, A. (2002). Heterogeneity of sodium current in atrial vs epicardial ventricular myocytes of adult guinea pig hearts. *J. Mol. Cell Cardiol.* 34 (9), 1185–1194. doi: 10.1006/jmcc.2002.2053

Limberg, S. H., Netter, M. F., Rolfes, C., Rinne, S., Schlichthorl, G., and Zuzarte, M. (2011). TASK-1 channels may modulate action potential duration of human atrial cardiomyocytes. *Cell Physiol. Biochem.* 28 (4), 613–624. doi: 10.1159/000335757

Lolicato, M., Riegelhaupt, P. M., Arrigoni, C., Clark, K. A., and Minor, D. L. Jr. (2014). Transmembrane helix straightening and buckling underlies activation of mechanosensitive and thermosensitive K(2P) channels. *Neuron* 84 (6), 1198–1212. doi: 10.1016/j.neuron.2014.11.017

Lolicato, M., Arrigoni, C., Mori, T., Sekioka, Y., Bryant, C., and Clark, K. A. (2017). K2P2.1 (TREK-1)-activator complexes reveal a cryptic selectivity filter binding site. *Nature* 547 (7663), 364–368. doi: 10.1038/nature22988

Miles, R. H., Passman, R., and Murdock, D. K. (2011). Comparison of effectiveness and safety of ranolazine versus amiodarone for preventing atrial fibrillation after coronary artery bypass grafting. *Am. J. Cardiol.* 108 (5), 673–676. doi: 10.1016/j.amjcard.2011.04.017

Miller, A. N., and Long, S. B. (2012). Crystal structure of the human two-pore domain potassium channel K2P1. *Science* 335 (6067), 432–436. doi: 10.1126/science.1213274

Mulkey, D. K., Talley, E. M., Stornetta, R. L., Siegel, A. R., West, G. H., and Chen, X. (2007). TASK channels determine pH sensitivity in select respiratory neurons but do not contribute to central respiratory chemosensitivity. *J. Neurosci.* 27 (51), 14049–14058. doi: 10.1523/JNEUROSCI.4254-07.2007

Nash, D. T., and Nash, S. D. (2008). Ranolazine for chronic stable angina. *Lancet* 372 (9646), 1335–1341. doi: 10.1016/S0140-6736(08)61554-8

Nesterenko, V. V., Zygmunt, A. C., Rajamani, S., Belardinelli, L., and Antzelevitch, C. (2011). Mechanisms of atrial-selective block of Na(+) channels by ranolazine: II. Insights from a mathematical model. *Am. J. Physiol. Heart Circ. Physiol.* 301 (4), H1615–H1624. doi: 10.1152/ajpheart.00243.2011

Nguyen, P. T., DeMarco, K. R., Vorobyov, I., Clancy, C. E., and Yarov-Yarovoy, V. (2019). Structural basis for antiarrhythmic drug interactions with the human cardiac sodium channel. *Proc. Natl. Acad. Sci. U.S.A.* 116 (8), 2945–2954. doi: 10.1073/pnas.1817446116

Olschewski, A., Li, Y., Tang, B., Hanze, J., Eul, B., and Bohle, R. M. (2006). Impact of TASK-1 in human pulmonary artery smooth muscle cells. *Circ. Res.* 98 (8), 1072–1080. doi: 10.1161/01.RES.0000219677.12988.e9

Putzke, C., Wemhoner, K., Sachse, F. B., Rinne, S., Schlichthorl, G., and Li, X. T. (2007). The acid-sensitive potassium channel TASK-1 in rat cardiac muscle. *Cardiovasc. Res.* 75 (1), 59–68. doi: 10.1016/j.cardiores.2007.02.025

Rajamani, S., Shryock, J. C., and Belardinelli, L. (2008). Rapid kinetic interactions of ranolazine with HERG K+ current. *J. Cardiovasc. Pharmacol.* 51 (6), 581–589. doi: 10.1097/FJC.0b013e3181799690

Ramirez, D., Arevalo, B., Martinez, G., Rinne, S., Sepulveda, F. V., and Decher, N. (2017). Side Fenestrations Provide anAnchorfor a Stable Binding of A1899 to the Pore of TASK-1 Potassium Channels. *Mol. Pharm.* 14 (7), 2197–2208. doi: 10.1021/acs.molpharmaceut.7b00005

Sakakibara, Y., Wasserstrom, J. A., Furukawa, T., Jia, H., Arentzen, C. E., and Hartz, R. S. (1992). Characterization of the sodium current in single human atrial myocytes. *Circ. Res.* 71 (3), 535–546. doi: 10.1161/01.RES.71.3.535

Sakakibara, Y., Furukawa, T., Singer, D. H., Jia, H., Backer, C. L., and Arentzen, C. E. (1993). Sodium current in isolated human ventricular myocytes. *Am. J. Physiol.* 265 (4 Pt 2), H1301–H1309. doi: 10.1152/ajpheart.1993.265.4.H1301

Salentin, S., Schreiber, S., Haupt, V. J., Adasme, M. F., and Schroeder, M. (2015). PLIP: fully automated protein-ligand interaction profiler. *Nucleic Acids Res.* 43 (W1), W443–W447. doi: 10.1093/nar/gkv315

Schmidt, C., Wiedmann, F., Schweizer, P. A., Becker, R., Katus, H. A., and Thomas, D. (2013). Class I antiarrhythmic drugs inhibit human cardiac two-pore-domain K(+) (K2 (2)p) channels. *Eur. J. Pharmacol.* 721 (1-3), 237–248. doi: 10.1016/j.ejphar.2013.09.029

Schmidt, C., Wiedmann, F., Voigt, N., Zhou, X. B., Heijman, J., and Lang, S. (2015). Upregulation of K(2P)3.1 K+ Current Causes Action Potential Shortening in Patients With Chronic Atrial Fibrillation. *Circulation* 132 (2), 82–92. doi: 10.1161/CIRCULATIONAHA.114.012657

Schmidt, C., Wiedmann, F., Zhou, X. B., Heijman, J., Voigt, N., and Ratte, A. (2017). Inverse remodelling of K2P3.1 K+ channel expression and action potential duration in left ventricular dysfunction and atrial fibrillation: implications for patient-specific antiarrhythmic drug therapy. *Eur. Heart J.* 38 (22), 1764–1774. doi: 10.1093/eurheartj/ehw559

Schmidt, C., Wiedmann, F., Gaubatz, A. R., Ratte, A., Katus, H. A., and Thomas, D. (2018). New Targets for Old Drugs: Cardiac Glycosides Inhibit Atrial-Specific K2P3.1 (TASK-1) Channels. *J. Pharmacol. Exp. Ther.* 365 (3), 614–623. doi: 10.1124/jpet.118.247692

Skarsfeldt, M. A., Jepps, T. A., Bomholtz, S. H., Abildgaard, L., Sorensen, U. S., and Gregers, E. (2016). pH-dependent inhibition of K(2)P3.1 prolongs atrial refractoriness in whole hearts. *Pflugers Arch.* 468 (4), 643–654. doi: 10.1007/s00424-015-1779-0

Sossalla, S., Kallmeyer, B., Wagner, S., Mazur, M., Maurer, U., and Toischer, K. (2010). Altered Na(+) currents in atrial fibrillation effects of ranolazine on arrhythmias and contractility in human atrial myocardium. *J. Am. Coll. Cardiol.* 55 (21), 2330–2342. doi: 10.1016/j.jacc.2009.12.055

Streit, A. K., Netter, M. F., Kempf, F., Walecki, M., Rinne, S., and Bollepalli, M. K. (2011). A specific two-pore domain potassium channel blocker defines the structure of the TASK-1 open pore. *J. Biol. Chem.* 286 (16), 13977–13984. doi: 10.1074/jbc.M111.227884

Trott, O., and Olson, A. J. (2010). AutoDock Vina: improving the speed and accuracy of docking with a new scoring function, efficient optimization, and multithreading. *J. Comput. Chem.* 31 (2), 455–461. doi: 10.1002/jcc.21334

Undrovinas, A. I., Belardinelli, L., Undrovinas, N. A., and Sabbah, H. N. (2006). Ranolazine improves abnormal repolarization and contraction in left ventricular myocytes of dogs with heart failure by inhibiting late sodium current. *J. Cardiovasc. Electrophysiol.* 17 Suppl 1, S169–s177. doi: 10.1111/j.1540-8167.2006.00401.x

Vu, M. T., Du, G., Bayliss, D. A., and Horner, R. L. (2015). TASK Channels on Basal Forebrain Cholinergic Neurons Modulate Electrocortical Signatures of Arousal by Histamine. *J. Neurosci.* 35 (40), 13555–13567. doi: 10.1523/JNEUROSCI.1445-15.2015

Wang, G. K., Calderon, J., and Wang, S. Y. (2008). State- and use-dependent block of muscle Nav1.4 and neuronal Nav1.7 voltage-gated Na+ channel isoforms by ranolazine. *Mol. Pharmacol.* 73 (3), 940–948. doi: 10.1124/mol.107.041541

Waterhouse, A., Bertoni, M., Bienert, S., Studer, G., Tauriello, G., and Gumienny, R. (2018). SWISS-MODEL: homology modelling of protein structures and complexes. *Nucleic Acids Res.* 46 (W1), W296–w303. doi: 10.1093/nar/gky427

Wiedmann, F., Kiper, A. K., Bedoya, M., Ratte, A., Rinne, S., and Kraft, M. (2019). Identification of the A293 (AVE1231) binding site in the cardiac two-pore-domain potassium channel task-1: a common low affinity antiarrhythmic drug binding site. *Cell Physiol. Biochem.* 52 (5), 1223–1235. doi: 10.33594/000000083

Wirth, K. J., Paehler, T., Rosenstein, B., Knobloch, K., Maier, T., and Frenzel, J. (2003). Atrial effects of the novel K(+)-channel-blocker AVE0118 in anesthetized pigs. *Cardiovasc. Res.* 60 (2), 298–306. doi: 10.1016/S0008-6363(03)00543-1

Wirth, K. J., Brendel, J., Steinmeyer, K., Linz, D. K., Rutten, H., and Gogelein, H. (2007). In vitro and *in vivo* effects of the atrial selective antiarrhythmic compound AVE1231. *J. Cardiovasc. Pharmacol.* 49 (4), 197–206. doi: 10.1097/FJC.0b013e318032002f

10

Handling of Ventricular Fibrillation in the Emergency Setting

Zoltán Szabó[1], Dóra Ujvárosy[1,2], Tamás Ötvös[1,2], Veronika Sebestyén[1,2] and Péter P. Nánási[3,4]*

[1] Department of Emergency Medicine, Faculty of Medicine, University of Debrecen, Debrecen, Hungary, [2] Doctoral School of Health Sciences, Faculty of Public Health, University of Debrecen, Debrecen, Hungary, [3] Department of Physiology, Faculty of Medicine, University of Debrecen, Debrecen, Hungary, [4] Department of Dental Physiology, Faculty of Dentistry, University of Debrecen, Debrecen, Hungary

***Correspondence:**
Zoltán Szabó
szaboz.med@gmail.com*

Ventricular fibrillation (VF) and sudden cardiac death (SCD) are predominantly caused by channelopathies and cardiomyopathies in youngsters and coronary heart disease in the elderly. Temporary factors, e.g., electrolyte imbalance, drug interactions, and substance abuses may play an additive role in arrhythmogenesis. Ectopic automaticity, triggered activity, and reentry mechanisms are known as important electrophysiological substrates for VF determining the antiarrhythmic therapies at the same time. Emergency need for electrical cardioversion is supported by the fact that every minute without defibrillation decreases survival rates by approximately 7%–10%. Thus, early defibrillation is an essential part of antiarrhythmic emergency management. Drug therapy has its relevance rather in the prevention of sudden cardiac death, where early recognition and treatment of the underlying disease has significant importance. Cardioprotective and antiarrhythmic effects of beta blockers in patients predisposed to sudden cardiac death were highlighted in numerous studies, hence nowadays these drugs are considered to be the cornerstones of the prevention and treatment of life-threatening ventricular arrhythmias. Nevertheless, other medical therapies have not been proven to be useful in the prevention of VF. Although amiodarone has shown positive results occasionally, this was not demonstrated to be consistent. Furthermore, the potential proarrhythmic effects of drugs may also limit their applicability. Based on these unfavorable observations we highlight the importance of arrhythmia prevention, where echocardiography, electrocardiography and laboratory testing play a significant role even in the emergency setting. In the following we provide a summary on the latest developments on cardiopulmonary resuscitation, and the evaluation and preventive treatment possibilities of patients with increased susceptibility to VF and SCD.

Keywords: ventricular fibrillation, sudden cardiac death, cardiopulmonary resuscitation, ventricular repolarization, electrocardiography

INTRODUCTION

Ventricular fibrillation (VF) is an emergency condition that, without immediate treatment, leads to death. In the event of this malignant ventricular arrhythmia chaotic, disorganized electrical activity appears in the ventricular myocardium. In such cases the heart is unable to transport blood effectively, which leads to circulatory collapse, clinical death, and if left unattended, biological death.

Sudden cardiac death (SCD) is a leading death cause all over the world, affecting some 5 million people a year (Berdowski et al., 2010; Glinge et al., 2016) with a low survival rate of approximately 10% (Kim et al., 2016). In the United States 300–400 thousand, while in Europe 700 thousand cases of sudden cardiac death are registered a year. Its incidence is 100/100000 in the case of 50-year-old men, it is as high as 800/100000 among men 75 years of age. SCD is more frequent among men than women (6.68/100000 vs. 1.4/100000) (Eckart et al., 2011; Priori et al., 2015). VF is the arrhythmia to manifest first and with the highest frequency in relation to registered circulatory collapses (Rea et al., 2004), which accounts for about 30% of the cases (Bourque et al., 2007).

PATHOLOGICAL CONDITIONS UNDERLYING VENTRICULAR FIBRILLATION

The most common factors that may contribute to the development of VF are acquired risk factors, e.g., ischemic heart disease, cardiomyopathies, electrolyte imbalances, certain drug therapies affecting myocardial repolarization, and less frequently inherited disorders, e.g., ion channel abnormalities (channelopathies), congenital valvular diseases, and coronary artery anomalies. (**Table 1**) (Garson and McNamara, 1985; Jouven et al., 1999; Thompson et al., 2000; Frothingham, 2001; Haddad and Anderson, 2002; Taylor, 2003; Yap and Camm, 2003; Vieweg and Wood, 2004; Owens and Ambrose, 2005; Haissaguerre et al., 2008; Priori et al., 2015; Aiba, 2019; Coutinho Cruz et al., 2019).

TABLE 1 | Etiology of ventricular fibrillation.

PATHOLOGICAL FACTORS THAT PLAY A ROLE IN THE DEVELOPMENT OF VENTRICULAR FIBRILLATION		
INHERITED	**ACQUIRED**	**TEMPORARY CAUSES**
long QT syndrome	ischemic heart disease	sepsis
short QT syndrome	chronic kidney disease	electrolyte disorders (especially K^+ and Mg^{++})
Brugada-syndrome	hypertension	electrocution
catecholaminergic polymorphic ventricular tachycardia	cardiomyopathies	drug abuse (cocaine, methamphetamine)
arrhythmogenic right ventricular dysplasia	acquired aortic disorders	provocative body posture in the case of structural heart disease
single nucleotide polymorphisms (e.g. on 21q21 and 2q24.2 loci)	prior aborted cardiac death	drugs affecting QT interval: antimicrobial agents antipsychotics
J-point elevation syndromes	post-valvular surgery, post-TGA surgery or other heart surgeries	antidepressants antiarrhythmic drugs: amiodarone, sotalol,
inherited structural heart diseases (tetralogy of Fallot, VSD, mitral prolapse, aortic disorders)	post-PCI or post-thrombolysis (reperfusion damage)	procainamide, quinidine, dofetilide, ibutilide

VSD, ventricular septal defect, TGA, transposition of the great arteries, PCI, primary coronary intervention.

Channelopathies listed under inherited primary arrhythmia syndromes, like long and short QT syndromes and Brugada-syndrome (BrS), are important pathogenetic factors (Aiba, 2019). In 70% of long QT syndromes (LQTS) the mutation of the *KCNQ1* or the *KCNH2* (*hERG*) genes have been clarified. These genes encode the potassium channels responsible for the slow (I_{Ks}) and rapid component (I_{Kr}) of the delayed rectifier repolarising potassium current, respectively. Beyond *KCNQ1* (LQT1) and *KCNH2* (LQT2), *SCN5A* (LQT3) is the third most frequently affected gene that plays a role in the genesis of LQTS. Mutation of the *SCNA5* contributes to an increase in the depolarising sodium inward current leading to the consequent prolongation of the QT interval (Priori et al., 2013). Furthermore, the role of mutations of the L-type calcium channel and other structural proteins was described in the pathogenesis of LQTS, however the triggering mutation has not been identified yet in many other cases (Schwartz et al., 2012). In the case of catecholaminergic polymorphic ventricular tachycardia (CPVT) the autosomal dominant inherited mutation of the type-2 cardiac ryanodine receptor has been identified as a possible cause. Moreover, the mutation of the Kir2.1 inward rectifier potassium channel encoded by *KCNJ2* gene can also lead to CPVT (Priori et al., 2013). The Brugada syndrome is known as a familial disease which is inherited in an autosomal dominant pattern with incomplete penetration, however in 60% of the cases occurs sporadically (Campuzano et al., 2010). Nearly 400 gene mutations have been described as a possible underlying factor in the genesis of this disease, nevertheless, in more than 80% of the cases the mutation and/or copy number variation of *SCN5A* gene encoding the Kv1.5 voltage gated sodium channel have been found (Kapplinger et al., 2010; Eastaugh et al., 2011). However, recently a thorough evaluation of the routine genetic testing panels was made. As a result, mutation of *SCNA5* gene was proven to be the only real, clinically valid disease-causing gene in case of BrS. Other gene-disease associations appeared to be debatable (Hosseini et al., 2018). The highest occurence of ECG alterations and cardiac events were reported in case of *SCNA5* mutation among BrS patients (Yamagata et al., 2017). Several gene polymorphisms, epigenetic factors and posttranslational modifications were also revealed as a pathogenic condition of BrS in the past few years (Kim et al., 2013; Webster et al., 2013) Arrhythmogenic right ventricular dysplasia (ARVD) may also have an effect in arrhythmogenesis and the development of SCD (Marcus et al, 2010). The single nucleotide polymorphisms (SNPs) located in the 21q21 and 2q24.2 loci also contribute to an increased risk for SCD (Bezzina et al., 2010; Arking et al., 2011).

THE ELECTROPHYSIOLOGICAL MECHANISMS UNDERLYING THE DEVELOPMENT OF VENTRICULAR FIBRILLATION

The electrical (repolarization) heterogeneity and secondary anisotropy of the ventricular myocardium play a crucial role in the genesis of VF. The monophasic action potentials (MAPs) characterising the electrical feature of a myocardial cell in the endocardial, mid-myocardial, and epicardial layers differ from each other, where types and expression levels of potassium channels responsible for transient outward currents (I_{to}) are also different. These dissimilarities can form a transmural voltage gradient during the activation of the ventricular myocardium. As a result, increased ventricular electrical anisotropy and an enhanced ventricular arrhythmia vulnerability may appear (Antzelevitch et al., 2000). Anisotropy can also be influenced by the differences in the distribution of intercellular electrical signal transducer gap junctions (Rohr, 2004). The macroscopic discontinuity of the myocardium (e.g., presence of septa, trabecula, papillary muscles), and the accumulation of connective tissue due to hypertrophy or infarction may also generate ventricular anisotropy (Antzelevitch et al., 2000). Scars and fibrotic tissues deposited parallel (not perpendicular) to the myocardial fibers can cease intercellular connections, consequently electrical conduction may turn irregular (Spach and Josephson, 1994). In the case of myocardial hypertrophy and heart failure (HF) the prolongation of action potential duration (APD) may consequently form early afterdepolarizations (EADs) (Nabauer and Kaab, 1998) Heart failure can cause a significant decrease in the repolarising I_{to} and delayed rectifier potassium currents (I_{Kr} and I_{Ks} currents of K channels encoded by *KCNH2* and *KCNQ1* genes) that may enhance the effect of proarrhythmic factors (e.g., hypokalemia, hypomagnesemia, class III antiarrhythmic drugs) (Nuss et al., 1996; Anumonwo and Lopatin, 2010). In the case of LQTS the mutation of potassium channels decreases their function by at least 50% leading to a prolonged repolarization, APD and QT interval. Class III antiarrhythmic drugs have a similar APD prolonging effect, that may contribute to an increased ventricular proarrhythmic susceptibility (Nuss et al, 1996; Peters et al., 2000). In the cases of heart failure and left ventricular hypertrophy, the downregulation of potassium channels, the decrease of transient outward currents (I_{to}) and the decrease of rapid and slow components of the delayed rectifier currents (I_{Kr}, I_{Ks}) can contribute to the prolongation of APD. Regarding HF, the overexpression of *HCN2* and *HCN4* genes can appear resulting in an increased pacemaker current (I_f) not only in the SA node, but in the ventricular tissue, too. The electrical remodeling of the heart can lead to a reduced ventricular repolarization reserve, increasing the risk of ventricular arrhythmias based on triggered activity, ectopic automaticity, and reentry mechanisms (Cerbai et al., 2001; Stillitano et al., 2008). ATP-sensitive potassium channels (K_{ATP} channels) localized in the sarcolemmal membrane may be activated by metabolic stress or ischemia causing the shortening of APD, preventing the heart from calcium overload and contraction abnormalities. Moreover, myocardial hypertrophy and ischemia can increase the expression levels of Kir 6.1 and Kir 6.2 K_{ATP} channels, leading to an increased risk for ventricular dysrhythmias based on heterogeneous shortening of the AP (Akrouh et al., 2009; Tinker et al., 2018). In 1998 repolarization reserve has been defined by Roden et al. as a defensive mechanism of the myocardium, which protects the heart from the emergence of arrhythmias in particular circumstances where APD has already been prolonged. For instance, enhanced inward Na^+ currents contributes to an increase in delayed rectifier outward potassium current (especially I_{Kr}) as a compensatory mechanism in order to prevent the prolongation of repolarization. Furthermore, congenital alterations in ion currents of the myocardium, heart failure, cardiac hypertrophy, bradycardia, increased sympathetic activation, female gender, recent pharmacological conversion from atrial fibrillation to sinus rhythm, use of diuretics, hypokalemia, hypomagnesemia, administration of class IA, IC or III antiarrhythmic drugs or agents with I_{Kr} blocking effect can decrease repolarization reserve. Co-occurence of certain conditions which affect more than one type of ion currents involved in regular repolarization may critically reduce repolarization reserve and can result in proarrhythmia (Roden, 1998; Varró and Baczkó, 2011).

The underlying electrophysiological mechanisms of ventricular fibrillation consequently include *ectopic automaticity*, *reentry* and *triggered activity* (due to early and late afterdepolarizations) (**Figure 1**) (Bayes De Luna et al., 1989; Peters et al., 2000).

Ectopic automaticity is the result of spontaneous diastolic depolarization, where current of injury (local alterations in K^+ gradient) due to acute ischemic damage is an important provoking mechanism (Thygesen and Uretsky, 2004). In the case of *ectopic automaticity* it is a ventricular premature beat caused by inherited or acquired ectopic impulse-generating foci that most frequently play a role in triggering VF (Van Camp, 1992; Singh and Noheria, 2018). Ventricular premature beats may arise from any part of the electrical conducting system of the heart, especially from the Purkinje fibers, and may also originate from the right or left ventricular outflow tract, or the papillary muscles. Nevertheless, monomorphic ventricular tachycardia or atrial fibrillation as part of a preexcitation syndrome may also contribute to VF (Viskin et al., 2013).

A frequent underlying cause of the unidirectional block serving as the basis of *reentry mechanism* may be the prolongation of the monophasic action potential of the myocyte and the consequential heterogeneity of ventricular repolarization. This process may be facilitated by myocardial ischemia and may trigger an increase in the monophasic AP duration restitution slope as well as changes in the amplitude of AP (electrical alternans) (Krummen et al., 2016).

Triggered activity may also appear as a consequence of early (EAD) or delayed afterdepolarization (DAD). EAD is caused by the early reactivation of L-type Ca-channels, a consequence of a decrease in repolarising potassium currents or an increase in the activity of positive currents toward the intracellular space (Roden, 2016). Furthermore, oxidative stress, hypokalemia may also play an additive role in the pathomechanism of EAD (Antzelevitch et al., 1991; Karagueuzian et al., 2013; Antzelevitch et al., 2014; Markandeya and Kamp, 2015). In contrast, DAD develops after the repolarization of the myocyte membrane due to intracellular calcium excess or an increased sensitivity of intracellular ryanodine receptors (Priori and Chen, 2011). Delayed after depolarizations often serve as a background

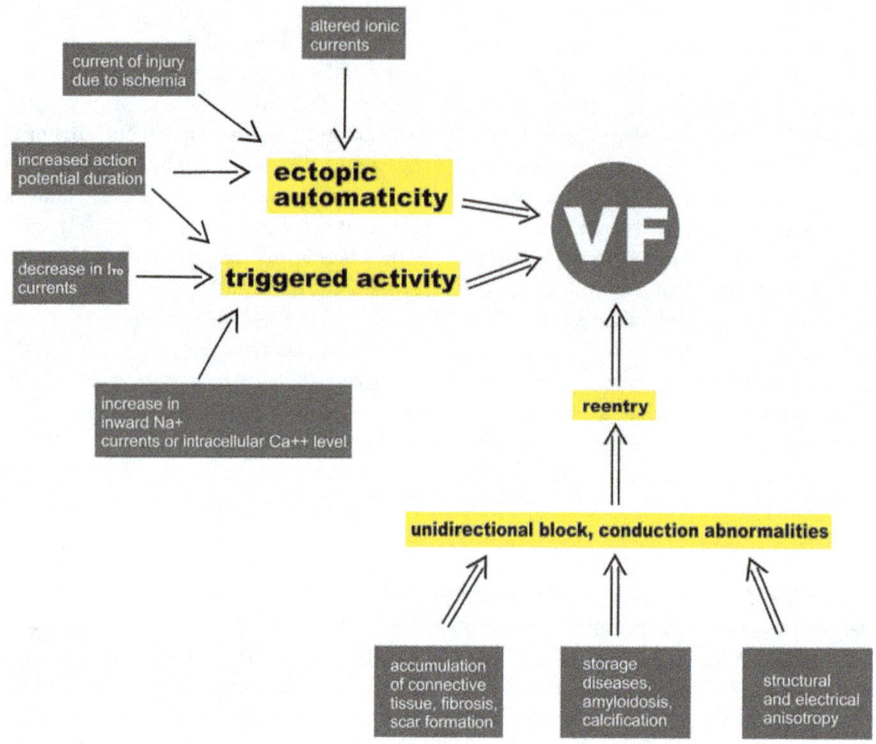

FIGURE 1 | Pathomechanism of ventricular fibrillation (VF).

for ventricular arrhythmias caused by heart failure or digoxin toxicity and can also play a role in the genesis of CPVT (Priori and Chen, 2011).

RISK ASSESSMENT OF VENTRICULAR FIBRILLATION

Several diagnostic tools are available for the risk stratification of ventricular arrhythmias and sudden cardiac death. Certain parameters of the 12-lead surface ECG (e.g., QT interval and dispersion, T wave peak-to-end interval, arrhythmogeneity index, epsilon wave, delta wave, Brugada sign, J point elevation, etc.) may be of help in predicting life-threatening ventricular dysrhythmias and clarifying the underlying arrhythmia mechanism. Holter ECG may be useful in arrhythmia risk stratification (by determining T wave alternans, heart rate variability, QT variability, etc.). Echocardiography is widely used to determine structural and functional abnormalities of the heart. Accumulation of connective tissue in the left ventricle (scar burden) and fatty tissue in the right ventricle (ARVD) can be examined by MRI. Coronary CT angiography and coronarography may be of help to recognize coronary artery disease as a possible underlying arrhythmogenic factor. Electrophysiological testing is suitable for the examination of VT/VF inducibility and for the definition of the arrhythmia foci. Serum level of certain biomarkers may also be taken into consideration as part of ventricular arrhythmia risk assessment (Deyell et al., 2015).

Laboratory Opportunities for Predicting Ventricular Arrhythmias

Considering laboratory biomarkers, in addition to the now more widely used NT-proBNP and the high-sensitive troponin T, osteopontin, galectin-3, and soluble ST2 can also be applied to determine the arrhythmia vulnerability of the ventricular myocardium (Pascual-Figal et al., 2009; Patton et al., 2011; Francia et al., 2014; Xu et al., 2019). NT-proBNP is a neurohormone produced by the brain, the left atrium, and the left ventricle, whose serum level significantly rises in the case of left ventricular dysfunction. Examining the population of the Cardiovascular Health Study Patton et al. found 289 cases of sudden cardiac death where the increased NT-proBNP value involved 4.2 times higher risk of the development of sudden cardiac death (Patton et al., 2011). Xu et al. examined 104 patients treated with aborted cardiac death where during the follow-up period a higher hsTnT level was measured in the case of patients who suffered repeated episodes of ventricular fibrillation (Xu et al., 2019). Osteopontin and galectin-3 are primarily ventricular myocardium-specific fibrosis markers whose increased serum-level implies enhanced myocardial fibrosis and thereby, due to the increased electrical heterogeneity, enhanced risk of ventricular arrhythmias (Francia et al., 2014). Soluble ST2 is a member of the interleukin-1 receptor family, produced by cardiomyocytes. Pascual-Figal et al. found that increased sST2 values involved 1.39 times higher risk of sudden cardiac death compared to persons with a regular serum level (Pascual-Figal et al., 2009). In a cohort study based on the clinical data of 72 patients, Scheirlynck et al. proved that mitral annulus disjunction (MAD) was linked to a higher sST2 level in the presence of ventricular arrhythmias. The focal fibrosis of the mitral apparatus has been shown to be associated with the electrical instability and the hypermobility of the mitral valve, which together can lead to an enhanced ventricular arrhythmia susceptibility. In contrary to the study of Patton et al., they found normal NT-proBNP and CRP levels in their population. In the same study TGFß1 was assumed to be responsible for the ventricular arrhythmogeneity (Scheirlynck et al., 2019). In the Physicians' Health Study a positive correlation was reported between high serum CRP levels and increased arrhythmia risk vulnerability, however in the Nurse's Health Study population similar connection could not be proven (Balla et al., 2019). In the Paris study, the increased serum concentration of non-esterified free fatty acids were described as an independent risk factor for SCD in middle-aged men (Balla et al., 2019). Furthermore, increased serum levels of matrix metalloproteinazes (MMPs) and their inhibitor molecules (TIMPs) - which may take part in the genesis of cardiac fibrosis - have also been shown to contribute to an increased risk of ventricular dysrhythmias (Klappacher et al., 1995). In another investigation by Benito et al. the elevated serum level of testosterone, and the decreased serum level of oestrogen were in correlation with an increased probability of malignant ventricular arrhythmias (Benito et al., 2008).

Estimating Arrhythmia Susceptibility With Imaging Methods

Left ventricular ejection fraction (EF) measured during echocardiography is suitable for predicting malignant ventricular arrhythmia and, according to current knowledge, is the only echocardiographic parameter with predictive value for an increased risk of sudden cardiac death in the case of ischemic heart disease and left ventricular dysfunction (Fogel, 2002; Moss et al., 2002; Alberte and Zipes, 2003). Echocardiographic examinations may also be of help in the detection of structural heart diseases (concentric and eccentric left ventricular hypertrophy, valvulopathies, chamber diameters, etc.) underlying ventricular arrhythmias (Cheitlin et al., 2003; Priori et al., 2015).

Another opportunity is to perform a cardiac MR, which thanks to its high resolution gives a more precise picture of wall motion disorders, is suitable for performing more refined volumetric measurements and provides a better approximation of the left ventricular mass than echocardiography, is at the same time much more expensive, less accessible, and may requires the administration of a contrast agent. It is of outstanding value in the diagnostics of patients with arrhythmogenic right ventricular dysplasia, in assessing the tissue structure of the ventricular wall (Priori et al., 2015).

Electrocardiographic Estimation of the Risk for Ventricular Arrhythmias

Determining the respective parameters of a 12-lead surface ECG is an inexpensive, easy to perform and reproducable method, which can be widely used in the everyday clinical practice for predicting ventricular arrhythmias.

Short QT interval (QT interval corrected to heart rate <300 ms) and *long QT interval* (QT interval corrected to heart rate, for men ≥ 451 ms, for women ≥471 ms) involve a confirmed increased risk of sudden cardiac death (Malik and Batchvarov, 2000; Boriani et al., 2006). Zhang et al. showed that the relative risk of SCD comparing patients with the longest and shortest QT interval was 1.44 (Zhang et al., 2011). Vink et al. proved that manual measurement of QT interval corrected according to Bazett formula has a specificity of 86% and a sensitivity of 85% simultaneously (Vink et al., 2018). QT dispersion is also a widely used ventricular arrhythmia risk marker; it is the difference between the longest and shortest QT intervals in the 12-lead electrocardiogram and can be used to estimate the spatial dispersion of ventricular repolarization. Increased QT dispersion, showing a repolarization heterogeneity, has been reported in several pathological conditions; its predictive value for an arrhytmia risk and SCD has been confirmed in the cases of amyloidosis, hyperlipidemia, systemic sclerosis, thyroid dysfunction, diabetes mellitus, and chronic kidney disease (Sgreccia et al., 1998; Lőrincz et al., 1999; Cardoso et al., 2001; Szabó et al., 2005; Bakiner et al., 2008; Gilotra et al., 2013; Tse and Yan, 2017). Interestingly, when compared to hemodiafiltration QT dispersion has been found to be significantly higher during hemodialysis (Barta et al., 2014). In the case of patients with coronary artery disease increased QT dispersion had 92% sensitivity and 81% specificity in the prediction of SCD (Darbar et al., 1996).

Short-term beat-to-beat variability of the QT interval (QTv) can be determined manually or by means of a computer software. Generally, 30 consecutive QT intervals in leads II and V5 are measured (Berger et al., 1997). Increased QTv has been described in patients with dilated cardiomyopathy (DCM), heart failure, drug-induced or congenital long QT syndromes, panic disorder, and even in the cases of young athletes with moderate left ventricular hypertrophy (Hinterseer et al., 2008; Hinterseer et al., 2009; Hinterseer et al., 2010; Lengyel et al., 2011; Varkevisser et al., 2012). Furthermore, QTv was shown to be useful in the detection of latent repolarization disorders. QT variability index (QTVI) can be calculated from the logarithmic ratio of the mean QTc interval and heart rate and the variability of QT interval and heart rate. Its increase indicates repolarization heterogeneity. QTVI may increase in many conditions, e.g., DCM, acute ischemia, HF, LQTS, renal failure, ventricular arrhythmias, and SCD (Dobson et al., 2013). However, its predictive and diagnostic value has not been clearly elucidated yet. Investigators agree that QTVI combined with QTc, QTv, and heart rate variability may improve the risk stratification of patients with enhanced arrhythmia susceptibility (Oosterhoff et al., 2011).

T wave peak-to-end interval (Tpe) and the arrhythmogeneity index (AIX, derived as the ratio of Tpe and corrected QT interval) are also suitable for estimating the danger of ventricular arrhythmias (Gupta et al., 2008; Kors et al., 2008). The normal value of Tpe in the case of men is <94 ms and for women <92 ms (Haarmark et al., 2010). The prolongation of Tpe has been observed in the case of several clinical conditions, e.g., acute myocardial infarction, sleep apnea syndrome, hypertrophic cardiomyopathy, and LQTS (Shimizu et al., 2002; Yamaguchi et al., 2003; Haarmark et al., 2009; Kilicaslan et al., 2012). In a population with liver cirrhosis Tpe value has been confirmed to have a sensitivity of 90% and a specificity of 60% in the prediction of SCD (Salgado et al., 2016). Another study with patients who underwent primary coronary intervention (PCI) showed, that the prolongation of Tpe interval with regard to SCD had a sensitivity of 90%, and a specificity of 55% with a positive predictive value of 0.18 and a negative predictive value of 0.98 (Haarmark et al., 2009). The physiological value of arrhythmogeneity index is approximately 0.19–0.2 (Zehir et al., 2015) and has proven to be even more precise than the corrected QT value in the prediction of torsades de pointes ventricular tachycardia and sudden cardiac death (Yamaguchi et al., 2003; Topilski et al., 2007; Wang et al., 2019). In another study the increase in Tpe and AIX were found to be significantly higher during hemodialysis compared to hemodiafiltration which indicates a pronounced risk for ventricular arrhythmia formation during the conventional renal replacement therapy (Páll et al., 2017). In a further investigation by Wang et al. in patients with vasospastic angina pectoris, AIX had a sensitivity of 84% and a specificity of 89.5% in the prediction of malignant ventricular arrhythmias (Wang et al., 2019).

T wave alternans is yet another electrocardiographic parameter that represents beat-to-beat changes in T wave morphology. Its examination may be suitable for expressing the spatial heterogeneity of ventricular repolarization (Narayan, 2006). T wave alterations measured on electrocardiogram enlarged to a microvolt scale referred to as *microvolt T wave alternans* have proven to be useful not only for estimating the risk of ventricular arrhythmia but for assessing the necessity of implantable cardioverter defibrillator (ICD) as well (Bloomfield et al., 2004; Burattini et al., 2009).

The prevalence of the *Brugada ECG*-pattern and the epsilon wave characteristic of arrhythmogenic right ventricular dysplasia both indicate an increased risk for arrhythmias (Issa et al., 2012). Priori et al. found that out of 176 Brugada-syndrome patients there were clear diagnostic signs in the resting ECG of only 90 patients (Priori et al., 2002). Therefore, in the case of clinical suspicion it is recommended to perform a provocation test using class IA or IC sodium channel blockers intravenously. Flecainide was one of the drugs that were used for this purpose, however it turned out to be ineffective in revealing the Brugada sign on the surface ECG in 30% of the examined Brugada patients (Therasse et al., 2017). Thus, ajmalin is the preferred drug with higher efficacy during provocation tests (Berne and Brugada, 2012). Procainamide can also be suitable for the triggering of not only type-1, but type-2 and -3 Brugada signs on the surface electrocardiogram. For the same purpose, disopyramide, propafenone and pilsicainide may be applied, too (Obeyesekere et al., 2011; Berne and Brugada, 2012).

Recently, growing clinical significance has been attributed to what is referred to as the J -point elevation syndrome which are the early repolarization syndromes together with Brugada syndrome (Nademanee et al., 2019). As a characteristic feature of this J-point elevation of above 0.1 mV can be measured in at least 2 related ECG leads, which manifests together with concave ST-segment elevation and peaked prominent T waves. Based on the leads with J-point alterations, 3 types of early repolarization patterns can be differentiated (**Table 2**) (Antzelevitch and Yan, 2010).

THE TREATMENT OF VENTRICULAR FIBRILLATION

The most effective therapies for ventricular fibrillation and pulseless ventricular tachycardia (pVT) are immediate high-quality chest compression as well as early defibrillation, which latter plays a key role in terminating these arrhythmias (**Figure 2**) (Neumar et al., 2015).

Survival rate by early defibrillation in the case of resuscitation performed by lay people is 37.4% (Benjamin et al., 2017). The necessity of earliest possible electrical treatment is underpinned by the fact that the rate of successful resuscitation falls by 7%–10% per min from the circulatory collapse (Larsen et al., 1993). The availability of automated external defibrillators (AED) in public spaces and broad-scale training for lay persons about the use of the device may increase the current survival rate of 10% (Berg et al., 2019). In Scandinavia, there have been experiments with simulation practices using drones for the speedy delivery of AEDs with positive results and applying this method in real situations in future may improve the success rate of life saving as well (Sanfridsson et al., 2019). During a practice simulating out-of-hospital circulatory collapse the results of resuscitations performed by elderly bystanders (average age: 75.5 years) were compared considering several aspects. The bystanders did not have any prior training and the primary goal was to find out how modern telecommunication tools (smartphones, drones, AED) would affect their performance. Results showed that from the time of the circulatory collapse AED was placed on the simulated patients within 10 min and resuscitation started within 2.25 min (Sanfridsson et al., 2019).

An improvement in the chance of long-term survival and the least neurological damage were found in the case when the initial

TABLE 2 | Types of early repolarization syndromes (ERS) according to ECG-alterations and anatomical localization (based on Antzelevitch and Yan, 2010).

	EARLY REPOLARIZATION SYNDROME (ERS)		
	TYPE 1	**TYPE 2**	**TYPE 3**
Location of J wave abnormalities (ECG leads)	I, V4-6	II, III, aVF	in all leads
Anatomical localization of repolarization disorder	the anterolateral part of the left ventricle	inferior part of left ventricle	left and right ventricle

ECG, electrocardiography.

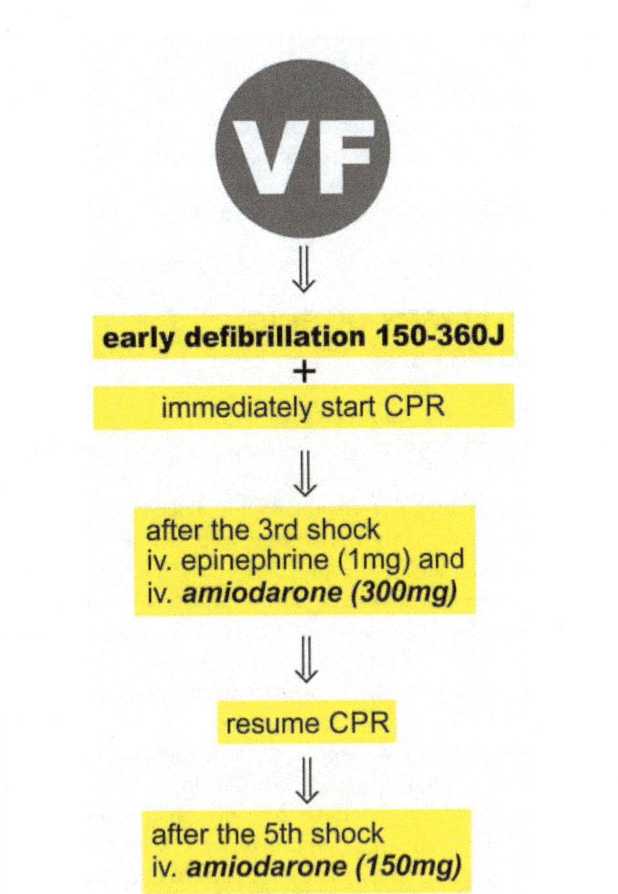

FIGURE 2 | Acute treatment of ventricular fibrillation. VF, ventricular fibrillation; CPR, cardiopulmonary resuscitation.

rhythm observed on site was ventricular fibrillation (Daya et al., 2015). Another important element of improving the neurological outcome is post-resuscitation care started in time, which includes coronary intervention and targeted temperature management (TTM) (Link et al., 2015). Based on the examination of 136 patients, the Hypothermia after Cardiac Arrest Study Group showed that the application of TTM clearly improved neurological outcome (based on CPC) and reduced mortality (Hypothermia after Cardiac Arrest Study Group, 2002). Stanger et al. examined 570 patients resuscitated after out-of-hospital sudden cardiac death who were administered TTM therapy in hospital. The patients were put into two groups depending on how many minutes after arrival in hospital TTM was started. The greatest difference between the early (20–81 min) and the late (167–319 min) groups was in survival. The early group had 1.59 times higher chance for survival compared to the late group, while they had only 1.49 times higher chance for a good neurological outcome, which did not prove clearly significant (Stanger et al., 2019). The 2015 resuscitation guideline recommends earliest possible PCI in the case of sudden cardiac death with acute coronary syndrome as the underlying cause (Nikolaou et al., 2015). Kahn et al. had found already that early PCI performed on patients who had suffered SCD due to STEMI could help survival with a good neurological outcome (Kahn et al., 1995). Examining 35 and 190 patients respectively, Nanjayya et al. and Bro-Jeppesen et al. compared patients who underwent and others who did not undergo immediate angiography and PCI in hospital, after out-of-hospital sudden death. Both studies found that early PCI had no significant positive effect on mortality (Bro-Jeppesen et al., 2012; Nanjayya and Nayyar, 2012). In contrast, Strote et al. found by retrospectively analyzing the data of 270 patients who had suffered sudden cardiac death that acute PCI (if performed within 6 h after the emergence of symptoms) ensured significantly better survival than PCI performed beyond 6 h (Strote et al., 2012).

CHEST COMPRESSION DEVICES

Research findings in recent years have confirmed that a most decisive element of successful resuscitation is high-quality chest compression interrupted for the briefest possible time (Levy et al., 2015). Due to the decreasing compression depth and the increasingly frequent interruptions, the manual sustainment of good-quality chest compression recommended as a target in the guidelines faces difficulties in the short run already. In view of the latter mechanical chest compression devices have become increasingly widespread and available as alternative solutions both in prehospital and in-hospital emergency care. With the help of these devices, high-quality compressions can be maintained even for a long time (Ujvárosy et al., 2018). Although the findings of the research performed have not yet confirmed significant differences in the outcome of resuscitations with the use of these devices, there are certain situations, e.g., continuous CPR during transport, when their application is clearly recommended by international guidelines (Soar et al., 2015).

According to the international resuscitation recommendation currently in force, the European Resuscitation Council ALS protocol, the application of mechanical devices is recommended if the sustainment of high-quality chest compressions is required for a longer time, e.g. during transportation, for a hypothermic patient or in the case of PCI during ongiong CPR (Soar et al., 2015).

There are currently two major types of mechanical devices available in trade, LUCAS (Lund University Cardiopulmonary Assist System) and AutoPulse (Load distributing band CPR). LUCAS is a system operating based on a piston principle and also plays a role in the active decompression of the chest; a silicone ring is to be pressed against the patient's chest, which thereafter exercises pressure in a depth of 5–6 cm with a frequency of 100/min, and helps the relaxation of the chest wall as well (Koster et al., 2017). In the case of AutoPulse, in contrast, a wide bandage is placed across the patient's chest, which thereafter implements pressure on the chest with a frequency of 80/min but does not take part in the relaxation of the chest (Koster et al., 2017). Research findings comparing resuscitations performed with the respective devices have not shown any differences as regards the success of resuscitation (Gates et al., 2015).

One of the greatest doubts arising in relation to the devices was potential injuries they could cause, but as has been confirmed by several autopsy findings, mechanical devices have not caused either other types of, or more serious or frequent injuries than manual chest compression. The most frequent injury they caused was similarly rib fracture (Koster et al., 2017).

In another study in relation to resuscitation performed using a LUCAS-2 mechanical chest compression device has similarly shown favourable results. The data of altogether 287 patients were investigated who suffered out-of-hospital non-traumatic circulatory collapse, out of which resuscitation using a LUCAS-2 device was performed in 55 cases, while manual chest compression was carried out in the others. Return of spontaneous circulation (ROSC) happened in 37% of the cases; in a slightly higher rate in the mechanical group ($p = 0.072$). Also, in cases of prolonged resuscitation, success rate was higher in the mechanical group ($p<0.05$). The number of traumatic injuries was not higher in the LUCAS-2 compared to the manual group (Ujvárosy et al., 2018).

CLINICAL FACTORS AFFECTING THE OUTCOME OF RESUSCITATION

The prognosis and long-term outcome of resuscitated patients who survived aborted cardiac death are significantly influenced by comorbidities (ischemic heart disease, hypertension), the extent of potential left ventricular hypertrophy and the mechanism of ventricular arrhythmogenesis. Koldobskiy et al. found that kidney failure, immunosuppression and obesity negatively influenced the outcome of resuscitation (Koldobskiy et al., 2014). Herlitz et al. examined the data of 33,453 patients and concluded that initial rhythm, lay resuscitation and the age of the patient very strongly influenced the outcome of CPR (Herlitz et al., 2005) Our own research findings have proven that the presence of left ventricular hypertrophy involved 5.1 times higher risk of the failure of resuscitation ($p = 0.0009$ $r = 0.1995$). We have also found that age and hypertension negatively influence success rate; in the case of hypertension there is a 1.82-time risk of a failed outcome ($p = 0.018$ $r = 0.143$) (Ujvárosy et al., 2018). Often the first and only 'symptom' of myocardial infarction is sudden cardiac death, and SCD was responsible for the death of almost half of the coronary patients and for nearly 325,000 deaths per year, in the USA (Myerburg et al., 1993; Singh and Noheria, 2018). Cardiological rehabilitation, favourable influence for the lipid profile, favourable medication and the management of comorbidities have nowadays significantly improved long-term prognosis in the case of SCD with ACS in the background (Bunch et al., 2005). Refractory VF, which is a relatively rare morbidity factor, involves expressly poor outcome (El-Sherif et al., 2017; Nas et al., 2019). Among the factors influencing long-term prognosis the most important one is neurological outcome, for characterising which the CPC (Cerebral Performance Category) scale is the most widely used method (**Table 3**) (Ajam et al., 2011).

In addition to the application of a mechanical device, a new opportunity for prehospital emergency diagnostics available is to perform echocardiography. This may help identify some of the reversible reasons (4H-4T) causing circulatory collapse and improve the efficiency of chest compression. For the confirmation of the further roles and efficiency of echocardiography during resuscitation as well as its effect on the outcome, further studies are requried (Teran et al., 2019).

DRUG THERAPY DURING RESUSCITATION

In international recommendations, therapy for VF and pVT includes the administration of epinephrine and amiodarone (Neumar et al., 2015). The mechanism of action of epinephrine in the case of cardiac arrest is the consequence to α-adrenergic effect, which, by directing systemic blood flow toward the heart increases myocardial blood supply, thus ensuring the minimum coronary perfusion pressure (CPP) required for successful defibrillation (Gough and Nolan, 2018). Proarrhythmic effect of epinephrine was described in both *ex vivo* and *in vitro* investigations. Epinephrine shortens sinus cycle length, decreases the effective refractory period of the ventricular myocardium and may also lead to increased atrial and ventricular automaticity and conduction abnormalities. Epinephrine was reported to be able to generate sinus tachycardia, supraventricular, and ventricular arrhythmias in a dose-dependent manner (Tisdale et al., 1995). Furthermore, the epicardial layer of the myocardium is more sensitive to sympathetic activation, than mid-myocardial, and the endocardial cells. Consequently, an additional heterogeneity in the APD and refractory period may appear resulting in an increased risk for ventricular arrhythmias (Antzelevitch et al., 1991; Antzelevitch and Yan, 2010). The platelet activator effect of α-adrenergic stimulation was also shown, hereby rising the possibility for microcirculatory myocardial damage (Hwang et al., 2019). Beyond its undoubtedly favorable effect with relation to cardiac arrest, its detrimental β-adrenergic activity can also be assumed. By the deterioration of systemic oxygen demand and the increase in myocardial oxygen consumption it

TABLE 3 | Cerebral performance category.

Cerebral Performance Category (CPC)	
CPC level 1	Normal ability or minimal disability (good cerebral performance, conscious, alert, able to work, and lead a normal life)
CPC level 2	Moderate cerebral disability (conscious, sufficient cerebral function for part-time work in a sheltered environment or independent activities of daily life. May have hemiplegia, seizures, ataxia, dysarthria, dysphasia, or permanent memory or mental changes).
CPC level 3	Severe disability (conscious, dependent on others for daily support because of impaired brain function).
CPC level 4	Severe disability (coma, vegetative state, no cognition, verbal or psychological interactions with the environment).
CPC level 5	Death (or brain death).

may further aggravate the lack of balance between oxygen supply and demand (Gough and Nolan, 2018), that has a special significance in the case of ventricular fibrillation.

Inhibition of the sympathetic activity contributes to the antiarrhythmic effect of β-adrenoceptor antagonists which manifests in the prolongation of AV-nodal refractory period. By reducing Ca^{++}, Na^{+} currents, and cAMP-dependent pacemaker currents (I_f), and by increasing K^{+} currents β-adrenoceptor antagonists cause negative chronotropy. Their classification is based on their chemical structure, β̃selectivity and pharmacokinetic properties. There are two subtypes of both α- and β-adrenoceptors. They have distinct distribution and density in different tissues. β_1-receptors have a more intense presence in the heart and β_2-receptors have a higher density in the smooth muscles and in the bronchi, however α1-, β_1-, and β_2-adrenoceptors occur on the surface of the cardiomyocytes. β-adrenoceptor antagonists mainly act on β_1-and β_2-adrenoceptors (Brodde, 2007; Schnee et al., 2008). Moreover, some of them have an intrinsic sympathomimetic activity caused by a partial β-agonist property, and others have vasodilator effects due to an associated α-blocker feature (Opie and Yusuf, 2001; Dorian, 2005). First generation β-adrenoceptor antagonists (such as propranolol, timolol, nadolol) inhibit β_1- and β_2-adrenoceptors equally, thus their antiarrhythmic effect is limited. Second generation of β-adrenoceptor antagonists (e.g., metoprolol, bisoprolol, atenolol, etc.) has a more pronounced β_1-selectivity especially in low doses. In this group bisoprolol is known as the most cardioselective agent with explicit antiarrhythmic activity. Third generation β-adrenoceptor antagonists (e.g., labetalol, carvedilol, nebivolol) has an additional vasodilating effect, hence they are usually ordered as antiarrhythmics mainly in hypertensive patients (do Vale et al., 2019). As effective antiarrhythmics, β-adrenoceptor antagonists decrease the mortality of patients with myocardial infarction by more than 30% (Norris et al.,1984; Teo et al.,1993; Hjalmarson, 1999). In the case of CPR and refractory VF, β-adrenoceptor antagonists (e.g., esmolol) were also reported to have moderating effect on the proarrhythmic property of epinephrine. Although success has been reported in relation to the administration of esmolol, considering the limited number of cases there are no straightforward recommendations regarding its use yet (Lee et al., 2016). In a study published in 2007, Bourque et al. summarized the results on the application of β-adrenoceptor antagonists. They presented the findings of experiments conducted between 1966 and 2006 on dogs and rats primarily, where the more favorable effects – compared to epinephrine – of β-adrenoceptor antagonists on myocardial oxygen demand were found among others (Bourque et al., 2007).

β_1-and β_2-adrenoceptors are also blocked by sotalol, however it also inhibits the rapid component of delayed rectifier potassium currents leading to a prolonged ventricular repolarization. Due to its combined mode of action, the racemic sotalol can be classified as a type II + III antiarrhythmic drug. The two enantiomers of sotalol display different pharmacodynamic activities and selectivities: D-sotalol blocks dominantly the rapid component of the delayed rectifier potassium current (I_{Kr}), while L-sotalol inhibits both I_{Kr} current and β-adrenoceptors (Funck-Brentano, 1993). In the SWORD trial, which had to be terminated prematurely due to the increased occurrence of ventricular arrhythmias, administration of D-sotalol was associated with a higher mortality rate among 3,121 patients with left ventricular EF ≤40% after myocardial infarction (Waldo et al., 1996). Therefore, D-sotalol is not used as an antiarrhythmic drug in the everyday clinical practice. D,L-sotalol (racemic sotalol containing equimolar amount of D and L enantiomers) inhibits mainly β-adrenoceptors and is appropriate for the treatment of malignant ventricular arrhythmias, especially in conditions with elevated serum catecholamine levels or increased sensitivity for catecholamines e.g. in the case of acute myocardial infarction, phaeochromocytoma, mitral prolapse, postoperative arrhythmias, and thyreotoxicosis. However, sotalol's torsadogenic effect limits its applicability (Opie and Yusuf, 2001). Although several animal experiments have been carried out to investigate the effect of sotalol on ventricular fibrillation so far, further data are needed to form recommendations in this indication (Jin et al., 2018). In the 2015 ESC Guideline for ventricular arrhythmias and SCD the application of sotalol is recommended for patients with coronary artery disease, but only in the case of implanted ICD due to its proarrhythmic effect (Priori et al., 2015).

According to our knowledge quinidine can play a life-saving role in patients with BrS, ERS, and idiopathic ventricular fibrillation (IVF). Quinidine is a class IA antiarrhythmic drug, that blocks α-adrenoceptors, muscarinic acetylcholine receptors and several types of voltage gated K channels beyond Kv1.5 Na channel. It reduces the frequency of impulse generation by prolonging spontaneous diastolic depolarization and elevates the threshold potential of action potentials. Oral quinidine is recommended for patients with ICD due to BrS, ERS, or IVF, while it decreases the number of ICD shocks and it also improves ICD-free survival (Malhi et al., 2019).

Amiodarone is an iodinated benzofuran, which was originally developed for the treatment of angina pectoris. Amiodarone prolongs the action potential duration and increases the refractory period of the atrial and ventricular myocardium, the AV-node and the Purkinje system (Mason, 1987). Amiodarone, a type III antiarrhythmic drug, having the qualities of all the four groups of antiarrhythmic agents-, blocks the activity of sodium and potassium channels, antagonises the functioning of both α- and β-adrenergic receptors and as a mild calcium antagonist it also has a blocking effect on the sinoatrial node, and the AV-nodal tissue (Lubic et al., 1994; Sampson and Kass, 2011). In the case of VF recurring after three defibrillations, the administration of 300 mg and later 150 mg of amiodarone is recommended (Neumar et al., 2015) It was based on the findings of two major studies, conducted in 1999 and 2002, that amiodarone replaced the earlier recommended lidocaine. In 2016, Laina et al. analyzed the findings of 1,663 studies conducted with amiodarone and found that amiodarone significantly increased short-term survival rate (OR = 1.42 p = 0.015). Findings with reference to the long-term effects of amiodarone affecting the neurological outcome primarily are not straightforward, although encouraging when compared to other antiarrhythmic agents (Laina et al., 2016; Karlis and Afantenou, 2018). In 2018, American Heart Association (AHA) recommended the further application of amiodarone or lidocaine in the case of VF/pVT due to their short-term positive effects (Panchal et al., 2018). The ROC-ALPS study investigated the short and long-term effects of captisol-based formulation of amiodarone and lidocain in the case of out-of hospital cardiac arrests. Both had a better short-term effect compared to the placebo, however, there have been no differences shown regarding long-term outcome, neurological status, and admission from hospital (Kudenchuk et al., 2016).

A synthetic amiodarone analogue, dronedarone is not iodinated, as it has been designed for avoiding the side effects of amiodarone. Dronedarone blocks L-type Ca, K, and Na channels. In animal studies the antiarrhythmic effect of dronaderone on the ventricular myocardium has been described (Finance et al., 1995). Additionally, in three human studies, it significantly decreased ventricular arrhythmogeneity, and the number of ICD shocks (Fink et al., 2011). However, in lack of widespread experiences it is still not applicable for the prevention and treatment of VF.

Taking all the available data into consideration it can be concluded that currently there is no appropriate antiarrhythmic agent that can safely prevent VF and would significantly improve the long-term outcome of patients with life-threatening ventricular arrhythmias (Panchal et al., 2018).

CONSIDERATIONS FOR THE TREATMENT OF REFRACTORY VENTRICULAR FIBRILLATION

In the case of refractory VF (refibrillation), the resuscitation recommendation suggests administering shocks of growing intensity up to 360 J (Soar et al., 2015). In case the ALS protocol fails, some authors recommend dual defibrillation (dual-sequential defibrillation [DSD]). In the latter case a second pair of electrodes in addition to the traditional pair is placed in an anteroposterior position and accordingly shock is administered with two defibrillators. The vector of the electric impulse administered changes compared to the original, which enables the defibrillation of larger parts of the cardiac muscle and may be more effective in the case of corpulent patients as well. In a retrospective study of 4 years, Cortez et al. found, out of 2,428 out-of-hospital circulatory collapses 12 cases of refractory VF where the application of the ALS protocol failed, the applied DSD was successful in 3 cases (ROSC and good CPC value) (Cortez et al., 2016). In order to enhance the chance of success Frye et al. combined the DSD protocol with administering lidocaine, as did the authors of other case studies as well (Frye et al, 2018). Although the ERC recommendation currently in force advises the administration of lidocaine during resuscitation only in the case of recurring VF or pregnancy, there are increasing attempts for using it in the case of refractory VF as well (Priori et al., 2015). While there is a wider use of devices, it is a disadvantage of DSD that uniform protocols are not available and there are no comprehensive large-scale studies on patients who have undergone DSD (Frye et al., 2018).

LONG-TERM TREATMENT AFTER ABORTED CARDIAC DEATH

Regarding long-term treatment of malignant ventricular arrhythmias, the application of implantable cardioverter defibrillator (ICD) is an important element, which releases an antitachycardia pacing or an electric shock at the occurrence of the rhythm disturbance (**Figure 3**).

In a study with 2,521 patients involved Bardy et al. found that the implantation of an ICD able to deliver only shocks, combined with conventional conservative therapy, reduced total mortality rate by 23% in the case of NYHA II and III heart failure patients with EF <35% compared to conservatively treated patients (Bardy et al., 2005). Antitachycardia pacing (ATP) is in fact meant to reduce the number of superfluous or inappropriate shocks, whereby patients' quality of life improves, and the lifetime of the device also grows. Most often the device delivers superfluous shocks due to supraventricular arrhythmias, which occurred in 8%–40% of the patients despite appropriate drug therapy. Moreover, ATP is also successful in stopping slow and fast ventricular tachycardia in almost 85%–90% of the cases, although it may happen in both cases if timing or setting are inappropriate that the ATP itself generates a malignant ventricular arrhythmia (Fisher et al., 1978;

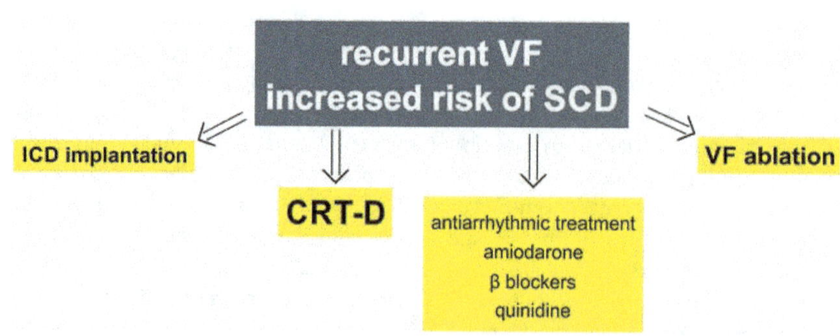

FIGURE 3 | Long-term therapy of ventricular fibrillation. ICD, implantable cardioverter defibrillator; SCD, sudden cardiac death; VF, ventricular fibrillation; CRT-D, cardiac resynchronization therapy combined with ICD.

Schuger et al., 2012). In the CASCADE study cardiac dysrhythmias due to ICD dysfunction have been shown to be significantly reduced by long-term administration of amiodarone (CASCADE study, 1991). This favourable effect of amiodarone is more pronounced compared to class IC antiarrhythmic drugs, e.g., quinidine, procainamide, and flecainide (Huang et al., 1991). However, there are cases reporting the effectiveness of long-term quinidine therapy administered shortly after intravenous infusion of β-adrenoceptor agonist isoproterenol in the case of VF storms in patients with BrS, when amiodarone was ineffective (Jongman et al., 2007; Dakkak et al., 2015). According to further observations the number of appropriate and inappropriate ICD shocks can be reduced by sotalol, nevertheless overall mortality seems not to improve compared to placebo (Kühlkamp et al., 1999; Bollmann et al., 2005). Azimilide, another class III antiarrhythmic drug equally inhibits the rapid and slow components of delayed rectifier K^+ currents. It has the same positive effects as amiodarone, but it is known to cause less proarrhythmic effect. Additionally, azimilide has not been proven to reduce left ventricular systolic function during long-term antiarrhythmic treatment (Dorian et al., 2004). Positive effects of dronaderone and dofetilide (blocker of the rapid component of delayed rectifier K^+ current) were also described, but less antiarrhythmic and mortality reducing effects were verified compared to amiodarone and sotalol (Bollmann et al., 2005). Recurrent VF episodes were registered in more than one third of ICD patients treated with amiodarone alone. Importantly, more favorable results were found in patients on combined β-adrenoceptor antagonist and amiodarone management (Connolly et al., 2006).

Newest ICDs are suitable for the purpose of cardiac resynchronization therapy (CRT) as well. Tang et al. examined 1798 patients, half of whom were grouped, in a randomized way, into the category 'only ICD', while the other half into the category ICD complemented by CRT. In the course of the 40-month examination period they found that the relative risk of cardiovascular death in the CRT group fell by 24% compared to the 'only ICD' group, and the frequency of hospitalization was also signifcantly lower (Tang et al., 2010).

The European Society of Cardiology has issued recommendations for subcutaneous ICDs as well. The malfunctioning of these devices develops rarely, although the application of ATP or cardiac resynchronization is not available.

The implantation of ICD's is mainly performed as secondary prevention combined with β-adrenoceptor antagonist therapy (e.g. metoprolol 100 mg/die, carvedilol 50 mg/die or bisoprolol 10 mg/die) for patients who suffered malignant ventricular arrhythmia episodes (Connolly et al., 2006). For the purpose of primary prevention ICD's are implanted primarily for patients with congenital heart diseases, but according to the AHA protocol currently in force it is to be considered for patients suffering from heart failure as well (Al-Khatib et al., 2018). MADIT, MADIT-II, and SCD-HeFT trials proved that populations suffering from heart failure and ischemic heart disease, ICD implanation significantly improved overall mortality without any additional therapies (Moss et al., 1996; Moss et al., 2002; Mark et al., 2006). Accordingly, ICD implantation as a primary prevention is recommended for NYHA I heart failure patients where left ventricular ejection fraction is under 30%, for NYHA II and III patients where EF is under 35% and in the case of ischemic heart disease where EF is less than 40% (Al-Khatib et al., 2018).

The administration of β-adrenoceptor antagonists has especially great significance in the case of congenital heart disease patients and primary ion channel diseases. Both the short- and long-term survival of inherited long QT syndrome patients is clearly positively influenced β-adrenoceptor antagonist therapy unless it is the LQT3 type. The suggested β-adrenoceptor antagonists are propranolol (2–4 mg/kg/die) or the long-acting nadolol (1.5 mg/kg/die), while other β-adrenoceptor antagonists, e.g., metoprolol or atenolol seem to be ineffective in this particular indication. Regarding LQT3, drugs decreasing the late sodium current, e.g., flecainide, dofetilide, mexiletine, or ranolazine can be administered (Schwartz et al., 2012; Antzelevitch et al., 2014). Wilde et al. examined 118 LQT3-type LQT syndrome patients who had suffered some cardiac event (SCD, syncope, aborted cardiac death). They found that the administration of β-adrenoceptor antagonist reduced the development of a similar cardiac event among these patients later on by 83% in the case of women, while no such difference was found in the case of men (Wilde et al., 2016). The study of Shimizu et al. also emphasises the difference between the two sexes. They sequenced the clinical genomes of 1,124 patients including the pathological mutations causing the long QT syndrome. The retrospective data and the genetic findings together highlight the fact that LQT1 and LQT2 mutations much more frequently involve malignant ventricular arrhythmias in the case of women, while as regards the other 3 major types of mutation no differences can be detected between the two sexes (Shimizu et al., 2019). This is one reason why a widening range of attempts have been made for the genetically based risk assessment of channelopathies as it may be of use in the selection of closer observation and specific drug therapy.

ACE-inhibitors and aldosterone antagonists (eplerenone), which protect from ventricular arrhythmias associated to ischemic heart disease primarily, reduce the heterogeneity of APD and left ventricular reverse remodelling and lower the risk of sudden cardiac death (Alberte and Zipes, 2003; Pitt et al., 2003). It was confirmed in the CONSENSUS study already that in the period examined the administration of enalapril in the case of 253 patients suffering from NYHA IV heart failure reduced the development of SCD by 27% (CONSENSUS Trial Study Group, 1987). In the SOLVD study examining 2569 patients Lam et al. found that the administration of 20 mg enalapril per day reduced overall mortality by 12% and cardiovascular mortality by 4% in the case of heart failure patients (Lam et al., 2018). In the SAVE trial on 2,231 patients the administration of 3x25 mg captopril daily reduced overall cardiovascular mortality by a few percent compared to the placebo group but it did not meaningfully affect the risk of sudden cardiac death (Pfeffer et al., 1992). In the HOPE study 9,297 patients with preserved left ventricular function, but high cardiovascular risk were examined. Patients taking 10 mg of ramipril daily had a relative risk of 0.62 for SCD compared to placebo group (The Heart Outcomes Prevention Evaluation Study (HOPE) Investigators, 2000). Based on PROGRESS, EUROPA and ASCOT-BLPA trials the administration of 4–10 mg perindopril daily (individual dose is required based on kidney function and other taken drugs) significantly reduced cardiovascular mortality and the occurence of sudden cardiac death (Campbell, 2006). On the contrary, in the IMAGINE study 2,553 patients with left ventricular ejection fraction ≥40% were examined who underwent CABG, where 40 mg quinapril were given daily early after the operation. Compared to the placebo group there were no significant positive effects on cardiovascular mortality and on the occurrence of ventricular arrhythmias up to 3 years after surgery. However, ACE-I treatment increased the incidence of adverse events, mainly early after CABG (Rouleau et al, 2008).

The angiotensin-receptor blocker candesartan was proven, based on the CHARM low LVEF study published in 2004, to signifcantly reduce overall mortality as well as cardiovascular mortality when added to the base therapy of chronic heart failure patients with left ventricular EF of lower than 40% (Young et al., 2004). The same was confirmed by the favorable findings of the RESOLVD study where candesartan was added to the ACE-inhibitor (enalapril) and β-adrenoceptor antagonist (metoprolol) and the triple combination produced more favorable prognosis (McKelvie et al., 2003). Based on the data of ONTARGET, PROFESS and TRANSCEND studies the positive effects of angiotensin receptor blocker telmisartan at the daily dose of 80 mg on cardiovascular mortality and on the occurence of ventricular arrhythmias were confirmed. At the same time the superior effects of ACE-Is (e.g., ramipril, perindopril) compared to telmisartan were also noted (DiNicolantonio and O'Keefe, 2014).

Statins are inhibitors of the hydroximethylglutaryl coenzyme A reductase, i.e., they reduce the serum cholesterole level, in addition to which, thanks also to their pleiotropic effect, they reduce the likelihood of malignant ventricular arrhythmias. The DEFINITE study examined 229 non-ischemic heart disease patients undergoing ICD therapy where the administration of statins significantly reduced ventricular arrhythmogenesis and sudden cardiac death compared to patients without statin administration (Goldberger et al., 2006).

Furthermore, in the case of arrhythmias triggered by EADs, inhibitors of the L-type Ca^{++} currents may be administered as part of the long-term therapy. Morita et al. found that the late type Na channel blocker ranolazine reduced repolarization heterogeneity, and increased the threshold potential value required for the development of VF. In addition, its non-selective blocking property on L-type Ca channels and I_{Kr}, I_{Ks} currents was detected, too. Ranolazine is also effective in the case of VF with underlying reentry mechanism (Morita et al., 2011) and has been furthermore proven to signifcantly reduce the delivery of inappropriate ICD shocks (Bunch et al., 2011; Zareba et al., 2018). However, further data are needed to clearly evaluate the exact role of ranolazine in the prevention of SCD. According to the latest ESC guideline, ranolazine is recommended only in the case of LQTS3 patients as a preventive treatment of ventricular fibrillation (Priori et al., 2015).

The cyclin-dependent kinase inhibitor roscovitine, originally developed as a chemotherapeutic agent, accelerated the inactivation of L-type Ca channels in the course of model experiments, thereby reducing the likelihood of the development of ventricular arrhythmias (Krummen et al., 2016). Further research is however needed with reference to these agents.

ABLATION OF VF TRIGGERS AND SUBSTRATES

In the cases of recurrent or refractory VF and ICD storms secondary to repeated VF episodes, ablation of VF triggers and substrates have to be taken into consideration. In these circumstances electrophysiological testing, and intracardiac mapping are performed (Cheniti et al., 2017). In order to clearly localize the ablation site, beyond classical pace mapping, entrainment and phase mapping, lately, activation, or substrate mapping have been accomplished (deBakker, 2019). Radiofrequency ablations of both VF triggers and subtrates have to be achieved. Endocardial data can be completed with epicardial maps served by electrocardiographic imaging (ECGI) method. During ECGI process a special vest with 252 surface electrodes is worn by the patients. Data of ECGI combined with computer tomography raise the opportunity of a more exact localization of arrhythmia foci. During ECGI procedure together with intracardiac mapping, both endo- and epicardial maps can be gained by the investigator (Singh and Noheria, 2018).

In VF patients with ischemic heart disease, non-ischemic cardiomyopathies, valvulopathies, amyloidosis, long QT syndromes and IVF, short-coupling triggering ventricular premature beats originating from the Purkinje system were identified and ablated (Cheniti et al., 2018; Singh and Noheria, 2018). In 2011, successful epicardial ablations of premature beats of the right ventricular outflow tract (RVOT) were published in patients with BrS. In 2019, another study provided data on the VF ablation of 52 ERS patients. These interventions were carried out in the right ventricle, RVOT and Purkinje fibres. In both studies, during a 3-year follow-up period, 90% of patients were reported to be free of recurrent VF episodes (Nademanee et al., 2011; Nademanee et al., 2019).

SUMMARY

Sudden cardiac death is a leading death cause in developed countries, its fast and effective treatment as well as prevention are therefore high priority tasks. There are several non-invasive diagnostic opportunities serving the timely detection of diseases increasing susceptibility to inherited and acquired ventricular arrhythmia, and earliest possible detection is followed, as part of a long-term therapeutic strategy, by the assessment and application of drug and device therapy on an individual basis. In the case of cardiopulmonary resuscitation early defibrillation in addition to minimally interrupted chest compression has been proven to improve the outcome of patients. Radiofrequency ablation of VF triggers and substrates is also a feasible and emerging therapeutical opportunity.

AUTHOR CONTRIBUTIONS

All authors confirm that they have read and approved the paper and they have met the criteria for authorship. ZS: wrote the manuscript. DU: took part in preparing the manuscript. TÖ: took part in preparing the manuscript. VS: took part in preparing the manuscript. PN: prepared and reviewed the manuscript before publication.

FUNDING

This work was funded by GINOP-2.3.2-15-2016-00062.

REFERENCES

Aiba, T. (2019). Recent understanding of clinical sequencing and gene-based risk stratification in inherited primary arrhythmia syndrome. *J. Cardiol.* 73 (5), 335–342. doi: 10.1016/j.jjcc.2019.01.009

Ajam, K., Gold, L. S., Beck, S. S., Damon, S., Phelps, R., and Rea, T. D. (2011). Reliability of the cerebral performance category to classify neurological status among survivors of ventricular fibrillation arrest: a cohort study. *Scand. J. Trauma Resusc Emerg Med.* 19, 38. doi: 10.1186/1757-7241-19-38

Akrouh, A., Halcomb, S. E., Nichols, C. G., and Sala-Rabanal, M. (2009). Molecular biology of K(ATP) channels and implications for health and disease. *IUBMB Life.* 61 (10), 971–978. doi: 10.1002/iub.246

Alberte, C., and Zipes, D. P. (2003). Use of nonantiarrhythmic drugs for prevention of sudden cardiac death. *J. Cardiovasc. Electrophysiol.* 14 (Suppl 9), S87–S95. doi: 10.1046/j.1540-8167.14.s9.23.x

Al-Khatib, S. M., Stevenson, W. G., Ackerman, M. J., Bryant, W. J., Callans, D. J., Curtis, A. B., et al. (2018). 2017 AHA/ACC/HRS guideline for management of patients with ventricular arrhythmias and the prevention of sudden cardiac death a report of the american college of cardiology/american heart association task force on clinical practice guidelines and the heart rhythm society. *Heart Rhythm.* 15 (10), e190–e252. doi: 10.1016/j.hrthm.2017.10.035

Antzelevitch, C., and Yan, G. X. (2010). J wave syndromes. *Heart Rhythm.* 7 (4), 549–558. doi: 10.1016/j.hrthm.2009.12.006

Antzelevitch, C., Sicouri, S., Litovsky, S. H., Lukas, A., Krishnan, S. C., Di Diego, J. M., et al. (1991). Heterogeneity within the ventricular wall. Electrophysiology and pharmacology of epicardial, endocardial, and M cells. *Circ. Res.* 69 (6), 1427–1449. doi: 10.1161/01.res.69.6.1427

Antzelevitch, C., Yan, G. X., Shimizu, W., and Burashnikov, A. (2000). "Electrical heterogeneity, the ECG, and cardiac arrhythmias," in *Ch 26 in Cardiac Electrophysiology from cell to bedside, 3rd ed.* Eds. D. P. Zipes and J. Jalife (Philadelphia: W. B. Saunders), 222–238.

Antzelevitch, C., Nesterenko, V., Shryock, J. C., Rajamani, S., Song, Y., and Belardinelli, L. (2014). The role of late I Na in development of cardiac arrhythmias. *Handb. Exp. Pharmacol.* 221, 137–168. doi: 10.1007/978-3-642-41588-3_7

Anumonwo, J. M., and Lopatin, A. N. (2010). Cardiac strong inward rectifier potassium channels. *J. Mol. Cell Cardiol.* 48 (1), 45–54. doi: 10.1016/j.yjmcc.2009.08.013

Arking, D. E., Junttila, M. J., Goyette, P., Huertas-Vazquez, A., Eijgelsheim, M., Blom, M. T., et al. (2011). Identification of a sudden cardiac death susceptibility locus at 2q24.2 through genome-wide association in European ancestry individuals. *PloS Genet.* 7 (6), e1002158. doi: 10.1371/journal.pgen.1002158

Bakiner, O., Ertorer, M. E., Haydardedeoglu, F. E., Bozkirli, E., Tutuncu, N. B., and Demirag, N. G. (2008). Subclinical hypothyroidism is characterized by increased QT interval dispersion among women. *Med. Princ Pract.* 17 (5), 390–394. doi: 10.1159/000141503

Balla, C., Vitali, F., Brieda, A., Gualandi, F., Ferlini, A., Bertini, M., et al. (2019). Predictors of cardiac arrhythmic events in non coronary artery disease patients. *BMC Cardiovasc. Disord.* 19 (1), 104. doi: 10.1186/s12872-019-1083-6

Bardy, G. H., Lee, K. L., Mark, D. B., Poole, J. E., Packer, D. L., Boineau, R., et al. (2005). Amiodarone or an implantable cardioverter-defibrillator for congestive heart failure. *N Engl. J. Med.* 352, 225–237. doi: 10.1056/NEJMoa043399

Barta, K., Czifra, Á., Kun, C., Páll, A., Kulcsár, J., Paragh, G., et al. (2014). Hemodiafiltration beneficially affects QT interval duration and dispersion compared to hemodialysis. *Clin. Exp. Nephrol.* 18 (6), 952–959. doi: 10.1007/s10157-014-0950-9

Bayes De Luna, A., Coumel, P., and Leclercq, J. F. (1989). Ambulatory sudden death: mechanisms of production of fatal arrhythmia on the basis of data from 157 cases. *Am. Heart. J.* 117, 151–159. doi:10.1016/0002-8703(89)90670-4

Benito, B., Sarkozy, A., Mont, L., Henkens, S., Berruezo, A., Tamborero, D., et al. (2008). Gender differences in clinical manifestations of Brugada syndrome. *J. Am. Coll. Cardiol.* 52 (19), 1567–1573. doi: 10.1016/j.jacc.2008.07.052

Benjamin, E. J., Blaha, M. J., Chiuve, S. E., Cushman, M., Das, S. R., Deo, R., et al. (2017). Heart disease and stroke statistics 2017 Update: a report from the American heart association. *Circulation* 135, e146–e603. doi: 10.1161/CIR.0000000000000485

Berdowski, J., Berg, R. A., Tijssen, J. G., and Koster, R. W. (2010). Global incidences of out-of-hospital cardiac arrest and survival rates: systematic review of 67 prospective studies. *Resuscitation* 81, 1479–1487. doi: 10.1016/j.resuscitation.2010.08.006

Berg, D. D., Bobrow, B. J., and Berg, R. A. (2019). Key components of a community response to out-of-hospital cardiac arrest. *Nat. Rev. Cardiol.* 16 (7), 407–416. doi: 10.1038/s41569-019-0175-4

Berger, R. D., Kasper, E. K., Baughman, K. L., Marban, E., Calkins, H., and Tomaselli, G. F. (1997). Beat-to-beat QT interval variability: novel evidence for repolarization lability in ischemic and nonischemic dilated cardiomyopathy. *Circulation* 96 (5), 1557–1565. doi: 10.1161/01.CIR.96.5.1557

Berne, P., and Brugada, J. (2012). Brugada syndrome. *Circ. J.* 76 (7), 1563–1571. doi: 10.1253/circj.cj-12-0717

Bezzina, C. R., Pazoki, R., Bardai, A., Marsman, R. F., de Jong, J. S., Blom, M. T., et al. (2010). Genome-wide association study identifies a susceptibility locus at 21q21 for ventricular fibrillation in acute myocardial infarction. *Nat. Genet.* 42, 688–691. doi: 10.1038/ng.623

Bloomfield, D. M., Steinman, R. C., Namerow, P. B., Parides, M., Davidenko, J., Kaufman, E. S., et al. (2004). Microvolt T wave alternans distinguishes between patients likely and patients not-likely to benefit from implanted cardiac defibrillator therapy: a solution to the multicentre automatic defibrillator implantation trial. *Circulation* 110, 1885–1889. doi: 10.1161/01.CIR.0000143160.14610.53

Bollmann, A., Husser, D., and Cannom, D. S. (2005). Antiarrhythmic drugs in patients with implantable cardioverter-defibrillators. *Am. J. Cardiovasc. Drugs* 5 (6), 371–378. doi: 10.2165/00129784-200505060-00004

Boriani, G., Biffi, M., Valzania, C., Bronzetti, G., and Martignani, C. (2006). Short QT syndrome and arrhythmogenic cardiac diseases in the young: the challenge of implantable cardioverter defibrillator therapy for children. *Eur. Heart J.* 27 (20), 2382–2384. doi: 10.1093/eurheartj/ehl223

Bourque, D., Daoust, R., Huard, V., and Charneux, M. (2007). Beta-blockers for the treatment of cardiac arrest from ventricular fibrillation. *Resuscitation* 75, 434–434. doi: 10.1016/j.resuscitation.2007.05.013

Brodde, O. E. (2007). Beta-adrenoceptor blocker treatment and the cardiac beta-adrenoceptor-G-protein(s)-adenylyl cyclase system in chronic heart failure. *Naunyn Schmiedebergs Arch. Pharmacol.* 374 (5-6), 361–372. doi: 10.1007/s00210-006-0125-7

Bro-Jeppesen, J., Kjaergaard, J., Wanscher, M., Pedersen, F., Holmvang, L., Lippert, F. K., et al. (2012). Emergency coronary angiography in comatose cardiac arrest patients: do real-life experiences support the guidelines? *Eur.*

Heart J. Acute Cardiovasc. Care 1 (4), 291–301. doi: 10.1177/2048872612465588

Burattini, L., Bini, S., and Burattini, R. (2009). Comparative analysis of methods for automatic detection and quantification of microvolt T-wave alternans. *Med. Eng. Phys.* 31 (10), 1290–8. doi: 10.1016/j.medengphy.2009.08.009

Bunch, T. J., Mahapatra, S., Murdock, D., Molden, J., Weiss, J. P., May, H. T., et al. (2011). Ranolazine reduces ventricular tachycardia burden and ICD shocks in patients with drug-refractory ICD shocks. *Pacing Clin. Electrophysiol.* 34 (12), 1600–1606. doi: 10.1111/j.1540-8159.2011.03208.x

Bunch, T. J., Hammill, S. C., and White, R. D. (2005). Outcomes after ventricular fibrillation out-of-hospital cardiac arrest: expanding the chain of survival. *Mayo Clin. Proc.* 80 (6), 774–782. doi: 10.1016/S0025-6196(11)61532-2

Campbell, D. J. (2006). A review of Perindopril in the reduction of cardiovascular events. *Vasc. Health Risk Manage.* 2 (2), 117–124. doi: 10.2147/vhrm.2006.2.2.117

Campuzano, O., Brugada, R., and Iglesias, A. (2010). Genetics of Brugada syndrome. *Curr. Opin. Cardiol.* 25 (3), 210–215. doi: 10.1097/HCO.0b013e32833846ee

Cardiac Arrest in Seattle: Conventional Versus Amiodarone Drug Evaluation (the CASCADE study). (1991). *Am. J. Cardiol.* 67 (7), 578–584. doi: 10.1016/0002-9149(91)90895-r

Cardoso, C., Salles, G., Bloch, K., Deccache, W., and Siqueira-Filho, A. G. (2001). Clinical determinants of increased QT dispersion in patients with diabetes mellitus. *Int. J. Cardiol.* 79 (2–3), 253–262. doi: 10.1016/s0167-5273(01)00443-0

Cerbai, E., Sartiani, L., DePaoli, P., Pino, R., Maccherini, M., Bizzarri, F., et al. (2001). The properties of the pacemaker current I(F)in human ventricular myocytes are modulated by cardiac disease. *J. Mol. Cell Cardiol.* 33 (3), 441–448. doi: 10.1006/jmcc.2000.1316

Cheitlin, M. D., Armstrong, W. F., Aurigemma, G. P., Beller, G. A., Bierman, F. Z., Davis, J. L., et al. (2003). ACC/AHA/ASE 2003 guideline update for the clinical application of echocardiography-summary article: a report of the american college of cardiology/american heart association task force on practice guidelines (ACC/AHA/ASE committee to update the 1997 guidelines for the clinical application of echocardiography). *J. Am. Coll. Cardiol.* 42, 954–970. doi: 10.1161/01.CIR.0000073597.57414.A9

Cheniti, G., Hocini, M., Martin, R., Sacher, F., Dubois, R., Haissaguerre, M., et al. (2017). Is VF an ablatable rhythm? *Curr. Treat Options Cardiovasc. Med.* (2), 14. doi: 10.1007/s11936-017-0511-0

Cheniti, G., Vlachos, K., Meo, M., Puyo, S., Thompson, N., Denis, A., et al. (2018). Mapping and ablation of idiopathic ventricular fibrillation. *Front. Cardiovasc. Med.* 5, 123. doi: 10.3389/fcvm.2018.00123

Connolly, S. J., Dorian, P., Roberts, R. S., Gent, M., Bailin, S., Fain, E. S., et al. (2006). Comparison of beta-blockers, amiodarone plus beta-blockers, or sotalol for prevention of shocks from implantable cardioverter defibrillators: the OPTIC Study: a randomized trial. *JAMA* 295 (2), 165–171. doi: 10.1001/jama.295.2.165

CONSENSUS Trial Study Group. (1987). Effects of enalapril on mortality in severe congestive heart failure. results of the cooperative north scandinavian enalapril survival study (CONSENSUS). *N Engl. J. Med.* 316 (23), 1429–1435. doi: 10.1056/NEJM198706043162301

Cortez, E., Krebs, W., Davis, J., Keseg, D. P., and Panchal, A. R. (2016). Use of double sequential external defibrillation for refractory ventricular fibrillation during out-of-hospital cardiac arrest. *Resuscitation* 108, 82–86. doi: 10.1016/j.resuscitation.2016.08.002

Coutinho Cruz, M., Viveiros Monteiro, A., Portugal, G., Laranjo, S., Lousinha, A., Valente, B., et al. (2019). Long-term follow-up of adult patients with congenital heart disease and an implantable cardioverter defibrillator. *Congenit. Heart. Dis.* 14 (4), 525–533. doi: 10.1111/chd.12767

Dakkak, M., Baxi, K., and Patel, A. (2015). Beneficial effects of isoproterenol and quinidine in the treatment of ventricular fibrillation in brugada syndrome. *Case Rep. Cardiol.* 2015, 753537. doi: 10.1155/2015/753537

Darbar, D., Luck, J., Davidson, N., Pringle, T., Main, G., McNeill, G., et al. (1996). Sensitivity and specificity of QTc dispersion for identification of risk of cardiac death in patients with peripheral vascular disease. *BMJ* 312 (7035), 874–8; discussion 878-9. doi: 10.1136/bmj.312.7035.874

Daya, M. R., Schmicker, R. H., Zive, D. M., Rea, T. D., Nichol, G., Buick, J. E., et al. (2015). Out-of-hospital cardiac arrest survival improving over time: results from the resuscitation outcomes consortium (ROC). *Resuscitation* 91, 108–115. doi: 10.1016/j.resuscitation.2015.02.003

deBakker, J. M. (2019). Electrogram recording and analyzing techniques to optimize selection of target sites for ablation of cardiac arrhythmias. *Pacing Clin. Electrophysiol.* 42 (12), 1503–1516. doi: 10.1111/pace.13817

Deyell, M. W., Krahn, A. D., and Goldberger, J. J. (2015). Sudden cardiac death risk stratification. *Circ. Res.* 116 (12), 1907–1918. doi: 10.1161/CIRCRESAHA.116.304493

DiNicolantonio, J. J., and O'Keefe, J. H. (2014). Perindopril for improving cardiovascular events. *Vasc. Health Risk Manage.* 10, 539–548. doi: 10.2147/VHRM.S68384

do Vale, G. T., Ceron, C. S., Gonzaga, N. A., Simplicio, J. A., and Padovan, J. C. (2019). Three generations of β-blockers: history, class differences and clinical applicability. *Curr. Hypertens. Rev.* 15 (1), 22–31. doi: 10.2174/1573402114666180918102735

Dobson, C. P., Kim, A., and Haigney, M. (2013). QT Variability Index. *Prog. Cardiovasc. Dis.* 56 (2), 186–194. doi: 10.1016/j.pcad.2013.07.004

Dorian, P., Borggrefe, M., Al-Khalidi, H. R., Hohnloser, S. H., Brum, J. M., Tatla, D. S., et al. (2004). Placebo-controlled, randomized clinical trial of azimilide for prevention of ventricular tachyarrhythmias in patients with an implantable cardioverter defibrillator. *Circulation* 110 (24), 3646–3654. doi: 10.1161/01.CIR.0000149240.98971.A8

Dorian, P. (2005). Antiarrhythmic action of β-Blockers: potential mechanisms. *Cardiovasc. Pharmacol. Therapeut* 10 (Suppl I), S15–S22. doi: 10.1177/10742484050100i403

Eastaugh, L. J., James, P. A., Phelan, D. G., and Davis, A. M. (2011). Brugada syndrome caused by a large deletion in SCN5A only detected by multiplex ligation-dependent probe amplification. *J. Cardiovasc. Electrophysiol.* 22 (9), 1073–1076. doi: 10.1111/j.1540-8167.2010.02003.x

Eckart, R. E., Shry, E. A., Burke, A. P., McNear, J. A., Appel, D. A., Castillo-Rojas, L. M., et al. (2011). Sudden death in young adults: an autopsy-based series of a population undergoing active surveillance. *J. Am. Coll. Cardiol.* 58 (12), 1254–1261. doi: 10.1016/j.jacc.2011.01.049

El-Sherif, N., Boutjdir, M., and Turitto, G. (2017). Sudden cardiac death in ischemic heart disease: pathophysiology and risk stratification. *Card Electrophysiol. Clin.* 9 (4), 681–691. doi: 10.1016/j.ccep.2017.08.003

Finance, O., Manning, A., and Chatelain, P. (1995). Effects of a new amiodarone-like agent, SR 33589, in comparison to amiodarone, D,L-sotalol, and lignocaine, on ischemia-induced ventricular arrhythmias in anesthetized pigs. *J. Cardiovasc. Pharmacol.* 26 (4), 570–576. doi: 10.1097/00005344-199510000-00010

Fink, A., Duray, G. Z., and Hohnloser, S. H. (2011). A patient with recurrent atrial fibrillation and monomorphic ventricular tachycardia treated successfully with dronedarone. *Europace* 13 (2), 284–285. doi: 10.1093/europace/euq365

Fisher, J. D., Mehra, R., and Furman, S. (1978). Termination of ventricular tachycardia with bursts of rapid ventricular pacing. *Am. J. Cardiol.* 41, 94–102. doi: 10.1016/0002-9149(78)90138-8

Fogel, M. A. (2002). Use of ejection fraction (or lack thereof), morbidity/mortality and heart failure drug trials: a review. *Int. J. Cardiol.* 84 (2–3), 119–132. doi: 10.1016/s0167-5273(02)00134-1

Francia, P., Adduci, C., Semprini, L., Borro, M., Ricotta, A., Sensini, I., et al. (2014). Osteopontin and galectin-3 predict the risk of ventricular tachycardia and fibrillation in heart failure patients with implantable defibrillators. *J. Cardiovasc. Electrophysiol.* 25 (6), 609–616. doi: 10.1111/jce.12364

Frothingham, R. (2001). Rates of torsades de pointes associated with ciprofloxacin, ofloxacin, levofloxacin, gatifloxacin, and moxifloxacin. *Pharmacotherapy* 21, 1468–1472. doi: 10.1592/phco.21.20.1468.34482

Frye, K. L., Adewale, A., Kennedy, E., and O'Grady, L. (2018). Beyond advanced cardiac life support: dual-sequential defibrillation for refractory ventricular fibrillation after witnessed cardiac arrest in the emergency department. *Cureus* 10 (12), e3717. doi: 10.7759/cureus.3717

Funck-Brentano, C. (1993). Pharmacokinetic and pharmacodynamic profiles of d-sotalol and d,l-sotalol. *Eur Heart J.* 14 (Suppl H), 30–35. doi: 10.1093/eurheartj/14.suppl_h.30

Garson, A., and McNamara, D. G. (1985). Sudden death in a pediatric cardiology population, 1958 to 1983: relation to prior arrhythmias. *J. Am. Coll. Cardiol.* 5 (Suppl), 134B–137B. doi: 10.1016/S0735-1097(85)80543-X

Gates, S., Quinn, T., Deakin, C. D., Blair, L., Couper, K., and Perkins, G. D. (2015). Mechanical chest compression for out of hospital cardiac arrest: systematic review and meta-analysis. *Resuscitation* 94, 91–97. doi: 10.1016/j.resuscitation.2015.07.002

Gilotra, N. A., Chow, G. V., and Cingolani, O. H. (2013). Cardiac amyloidosis presenting with prolonged QT interval and recurrent polymorphic ventricular tachycardia. *Tex Heart Inst. J.* 40 (2), 193–195.

Glinge, C., Sattler, S., Jabbari, R., and Tfelt-Hansen, J. (2016). Epidemiology and genetics of ventricular fibrillation during acute myocardial infarction. *J. Geriatr. Cardiol.* 13 (9), 789–797. doi: 10.11909/j.issn.1671-5411.2016.09.006

Goldberger, J. J., Subacius, H., Schaechter, A., Howard, A., Berger, R., Shalaby, A., et al. (2006). Effects of statin therapy on arrhythmic events and survival in patients with nonischemic dilated cardiomyopathy. *J. Am. Coll. Cardiol.* 48 (6), 1228–1233. doi: 10.1016/j.jacc.2006.05.053

Gough, C. J. R., and Nolan, J. P. (2018). The role of adrenaline in cardiopulmonary resuscitation. *Crit. Care* 22 (1), 139. doi: 10.1186/s13054-018-2058-1

Gupta, P., Patel, C., Patel, H., Narayanaswamy, S., Malhotra, B., Green, J. T., et al. (2008). T(p-e)/QT ratio as an index of arrhythmogenesis. *J. Electrocardiol.* 41, 567–574. doi: 10.1016/j.jelectrocard.2008.07.016

Haarmark, C., Hansen, P. R., Vedel-Larsen, E., Pedersen, S. H., Graff, C., Andersen, M. P., et al. (2009). The prognostic value of the T peak-T end interval in patients undergoing primary percutaneous coronary intervention for ST segment elevation myocardial infarction. *J. Electrocardiol.* 42, 555–560. doi: 10.1016/j.jelectrocard.2009.06.009

Haarmark, C., Graff, C., Andersen, M. P., Hardahl, T., Struijk, J. J., Toft, E., et al. (2010). Reference values of electrocardiogram repolarization variables in a healthy population. *J. Electrocardiol.* 43 (1), 31–39. doi: 10.1016/j.jelectrocard.2009.08.001

Haddad, P. M., and Anderson, I. M. (2002). Antipsychotic-related QTc prolongation, torsade de pointes and sudden death. *Drugs* 62, 1649–1671. doi: 10.2165/00003495-200262110-00006

Haissaguerre, M., Derval, N., Sacher, F., Jesel, L., Deisenhofer, I., de Roy, L., et al. (2008). Sudden cardiac arrest associated with early repolarization. *N Engl. J. Med.* 358, 2016. doi: 10.1056/NEJMoa071968

Herlitz, J., Engdahl, J., Svensson, L., Angquist, K. A., Young, M., and Holmberg, S. (2005). Factors associated with an increased chance of survival among patients suffering from an out-of-hospital cardiac arrest in a national perspective in Sweden. *Am. Heart J.* 149 (1), 61–66. doi: 10.1016/J.Ahj.2004.07.014

Hinterseer, M., Thomsen, M. B., Beckmann, B. M., Pfeufer, A., Schimpf, R., Wichmann, H. E., et al. (2008). Beat-to-beat variability of QT intervals is increased in patients with drug-induced long-QT syndrome: a case control pilot study. *Eur. Heart J.* 29 (2), 185–190. doi: 10.1093/eurheartj/ehm586

Hinterseer, M., Beckmann, B. M., Thomsen, M. B., Pfeufer, A., Dalla Pozza, R., Loeff, M., et al. (2009). Relation of increased short-term variability of QT interval to congenital long-QT syndrome. *Am. J. Cardiol.* 103 (9), 1244–1248. doi: 10.1016/j.amjcard.2009.01.011

Hinterseer, M., Beckmann, B. M., Thomsen, M. B., Pfeufer, A., Ulbrich, M., Sinner, M. F., et al. (2010). Usefulness of short-term variability of QT intervals as a predictor for electrical remodeling and proarrhythmia in patients with nonischemic heart failure. *Am. J. Cardiol.* 106 (2), 216–220. doi: 10.1016/j.amjcard.2010.02.033

Hjalmarson, A. (1999). Prevention of sudden cardiac death with beta blockers. *Clin. Cardiol.* 22 Suppl 5, V11–V15.

Hosseini, S. M., Kim, R., Udupa, S., Costain, G., Jobling, R., Liston, E., et al. (2018). Reappraisal of reported genes for sudden arrhythmic death. *Circulation* 138 (12), 1195–1205. doi: 10.1161/CIRCULATIONAHA.118.035070

Huang, S. K., Tan de Guzman, W. L., Chenarides, J. G., Okike, N. O., and Vander Salm, T. J. (1991). Effects of long-term amiodarone therapy on the defibrillation threshold and the rate of shocks of the implantable cardioverter-defibrillator. *Am. Heart J.* 122 (3 Pt 1), 720–727. doi: 10.1016/0002-8703(91)90517-l

Hwang, C. W., Gamble, G., Marchick, M., and Becker, T. K. (2019). A case of refractory ventricular fibrillation successfully treated with low-dose esmolol. *BMJ Case Rep.* 12, e228208. doi: 10.1136/bcr-2018-228208

Hypothermia after Cardiac Arrest Study Group. (2002). Mild therapeutic hypothermia to improve the neurologic outcome after cardiac arrest. *N Engl. J. Med.* 346 (8), 549–556. doi: 10.1056/NEJMoa012689

Issa, Z. F., Miller, J. M., and Zipes, D. P. (2012). "Ventricular arrhythmias in inherited channelopathies." in: *Ch 31 in clinical arrhythmology and electrophysiology: a companion to Braunwald's heart disease. 2nd edition.* Eds. Z. F. Issa, J. M. Miller and D. P. Zipes (Philadelphia: W.B. Saunders), 645–684. doi: 10.1016/B978-1-4557-1274-8.00031-2

Jin, Q., Wu, L., Dosdall, D. J., Li, L., Rogers, J. M., Ideker, R. E., et al. (2018). Effects of combination of sotalol and verapamil on initiation, maintenance and termination of ventricular fibrillation in swine hearts. *Cardiovasc. Ther.* 36 (3), e12326. doi: 10.1111/1755-5922.12326

Jongman, J. K., Jepkes-Bruin, N., Ramdat Misier, A. R., Beukema, W. P., Delnoy, P. P., Oude Luttikhuis, H., et al. (2007). Electrical storms in Brugada syndrome successfully treated with isoproterenol infusion and quinidine orally. *Neth. Heart J.* 15 (4), 151–155. doi: 10.1007/bf03085972

Jouven, X., Desnos, M., Guerot, C., and Ducimetière, P. (1999). Predicting sudden death in the population: the Paris prospective study I. *Circulation* 99, 1978–1983. doi: 10.1161/01.cir.99.15.1978

Kahn, J. K., Glazier, S., Swor, R., Savas, V., and O'Neill, W. W. (1995). Primary coronary angioplasty for acute myocardial infarction complicated by out-of-hospital cardiac arrest. *Am. J. Cardiol.* 75 (15), 1069–1070. doi: 10.1016/s0002-9149(99)80727-9

Kapplinger, J. D., Tester, D. J., Alders, M., Benito, B., Berthet, M., Brugada, J., et al. (2010). An international compendium of mutations in the SCN5A-encoded cardiac sodium channel in patients referred for Brugada syndrome genetic testing. *Heart Rhythm.* 7 (1), 33–46. doi: 10.1016/j.hrthm.2009.09.069

Karagueuzian, H. S., Nguyen, T. P., Qu, Z., and Weiss, J. N. (2013). Oxidative stress, fibrosis, and early afterdepolarization-mediated cardiac arrhythmias. *Front. Physiol.* 4, 19. doi: 10.3389/fphys.2013.00019 eCollection 2013.

Karlis, G., and Afantenou, S. (2018). Drugs in cardiac arrest: the rise and fall of antiarrhythmics. *Acta Cardiol.* 73 (4), 325–327. doi: 10.1080/00015385.2017.1389803

Kilicaslan, F., Tokatli, A., Ozdag, F., Uzun, M., Uz, O., Isilak, Z., et al. (2012). Tp-e interval, Tp-e/QT ratio and Tp-e/QTc ratio are prolonged in patients with moderate and severe obstructive sleep apnea. *Pacing Clin. Electrophysiol.* 35, 966–972. doi: 10.1111/j.1540-8159.2012.03439.x

Kim, G. H., Ryan, J. J., and Archer, S. L. (2013). The role of redox signaling in epigenetics and cardiovascular disease. *Antioxid. Redox Signal.* 18 (15), 1920–1936. doi: 10.1089/ars.2012.4926

Kim, T. H., Hong, K. J., Shin, S. D., Kim, C. H., Song, S. W., Song, K. J., et al. (2016). Quality between mechanical compression on reducible stretcher versus manual compression on standard stretcher in small elevator. *Am. J. Emerg Med.* 34, 1604–1609. doi: 10.1016/j.ajem.2016.05.072

Klappacher, G., Franzen, P., Haab, D., Mehrabi, M., Binder, M., Plesch, K., et al. (1995). Measuring extracellular matrix turnover in the serum of patients with idiopathic or ischemic dilated cardiomyopathy and impact on diagnosis and prognosis. *Am. J. Cardiol.* 75 (14), 913–918. doi: 10.1016/s0002-9149(99)80686-9

Koldobskiy, D., Groves, S., Scharf, S. M., and Cowan, M. J. (2014). Validation of factors affecting the outcome of cardiopulmonary arrest in a large, urban, academic medical center. *Hindawi Publishing Corp. J. Crit. Care Med.* 2014, 7 pages. doi: 10.1155/2014/168132

Kors, J. A., Ritsema van Eck, H. J., and van Herpen, G. (2008). The meaning of the Tp-Te interval and its diagnostic value. *J. Electrocardiol.* 41, 575–580. doi: 10.1016/j.jelectrocard.2008.07.030

Koster, R. W., Beenen, L. F., van der Boom, E. B., Spijkerboer, A. M., Tepaske, R., van der Wal, A. C., et al. (2017). Safety of mechanical chest compression devices AutoPulse and LUCAS in cardiac arrest: a randomized clinical trial for non-inferiority. *Eur. Heart J.* 38 (40), 3006–3013. doi: 10.1093/eurheartj/ehx318

Krummen, D. E., Ho, G., Villongco, C. T., Hayase, J., and Schricker, A. A. (2016). Ventricular fibrillation: triggers, mechanisms and therapies. *Future Cardiol.* 12 (3), 373–390. doi: 10.2217/fca-2016-0001

Kudenchuk, P. J., Brown, S. P., Daya, M., Rea, T., Nichol, G., Morrison, L. J., et al. (2016). Amiodarone, lidocaine, or placebo in out-of-hospital cardiac arrest. *N Eng. J. Med.* 374, 1711–1722. doi: 10.1056/NEJMoa1514204

Kühlkamp, V., Mewis, C., Mermi, J., Bosch, R. F., and Seipel, L. (1999). Suppression of sustained ventricular tachyarrhythmias: a comparison of d,l-sotalol with no antiarrhythmic drug treatment. *J. Am. Coll. Cardiol.* 33 (1), 46–52. doi: 10.1016/s0735-1097(98)00521-x

Laina, A., Karlis, G., Liakos, A., Georgiopoulos, G., Oikonomou, D., Kouskouni, E., et al. (2016). Amiodarone and cardiac arrest: Systematic review and meta-analysis. *Int. J. Cardiol.* 221, 780–788. doi: 10.1016/j.ijcard.2016.07.138

Lam, P. H., Dooley, D. J., Fonarow, G. C., Butler, J., Bhatt, D. L., Filippatos, G. S., et al. (2018). Similar clinical benefits from below-target and target dose enalapril in patients with heart failure in the SOLVD Treatment trial. *Eur. J. Heart Fail.* 20 (2), 359–369. doi: 10.1002/ejhf.937

Larsen, M. P., Eisenberg, M. S., Cummins, R. O., and Hallstrom, A. P. (1993). Predicting survival from out-of-hospital cardiac arrest: a graphic model. *Ann. Emerg Med.* 22, 1652–1658. doi: 10.1016/s0196-0644(05)81302-2

Lee, Y. H., Lee, K. J., Min, Y. H., Ahn, H. C., Sohn, Y. D., Lee, W. W., et al. (2016). Refractory ventricular fibrillation treated with esmolol. *Resuscitation* 107, 150–155. doi: 10.1016/j.resuscitation.2016.07.243

Lengyel, C., Orosz, A., Hegyi, P., Komka, Z., Udvardy, A., Bosnyák, E., et al. (2011). Increased short-term variability of the QT interval in professional soccer players: possible implications for arrhythmia prediction. *PloS One* 6 (4), e18751. doi: 10.1371/journal.pone.0018751

Levy, M., Yost, D., Walker, R. G., Scheunemann, E., and Mendive, S. R. (2015). A quality improvement initiative to optimize use of a mechanical chest compression device wihin a high-performance CPR approach to out-of-hospital cardiac arrest resuscitation. *Resuscitation* 92, 32–37. doi: 10.1016/j.resuscitation.2015.04.005

Link, M. S., Berkow, L. C., Kudenchuk, P. J., Halperin, H. R., Hess, E. P., Moitra, V. K., et al. (2015). Part 7: adult advanced cardiovascular life support:2015 American heart association guidelines update for cardiopulmonary resuscitation and emergency cardiovascular care. *Circulation* 132, S444–S464. doi: 10.1161/CIR.0000000000000261

Lőrincz, I., Mátyus, J., Zilahi, Z., Kun, C., Karányi, Z., and Kakuk, G. (1999). QT dispersion in patients with end-stage renal failure and during hemodialysis. *J. Am. Soc. Nephrol.* 10, 1297–1302.

Lubic, S. P., Nguyen, K. P., Dave, B., and Giacomini, J. C. (1994). Antiarrhythmic agent amiodarone possesses calcium channel blocker properties. *J. Cardiovasc. Pharmacol.* 24 (5), 707–714. doi: 10.1097/00005344-199424050-00004

Malhi, N., Cheung, C. C., Deif, B., Roberts, J. D., Gula, L. J., Green, M. S., et al. (2019). Challenge and impact of Quinidine access in sudden death syndromes. *JACC: Clin. Electrophysiol.* 5 (3), 376–382. doi: 10.1016/j.jacep.2018.10.007

Malik, M., and Batchvarov, V. N. (2000). Measurement, interpretation and clinical potential of QTdispersion. *J. Am. Coll. Cardiol.* 36 (6), 1749–1766. doi: 10.1016/s0735-1097(00)00962-1

Marcus, F. I., McKenna, W. J., Sherrill, D., Basso, C., Bauce, B., Bluemke, D. A., et al. (2010). Diagnosis of arrhythmogenic right ventricular cardiomyopathy/dysplasia: proposed modification of the task force criteria. *Circulation* 121 (13), 1533–1541. doi: 10.1093/eurheartj/ehq025

Mark, D. B., Nelson, C. L., Anstrom, K. J., Al-Khatib, S. M., Tsiatis, A. A., Cowper, P. A., et al. (2006). Cost-Effectiveness of defibrillator therapy or amiodarone in chronic stable heart failure results from the sudden cardiac death in heart failure trial (SCD-HeFT). *Circulation* 114 (2), 135–142. doi: 10.1161/CIRCULATIONAHA.105.581884

Markandeya, Y. S., and Kamp, T. J. (2015). Rational strategy to stop arrhythmias: early afterdepolarizations and L-type Ca2+ current. *J. Gen. Physiol.* 145 (6), 475–479. doi: 10.1085/jgp.201511429

Mason, J. W. (1987). Amiodarone. *N Engl. J. Med.* 316 (8), 455–466. doi: 10.1056/NEJM198702193160807

McKelvie, R. S., Rouleau, J. L., White, M., Afzal, R., Young, J. B., Maggioni, A. P., et al. (2003). Comparative impact of enalapril, candesartan or metoprolol alone or in combination on ventricular remodelling in patients with congestive heart failure. *Eur. Heart J.* 24, 1727–1734. doi: 10.1016/s0195-668x(03)00477-9

Morita, N., Lee, J. H., Xie, Y., Sovari, A., Qu, Z., Weiss, J. N., et al. (2011). Suppression of re-entrant and multifocal ventricular fibrillation by the late sodium current blocker ranolazine. *J. Am. Coll. Cardiol.* 57 (3), 366–375. doi: 10.1016/j.jacc.2010.07.045

Moss, A. J., Hall, W. J., Cannom, D. S., Daubert, J. P., Higgins, S. L., Klein, H., et al. (1996). Improved survival with an implanted defibrillator in patients with coronary disease at high risk for ventricular arrhythmia. multicenter automatic defibrillator implantation trial investigators. *N. Engl. J. Med.* 335 (26), 1933–1940. doi: 10.1056/NEJM199612263352601

Moss, A. J., Zareba, W., Hall, W. J., Klein, H., Wilber, D. J., Cannom, D. S., et al. (2002). Multicenter automatic defibrillator implantation trial ii investigators: prophylactic implantation of a defibrillator in patients with myocardial infarction and reduced ejection fraction. *N. Engl. J. Med.* 346 (12), 877–883. doi: 10.1056/NEJMoa013474

Myerburg, R. J., Kessler, K. M., and Castellanos, A. (1993). Sudden cardiac death: epidemiology, transient risk, and intervention assessment. *Ann. Intern Med.* 119 (12), 1187–1197. doi: 10.7326/0003-4819-119-12-199312150-00006

Nabauer, M., and Kaab, S. (1998). Potassium channel down-regulation in heart failure. *Cardiovasc. Res.* 37 (2), 324–334. doi: 10.1016/s0008-6363(97)00274-5

Nademanee, K., Veerakul, G., Chandanamattha, P., Chaothawee, L., Ariyachaipanich, A., Jirasirirojanakorn, K., et al. (2011). Prevention of ventricular fibrillation episodes in brugada syndrome by catheter ablation over the anterior right ventricular outflow tract epicardium. *Circulation* 123 (12), 1270–1279. doi: 10.1161/CIRCULATIONAHA.110.972612

Nademanee, K., Haissaguerre, M., Hocini, M., Nogami, A., Cheniti, G., Duchateau, J., et al. (2019). Mapping and ablation of ventricular fibrillation associated with early repolarization syndrome. *Circulation.* 140 (18), 1477–1490. doi: 10.1161/CIRCULATIONAHA.118.039022

Nanjayya, V. B., and Nayyar, V. (2012). Immediate coronary angiogram in comatose survivors of out-of-hospital cardiac arrest–an australian study. *Resuscitation* 83 (6), 699–704. doi: 10.1016/j.resuscitation.2011.12.004

Narayan, S. M. (2006). T wave alternans and the susceptibility to ventricular arrhythmias. *J. Am. Coll. Cardiol.* 47, 269–281. doi: 10.1016/j.jacc.2005.08.066

Nas, J., Thannhauser, J., Bonnes, J. L., and Brouwer, M. A. (2019). Importance of the distinction between recurrent and shock-resistant ventricular fibrillation: call for a uniform definition of refractory VF, resuscitation. *Resuscitation.* 138, 312–313. doi: 10.1016/j.resuscitation.2019.01.042

Neumar, R. W., Shuster, M., Callaway, C. W., Gent, L. M., Atkins, D. L., Bhanji, F., et al. (2015). Part 1: Executive summary: 2015 american heart association guidelines for cardiopulmonary resuscitation and emergency cardiovascular care. *Circulation* 132, S315–S367. doi: 10.1161/CIR.0000000000000252

Nikolaou, N. I., Welsford, M., Beygui, F., Bossaert, L., Ghaemmaghami, C., Nonogi, H., et al. (2015). Part 5: acute coronary syndromes: 2015 international consensus on cardiopulmonary resuscitation and emergency cardiovascular care science with treatment recommendations. *Resuscitation* 95, e121–e146. doi: 10.1016/j.resuscitation.2015.07.043

Norris, R. M., Barnaby, P. F., Brown, M. A., Geary, G. G., Clarke, E. D., Logan, R. L., et al. (1984). Prevention of ventricular fibrillation during acute myocardial infarction by intravenous propranolol. *Lancet* 2 (8408), 883–886. doi: 10.1016/s0140-6736(84)90651-2

Nuss, H. B., Johns, D. C., Kääb, S., Tomaselli, G. F., Kass, D., Lawrence, J. H., et al. (1996). Reversal of potassium channel deficiency in cells from failing hearts by adenoviral gene transfer: a prototype for gene therapy for disorders of cardiac excitability and contractility. *Gene Ther.* 3 (10), 900–912.

Obeyesekere, M. N., Klein, G. J., Modi, S., Leong-Sit, P., Gula, L. J., Yee, R., et al. (2011). How to perform and interpret provocative testing for the diagnosis of brugada syndrome, long-QT syndrome, and catecholaminergic polymorphic ventricular Tachycardia. *Circ.: Arrhythmia Electrophysiol.* 4, 958–964. doi: 10.1161/CIRCEP.111.965947

Oosterhoff, P., Tereshchenko, L. G., van der Heyden, M. A., Ghanem, R. N., Fetics, B. J., Berger, R. D., et al. (2011). Short-term variability of repolarization predicts ventricular tachycardia and sudden cardiac death in patients with structural heart disease: a comparison with QT variability index. *Heart Rhythm.* 8 (10), 1584–1590. doi: 10.1016/j.hrthm.2011.04.033

Opie, L. H., and Yusuf, S. (2001). "β-blocking agents. Ch 1," in *Drugs for the heart, 5th ed.* Eds. L. H. Opie (Philadelphia: WB Saunders), 1–60.

Owens, R. C., and Ambrose, P. G. (2005). Antimicrobial safety: focus on fluoroquinolones. *Clin. Infect. Dis. Off Publ Infect. Dis. Soc. Am.* 41Suppl 2, S144–S157. doi: 10.1086/428055

Páll, A., Sebestyén, V., Czifra, Á., Becs, G., Agarwal, A., Abolfazl, Z., et al. (2017). The disparate effect of hemodialysis and hemodiafiltration on T-wave-peak-to-end interval (Tpe) and Tpe/QT ratio of the surface electrocardiogram. *Trauma Emerg Care* 2 (5), 1–6. doi: 10.15761/TEC.1000142

Panchal, A. R., Berg, K. M., Kudenchuk, P. J., Del Rios, M., Hirsch, K. G., Link, M. S., et al. (2018). 2018 American heart association focused update on advanced cardiovascular life support use of antiarrhythmic drugs during and immediately after cardiac arrest: an update to the american heart association guidelines for cardiopulmonary resuscitation and emergency cardiovascular care. *Circulation* 138, e740–e749. doi: 10.1161/CIR.0000000000000613

Pascual-Figal, D. A., Ordoñez-Llanos, J., Tornel, P. L., Vázquez, R., Puig, T., Valdés, M., et al. (2009). Soluble ST2 for predicting sudden cardiac death in patients with chronic heart failure and left ventricular systolic dysfunction. *J. Am. Coll. Cardiol.* 54 (23), 2174–2179. doi: 10.1016/j.jacc.2009.07.041

Patton, K. K., Sotoodehnia, N., DeFilippi, C., Siscovick, D. S., Gottdiener, J. S., and Kronmal, R. A. (2011). N-terminal pro-B-type natriuretic peptide is associated with sudden cardiac death risk: the Cardiovascular Health Study. *Heart Rhythm.* 8, 228–233. doi: 10.1016/j.hrthm.2010.10.038

Peters, N. S., Cabo, C., and Wit, A. L. (2000). "Arrhythmogenic mechanisms: Automaticity, Triggered activity, and Reentry," in *Ch 40 in Cardiac Electrophysiology from cell to bedside, 3rd Ed.* Eds. D. P. Zipes and J. Jalife (Philadelphia: W. B. Saunders), 345–355.

Pfeffer, M. A., Braunwald, E., Moye, L. A., Basta, L., Brown, E. J., Cuddy, T. E., et al. (1992). Effect of captopril on mortality and morbidityin patients with left ventricular dysfunction after myocardial infarction. Results of the survival and ventricular enlargement trial. *N Engl. J. Med.* 327, 669–677. doi: 10.1056/NEJM199209033271001

Pitt, B., Remme, W., Zannad, F., Neaton, J., Martinez, F., Roniker, B., et al. (2003). Eplerenone Eplerenone, a selective aldosterone blocker, in patients with left ventricular dysfunction after myocardial infarction. *N Engl. J. Med.* 348, 1309–1321. doi: 10.1016/j.jacc.2005.04.038

Priori, S. G., and Chen, S. R. (2011). Inherited dysfunction of sarcoplasmic reticulum Ca2+ handling and arrhythmogenesis. *Circ. Res.* 108, 871–883. doi: 10.1161/CIRCRESAHA.110.226845

Priori, S. G., Napolitano, C., Gasparini, M., Pappone, C., Della Bella, P., Giordano, U., et al. (2002). Natural history of Brugada syndrome: insights for risk stratification and management. *Circulation* 105, 1342–1347. doi: 10.1161/hc1102.105288

Priori, S. G., Wilde, A. A., Horie, M., Cho, Y., Behr, E. R., Berul, C., et al. (2013). HRS/EHRA/APHRS expert consensus statement on the diagnosis and management of patients with inherited primary arrhythmia syndromes: document endorsed by HRS, EHRA, and APHRS in May 2013 and by ACCF, AHA, PACES, and AEPC in June 2013. *Heart Rhythm.* 10, 1932–1963. doi: 10.1016/j.hrthm.2013.05.014

Priori, S. G., Blomström-Lundqvist, C., Mazzanti, A., Blom, N., Borggrefe, M., Camm, J., et al. (2015). 2015 ESC guidelines for the management of patients with ventricular arrhythmias and the prevention of sudden cardiac death: the task force for the management of patients with ventricular arrhythmias and the prevention of sudden cardiac death of the european society of cardiology (ESC). Endorsed by: association for European paediatric and congenital cardiology (AEPC). *Eur. Heart J.* 36 (41), 2793–2867. doi: 10.1093/eurheartj/ehv316

Rea, T. D., Eisenberg, M. S., Sinibaldi, G., and White, R. D. (2004). Incidence of EMS-treated out-of-hospital cardiac arrest in the United States. *Resuscitation* 63, 17–24. doi: 10.1016/j.resuscitation.2004.03.025

Roden, D. M. (1998). Taking the "idio" out of "idiosyncratic": predicting torsades de pointes. *Pacing Clin. Electrophysiol.* 21 (5), 1029–1034. doi: 10.1111/j.1540-8159.1998.tb00148.x

Roden, D. M. (2016). Predicting drug-induced QT prolongation and torsades de pointes. *J. Physiol.* 594, 2459–2468. doi: 10.1113/JP270526

Rohr, S. (2004). Role of gap junctions in the propagation of the cardiac action potential. *Cardiovasc. Res.* 62 (2), 309–322. doi: 10.1016/j.cardiores.2003.11.035

Rouleau, J. L., Warnica, W. J., Baillot, R., Block, P. J., Chocron, S., Johnstone, D., et al. (2008). Effects of angiotensin-converting enzyme inhibition in low-risk patients early after coronary artery bypass surgery. *Circulation* 117 (1), 24–31. doi: 10.1161/CIRCULATIONAHA.106.685073

Salgado, A. A., Barbosa, P. R., Ferreira, A. G., Reis, C. A., and Terra, C. (2016). Prognostic value of a new marker of ventricular repolarization in cirrhotic patients. *Arq. Bras. Cardiol.* 107 (6), 523–531. doi: 10.5935/abc.20160181

Sampson, K. J., and Kass, R. S. (2011). "Antiarrhythmic drugs," in *Goodman & Gilman's the pharmacological basis of therapeutics, 12th ed.* Eds. L. L. Brunton, B. A. Chabner and B. C. Knollman (New York: McGraw-Hill), 815–848.

Sanfridsson, J., Sparrevik, J., Hollenberg, J., Nordberg, P., Djärv, T., Ringh, M., et al. (2019). Drone delivery of an automated external defibrillator - a mixed method simulation study of bystander experience. *Scand. J. Trauma Resusc Emerg Med.* 27 (1), 40. doi: 10.1186/s13049-019-0622-6

Scheirlynck, E., Dejgaard, L. A., Skjølsvik, E., Lie, O. H., Motoc, A., Hopp, E., et al. (2019). Increased levels of sST2 in patients with mitral annulus disjunction and ventricular arrhythmias. *Open Heart.* 6 (1), e001016. doi: 10.1136/openhrt-2019-001016

Schnee, P. M., Shah, N., Bergheim, M., Poindexter, B. J., Buja, L. M., Gemmato, C., et al. (2008). Location and density of alpha- and beta-adrenoreceptor sub-types in myocardium after mechanical left ventricular unloading. *J. Heart Lung Transplant* 27 (7), 710–717. doi: 10.1016/j.healun.2008.03.015

Schuger, C., Daubert, J. P., Brown, M. W., Cannom, D., Estes, N. A., Hall, W. J., et al. (2012). Multicenter automatic defibrillator implantation trial: reduce inappropriate therapy (MADIT-RIT): background, rationale, and clinical protocol. *Ann. Noninvasive Electrocardiol.* 17 (3), 176–185. doi: 10.1111/j.1542-474X.2012.00531.x

Schwartz, P. J., Crotti, L., and Insolia, R. (2012). Long-QT syndrome: from genetics to management. *Circ. Arrhythm Electrophysiol.* 5 (4), 868–877. doi: 10.1161/CIRCEP.111.962019

Sgreccia, A., Morelli, S., Ferrante, L., Perrone, C., De Marzio, P., De Vincentiis, G., et al. (1998). QT interval and QT dispersion in systemic sclerosis (scleroderma). *J. Intern Med.* 243 (2), 127–132.

Shimizu, M., Ino, H., Okeie, K., Yamaguchi, M., Nagata, M., Hayashi, K., et al. (2002). T peak to T end interval may be a better predictor of highrisk patients with hypertrophic cardiomyopathy associated with a cardiac troponin I mutation than QT dispersion. *Clin. Cardiol.* 25, 335–339. doi: 10.1002/clc.4950250706

Shimizu, W., Makimoto, H., Yamagata, K., Kamakura, T., Wada, M., Miyamoto, K., et al. (2019). Genetics and clinical aspects of congenital long-QT syndrome: results from the Japanese multicenter registry. *JAMA Cardiol.* 4 (3), 246–254. doi: 10.1001/jamacardio.2018.4925

Singh, P., and Noheria, A. (2018). Ablation approaches for ventricular fibrillation. *Curr. Treat Options Cardiovasc. Med.* 20 (3), 21. doi: 10.1007/s11936-018-0612-4

Soar, J., Nolan, J. P., Böttiger, B. W., Perkins, G. D., Lott, C., Carli, P., et al. (2015). European resuscitation council guidelines for resuscitation 2015, section 3. *Adult adv. Life support Resuscitation* 95, 100–147. doi: 10.1016/j.resuscitation.2015.07.016

Spach, M. S., and Josephson, M. E. (1994). Initiating reentry: the role of nonuniform anisotropy in small circuits. *J. Cardiovasc. Electrophysiol.* 5 (2), 182–209. doi: 10.1111/j.1540-8167.1994.tb01157.x

Stanger, D., Kawano, T., Malhi, N., Grunau, B., Tallon, J., Wong, G. C., et al. (2019). Door-to-targeted temperature management initiation time and outcomes in out-of-hospital cardiac arrest: insights from the continuous chest compressions trial. *J. Am. Heart Assoc.* 8 (9), e012001. doi: 10.1161/JAHA.119.012001

Stillitano, F., Lonardo, G., Zicha, S., Varro, A., Cerbai, E., Mugelli, A., et al. (2008). Molecular basis of funny current (If) in normal and failing human heart. *J. Mol. Cell Cardiol.* 45 (2), 289–299. doi: 10.1016/j.yjmcc.2008.04.013

Strote, J. A., Maynard, C., Olsufka, M., Nichol, G., Copass, M. K., Cobb, L. A., et al. (2012). Comparison of role of early (less than six hours) to later (more than six hours) or no cardiac catheterization after resuscitation from out-of-hospital cardiac arrest. *Am. J. Cardiol.* 109 (4), 451–454. doi: 10.1016/j.amjcard.2011.09.036

Szabó, Z., Harangi, M., Lörincz, I., Seres, I., Katona, E., Karányi, Z., et al. (2005). Effect of hyperlipidemia on QT dispersion in patients without ischemic heart disease. *Can. J. Cardiol.* 21 (10), 847–850.

Tang, A. S., Wells, G. A., Talajic, M., Arnold, M. O., Sheldon, R., Connolly, S., et al. (2010). Cardiac-resynchronization therapy for mild-to-moderate heart failure. *N Engl. J. Med.* 363 (25), 2385–2395. doi: 10.1056/NEJMoa1009540

Taylor, D. M. (2003). Antipsychotics and QT prolongation. *Acta Psychiatr. Scand.* 107, 85–95. doi: 10.1034/j.1600-0447.2003.02078.x

Teo, K. K., Yusuf, S., and Furberg, C. D. (1993). Effects of prophylactic antiarrhythmic drug therapy in acute myocardial infarction. an overview of results from randomized controlled trials. *JAMA* 270 (13), 1589–1595.

Teran, F., Dean, A. J., Centeno, C., Panebianco, N. L., Zeidan, A. J., Chan, W., et al. (2019). Evaluation of out-of-hospital cardiac arrest using transesophagea echocardiography in the emergency department. *Resuscitation* 137, 140–147. doi: 10.1016/j.resuscitation.2019.02.013

The Heart Outcomes Prevention Evaluation Study (HOPE) Investigators. (2000). Effects of an angiotensin-converting-enzyme inhibitor, ramipril, on cardiovascular events in high-risk patients. *N Engl. J. Med.* 342 (3), 145–153. doi: 10.1056/NEJM200001203420301

Therasse, D., Sacher, F., Petit, B., Babuty, D., Mabo, P., Martins, R., et al. (2017). Sodium-channel blocker challenge in the familial screening of Brugada syndrome: safety and predictors of positivity. *Heart Rhythm.* 14 (10), 1442–1448. doi: 10.1016/j.hrthm.2017.06.031

Thompson, C. A., Yarzebski, J., Goldberg, R. J., Lessard, D., Gore, J. M., and Dalen, J. E. (2000). Changes over time in the incidence and case-fatality rates of primary ventricular fibrillation complicating acute myocardial infarction: perspectives from the worcester heart attack study. *Am. Heart J.* 139, 1014. doi: 10.1067/mhj.2000.106160

Thygesen, K., and Uretsky, B. F. (2004). Acute ischaemia as a trigger of sudden cardiac death. *Eur. Heart J. Suppl.* 6 (SupplD), 88–90. doi: 10.1016/j.ehjsup.2004.05.006

Tinker, A., Aziz, Q., Li, Y., and Specterman, M. (2018). ATP-Sensitive potassium channels and their physiological and pathophysiological roles. *Compr. Physiol.* 8 (4), 1463–1511. doi: 10.1002/cphy.c170048

Tisdale, J. E., Patel, R. V., Webb, C. R., Borzak, S., and Zarowitz, B. J. (1995). Proarrhythmic effects of intravenous vasopressors. *Ann. Pharmacother.* 29 (3), 269–281. doi: 10.1177/106002809502900309

Topilski, I., Rogowski, O., Rosso, R., Justo, D., Copperman, Y., Glikson, M., et al. (2007). The morphology of the QT interval predict torsades de pointes during acquired bradyarrhythmias. *J. Am. Coll. Cardiol.* 49, 320–328. doi: 10.1016/j.jacc.2006.08.058

Tse, G., and Yan, B. P. (2017). Traditional and novel electrocardiographic conduction and repolarization markers of sudden cardiac death. *Europace* 19 (5), 712–721. doi: 10.1093/europace/euw280

Ujvárosy, D., Sebestyén, V., Pataki, T., Ötvös, T., Lőrincz, I., Paragh, G., et al. (2018). Cardiovascular risk factors differently affect the survival of patients undergoing manual or mechanical resuscitation. *BMC Cardiovasc. Disord.* 18 (1), 227. doi: 10.1186/s12872-018-0962-6

Van Camp, S. P. (1992). Sudden death. *Clin. Sports Med.* 11, 273–289.

Varkevisser, R., Wijers, S. C., van der Heyden, M. A., Beekman, J. D., Meine, M., and Vos, M. A. (2012). Beat-to-beat variability of repolarization as a new biomarker for proarrhythmia *in vivo*. *Heart Rhythm.* 9 (10), 1718–1726. doi: 10.1016/j.hrthm.2012.05.016

Varró, A., and Baczkó, I. (2011). Cardiac ventricular repolarization reserve: a principle for understanding drug-related proarrhythmic risk. *Br. J. Pharmacol.* 164 (1), 14–36. doi: 10.1111/j.1476-5381.2011.01367.x

Vieweg, W. V., and Wood, M. A. (2004). Tricyclic antidepressants, QT interval prolongation, and torsade de pointes. *Psychosomatics* 45, 371–377. doi: 10.1176/appi.psy.45.5.371

Vink, A. S., Neumann, B., Lieve, K. V., Sinner, M. F., Hofman, N., El Kadi, S., et al. (2018). Determination and interpretation of the QT interval. *Circulation* 138 (21), 2345–2358. doi: 10.1161/CIRCULATIONAHA.118.033943

Viskin, S., Adler, A., and Belhassen, B. (2013). "Idiopathic ventricular fibrillation," in *Electrical disease of the heart, volume 1. 2nd ed.* Eds. I. Gussak and C. Antzelevitch (London: Springer;), 629–646.

Waldo, A. L., Camm, A. J., deRuyter, H., Friedman, P. L., MacNeil, D. J., Pauls, J. F., et al. (1996). Effect of d-sotalol on mortality in patients with left ventricular dysfunction after recent and remote myocardial infarction. the SWORD investigators. survival with oral d-sotalol. *Lancet* 348, 7–12. doi: 10.1016/s0140-6736(96)02149-6

Wang, X., Zhang, L., Gao, C., Wu, S., and Zhu, J. (2019). ST-segment elevation and the Tpeak-Tend/QT ratio predict the occurrence of malignant arrhythmia events in patients with vasospastic angina. *J. Electrocardiol.* 53, 52–56. doi: 10.1016/j.jelectrocard.2019.01.001

Webster, A. L., Yan, M. S., and Marsden, P. A. (2013). Epigenetics and cardiovascular disease. *Can. J. Cardiol.* 29 (1), 46–57. doi: 10.1016/j.cjca.2012.10.023

Wilde, A. A., Moss, A. J., Kaufman, E. S., Shimizu, W., Peterson, D. R., Benhorin, J., et al. (2016). Clinical aspects of type 3 long-qt syndrome: an international multicenter study. *Circulation* 134 (12), 872–882. doi: 10.1161/CIRCULATIONAHA.116.021823

Xu, J., Hee, L., Hopkins, A., Juergens, C. P., Lo, S., French, J. K., et al. (2019). Clinical and angiographic predictors of mortality in sudden cardiac arrest patients having cardiac catheterization: a single centre registry. *Heart Lung Circ.* 28 (3), 370–378. doi: 10.1016/j.hlc.2018.01.005

Yamagata, K., Horie, M., Aiba, T., Ogawa, S., Aizawa, Y., Ohe, T., et al. (2017). Genotype-Phenotype correlation of SCN5A mutation for the clinical and electrocardiographic characteristics of probands with brugada syndrome: a japanese multicenter registry. *Circulation* 135 (23), 2255–2270. doi: 10.1161/CIRCULATIONAHA.117.027983

Yamaguchi, M., Shimizu, M., Ino, H., Terai, H., Uchiyama, K., Oe, K., et al. (2003). T wave peak-to-end interval and QT dispersion in acquired long QT syndrome: a new index for arrhythmogenicity. *Clin. Sci.* 105, 671–676. doi: 10.1042/CS20030010

Yap, Y. G., and Camm, A. J. (2003). Drug induced QT prolongation and torsades de pointes. *Heart Br. Card Soc* 89:, 1363–1372. doi: 10.1136/heart.89.11.1363

Young, J. B., Dunlap, M. E., Pfeffer, M. A., Probstfield, J. L., Cohen-Solal, A., Dietz, R., et al. (2004). Mortality and morbidity reduction with Candesartan in patients with chronic heart failure and left ventricular systolic dysfunction: results of the CHARM low-left ventricular ejection fraction trials. *Circulation* 110 (17), 2618–2626. doi: 10.1161/01.CIR.0000146819.43235.A9

Zareba, W., Daubert, J. P., Beck, C. A., Huang, D. T., Alexis, J. D., and Brown, M. W. (2018). Ranolazine in high-risk patients with implanted cardioverter-defibrillators: The RAID trial. *J. Am. Coll. Cardiol.* 72 (6), 636–645. doi: 10.1016/j.jacc.2018.04.086

Zehir, R., Karabay, C. Y., Kalaycı, A., Akgün, T., Kılıçgedik, A., and Kırma, C. (2015). Evaluation of Tpe interval and Tpe/QT ratio in patients with slow coronary flow. *Anatol. J. Cardiol.* 15 (6), 463–467. doi: 10.5152/akd.2014.5503

Zhang, Y., Post, W. S., Blasco-Colmenares, E., Dalal, D., Tomaselli, G. F., and Guallar, E. (2011). Electrocardiographic QT interval and mortality: a meta-analysis. *Epidemiology* 22 (5), 660–670. doi: 10.1097/EDE.0b013e318225768b

11

Electrical Restitution and Its Modifications by Antiarrhythmic Drugs in Undiseased Human Ventricular Muscle

Tamás Árpádffy-Lovas [1,2], István Baczkó [1,2], Beáta Baláti [1], Miklós Bitay [3], Norbert Jost [1,2,4], Csaba Lengyel [5], Norbert Nagy [1,4], János Takács [1], András Varró [1,2,4†] and László Virág [1,2†]*

[1] Department of Pharmacology and Pharmacotherapy, Faculty of Medicine, University of Szeged, Szeged, Hungary, [2] Department of Pharmacology and Pharmacotherapy, Interdisciplinary Excellence Centre, University of Szeged, Szeged, Hungary, [3] Department of Cardiac Surgery, Faculty of Medicine, University of Szeged, Szeged, Hungary, [4] MTA-SZTE Research Group for Cardiovascular Pharmacology, Hungarian Academy of Sciences, Szeged, Hungary, [5] First Department of Internal Medicine, University of Szeged, Szeged, Hungary

***Correspondence:**
András Varró
varro.andras@med.u-szeged.hu

†These authors share senior authorship

Introduction: Re-entry is a basic mechanism of ventricular fibrillation, which can be elicited by extrasystolic activity, but the timing of an extrasystole can be critical. The action potential duration (APD) of an extrasystole depends on the proximity of the preceding beat, and the relation between its timing and its APD is called electrical restitution. The aim of the present work was to study and compare the effect of several antiarrhythmic drugs on restitution in preparations from undiseased human ventricular muscle, and other mammalian species.

Methods: Action potentials were recorded in preparations obtained from rat, guinea pig, rabbit, and dog hearts; and from undiseased human donor hearts using the conventional microelectrode technique. Preparations were stimulated with different basic cycle lengths (BCLs) ranging from 300 to 5,000 ms. To study restitution, single test pulses were applied at every 20th beat while the preparation was driven at 1,000 ms BCL.

Results: Marked differences were found between the animal and human preparations regarding restitution and steady-state frequency dependent curves. In human ventricular muscle, restitution kinetics were slower in preparations with large phase 1 repolarization with shorter APDs at 1000 ms BCL compared to preparations with small phase 1. Preparations having APD longer than 300 ms at 1000 ms BCL had slower restitution kinetics than those having APD shorter than 250 ms. The selective I_{Kr} inhibitors E-4031 and sotalol increased overall APD and slowed the restitution kinetics, while I_{Ks} inhibition did not influence APD and electrical restitution. Mexiletine and nisoldipine shortened APD, but only mexiletine slowed restitution kinetics.

Discussion: Frequency dependent APD changes, including electrical restitution, were partly determined by the APD at the BCL. Small phase 1 associated with slower restitution suggests a role of I_{to} in restitution. APD prolonging drugs slowed restitution, while mexiletine, a known inhibitor of I_{Na}, shortened basic APD but also slowed restitution.

These results indicate that although basic APD has an important role in restitution, other transmembrane currents, such as I_{Na} or I_{to}, can also affect restitution kinetics. This raises the possibility that ion channel modifier drugs slowing restitution kinetics may have antiarrhythmic properties by altering restitution.

Keywords: arrhythmia, action potential, electrical restitution, human ventricle, cardiac electrophysiogy

INTRODUCTION

Cardiovascular diseases are the leading causes of mortality in Western countries including the USA, Germany, France, and the UK. In approximately 50% of the cases the cause of death in cardiac patients is sudden cardiac death due to ventricular fibrillation (Jazayeri and Emert, 2019). The underlying mechanisms of ventricular fibrillation are complex, often multi-factorial, and are still not fully understood, therefore, they are subjects of current investigations. In general, arrhythmias can be explained by impaired impulse conduction and/or abnormal automaticity within the heart. The cellular cause of impulse conduction defects can have a distinct anatomical cause exhibiting a fixed pathway, usually determined by ischemic or fibrotic injury (Nguyen et al., 2017; Himel et al., 2019). Alternatively, the re-entry pathway can form without such injuries, due to enhanced dispersion of repolarization and consequently enhanced dispersion of refractoriness (Himel et al., 2019). The latter determines the ability of the ventricular muscle to be re-excited following a previous beat. In case the differences in action potential duration (APD), and consequently the effective refractory period (ERP) are enhanced, i.e. dispersion of APD or repolarization is augmented, the propagation of an early extra beat can be delayed or blocked in the direction that has myocytes with longer APDs, but conducted normally to the direction that has myocytes with shorter APDs. Therefore, in such an area, the extra beat can travel in a zig-zag pattern and can re-enter into areas that have been previously excited, eliciting chaotic rhythm or even fibrillation. Accordingly, the timing of an extrasystole is critical for arrhythmogenesis (Akar et al., 2002; Tran et al., 2007; Zaniboni, 2019). It has been known for a long time that the APD/ERP of an extrasystole depends on the proximity of the preceding beat, called diastolic interval; and as the diastolic intervals increase, the APDs/ERPs of the extra beats also increase. This process is called electrical restitution and had been described long ago (Nolasco and Dahlen, 1968; Boyett and Jewell, 1978; Elharrar and Surawicz, 1983), but its importance in arrhythmia research gained particular attention again in the past two decades (Gilmour, 2002; Franz, 2003; Kalb et al., 2004; Gilmour, 2009; Orini et al., 2016; Osadchii, 2017a; Osadchii, 2017b; Shattock et al., 2017; Orini et al., 2019; Osadchii, 2019). According to the restitution hypothesis, as diastolic intervals increase due to propagation of an extrasystole, the next following possible extrasystole would encounter prolonged APD/ERP and local conduction defect can occur. A steeper or faster restitution curve would favor such an effect and would be considered proarrhythmic; flattened or slower electrical restitution would have the opposite effect (Garfinkel et al., 2000; Qu et al., 2014; Shattock et al., 2017; Osadchii, 2017a; Osadchii, 2017b). Several studies in different preparations investigated the effects of antiarrhythmic drugs on the cardiac electric restitution properties (Varró et al., 1985; Hsieh et al., 2013; Osadchii, 2017a; Osadchii, 2017b; Shattock et al., 2017). These studies yielded different results depending on the protocols (dynamic or standard), on the basic stimulation frequencies, on the preparations (ventricular muscle or Purkinje fibers), and on the species (guinea-pig, rabbit, rat, or dog) used in their experimental approaches (Elharrar and Surawicz, 1983; Kalb et al., 2004; Orini et al., 2016; Shattock et al., 2017; Osadchii, 2019). The species used may have special significance, since, as **Figure 2** shows, there are marked differences between restitution curves measured in ventricular papillary muscle from different species (in rat, guinea-pig, rabbit, dog or human preparations) with the same experimental restitution pacing protocol and basic stimulation frequency. Therefore, the aim of the present work was to study the effect of several antiarrhythmic drugs on undiseased human ventricular muscle to better understand the possible implications of drug effects on electrical restitution, and understand these effects in human arrhythmogenesis.

Abbreviations: APA, action potential amplitude; APD, action potential duration; APD50, APD measured at 50% of repolarization; APD90, APD measured at 90% of repolarization; ERP, effective refractory period; Vmax, maximum upstroke velocity; RP, resting membrane potential.

METHODS

Human General Donor Cardiac Tissue Ethics Statement

Hearts were obtained from general organ donors whose undiseased hearts were explanted to obtain pulmonary and aortic valves for transplant surgery. Before cardiac explantation, organ donors did not receive medication apart from dobutamine, furosemide, and plasma expanders. According to the Hungarian law to obtain samples from donors, the consent of the patients or relatives is not needed. Therefore, consent is waived under local legislation. The investigations conformed to the principles of the Declaration of Helsinki. Experimental protocols were approved by the National Scientific and Research Ethical Review Boards (4991-0/2010-1018EKU [339/PI/010]).

Animals

All experiments were carried out in compliance with the Guide for the Care and Use of Laboratory Animals (USA NIH publication NO 85-23, revised 1996) and conformed to the Directive 2010/63/EU of the European Parliament. The protocols have been approved by the Ethical Committee for the Protection of Animals in Research of the University of Szeged, Szeged, Hungary (approval number: I-74-24-2017) and by the Department of Animal Health and Food Control of the Ministry of Agriculture and Rural Development (authority approval number XIII/3331/2017).

Conventional Microelectrode Technique

Action potentials were recorded in right ventricular trabeculae or papillary muscle preparations obtained from rat, guinea pig, rabbit, dog hearts, and from undiseased human donor hearts using the conventional microelectrode technique.

Rats (either sex, 200–400 g), guinea-pigs (either sex, 400–600 g), rabbits (either sex, 2.5–3.5 kg) and dogs (either sex, 10–15 kg) were anesthetized by sodium pentobarbitone (30 mg/kg i.p. for rat and guinea pig, i.v. for rabbit and dog) following sedation (xylazine 1 mg/kg). The animals also received intravenous injection of 400 U/kg heparin. In case of human donor hearts, immediately after explantation, each heart was perfused with cardioplegic solution and kept cold (4–6°C) for 2–4 hours before dissection.

Preparations were individually mounted in a tissue chamber with a volume of 50 ml. During experiments, modified Locke's solution was used, containing (in mM): NaCl, 128.3; KCl, 4; $CaCl_2$, 1.8; $MgCl_2$, 0.42; $NaHCO_3$, 21.4; and glucose, 10. The pH of this solution was set between 7.35 and 7.4 when gassed with the mixture of 95% O_2 and 5% CO_2 at 37°C. Each preparation was stimulated through a pair of platinum electrodes in contact with the preparation using rectangular current pulses of 1 to 3 ms duration at twice of the threshold strength at a constant basic cycle length of 1000 ms (S1). These stimuli were delivered for at least 60 min allowing the preparation to equilibrate before the measurements were initiated. Transmembrane potentials were recorded using conventional glass microelectrodes, filled with 3 M KCl, and having tip resistances of 5–20 MΩ, connected to the input of a high impedance electrometer (Experimetria, type 309, Budapest, Hungary) which was coupled to a dual beam oscilloscope.

The resting potential (RP), action potential amplitude (APA), maximum upstroke velocity (V_{max}), and APD measured at 50% and 90% of repolarization (APD_{50} and APD_{90}, respectively) were determined off-line using an in-house developed software (APES) running on a computer equipped with an ADA 3300 analog-to-digital data acquisition board (Real Time Devices, Inc., State College, Pennsylvania) having a maximum sampling frequency of 40 kHz.

The following types of stimulations were applied in the course of the experiments: stimulation with a constant cycle length of 1000 ms; stimulation with different constant cycle lengths ranging from 300 to 5000 ms. To determine the recovery kinetics of APD_{90} (APD_{90} restitution), extra test action potentials were elicited by using single test pulses (S2) in a preparation driven at a basic cycle length of 1000 ms. The S1–S2 coupling interval was increased progressively from the end of the refractory period. The effective refractory period was defined as the longest S1–S2 interval at which S2 failed to elicit a propagated response. The diastolic intervals preceding the test action potential were measured from the point corresponding to 90% of repolarization of the preceding basic beat to the upstroke of the test action potential and were increased progressively.

Attempts were made to maintain the same impalement throughout each experiment. In case an impalement became dislodged, adjustment was attempted, and if the action potential characteristics of the re-established impalement deviated by less than 5% from the previous measurement, the experiment continued. All measurements were performed at 37°C.

Data Analysis

All data are expressed as means ± SEM. The "n" number refers to the number of experiments (i.e. the number of ventricular muscle preparations). Data points of restitution curves were fitted by a mono-exponential function in order to calculate the kinetic time constant of the APD_{90} restitution process:

$$APD = APD_{ss} - A * \exp(-DI/\tau)$$

where APD_{ss} is the maximal action potential duration (APD_{90}), A is the amplitude of the exponential function, DI is the diastolic interval, and τ is the time constant.

RESULTS

In **Figure 1**, frequency dependent APD changes are shown in different species including human following various constant steady-state (S1–S1) and abrupt changes of cycle lengths (S1–S2). The figure shows that there are marked differences both in the electrical restitution and steady-state frequency dependent curves. The nature and mechanism of the frequency dependent APD changes (Carmeliet, 1977; Elharrar and Surawicz, 1983; Obreztchikova et al., 2006; Qu et al., 2014; Ni et al., 2019) including electrical restitution are not fully resolved yet. A recent study of Schattock et al. (2017) suggested that the slope of the restitution curve depends on the APD of the basic heart rate. Therefore, as **Figure 2** shows, human ventricular electrical restitution curves separated according to their action potential durations at basic cycle length of 1000 ms. In preparations with APD_{90} shorter than 250 ms, the time constant (τ) was 63.9 ± 6.0 ms (n = 10), while in preparations with APD_{90} longer than 300 ms τ was 125.5 ± 9.1 ms (n = 17). **Figure 2** indicates that electrical restitution kinetics are slower as action potential durations increase, suggesting that restitution kinetics, at least partly, indeed depend on intrinsic behavior of the repolarization process. In addition, as shown in **Figure 3**, human ventricular APD restitution curves have somewhat slower restitution kinetics where the basic action potentials showed prominent phase 1 repolarization during the plateau phase (τ = 126.1 ± 8.1 ms, n = 16) compared to those that had no strong phase 1 repolarization (τ = 98.5 ± 10.0 ms, n = 10), suggesting a possible role of I_{to} in the restitution process. In this respect, it is worth to note that APDs in preparations having prominent phase 1 repolarization were shorter than those having no or small phase 1 repolarization. Also, rabbit restitution curves and steady-state frequency-dependent APD have a declining slope

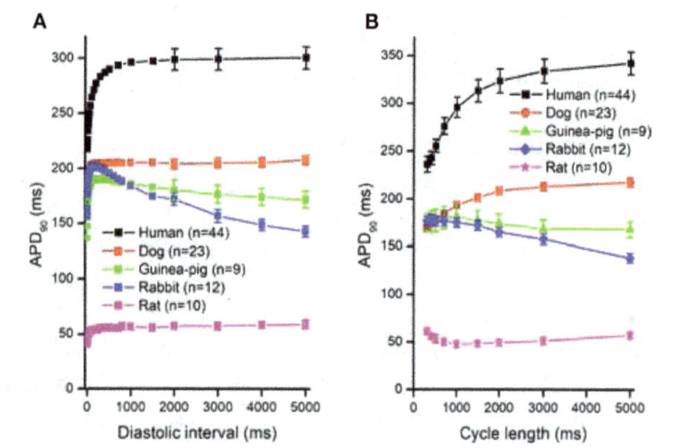

FIGURE 1 | Action potential duration (APD_{90}) restitution curves (panel **A**) and the steady-state cycle length dependence of the action potential duration (panel **B**) in human, dog, guinea pig, rabbit, and rat right ventricular muscle preparations. For the sake of clarity, the SEM values were indicated in case of diastolic intervals 2000 – 5000 ms in (panel **A**).

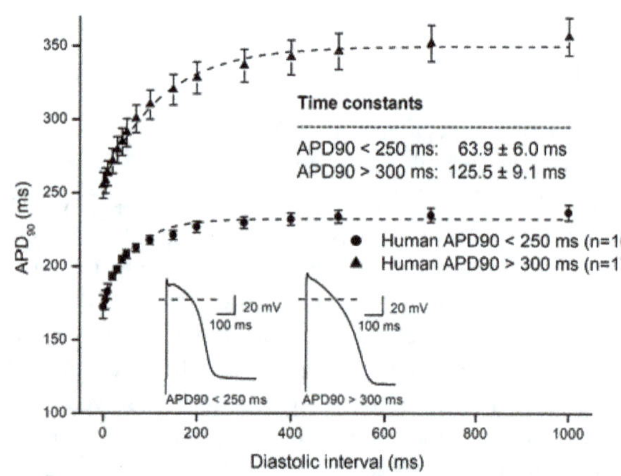

FIGURE 2 | Comparing human ventricular electrical restitution curves based on the action potential duration. Human APD_{90} restitution curves were separated into short APD ($APD_{90} < 250$ ms) and long APD ($APD_{90} > 300$ ms) groups. The data points up to 1000 ms diastolic interval were fitted by single exponential function. The inset shows the kinetical time constants for the two groups.

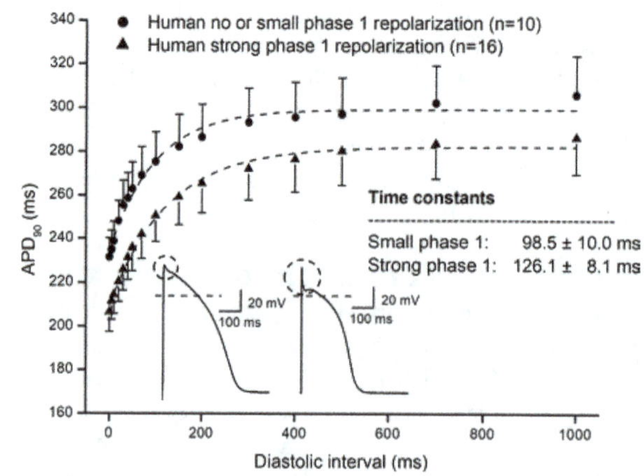

FIGURE 3 | Comparing human ventricular action potential duration restitution curves based on the amplitude of phase 1 repolarization. Human APD_{90} restitution curves were separated into two groups, one showed prominent phase 1 repolarization and another one had no or small phase 1 repolarization. The data points up to 1000 ms diastolic interval were fitted by single exponential function. The inset shows the kinetical time constants for the two groups.

at diastolic intervals and cycle lengths longer than 1000 ms. Since in rabbit I_{to} is characterized by slow recovery (Fermini et al., 1992; Sánchez-Chapula et al., 1994), these results also suggest a possible role of I_{to} in the cycle length dependent APD changes including restitution.

In further experiments, the effects of several antiarrhythmic drugs were studied on the electrical restitution curves in human undiseased ventricular muscle preparations. **Figure 4** shows that the selective rapid delayed rectifier potassium current (I_{Kr}) inhibitor E-4031 and sotalol increased overall APD and slowed the kinetics of the restitution curve (from $\tau = 82.6 \pm 5.5$ ms to $\tau = 160.3 \pm 11.1$ ms, n = 5; and from $\tau = 95.8 \pm 10.7$ ms to $\tau = 152.7 \pm 8.7$ ms, n = 5, respectively). **Figure 5** illustrates that L-735,821, a specific inhibitor of the slow delayed rectifier potassium current (I_{Ks}) does not influence APD and electrical restitution curves ($\tau = 113.1 \pm 8.4$ ms vs. $\tau = 111.9 \pm 7.3$ ms, n = 7). In further experiments, the effects of the inward sodium current (I_{Na}) inhibitor mexiletine and the inward L-type calcium current blocker nisoldipine were studied on human ventricular electrical restitution curves. **Figure 6** shows that both mexiletine and nisoldipine shortened APD but only mexiletine slowed restitution kinetics in human ventricular muscle preparations (from $\tau = 98.1 \pm 10.9$ ms to $\tau = 133.2 \pm 13.1$ ms, n = 6; from $\tau = 111.1 \pm 9.2$ ms to $\tau = 113.1 \pm 7.4$ ms, n = 6, respectively).

DISCUSSION

In this study, the electrical restitution of APD and its possible influence by several antiarrhythmic drugs in human ventricular muscle was investigated. Notwithstanding plentiful data in different animal experiments, according to our best knowledge, there is no systemic study on electrical restitution available in undiseased human ventricular muscle with the conventional microelectrode technique.

The main novel findings in the present work are as follows;

1. Human ventricular APD restitution differs from those reported in other species.
2. In spite of the marked species differences in the ventricular restitution curve, in human ventricle, similar to those reported earlier in other mammalian species (Shattock et al., 2017), longer repolarization is associated with slower restitution kinetics.
3. However, human ventricle exhibiting prominent phase 1 repolarization, presumably due to high level of I_{to}

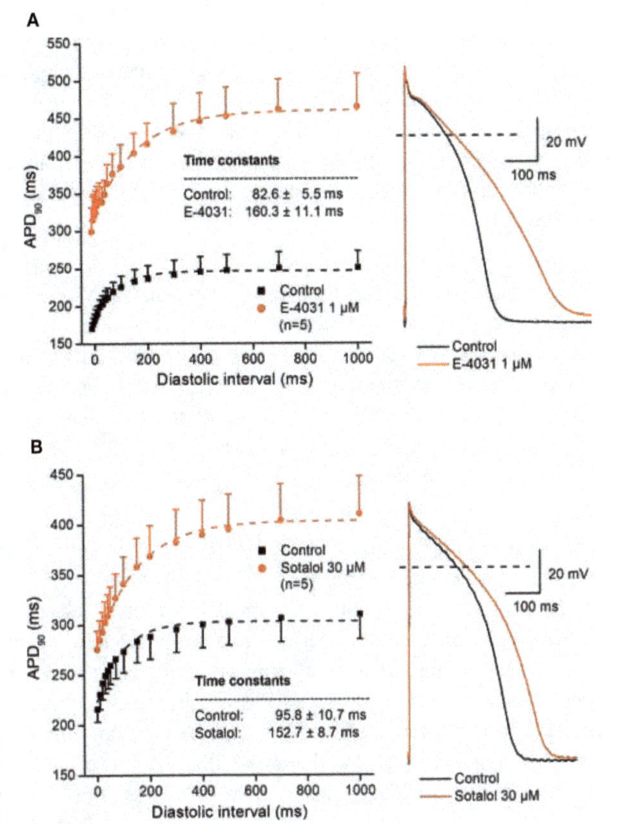

FIGURE 4 | Effect of two selective rapid delayed rectifier inhibitor antiarrhythmic drugs – E-4031 (panel **A**) and sotalol (panel **B**) – on the human electrical restitution curve. The data points up to 1000 ms diastolic interval were fitted by single exponential function. The inset shows the kinetical time constants in control conditions and after drug application. On the right part of the figure original action potential traces are shown before and after drug application at basic cycle length of 1000 ms.

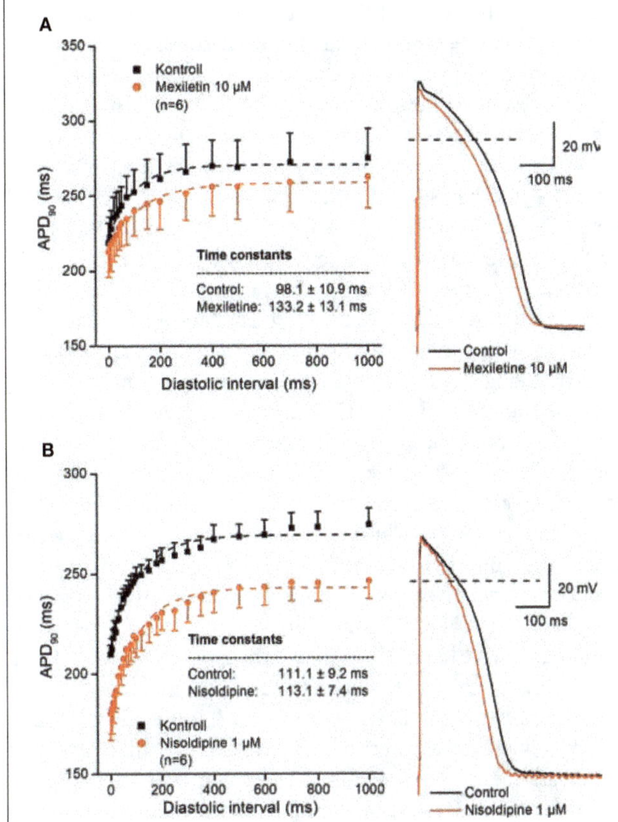

FIGURE 6 | Effect of the sodium channel inhibitor mexiletine (panel **A**) and the L-type calcium current blocker nisoldipine (panel **B**) on the human electrical restitution curve. The data points up to 1000 ms diastolic interval were fitted by single exponential function. The inset shows the kinetical time constants in control conditions and after drug application. On the right part of the figure original action potential traces are shown before and after drug application at basic cycle length of 1000 ms.

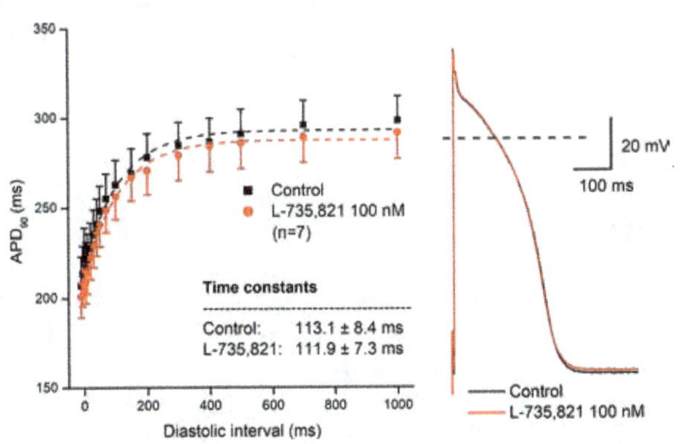

FIGURE 5 | Lack of effect of the selective slow delayed rectifier inhibitor L-735,821 on the human electrical restitution curve. The data points up to 1000 ms diastolic interval were fitted by single exponential function. The inset shows the kinetical time constants in control conditions and after application of L-735,821. On the right part of the figure original action potential traces are shown before and after drug application at basic cycle length of 1000 ms.

expression, was associated with shorter APD but slower restitution kinetics.

4. Drugs that inhibit I_{Kr} and I_{Na} slow restitution kinetics of APD restitution curve but drugs inhibiting I_{Ks} do not influence electrical APD restitution curves in human ventricular muscle.

APD restitution is an important process in the adaptation of the action potential to abrupt changes in cycle length and has been postulated playing an important role in the susceptibility to re-entrant arrhythmias, such as ventricular fibrillation (Garfinkel et al., 2000; Gilmour, 2002; Toal et al., 2009; Qu et al., 2014; Orini et al., 2016; Osadchii, 2017a; Osadchii, 2017b). Accordingly, it is generally agreed that slower restitution kinetics and a less steep restitution slope would result in antiarrhythmic effects, while steeper and faster restitution would be proarrhythmic (Garfinkel et al., 2000; Gilmour, 2002; Qu et al., 2014; Osadchii, 2017a; Osadchii, 2017b; Shattock et al., 2017; Zaniboni, 2019). As diastolic intervals are increasing due to propagation of an extra beat, a next short coupled extra beat would encounter longer

APD or ERP and, as a result of this, local conduction block can develop. A steeper restitution curve would facilitate this possibility with potential proarrhythmic consequences, but a flattened restitution curve would have the opposite effect.

Repolarization of cardiac ventricular muscle has been known for long to be dependent on species and stimulation frequency (Carmeliet, 1977; Boyett and Jewell, 1978). The cellular and subcellular mechanisms of APD restitution have been studied extensively. However, they are still subjects of debate (Boyett and Jewell, 1978; Elharrar and Surawicz, 1983; Hsieh et al., 2013; Osadchii, 2017a; Osadchii, 2017b; Shattock et al., 2017; Zaniboni, 2019). Frequency dependent APD changes including APD restitution in case the cycle length or diastolic interval ranges are sufficiently long can be characterized by multiple exponential fits (Elharrar and Surawicz, 1983; Varró et al., 1985). The rapid exponential components of these fits are generally attributed to deactivation and recovery from inactivation properties of various ion channels activated during the previous baseline beats, as well as intracellular and extracellular ion concentration changes, which directly or indirectly alter electrogenic pumps and exchangers, often called collectively as "short term memory" (Elharrar and Surawicz, 1983; Toal et al., 2009). Changes in the expression of ion channels can cause the so-called long-term memory (Obreztchikova et al., 2006), which was not investigated in our experiments.

In a recent study by Shattock et al. (2017) it was suggested that APD restitution kinetics were determined by the length of the APD of the basic beat. This speculation was based on guinea pig and rabbit experiments in Langendorff preparation measuring monophasic APD with a Franz catheter, or with the sharp microelectrode technique in single isolated guinea-pig myocytes applying the dynamic restitution protocol (Shattock et al., 2017). In this study, a wide range of drugs that all prolong APD by different modes of actions (such as clofilium, Bay K 8644, veratridine, catecholamines; and interventions such as low extracellular Ca^{2+} and transverse aortic constriction induced heart failure) slowed the kinetics or flattened the restitution curves. Based on these results, in agreement with the hypothesis of Zaza (Zaza and Varró, 2006; Zaza, 2010) and later by others (Bányász et al., 2009; Virág et al., 2009; Bárándi et al., 2010), it was argued that frequency dependent APD changes, including electrical restitution, were determined by the APD at the basic cycle length. The results of the present study partly support this idea, since all of the drugs studied with an APD prolonging effect slowed the restitution curve. Also, longer intrinsic APD was associated with slower restitution in human ventricular muscle. However, mexiletine and nisoldipine shortened basic APD but slowed or did not change the restitution curve. In addition, in the present study, the human ventricular muscle preparations with strong phase 1 repolarization showed slower restitution kinetics with shorter APD at the basic cycle lengths than those that showed no prominent phase 1 repolarization. Rabbit ventricular APD restitution curves showed a declining slope at diastolic intervals longer than 1000 ms. In human ventricular muscle, I_{to} recovers relatively rapidly, with a time constant of 10 ms (our own unpublished observation), but in rabbit the recovery of I_{to} is slower with time constant more than 1 s (Fermini et al., 1992; Sánchez-Chapula et al., 1994). These results suggest that although basic APD has important role in determining restitution slope and kinetics, other transmembrane currents, such as I_{Na} or I_{to}, can also play a role in restitution kinetics. This is also in agreement with earlier work in dog Purkinje fibers, where several drugs with I_{Na} and $I_{Ca\text{-}L}$ inhibition properties slowed APD restitution (Elharrar et al., 1984). It is also important to note that the basic stimulation frequency, which was 5 times higher in the study of Shattock et al. (2017), can partly explain the differences between their and our present works.

In our study, we used only undiseased donor cardiac ventricular preparations and did not study diseased tissue and atrial muscle. To the best of our knowledge there are no reported *in vitro* drug studies available with the latter preparations. Since APD restitution can be important phenomenon in the mechanism of atrial fibrillation this may be a limitation of our present investigations as such it would be worth to study in the future.

In conclusion, it should be recognized that important species differences exist in the ventricular restitution process including human. Our results indicate that the mechanism of the electrical restitution, at least in undiseased human ventricle, seems complex; and to understand it properly, further studies are needed. Based on our results, in addition to the basic APD, other factors, such as transmembrane ion currents, can influence restitution. The latter raises the possibility that ion channel modifier drugs slowing restitution kinetics may have antiarrhythmic properties by affecting electrical restitution, which may be considered in future drug development projects.

AUTHOR CONTRIBUTIONS

Conception and design of the experiments: AV, LV. Collection, analysis and interpretation of data: TÁ-L, CL, BB, MB, NN, JT. Drafting the article and revising it critically for intellectual content: IB, NJ, AV, LV.

FUNDING

This work was funded by the National Research Development and Innovation Office (NKFIH K-119992 (for AV), K-128851 (for IB), FK-129117 (for NN), and GINOP-2.3.2.-15-2016-00047), the Ministry of Human Capacities Hungary (20391-3/2018/FEKUSTRAT and EFOP-3.6.2-16-2017-00006), the UNKP-19-3-SZTE-5 (New National Excellence Program of the Ministry for Innovation and Technology; for TÁ-L) and János Bolyai Research Scholarship of the Hungarian Academy of Sciences (for NN). The GINOP and EFOP projects are co-financed by the European Union and the European Regional Development Fund.

REFERENCES

Akar, F. G., Yan, G.-X., Antzelevitch, C., and Rosenbaum, D. S. (2002). Unique topographical distribution of M cells underlies reentrant mechanism of torsade de pointes in the long-QT syndrome. *Circulation* 105, 1247–1253. doi: 10.1161/hc1002.105231

Bányász, T., Horváth, B., Virág, L., Bárándi, L., Szentandrássy, N., Harmati, G., et al. (2009). Reverse rate dependency is an intrinsic property of canine cardiac preparations. *Cardiovasc. Res.* 84, 237–244. doi: 10.1093/cvr/cvp213

Bárándi, L., Virág, L., Jost, N., Horváth, Z., Koncz, I., Papp, R., et al. (2010). Reverse rate-dependent changes are determined by baseline action potential duration in mammalian and human ventricular preparations. *Basic Res. Cardiol.* 105, 315–323. doi: 10.1007/s00395-009-0082-7

Boyett, M. R., and Jewell, B. R. (1978). A study of the factors responsible for rate-dependent shortening of the action potential in mammalian ventricular muscle. *J. Physiol. (Lond.)* 285, 359–380. doi: 10.1113/jphysiol.1978.sp012576

Carmeliet, E. (1977). Repolarisation and frequency in cardiac cells. *J. Physiol. (Paris)* 73, 903–923.

Elharrar, V., and Surawicz, B. (1983). Cycle length effect on restitution of action potential duration in dog cardiac fibers. *Am. J. Physiol.* 244, H782–H792. doi: 10.1152/ajpheart.1983.244.6.H782

Elharrar, V., Atarashi, H., and Surawicz, B. (1984). Cycle length-dependent action potential duration in canine cardiac Purkinje fibers. *Am. J. Physiol.* 247, H936–H945. doi: 10.1152/ajpheart.1984.247.6.H936

Fermini, B., Wang, Z., Duan, D., and Nattel, S. (1992). Differences in rate dependence of transient outward current in rabbit and human atrium. *Am. J. Physiol.* 263, H1747–H1754. doi: 10.1152/ajpheart.1992.263.6.H1747

Franz, M. R. (2003). The electrical restitution curve revisited: steep or flat slope–which is better? *J. Cardiovasc. Electrophysiol.* 14, S140–S147. doi: 10.1046/j.1540.8167.90303.x

Garfinkel, A., Kim, Y. H., Voroshilovsky, O., Qu, Z., Kil, J. R., Lee, M. H., et al. (2000). Preventing ventricular fibrillation by flattening cardiac restitution. *Proc. Natl. Acad. Sci. U. S. A.* 97, 6061–6066. doi: 10.1073/pnas.090492697

Gilmour, R. F. (2002). Electrical restitution and ventricular fibrillation: negotiating a slippery slope. *J. Cardiovasc. Electrophysiol.* 13, 1150–1151. doi: 10.1046/j.1540-8167.2002.01150.x

Gilmour, R. F. (2009). Restitution, heterogeneity and unidirectional conduction block: New roles for old players. *Heart Rhythm* 6, 544–545. doi: 10.1016/j.hrthm.2009.01.036

Himel, H. D., Cupelli, M., Gantt, M., Boutjdir, M., and El-Sherif, N. (2019). Role of spatial dispersion of repolarization in reentry around a functional core versus reentry around a fixed anatomical core. *Ann. Noninvasive Electrocardiol.* 24, e12647. doi: 10.1111/anec.12647

Hsieh, Y.-C., Chang, P.-C., Hsueh, C.-H., Lee, Y. S., Shen, C., Weiss, J. N., et al. (2013). Apamin-sensitive potassium current modulates action potential duration restitution and arrhythmogenesis of failing rabbit ventricles. *Circ. Arrhythmia Electrophysiol.* 6, 410–418. doi: 10.1161/CIRCEP.111.000152

Jazayeri, M.-A., and Emert, M. P. (2019). Sudden Cardiac Death: Who Is at Risk? *Med. Clin. North Am.* 103, 913–930. doi: 10.1016/j.mcna.2019.04.006

Kalb, S. S., Dobrovolny, H. M., Tolkacheva, E. G., Idriss, S. F., Krassowska, W., and Gauthier, D. J. (2004). The restitution portrait: a new method for investigating rate-dependent restitution. *J. Cardiovasc. Electrophysiol.* 15, 698–709. doi: 10.1046/j.1540-8167.2004.03550.x

Nguyen, M.-N., Kiriazis, H., Gao, X.-M., and Du, X.-J. (2017). Cardiac Fibrosis and Arrhythmogenesis. *Compr. Physiol.* 7, 1009–1049. doi: 10.1002/cphy.c160046

Ni, H., Zhang, H., Grandi, E., Narayan, S. M., and Giles, W. R. (2019). Transient outward K+ current can strongly modulate action potential duration and initiate alternans in the human atrium. *Am. J. Physiol. Heart Circ. Physiol.* 316, H527–H542. doi: 10.1152/ajpheart.00251.2018

Nolasco, J. B., and Dahlen, R. W. (1968). A graphic method for the study of alternation in cardiac action potentials. *J. Appl. Physiol.* 25, 191–196. doi: 10.1152/jappl.1968.25.2.191

Obreztchikova, M. N., Patberg, K. W., Plotnikov, A. N., Ozgen, N., Shlapakova, I. N., Rybin, A. V., et al. (2006). I(Kr) contributes to the altered ventricular repolarization that determines long-term cardiac memory. *Cardiovasc. Res.* 71, 88–96. doi: 10.1016/j.cardiores.2006.02.028

Orini, M., Taggart, P., Srinivasan, N., Hayward, M., and Lambiase, P. D. (2016). Interactions between Activation and Repolarization Restitution Properties in the Intact Human Heart: In-Vivo Whole-Heart Data and Mathematical Description. *PLoS One* 11, e0161765. doi: 10.1371/journal.pone.0161765

Orini, M., Yanni, J., Taggart, P., Hanson, B., Hayward, M., Smith, A., et al. (2019). Mechanistic insights from targeted molecular profiling of repolarization alternans in the intact human heart. *Europace* 21, 981–989. doi: 10.1093/europace/euz007

Osadchii, O. E. (2017a). Effects of Na+ channel blockers on the restitution of refractory period, conduction time, and excitation wavelength in perfused guinea-pig heart. *PLoS One* 12, e0172683. doi: 10.1371/journal.pone.0172683

Osadchii, O. E. (2017b). Role of abnormal repolarization in the mechanism of cardiac arrhythmia. *Acta Physiol.* 220, 1–71. doi: 10.1111/apha.12902

Osadchii, O. E. (2019). Effects of antiarrhythmics on the electrical restitution in perfused guinea-pig heart are critically determined by the applied cardiac pacing protocol. *Exp. Physiol.* 104, 490–504. doi: 10.1113/EP087531

Qu, Z., Hu, G., Garfinkel, A., and Weiss, J. N. (2014). Nonlinear and Stochastic Dynamics in the Heart. *Phys. Rep.* 543, 61–162. doi: 10.1016/j.physrep.2014.05.002

Sánchez-Chapula, J., Elizalde, A., Navarro-Polanco, R., and Barajas, H. (1994). Differences in outward currents between neonatal and adult rabbit ventricular cells. *Am. J. Physiol.* 266, H1184–H1194. doi: 10.1152/ajpheart.1994.266.3.H1184

Shattock, M. J., Park, K. C., Yang, H.-Y., Lee, A. W. C., Niederer, S., MacLeod, K. T., et al. (2017). Restitution slope is principally determined by steady-state action potential duration. *Cardiovasc. Res.* 113, 817–828. doi: 10.1093/cvr/cvx063

Toal, S. C., Farid, T. A., Selvaraj, R., Chauhan, V. S., Masse, S., Ivanov, J., et al. (2009). Short-term memory and restitution during ventricular fibrillation in human hearts: an in vivo study. *Circ. Arrhythmia Electrophysiol.* 2, 562–570. doi: 10.1161/CIRCEP.108.833442

Tran, D. X., Yang, M.-J., Weiss, J. N., Garfinkel, A., and Qu, Z. (2007). Vulnerability to re-entry in simulated two-dimensional cardiac tissue: effects of electrical restitution and stimulation sequence. *Chaos* 17, 043115. doi: 10.1063/1.2784387

Varró, A., Elharrar, V., and Surawicz, B. (1985). Effect of antiarrhythmic drugs on the premature action potential duration in canine cardiac Purkinje fibers. *J. Pharmacol. Exp. Ther.* 233, 304–311.

Virág, L., Acsai, K., Hála, O., Zaza, A., Bitay, M., Bogáts, G., et al. (2009). Self-augmentation of the lengthening of repolarization is related to the shape of the cardiac action potential: implications for reverse rate dependency. *Br. J. Pharmacol.* 156, 1076–1084. doi: 10.1111/j.1476-5381.2009.00116.x

Zaniboni, M. (2019). Restitution and Stability of Human Ventricular Action Potential at High and Variable Pacing Rate. *Biophys. J.* 117, 2382–2395. doi: 10.1016/j.bpj.2019.08.020

Zaza, A., and Varró, A. (2006). Rate-dependent modulation of repolarization: biology or math? (Abstract). *Eur. Heart J.* 27, 412.

Zaza, A. (2010). Control of the cardiac action potential: The role of repolarization dynamics. *J. Mol. Cell. Cardiol.* 48, 106–111. doi: 10.1016/j.yjmcc.2009.07.027

12

The Antimalarial Chloroquine Reduces the Burden of Persistent Atrial Fibrillation

Catalina Tobón[1†], Laura C. Palacio[1†], Bojjibabu Chidipi[2†], Diana P. Slough[3†], Thanh Tran[4], Nhi Tran[4], Michelle Reiser[2], Yu-Shan Lin[3], Bengt Herweg[4], Dany Sayad[4], Javier Saiz[5] and Sami Noujaim[2]*

[1] MATBIOM, Universidad de Medellín, Medellín, Colombia, [2] Molecular Pharmacology and Physiology Department, University of South Florida Morsani College of Medicine, Tampa, FL, United States, [3] Department of Chemistry, Tufts University, Medford, MA, United States, [4] Cardiology Department, University of South Florida Morsani College of Medicine, Tampa, FL, United States, [5] CI²B, Universitat Politècnica de València, Valencia, Spain

***Correspondence:**
Sami Noujaim
snoujaim@usf.edu

[†]These authors have contributed equally to this work

In clinical practice, reducing the burden of persistent atrial fibrillation by pharmacological means is challenging. We explored if blocking the background and the acetylcholine-activated inward rectifier potassium currents (I_{K1} and I_{KACh}) could be antiarrhythmic in persistent atrial fibrillation. We thus tested the hypothesis that blocking I_{K1} and I_{KACh} with chloroquine decreases the burden of persistent atrial fibrillation. We used patch clamp to determine the IC_{50} of I_{K1} and I_{KACh} block by chloroquine and molecular modeling to simulate the interaction between chloroquine and Kir2.1 and Kir3.1, the molecular correlates of I_{K1} and I_{KACh}. We then tested, as a proof of concept, if oral chloroquine administration to a patient with persistent atrial fibrillation can decrease the arrhythmia burden. We also simulated the effects of chloroquine in a 3D model of human atria with persistent atrial fibrillation. In patch clamp the IC_{50} of I_{K1} block by chloroquine was similar to that of I_{KACh}. A 14-day regimen of oral chloroquine significantly decreased the burden of persistent atrial fibrillation in a patient. Mathematical simulations of persistent atrial fibrillation in a 3D model of human atria suggested that chloroquine prolonged the action potential duration, leading to failure of reentrant excitation, and the subsequent termination of the arrhythmia. The combined block of I_{K1} and I_{KACh} can be a targeted therapeutic strategy for persistent atrial fibrillation.

Keywords: chloroquine, persistent atrial fibrillation, potassium inward rectifiers, I_{KACh}, I_{K1}

INTRODUCTION

Atrial fibrillation (AF) is the most common heart rhythm abnormality and its incidence and prevalence are increasingly alarming. In addition to increasing mortality, AF is a known risk factor for stroke (Wolf et al., 1991), dementia (Liao et al., 2015; Singh-Manoux et al., 2017), and cardiac contractile dysfunction (Schotten et al., 2002). Pharmacological rhythm control therapy for AF remains attractive, however, when AF becomes persistent, pharmacotherapy is frequently ineffective (Zimetbaum, 2012).

Chloroquine, an antimalarial 4-aminoquinoline, has been suggested to have antiarrhythmic properties through unknown mechanisms (Burrell and Martinez, 1958; Harris et al., 1988), and was shown to have a safe cardiac electrophysiological profile (Wozniacka et al., 2006; Teixeira et al.,

2014). Our previous work suggested that chloroquine terminates different forms of AF in animal models, in part, due to its ability to block potassium inward rectifiers (Noujaim et al., 2010; Filgueiras-Rama et al., 2012; Takemoto et al., 2018).

In persistent AF, the acetylcholine-activated inward rectifier potassium current I_{KACh} (molecular correlates are Kir3.1 and Kir3.4) was shown to be constitutively active and the inward rectifier potassium current I_{K1} (molecular correlates Kir2.1 and Kir2.3) has been shown to be upregulated (Voigt et al., 2010; Dobrev and Nattel, 2011). The constitutively active I_{KACh} could be considered as a background inward rectifier, which along with the increased I_{K1} may contribute to the shortening of the action potential duration and to create a substrate for the formation of stable, high frequency electrical rotors that maintain fibrillation (Atienza and Jalife, 2007; Noujaim et al., 2007). Consequently, blocking inward rectifiers could potentially be antiarrhythmic in the setting of persistent AF.

Recently, we used structural biology approaches to map the binding pocket of chloroquine in the intracellular domain of Kir3.1 (Takemoto et al., 2018). Chloroquine blocked I_{KACh} by binding at a specific site in the Kir3.1 intracellular ion permeation pathway (Takemoto et al., 2018). Previous work by us and others showed that chloroquine also blocks I_{k1} (Rodriguez-Menchaca et al., 2008; Noujaim et al., 2010). In this study, we tested in a patient with persistent AF whether chloroquine can reduce the arrhythmia burden, and we further explored the antiarrhythmic effects of chloroquine in a 3D model of the human atria with persistent AF.

METHODS

Patch Clamp

Experiments were performed as described earlier (Noujaim et al., 2011; Takemoto et al., 2018). HEK293 cells stably co-transfected with Kir3.1 and Kir3.4 were generously provided by the Bayliss Laboratory (University of Virginia), and HEK293 cells stably transfected with Kir2.1 were generously provided by the Jalife Laboratory (University of Michigan). Currents were recorded using EPC 800 amplifier (HEKA Elektronik, Lambrecht/Pfalz), A/D converter (Digidata 1550B plus Hum Silencer, Molecular Devices, San Jose, CA), and the pClamp 10.6 PC software (Molecular Devices). Analysis was performed with Clampfit 10.6 (pClamp, Molecular Devices) and OriginPro software packages (version 2018, Microcal). The patch pipettes had a resistance of 2.5–3MΩ. After GΩ seal formation, whole cell recordings were performed at room temperature (around 24°C). For I_{KACh}, the bath solution contained (in mM) 90 NaCl, 50 KCl, 1 $CaCl_2$, 2 $MgCl_2$, 10 HEPES, 10 glucose, and the pH adjusted to 7.4. The pipette internal solution contained (in mM) 100 K-aspartate, 10 NaCl, 40 KCl, 5 Mg-ATP, 2 EGTA, 0.1 GTP-Tris, and 10 HEPES at pH 7.2. For I_{K1}, the bath solution contained (in mM) 148 NaCl, 0.4 NaH_2PO_4, 1 $MgCl_2$, 5.4 KCl, 1.8 $CaCl_2$, 5.5 glucose, 15 HEPES, pH 7.4, and the pipette internal solution contained (in mM), 150 KCl, 1 $MgCl_2$, 5 EGTA, 5 HEPES, 5 phosphocreatine, 4.4 K_2ATP, and pH 7.2. I_{KACh} and I_{K1} were measured as the 1mM $BaCl_2$ sensitive current. Concentration–response curves and IC_{50} for currents inhibition at −140mV were determined with Prism 7 software using the standard variable slope equation $Y = 1/(1 + 10^{(LogIC50\ -\ X)*\mathrm{Slope}})$.

Molecular Docking of Chloroquine Into Kir2.1 and Kir3.1

As we previously described, the intracellular domain of tetrameric Kir2.1 (PDB: 1U4F) (Pegan et al., 2005) and Kir3.1 (PDB: 1U4E) (Pegan et al., 2005) were used for the docking simulations. The SMILES string for chloroquine was obtained from Drugbank (Wishart et al., 2008) (Accession Number: DB00608). The Kir2.1 and Kir3.1 proteins, and chloroquine were prepared using the Protein Preparation Wizard and LigPrep in Schrodinger's Maestro (Sastry et al., 2013), respectively. The protonation state of the drug was generated at a target pH of 7.0 in Epik (Shelley et al., 2007; Greenwood et al., 2010). The ligand was energy minimized with the OPLS_2005 force field (Shivakumar et al., 2010). A set of grids was created to map the proteins topologies before docking. The grids were generated using 60 × 60 × 60 points in the *x*, *y*, and *z* directions and centered around the aqueous channel with a spacing of 0.375 Å. Docking was performed with the Lamarckian genetic algorithm, with the population size set to 150, the number of generations set to 27,000 and the number of energy evaluations set to 2,500,000. Using Autodock 4.2 (Morris et al., 2009), one thousand runs were performed. The lowest energy poses from molecular docking were analyzed. Hydrogen bond analysis was performed using Visual Molecular Dynamics (Humphrey et al., 1996).

Estimation of Blocking Ability of Chloroquine

A voxel grid was generated using the atomic coordinates of the lowest energy pose from molecular docking of the tetrameric Kir2.1 or Kir3.1 bound to chloroquine. In this grid, each voxel was a cube of 0.2 × 0.2 × 0.2 Å. The van der Waals radius of each atom (Iijima et al., 1987) was used to fill the corresponding number of cubes. The use of the discrete grid allowed for a probe to search the space in the aqueous ion-permeation pathway. The probes were Voxel-approximated spheres with radii ranging from 1.4 Å (the ionic radius of a bare K^+ ion) to 3.9 Å in 0.1 Å increments. Three ångströms is the radius of a solvated K^+ ion up to its first hydration shell (Mahler and Persson, 2012). Originating from the extracellular opening of the channel, the probes were pushed longitudinally through the channel towards the intracellular side. If, at any point in the pathway, the probe was unable to proceed further, the probe's lateral position was adjusted in order to search all possible paths through the channel. The channel was considered blocked at a given probe radius if the probe was unable to find a path to move past chloroquine.

Human Study

A 67 year old female with history of tobacco use, persistent AF (AF sustained for more than seven days, and less than a year), and no other significant past medical history including no known coronary artery disease, was enrolled in this study. Institutional Review Board approval was obtained at the University of South Florida, Tampa, USA, and the study conformed to the principles outlined in the Declaration of Helsinki. Prior workup revealed normal blood pressure. Her laboratory values showed normal kidney and liver function tests. Echocardiography was unremarkable for structural heart disease, with an ejection fraction >50%. The patient has been on Apixaban and Metoprolol, and continued to be on these medications during the study. The patient gave informed consent, was equipped with a Cardionet monitor, and received the chloroquine regimen for amebiasis treatment, consisting of 600 mg chloroquine base once daily for 2 days, followed by 300 mg daily for 12 days. She was continuously monitored for the duration of chloroquine treatment. A previous Holter monitor recording (ZIO XT Patch) for 12 days obtained two months prior, was reviewed and showed that the patient had been continuously in AF, with a burden of 100%. Additionally, 12 lead ECG was recorded 3 days before and on the day of chloroquine regimen initiation, confirming that the patient was in AF in both instances.

Mathematical Simulations of Persistent Atrial Fibrillation in a 3D Model of Human Atria

The Courtemanche-Ramirez-Nattel membrane formalism (Courtemanche et al., 1998) was implemented to simulate the human atrial cell action potential. Cholinergic activity, a factor that promotes AF, was included in the model by implementing the following I_{KACh} equation developed by Kneller (Kneller et al., 2002):

$$I_{KACh} = \left(\frac{10}{1+9.13652/ACh^{0.477811}} \right) \left(0.0517 + \frac{0.4516}{1+e^{V_m+59.53}/17.18} \right) (V - E_K)$$

where V_m is the membrane potential, ACh is the acetylcholine concentration and E_K is the potassium equilibrium potential.

Based on experimental data (Workman et al., 2001; Van Wagoner, 2003), the cell model was modified in order to reproduce electrophysiological conditions of persistent AF: the maximum conductance of I_{K1} was increased by 100%, the maximum conductance of transient potassium current (I_{to}) and delayed rectifier potassium current (I_{Kur}) were decreased by 50%, and the maximum conductance of L-type calcium current (I_{CaL}) was decreased by 70% and for the constitutively active I_{KACh}, 5 nM of acetylcholine was simulated.

A realistic three-dimensional (3D) model of human atria including the main anatomical structures: left and right atria, twenty pectinate muscles, fossa ovalis, Bachmann's bundle, crista terminalis, left and right appendages, pulmonary veins, caval veins, atrioventricular rings and coronary sinus, was previously developed (Tobon et al., 2013). The model also includes three different pathways for the inter-atrial conduction, specific fiber orientations in 42 different atrial regions, heterogeneous tissue conductivity, anisotropy ratios and heterogeneous cellular properties. The wall of the atrial model is a monolayer surface, except the Bachmann's bundle and the pectinate muscles, which are solid structures. The model is composed of 52,906 hexahedral elements with a spatial resolution ranging from 300 to 700 μm.

The mathematical atrial cell model coupled with the 3D model was used to simulate a persistent AF episode. AF was generated with an S1–S2 stimulation protocol. S1 consisted of a train of ten stimuli with a basic cycle length of 1,000 ms, applied to the sinus node area, simulating sinus rhythm. After the last S1 stimulus, 6 ectopic S2 beats at 130 ms cycle length were delivered to the right superior pulmonary vein. Action potential propagation in the tissue was modeled using the monodomain reaction–diffusion equation:

$$\frac{1}{S_v} \nabla \cdot (\mathbf{D} \nabla V_m) = C_m \frac{\partial V_m}{\partial t} + I_{ion} - I_{stim}$$

where, S_v corresponds to the surface-to-volume ratio (range from 0.0086 to 0.02), D is the conductivity tensor, C_m is the membrane capacitance (100 pF), I_{ion} is the total ionic current that crosses the cell membrane and I_{stim} is the stimulus current (28 pA/pF). Equations were numerically solved using EMOS software (Heidenreich et al., 2010), which is a parallel code that implements the finite element method and operator splitting for solving the monodomain model. The time step was fixed to 0.001 ms. Simulation of 2 s of atrial activity required 32 h on a computing node with 12 dual core AMD Opteron Processors 2,218 clocked at 2.6 GHz.

Pseudo-unipolar atrial electrograms (EGMs) in the 3D model at 0.2 mm from the surface were simulated. The extracellular potential (Φ_e) in the endocardial atrial surface was computed using the large volume conductor approximation

$$\phi_e(r) = -K \int\int\int \nabla' V_m(r') \cdot \nabla' \left[\frac{1}{r' - r} \right] dv$$

where K (−0.0398) is a constant that includes the ratio of intracellular and extracellular conductivities, $\nabla' V_m$ is the spatial gradient of transmembrane potential, r is the distance from the source point (x, y, z) to the measuring point (x', y', z') and dv is the differential volume. EGMs at different points were visually inspected in order to analyze their morphologies as single, double or fractionated potentials. Double potentials were defined as EGMs with two negative or positive deflections and fractionated electrograms were defined as those exhibiting multiple (more than two) deflections. EGMs were processed with a 40–250 Hz band-pass filter, rectified and low-pass filtered at 20 Hz. Subsequently, spectral analysis of the signals was performed with a fast Fourier transform. The dominant frequency (DF) defined as the frequency corresponding to the highest peak of the power spectrum was calculated.

Modeling the Effect of Chloroquine on Potassium Currents

To develop a basic model of the effect of chloroquine on the major potassium currents that this drug has been shown to block (I_{KACh}, I_{K1}, and I_{Kr}) (Sanchez-Chapula et al., 2001), we used the steady state fraction of block (f), as done previously (Duarte M et al., 2013):

$$f = 1/(1 + IC_{50}/[C])$$

where C is the chloroquine concentration. The Hill equation was used to fit the Concentration–response relationships for chloroquine block. In this model, the channels kinetics were considered unchanged in the presence of the chloroquine. The IC_{50} for I_{KACh} and I_{K1} block by chloroquine were used from **Figures 1** and **2** and our earlier work (Noujaim et al., 2010) (0.97 μM for I_{K1} and 1.0 μM for I_{KACh}). For I_{Kr}, we used an IC_{50} of 2.5 μM as reported by Traebert et al in HEK293 cells (Traebert et al., 2004). The simulated fraction of block curve for I_{KACh} current fit well the experimental data shown in **Figures 1** and **2**, where $(1 - f) \cdot 100\%$ is the remaining current. After 5 s of baseline AF simulation, chloroquine was applied at increasing concentrations, from 1.0 μM to 8.7 μM, in order to simulate ~50% to ~90% block of I_{K1} and I_{KACh}, and from 1.0 μM to 25 μM, in order to simulate 30% to 90% block of I_{Kr}. We investigated the effects of chloroquine on AF dynamics by blocking either I_{K1}, I_{KACh} or I_{Kr} alone, or by blocking both I_{K1} and I_{KACh}, or by blocking the three currents. Action potential duration at 90% repolarization (APD_{90}) and the resting membrane potential (RMP) in a left atrial single cell were measured. All simulations were halted 2 s after chloroquine application.

RESULTS

Chloroquine Block of I_{K1} and I_{KACh}

Our earlier study using modeling, and protein NMR, suggested that chloroquine binds the intracellular domain of Kir3.1, at the level of amino acids F255 and D260 (Takemoto et al., 2018). Here, we conducted similar molecular docking simulations in order to compare the binding of chloroquine to Kir2.1 and Kir3.1. For each complex, one thousand docking runs were performed. The lowest energy poses for ligand–protein interactions were further studied. **Figures 1A** and **2A**, left panels, are zoomed in views of the tetrameric Kir2.1 (**Figure 1A**) and Kir3.1 (**Figure 2A**) channels, represented by gray ribbons, with the docked chloroquine depicted in cyan. In Kir2.1 (**Figure 1A**), the tertiary amine of chloroquine hydrogen-bonded to residue E224 of subunit B (black circles), and the aminoquinoline ring formed a hydrogen bond with the carbonyl oxygen of the diametrically opposed E224 of subunit D. The binding energy of chloroquine to Kir2.1 was -6.09 Kcal/mol. In Kir3.1 (**Figure 2A**), the tertiary amine of chloroquine hydrogen-bonded to residue D260 of subunit B (black circles), and the aminoquinoline ring was in proximity to the F255 ring of the adjacent subunit A. The binding energy of the ligand to the channel was -6.37 Kcal/mol. The Van der Waals representations of the Kir2.1 and Kir3.1 in complex with chloroquine are shown from the extracellular bird's eye views (**Figures 1A** and **2A**, bottom panels). The ion permeation pathways are in the middle, and the white arrows point to chloroquine which is shown in cyan. We then used patch clamp to compare the IC_{50} for chloroquine block of I_{K1} (**Figure 1B**) and I_{KACh} (**Figure 2B**). Top panels are representative

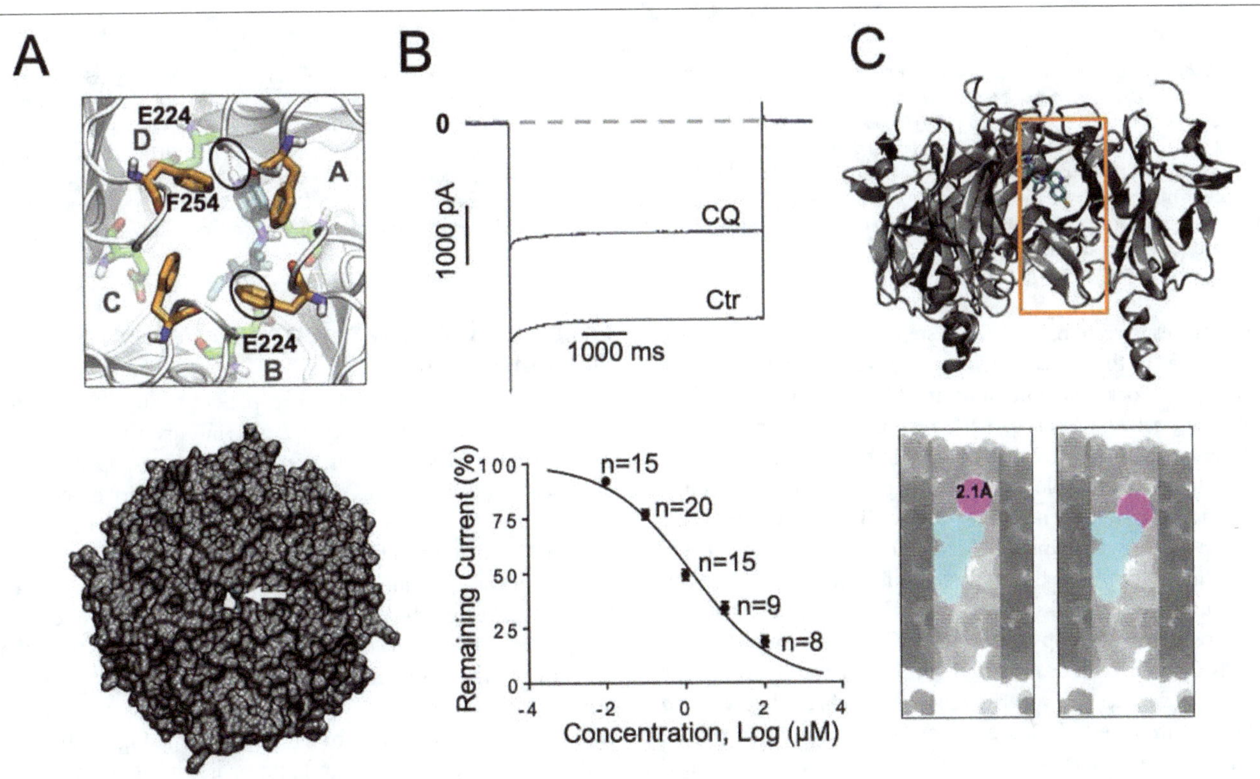

FIGURE 1 | I_{K1} block with chloroquine. **(A)** Docking of chloroquine in the intracellular domain of Kir2.1. The lowest energy pose is shown. Chloroquine makes hydrogen bonds with residue E224 from subunit B and with E224 from subunit D (black circles). Bottom panel: Extracellular bird's eye views of the van der Waals representation of the channel (gray) in complex with chloroquine (cyan). Chloroquine blocks the ion permeation pathway. **(B)** Barium sensitive I_{K1} traces in response to −140mV step pulses from a holding potential of 0 mV in the presence of 1 μM chloroquine (CQ). Concentration–response curves. IC_{50} for chloroquine block of I_{K1}: 1.3 μM, Hill Slope = −0.42, R^2=0.9. **(C)** Top panel: Longitudinal view of chloroquine bound to Kir2.1. Orange box denotes the voxelated part of the channel shown below. Bottom panel: Voxelation of Kir2.1 ion permeation pathway (grey) in complex with chloroquine (cyan). A probe (magenta) of radius 2.1 Å or larger, is blocked by chloroquine.

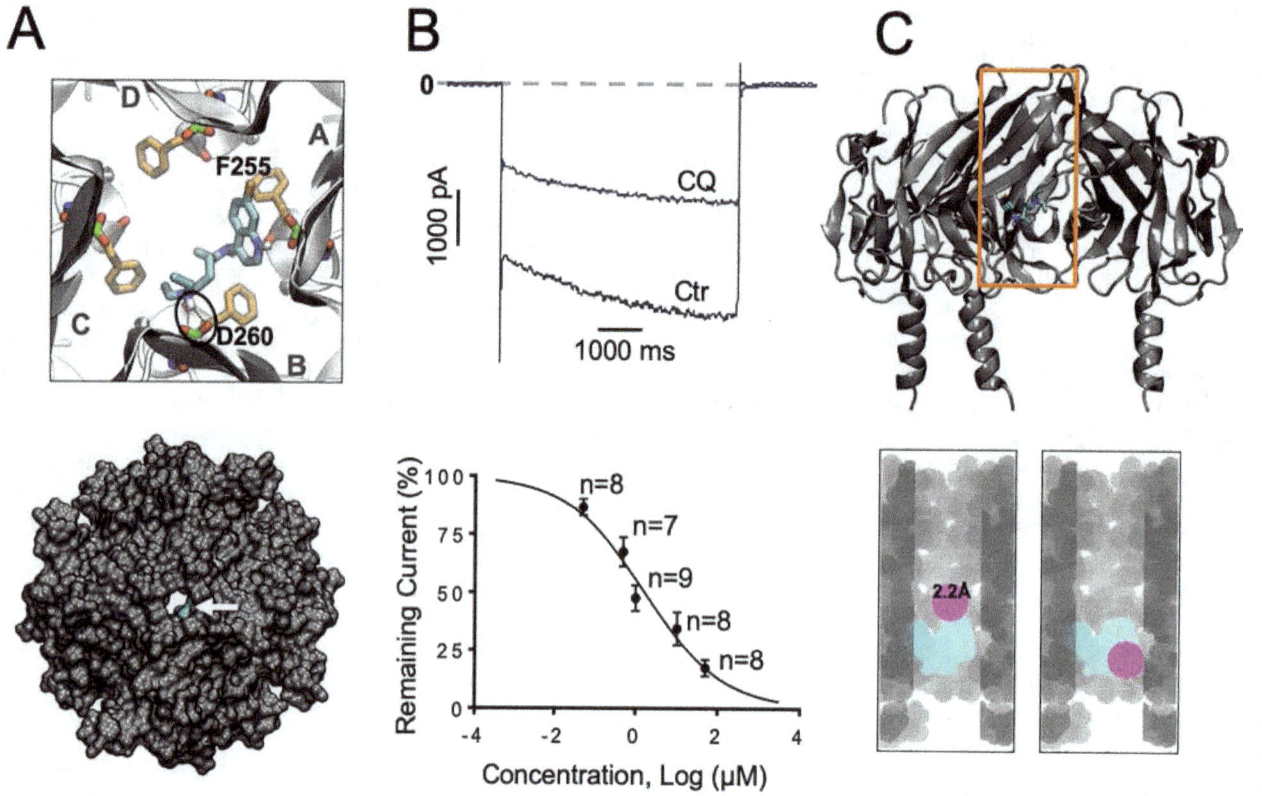

FIGURE 2 | I_{KACh} block with chloroquine. **(A)** Docking of chloroquine in the intracellular domain of Kir3.1. The lowest energy pose is shown. The D260 and F255 residues from each of the four Kir3.1 subunits are shown in green and orange sticks respectively. The tertiary amine nitrogen of chloroquine (cyan sticks) forms a hydrogen bond (black circle) with the side chain of D260 in the B subunit, while the aminoquinoline ring of chloroquine is in close proximity to the phenylalanine ring of F255 in the A subunit. Van der Waals representations of the channel bound to the drugs (cyan) viewed from the extracellular side is shown in the bottom panel. **(B)** Barium sensitive I_{KACh} traces in response to −140mV step pulses from a holding potential of −20 mV in the presence of 1 μM chloroquine (CQ). **(B)** Concentration–response curves. IC50 for chloroquine block of I_{KACh}: 1.2 μM, Hill Slope = −0.48, R^2=0.74. **(C)** Top panel: Longitudinal view of chloroquine bound to Kir3.1. Orange box denotes the voxelated part of the channel shown below. Bottom panel: Voxelation of Kir3.1 ion permeation pathway (grey) in complex with chloroquine (cyan). A probe (magenta) of radius 2.2 Å or larger, is blocked by chloroquine.

current traces in response to voltage steps in the presence of 1 μM chloroquine. In the concentration–response curves, the IC_{50}s of I_{K1} and I_{KACh} block by chloroquine at −140 mV were 1.3 μM and 1.2 μM respectively. Subsequently, we voxelated the models for Kir2.1 and Kir3.1 in order to verify that in the docked structures, chloroquine is able to block the flow of potassium ions through the intracellular ion permeation pathway (**Figures 1C** and **2C**). The intracellular domains of Kir2.1 and 3.1 are shown in the longitudinal view, with the front subunit removed, and bound chloroquine (cyan sticks) is exposed. In Kir2.1, chloroquine binds closer to the G loop area, while in Kir3.1, chloroquine binds towards the intracellular mouth of the permeation pathway. The orange box denotes the voxelated part of the channels presented in the bottom panels of **Figures 1C** and **2C**. It was found that in Kir2.1, a probe (magenta sphere) of radius ≥2.1 Å was blocked by the drug, while probes with radii <2.1 Å passed through. In Kir3.1, a probe of radius ≥2.2 Å was blocked by the drug, while probes with radii <2.2 Å passed through. 3.0 Å is the radius of a solvated K^+ ion up to its first hydration shell. These results are in agreement with the patch clamp experiments which showed similar IC_{50} for chloroquine block of Kir2.1 and Kir3.1.

Chloroquine Treatment in a Patient With Persistent AF

As proof of concept, we tested in a patient with persistent atrial fibrillation, whether chloroquine can modify the AF burden. This 67 year old female was non-diabetic, non-hypertensive, a previous smoker, with no known structural heart or coronary artery disease but with known persistent AF. **Figure 3A** shows the daily AF burden extracted from Holter monitoring. At baseline, the patient was in uninterrupted, persistent AF. **Figure 3B** is a 12 lead ECG taken on the day of study initiation in order to confirm the presence of AF. After initiation of chloroquine treatment, AF burden was significantly reduced, with extensive periods of normal sinus rhythm, and the first conversion to normal sinus rhythm happened on the third day of treatment. **Figure 3C** shows Holter traces at baseline (top), immediately before treatment initiation (middle), where the patient was in AF, and during sinus rhythm on the third day of the oral chloroquine regimen (bottom). The patient did not have premature ventricular contractions while on chloroquine. The QT and QTc intervals while in AF, at the beginning of the study, were 418 ms and 428 ms respectively, and at the end of study, the QT and QTc intervals while in sinus

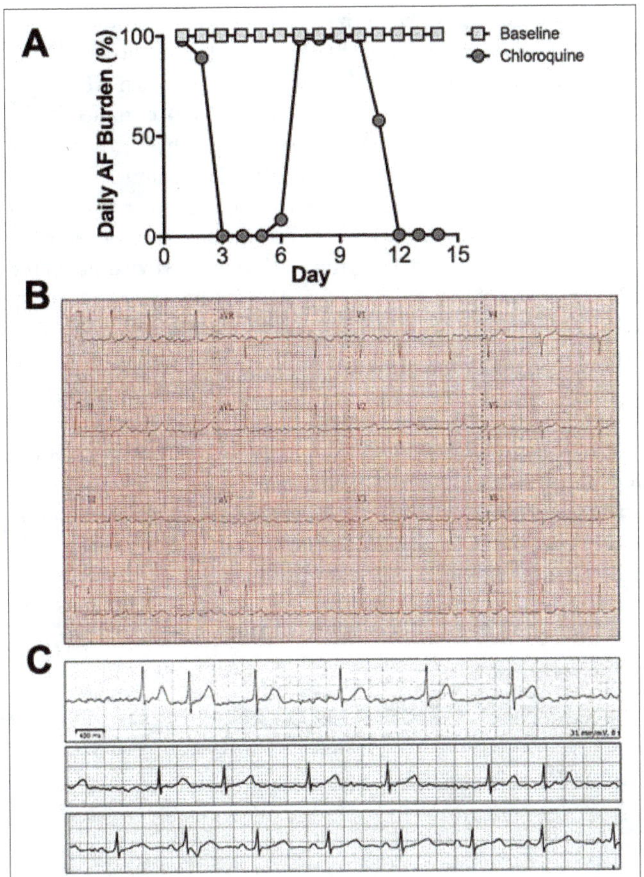

FIGURE 3 | Chloroquine effects on persistent AF. **(A)** Daily AF burden for 14 days in Holter monitoring at baseline, and for 14 days upon initiation of oral chloroquine (amebiasis treatment regimen). **(B)** 12 lead ECG on the day of chloroquine initiation, confirming the presence of AF. **(C)** Holter ECG strips from baseline (top), right before treatment initiation (middle), and on the 3rd day of treatment when AF converted to sinus rhythm (bottom).

rhythm were 450 ms and 461 ms. After the chloroquine regimen was completed, and upon follow up, the patient was back in atrial fibrillation as documented by a 12 lead ECG.

Effects of Chloroquine on Persistent AF in a 3D Model of Human Atria

A model of persistent AF was initiated by ectopic activity in the right superior pulmonary vein, and the arrhythmia was maintained by two stable rotors located in the posterior wall of the left atrium, near the left superior pulmonary vein and in the superior vena cava (**Figure 4A**). The calculated EGMs at sites 1, and 3, where the rotors were localized, showed double and fractionated potentials with low amplitude (**Figure 4B**). This occurred when the tip of the rotors pivoted at these locations, where the excitable but unexcited core resulted in multiple low amplitude deflections in the EGM. EGMs with single and double potentials were observed at sites 2 and 4 and were generated by wavefronts emanating from rotors and by wavebreaks at anatomical structures such as the crista terminalis and pectinate muscles. The DF was about 11 Hz (**Figure 4B**).

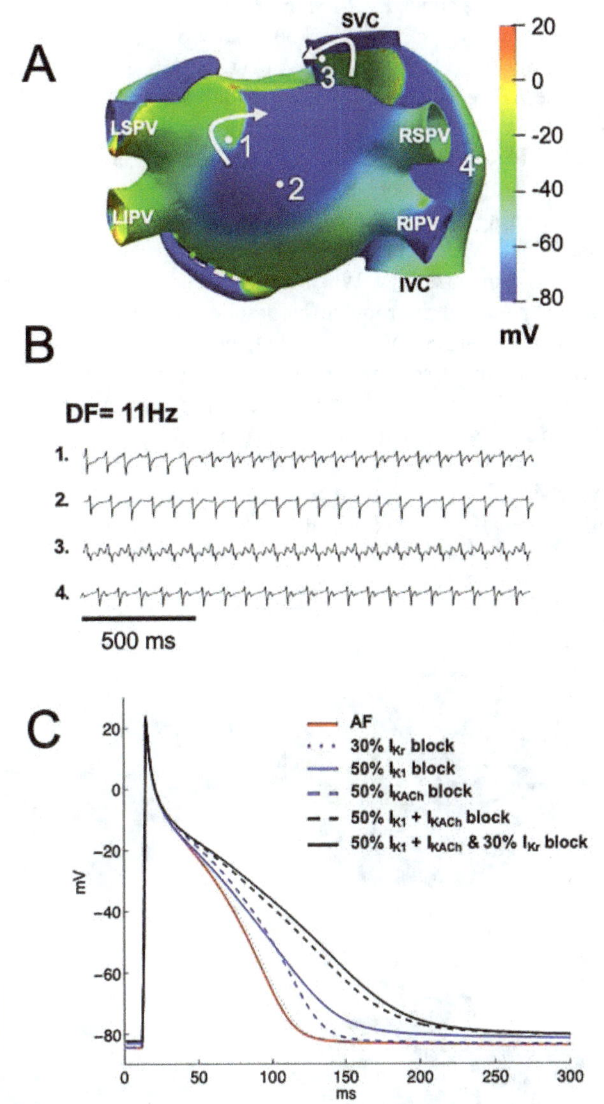

FIGURE 4 | Computational simulations of persistent AF in a 3D model of the human atria. **(A)** Snapshots of membrane voltage during persistent AF maintained by 2 rotors (curved arrows indicate rotation direction) in the posterior left atrium and the superior vena cava (SVC). Numbered dots indicate the locations of EGM recordings. **(B)** EGM traces displaying single (trace 2), double (traces 1 and 4) and fractionated (trace 3) potentials with low amplitude and high frequency of activation (DF of 11 Hz). **(C)** Single cell left atrial action potentials, at baseline AF (red trace), when I_{Kr} (blue dotted line), I_{K1} (blue solid line), I_{KACh} (blue dashed line), I_{K1} and I_{KACh} together (black dashed line), or the three currents together (black solid line) were blocked by 1 μM of chloroquine. LIPV, and LSPV: left inferior and superior pulmonary vein. RIPV, and RSPV: right inferior and superior pulmonary vein. SVC, and IVC: superior and inferior vena cava.

Chloroquine blocks I_{K1} and I_{KACh} with a similar IC_{50} of about 1 μM (0.97 μM for I_{K1} and 1.0 μM for I_{KACh}), this is around the plasma concentration that is achieved in patients. Additionally, chloroquine blocks I_{Kr} with an IC_{50} of 2.5 μM. We thus tested if chloroquine block of either I_{K1}, I_{KACh}, I_{Kr} alone, or I_{K1} and I_{KACh} together, or the three currents together terminates persistent AF. **Figure 4C** shows single cell left atrial action potentials when chloroquine was applied at 1 μM in order to simulate ~50% block of the I_{K1} and I_{KACh} currents and 30% block of I_{Kr}. When I_{Kr} was blocked by 30% (blue dotted line), APD_{90} prolonged from 98 ms (baseline AF, red line) to 101 ms, without changes in the RMP (−84.6 mV). When either I_{K1} or I_{KACh} were blocked by ~50% (blue solid and blue dashed lines), APD_{90} prolonged to 133 ms and 118 ms, with RMP values of −83.0 mV and −84.4 mV, respectively. When both I_{K1} and I_{KACh} currents were blocked by ~50% (black dashed line), APD_{90} prolonged to 170 ms and the RMP slightly depolarized to −82.3 mV. When I_{K1}, I_{KACh} and I_{Kr} currents were blocked by 1 μM of chloroquine (black solid line), the RMP slightly depolarized to −82.3 mV, but the APD_{90} prolonged to 179 ms.

When we increased the chloroquine concentration to 2.5 μM in order to simulate ~70% block of the I_{K1} and I_{KACh} currents and 50% block of the I_{Kr} current, APD_{90} prolonged to 164 ms, 128 ms and 103 ms, with RMP of −81.2 mV, −84.3 mV and −84.6 mV, when I_{K1}, or I_{KACh} or I_{Kr} was blocked respectively. When both I_{K1} and I_{KACh} were blocked by ~70%, APD_{90} prolonged to 259 ms and the RMP depolarized to −78.6 mV. Finally, when the three currents were blocked by 2.5 μM of chloroquine, APD_{90} prolonged to 291 ms, which corresponds to a 197% increase.

The two rotors maintaining AF at baseline continued to be present with up to 80% I_{K1} or 60% I_{KACh} block. In such scenarios, the rotor located in the posterior wall of the left atrium near the left pulmonary vein drifted to the inferior wall and the rotor located in the superior vena cava migrated to the free wall of the right atrium. Up to 90% block of I_{Kr} did not change the dynamics of the two rotors maintaining AF at baseline. However, when the block of I_{K1} reached 90% (**Figure 5A**) or I_{KACh} was blocked from 70 to 90% (**Figure 5B**), persistent AF converted into a stable reentrant tachycardia located at the free wall of the right atrium. In both cases, the EGMs presented single potentials generated by the wavefront emanating from the reentry and only in the posterior wall of the left atrium where the rotor wavefront pivots, some double EGMs generated by the passage of the rotor's core were observed in this area (**Figures 5A, B**). The DF was reduced to values between 8 Hz

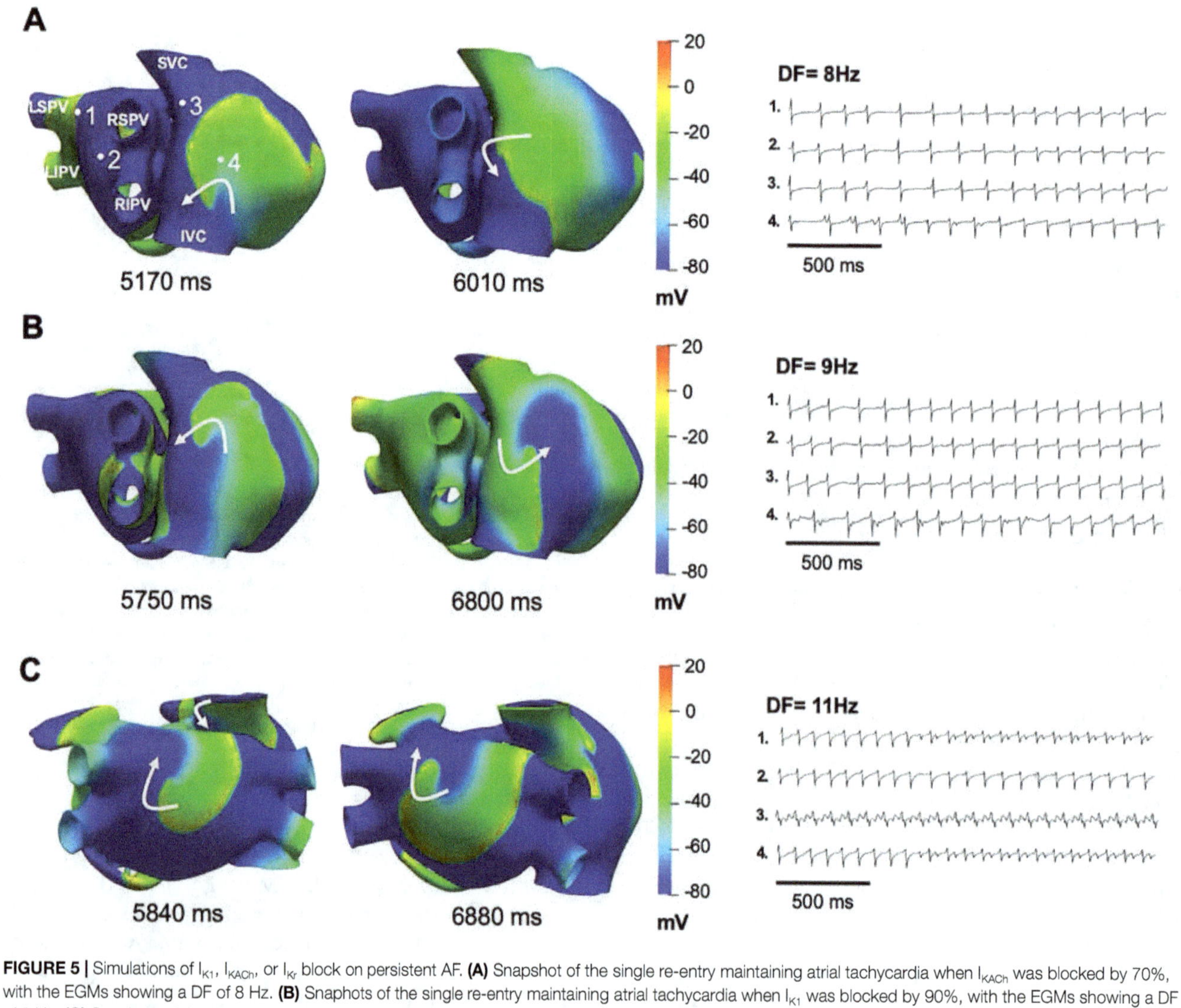

FIGURE 5 | Simulations of I_{K1}, I_{KACh}, or I_{Kr} block on persistent AF. **(A)** Snapshot of the single re-entry maintaining atrial tachycardia when I_{KACh} was blocked by 70%, with the EGMs showing a DF of 8 Hz. **(B)** Snaphots of the single re-entry maintaining atrial tachycardia when I_{K1} was blocked by 90%, with the EGMs showing a DF of 9 Hz. **(C)** Snaphots of the 2 rotors maintaining AF when I_{Kr} was blocked by 90%, with the EGMs showing a DF of 11 Hz.

and 9 Hz throughout the atria. **Figure 5C** shows that AF dynamics did not change appreciably when I_{Kr} was blocked by 90%.

When the effects of chloroquine on both I_{K1} and I_{KACh} together were simulated, termination of persistent AF was achieved with ~50% block of I_{K1} and I_{KACh} (**Figure 6A**). AF terminated 600 ms after the drug application, due to wavefront–wavetail interaction. Similarly, when the effects of chloroquine on the three currents together were simulated, termination of persistent AF was achieved with ~50% block of I_{K1} and I_{KACh} and 30% block of I_{Kr} (**Figure 6B**). AF terminated 380 ms after the drug application. AF terminated earlier when higher concentrations of chloroquine were simulated.

DISCUSSION

Our results showed that the aminoquinoline chloroquine blocks I_{K1} and I_{KACh}V by binding a pocket in the Kir2.1 and Kir3.1 channels intracellular ion permeation pathways. Moreover, chloroquine significantly reduced the burden of persistent AF in an otherwise healthy female patient. This was likely due to the ability of the drug to prolong the action potential duration, leading to a slowing down of the arrhythmia's dominant frequency, and subsequent failure of reentrant excitation due to wavefront–wavetail interaction.

Our molecular modeling suggested that chloroquine blocks I_{K1} and I_{KACh} by binding to a pocket in the intracellular water filled vestibule of Kir2.1 and Kir3.1. The drug appeared to hydrogen bond with electronegative residue D260 in Kir3.1, and E224 in Kir2.1, in proximity to residue F255 in Kir3.1 and the equivalent Kir2.1 residue F254.

At baseline AF, our simulations showed EGMs with double and fractionated potentials with low amplitude and high frequency when the tip of the rotors pivoted on the recording points (pivot point). Experimental and clinical studies of AF have documented intracardiac polymorphic EGMs in high frequency areas with fibrillatory conduction (Ryu et al., 2006; Kalifa et al., 2006; Narayan and Krummen, 2012; Narayan et al., 2012a; Narayan et al., 2012b; Narayan et al., 2012c; Narayan et al., 2012d) and fractionated EGMs when the rotor core passes at the recording point (Zlochiver et al., 2008). When I_{K1} or I_{KACh} were individually blocked with increasing concentrations of chloroquine AF organized into reentrant atrial tachycardia due to APD prolongation. EGMs with single potentials in the atria were observed, characteristic of EGMs recorded during atrial tachycardias (Ryu et al., 2006). Double potentials were generated by the passage of the reentry core at the recording point in the free wall of the right atrium. It has been reported that atrial potentials consisting of two or more deflections can be recorded during atrial tachycardias in sites of earliest activation such as the crista terminalis (De Groot and Schalij, 2006). When only I_{Kr} was blocked, AF dynamics did not change

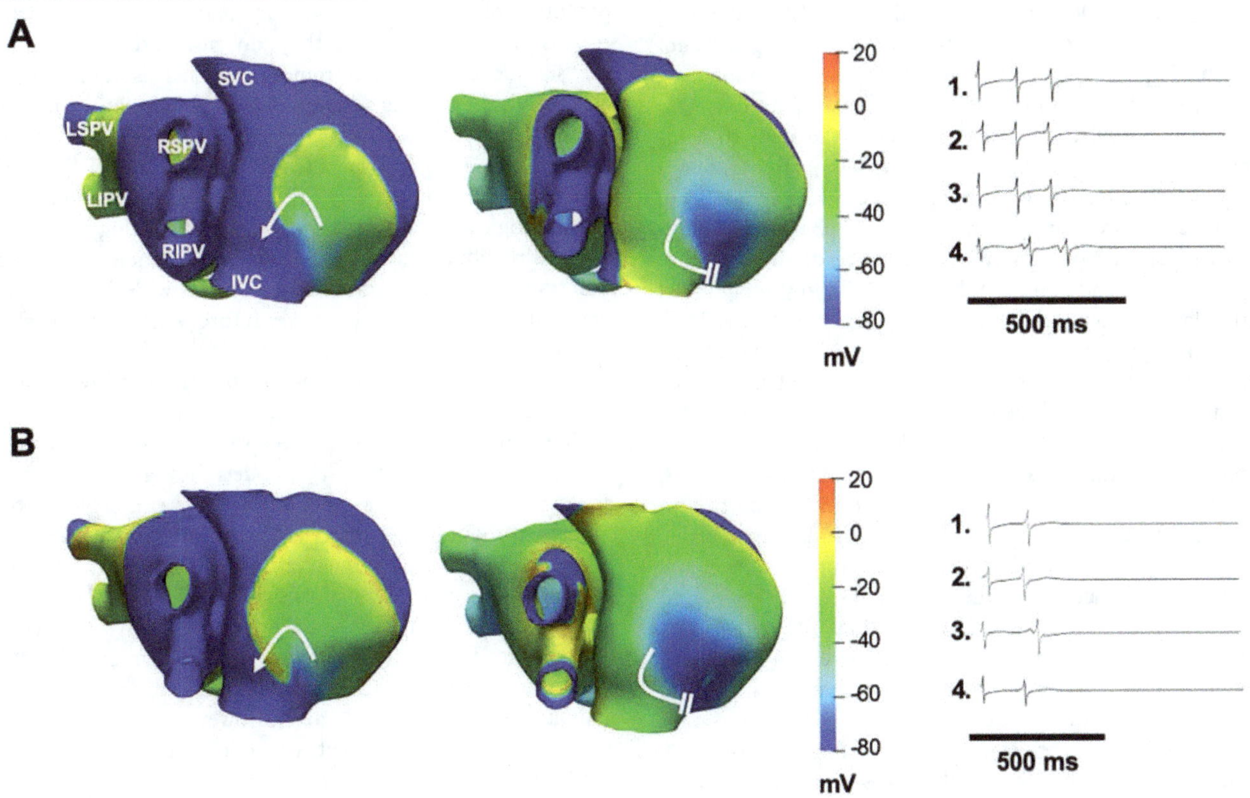

FIGURE 6 | Simulations of 1 μM chloroquine terminating AF by dual block of I_{K1} and I_{KACh} by 50% **(A)**, or by block of I_{Kr} by 30% and block of I_{K1} and I_{KACh} by 50% **(B)**. Voltage maps are snapshots of the last rotation of the re-entrant wave, where AF terminates after the wavefront interacts with the wavetail (white parallel lines). Curved white arrows: rotation direction. EGMs show arrhythmia termination.

(**Figure 5C**) because I_{Kr} block had a minimal effect on the APD (**Figure 4C**). While it has been reported that chloroquine is an I_{Kr} blocker (Sanchez-Chapula et al., 2002; Traebert et al., 2004), and can prolong the QT interval (White, 2007; Stas et al., 2008), in our simulations I_{Kr} block did not contribute substantially to the atrial antiarrhythmic properties. This could be in part due to the lower expression of hERG channels in the atria compared to the ventricles (Pond et al., 2000). When both I_{K1} and I_{KACh} (**Figure 6A**) or I_{K1}, I_{KACh} and I_{Kr} (**Figure 6B**) were blocked by 1 μM chloroquine, AF terminated.

The oral chloroquine regimen which we administered to a patient with persistent AF consisted of 600 mg chloroquine base once daily, for 2 days, followed by 300 mg once daily for 12 days. Therapeutic doses of chloroquine typically result in plasma concentrations around 1 μM (Karunajeewa et al., 2010), within the range of IC_{50} of I_{KACh} and I_{K1} block by the drug. The cardiac safety of chloroquine when used correctly is well documented. For instance, from cardiac electrophysiological safety standpoint, chloroquine is safe. This was shown in a large cohort of patients with systemic lupus erythematosus who have been treated with chloroquine for an average of 8 years. Chloroquine was found to be not only electrophysiologically safe, but to also have antiarrhythmic activity in those patients with autoimmune disease (Wozniacka et al., 2006; Teixeira et al., 2014). Chloroquine poisoning occurs with ingestion of more than 5 g of chloroquine per dose (Riou et al., 1988).

Presently, the treatment of persistent AF remains inadequate (Rietbrock et al., 2008; Shukla and Curtis, 2014). Clinical studies demonstrated that antiarrhythmics, or ablation strategies do not result in complete freedom from AF, thus antiarrhythmic drug therapy remains an important line of defense. With currently used antiarrhythmics, the rate of conversion to sinus rhythms is not optimal (Zimetbaum, 2012). Additionally, toxicities including life threatening arrhythmogenesis are a significant risk in antiarrhythmic rhythm control pharmacotherapy. Nevertheless, pharmacological maintenance of sinus rhythm offers secondary end point benefits such as improvement in left ventricular function, walking distance, in addition to atrial size reduction (Chung et al., 2005; Hagens et al., 2005; Rienstra et al., 2005). Hence, there is a need to improve the antiarrhythmic armamentarium, and to generate novel antiarrhythmics that are safe and that can reduce the burden of persistent AF or restore sinus rhythm. Based on this study and those of others, chloroquine appears to have antiarrhythmic properties in patients with AF (Burrell and Martinez, 1958; Harris et al., 1988). On the other hand, chloroquine's known side effects include QT prolongation (White, 2007; Stas et al., 2008), and retinal and gastrointestinal adverse reactions (Al-Bari, 2015). Therefore, using rational design to discover novel inward rectifier blockers based on small aminoquinolines such as chloroquine, but with an improved safety profile, could offer new avenues in the search of new pharmacotherapies for AF.

The combination of 3D virtual models of atrial fibrillation with modeling of ion channel block by small molecules opens the door for the simulation of antiarrhythmic drug effects, leading the way for the development of a more effective and safer generation of anti AF agents.

LIMITATIONS

Atrial remodeling in persistent AF is complex, with many changes occurring from the transcriptional to post-translational levels (Anisimov and Boheler, 2003; Volkova et al., 2005). In addition, autonomic, anatomical, sarcolemmal, and subsarcolemmal electrophysiological remodeling has been described in persistent AF, resulting in slow and discontinuous electrical propagation, and aberrant excitation–contraction coupling, as well as increased perpetuation of AF (Kumar et al., 2012). For instance, increased fibrosis (Koura et al., 2002), reduced I_{CaL}, increased background inward rectifiers currents (I_{K1} and constitutively active I_{KACh}) in addition to mitochondrial (Moslehi et al., 2012), and calcium handling abnormalities (Vest et al., 2005) are present in persistent AF. Such changes can play a significant role in creating the complex structural and functional substrates which promote the initiation and maintenance of high speed rotors responsible for atrial fibrillation. Therefore, it not unlikely that chloroquine's effect is not exclusively due to the block of I_{KACh} and I_{K1}. At the therapeutic chloroquine plasma concentration, which is around 1 μM, the drug blocks about 14% of the I_{Na} current, 7% of the I_{CaL}, and 9% of I_{Ks} (Sanchez-Chapula et al., 2001). It thus becomes conceivable that the multi-target effect of chloroquine contributed to its antiarrhythmic properties in persistent AF.

Although the electrophysiological remodeling conditions that we used in our simulations can reproduce the action potential phenotype observed in patients with persistent AF, as mentioned above, they do not take into account the significant structural remodeling that is found in the chronically fibrillating atria, which increases the complexity of the arrhythmia. Additionally, our numerical results were obtained using a specific virtual atria model that lacks fibrosis, albeit it includes a great number of anatomical and morphological details including electrophysiology, anatomy, fiber direction, anisotropy, and heterogeneity. Although functional reentries and rotors have been widely reported as maintenance mechanisms of AF, future works must include structural remodeling in order to address how chloroquine may be antiarrhythmic when ionic and structural remodeling are the driving mechanisms of persistent AF.

The simulated results may be atrial cell model-dependent. For instance, other human atrial models show a more triangular action potential and have a flatter restitution curve, however, all models introduce ionic remodeling in a similar way, resulting in effects on the action potential that are similar to what our simulations suggest. These models generally include decreases in I_{to}, I_{CaL} and I_{Kur}, and increased I_{K1}. More recently, AF models that also account for the remodeling of intracellular Ca^{2+} handling have been developed (Grandi et al., 2011; Skibsbye et al., 2016; Colman et al., 2017; Bai et al., 2018). However, the simpler I_{to}/ I_{CaL}/ I_{Kur}/ I_{K1} approach of persistent AF modeling remains commonly used, and we do not think that the use of a more complex model would substantially change the main results of our work. For modeling the effects of I_{Kr} block by chloroquine, we did not perform a concentration–response curve of the current block by the drug. We relied instead on the literature reported IC_{50} of 2.5

μM (Traebert et al., 2004), and thus, it is possible that variations around this value could affect the simulation results.

Two studies have reported that a benzopyrene derivative (Podd et al., 2016) and a benzamide related compound (Walfridsson et al., 2015) selectively inhibited I_{KACh}. However, the drugs failed in patients with paroxysmal AF and atrial flutter (Walfridsson et al., 2015; Podd et al., 2016). This could be because I_{KACh} is not constitutively active in paroxysmal AF (Voigt et al., 2007) and mechanistically, atrial flutter is very different from AF (Olshansky, 2004). Consequently, inhibiting I_{KACh} as part of an antiarrhythmic pharmaco-strategy should be reserved for the patient population in which the current is known to play a role. On the other hand, it is possible that chloroquine would reduce the burden of paroxysmal AF. It was shown that in patients with paroxysmal AF, a left/ right atrial gradient in I_{K1} exists (Voigt et al., 2010). This gradient could contribute to the ionic mechanism of paroxysmal AF, and therefore block of I_{K1} by chloroquine might be antiarrhythmic. Chloroquine might have limited antiarrhythmic effects in atrial flutter since its mechanisms are distinct from those of AF (Olshansky, 2004).

This is a proof of concept study which showed that chloroquine reduced persistent AF burden in a single patient. I_{K1} and I_{KACh} block is proposed as a plausible mechanism for this reduction as suggested by the numerical simulations. Further studies are needed in order to demonstrate a relation between I_{KACh} and I_{K1} block and reduction of persistent AF burden.

AUTHOR CONTRIBUTIONS

Designed Research: CT, LP, BC, DPS, TT, NT, MR, Y-SL, BH, DS, JS, and SN. Analyzed data: CT, LP, BC, DPS, Y-SL, BH, DS, JS, and SN. Wrote manuscript: CT, LP, BC, DPS, BH, JS, and SN.

FUNDING

This work was supported in part by National Institutes of Health grants R21HL138064, R01HL129136, by the Dirección General de Política Científica de la Generalitat Valenciana (PROMETEO 2016/088), and by the ACM SIGHPC/Intel Computational & Data Science fellowship.

REFERENCES

Al-Bari, M. A. (2015). Chloroquine analogues in drug discovery: new directions of uses, mechanisms of actions and toxic manifestations from malaria to multifarious diseases. *J. Antimicrob. Chemother.* 70, 1608–1621. doi: 10.1093/jac/dkv018

Anisimov, S. V., and Boheler, K. R. (2003). Aging-associated changes in cardiac gene expression: large scale transcriptome analysis. Advances in gerontology = Uspekhi gerontologii / Rossiiskaia akademiia nauk. *Gerontol. Obshchestvo* 11, 67–75.

Atienza, F., and Jalife, J. (2007). Reentry and atrial fibrillation. *Heart Rhythm.: Off. J. Heart Rhythm. Soc.* 4, S13–S16. doi: 10.1016/j.hrthm.2006.12.004

Bai, J., Gladding, P. A., Stiles, M. K., Fedorov, V. V., and Zhao, J. (2018). Ionic and cellular mechanisms underlying TBX5/PITX2 insufficiency-induced atrial fibrillation: Insights from mathematical models of human atrial cells. *Sci. Rep.* 8, 15642. doi: 10.1038/s41598-018-33958-y

Burrell, Z. L. Jr., and Martinez, A. C. (1958). Chloroquine and hydroxychloroquine in the treatment of cardiac arrhythmias. *New Engl. J. Med.* 258, 798–800. doi: 10.1056/NEJM195804172581608

Chung, M. K., Shemanski, L., Sherman, D. G., Greene, H. L., Hogan, D. B., Kellen, J. C., et al. (2005). Functional status in rate- versus rhythm-control strategies for atrial fibrillation: results of the Atrial Fibrillation Follow-Up Investigation of Rhythm Management (AFFIRM) Functional Status Substudy. *J. Am. Coll. Cardiol.* 46, 1891–1899. doi: 10.1016/j.jacc.2005.07.040

Colman, M. A., Pinali, C., Trafford, A. W., Zhang, H., and Kitmitto, A. (2017). A computational model of spatio-temporal cardiac intracellular calcium handling with realistic structure and spatial flux distribution from sarcoplasmic reticulum and t-tubule reconstructions. *PloS Comput. Biol.* 13, e1005714. doi: 10.1371/journal.pcbi.1005714

Courtemanche, M., Ramirez, R. J., and Nattel, S. (1998). Ionic mechanisms underlying human atrial action potential properties: insights from a mathematical model. *Am. J. Physiol.* 275, H301–H321. doi: 10.1152/ajpheart.1998.275.1.H301

De Groot, N. M., and Schalij, M. J. (2006). Fragmented, long-duration, low-amplitude electrograms characterize the origin of focal atrial tachycardia. *J. Cardiovasc. Electrophysiol.* 17, 1086–1092. doi: 10.1111/j.1540-8167.2006.00568.x

Dobrev, D., and Nattel, S. (2011). New insights into the molecular basis of atrial fibrillation: mechanistic and therapeutic implications. *Cardiovasc. Res.* 89, 689–691. doi: 10.1093/cvr/cvr021

Duarte M, R. A., Tobón, C., Cardona, K., and Saiz, J. (2013). *Chloroquine effect on human atrial action potential under normal conditions and during paroxysmal and chronic atrial fibrillation.* Columbia:A simulation study, PAHCE, 71–75. doi: 10.1109/PAHCE.2013.6568230

Filgueiras-Rama, D., Martins, R. P., Mironov, S., Yamazaki, M., Calvo, C. J., Ennis, S. R., et al. (2012). Chloroquine terminates stretch-induced atrial fibrillation more effectively than flecainide in the sheep heart. *Circ. Arrhythmia Electrophysiol.* 5, 561–570. doi: 10.1161/CIRCEP.111.966820

Grandi, E., Pandit, S. V., Voigt, N., Workman, A. J., Dobrev, D., Jalife, J., et al. (2011). Human atrial action potential and Ca2+ model: sinus rhythm and chronic atrial fibrillation. *Circ. Res.* 109, 1055–1066. doi: 10.1161/CIRCRESAHA.111.253955

Greenwood, J. R., Calkins, D., Sullivan, A. P., and Shelley, J. C. (2010). Towards the comprehensive, rapid, and accurate prediction of the favorable tautomeric states of drug-like molecules in aqueous solution. *J. Computer-aided Mol. Design* 24, 591–604. doi: 10.1007/s10822-010-9349-1

Hagens, V. E., Van Veldhuisen, D. J., Kamp, O., Rienstra, M., Bosker, H. A., Veeger, N. J., et al. (2005).Effect of rate and rhythm control on left ventricular function and cardiac dimensions in patients with persistent atrial fibrillation: results from the RAte Control versus Electrical Cardioversion for Persistent Atrial Fibrillation (RACE) study. *Heart Rhythm.: Off. J. Heart Rhythm. Soc.* 2, 19–24. doi: 10.1016/j.hrthm.2004.09.028

Harris, L., Downar, E., Shaikh, N. A., and Chen, T. (1988). Antiarrhythmic potential of chloroquine: new use for an old drug. *Can. J. Cardiol.* 4, 295–300.

Heidenreich, E. A., Ferrero, J. M., Doblare, M., and Rodriguez, J. F. (2010).Adaptive macro finite elements for the numerical solution of monodomain equations in cardiac electrophysiology. *Ann. Biomed. Eng.* 38, 2331–2345. doi: 10.1007/s10439-010-9997-2

Humphrey, W., Dalke, A., and Schulten, K. (1996). VMD: visual molecular dynamics. *J. Mol. Graphics* 14, 33–8, 27-8. doi: 10.1016/0263-7855(96)00018-5

Iijima, H., Dunbar, J. B. Jr., and Marshall, G. R. (1987). Calibration of effective van der Waals atomic contact radii for proteins and peptides. *Proteins* 2, 330–339. doi: 10.1002/prot.340020408

Kalifa, J., Tanaka, K., Zaitsev, A. V., Warren, M., Vaidyanathan, R., Auerbach, D., et al. (2006). Mechanisms of wave fractionation at boundaries of high-frequency excitation in the posterior left atrium of the isolated sheep heart during atrial fibrillation. *Circulation* 113, 626–633. doi: 10.1161/CIRCULATIONAHA.105.575340

Karunajeewa, H. A., Salman, S., Mueller, I., Baiwog, F., Gomorrai, S., Law, I., et al. (2010). Pharmacokinetics of chloroquine and monodesethylchloroquine in pregnancy. *Antimicrob. Agents Chemother.* 54, 1186–1192. doi: 10.1128/AAC.01269-09

Kneller, J., Zou, R., Vigmond, E. J., Wang, Z., Leon, L. J., and Nattel, S. (2002). Cholinergic atrial fibrillation in a computer model of a two-dimensional sheet of canine atrial cells with realistic ionic properties. *Circ. Res.* 90, E73–E87. doi: 10.1161/01.RES.0000019783.88094.BA

Koura, T., Hara, M., Takeuchi, S., Ota, K., Okada, Y., Miyoshi, S., et al. (2002). Anisotropic conduction properties in canine atria analyzed by high-resolution optical mapping: preferential direction of conduction block changes from longitudinal to transverse with increasing age. *Circulation* 105, 2092–2098. doi: 10.1161/01.CIR.0000015506.36371.0D

Kumar, S., Teh, A. W., Medi, C., Kistler, P. M., Morton, J. B., and Kalman, J. M. (2012). Atrial remodeling in varying clinical substrates within beating human hearts: relevance to atrial fibrillation. *Prog. In Biophys. Mol. Biol.* 110, 278–294. doi: 10.1016/j.pbiomolbio.2012.07.011

Liao, J. N., Chao, T. F., Liu, C. J., Wang, K. L., Chen, S. J., Tuan, T. C., et al. (2015). Risk and prediction of dementia in patients with atrial fibrillation–a nationwide population-based cohort study. *Int. J. Cardiol.* 199, 25–30. doi: 10.1016/j.ijcard.2015.06.170

Mahler, J., and Persson, I. (2012). A study of the hydration of the alkali metal ions in aqueous solution. *Inorg. Chem.* 51, 425–438. doi: 10.1021/ic2018693

Morris, G. M., Huey, R., Lindstrom, W., Sanner, M. F., Belew, R. K., Goodsell, D. S., et al. (2009). AutoDock4 and AutoDockTools4: Automated docking with selective receptor flexibility. *J. Comput. Chem.* 30, 2785–2791. doi: 10.1002/jcc.21256

Moslehi, J., DePinho, R. A., and Sahin, E. (2012). Telomeres and mitochondria in the aging heart. *Circ. Res.* 110, 1226–1237. doi: 10.1161/CIRCRESAHA.111.246868

Narayan, S. M., and Krummen, D. E. (2012). Targeting Stable Rotors to Treat Atrial Fibrillation. *Arrhythm Electrophysiol. Rev.* 1, 34–38. doi: 10.15420/aer.2012.1.34

Narayan, S. M., Krummen, D. E., Enyeart, M. W., and Rappel, W. J. (2012a). Computational mapping identifies localized mechanisms for ablation of atrial fibrillation. *PloS One* 7, e46034. doi: 10.1371/journal.pone.0046034

Narayan, S. M., Krummen, D. E., and Rappel, W. J. (2012b). Clinical mapping approach to diagnose electrical rotors and focal impulse sources for human atrial fibrillation. *J. Cardiovasc. Electrophysiol.* 23, 447–454. doi: 10.1111/j.1540-8167.2012.02332.x

Narayan, S. M., Krummen, D. E., Shivkumar, K., Clopton, P., Rappel, W. J., and Miller, J. M. (2012c). Treatment of atrial fibrillation by the ablation of localized sources: CONFIRM (Conventional Ablation for Atrial Fibrillation With or Without Focal Impulse and Rotor Modulation) trial. *J. Am. Coll. Cardiol.* 60, 628–636. doi: 10.1016/j.jacc.2012.05.022

Narayan, S. M., Patel, J., Mulpuru, S., and Krummen, D. E. (2012d). Focal impulse and rotor modulation ablation of sustaining rotors abruptly terminates persistent atrial fibrillation to sinus rhythm with elimination on follow-up: a video case study. *Heart Rhythm.: Off. J. Heart Rhythm. Soc.* 9, 1436–1439. doi: 10.1016/j.hrthm.2012.03.055

Noujaim, S. F., Pandit, S. V., Berenfeld, O., Vikstrom, K., Cerrone, M., Mironov, S., et al. (2007). Up-regulation of the inward rectifier K+ current (I K1) in the mouse heart accelerates and stabilizes rotors. *J. Physiol.* 578, 315–326. doi: 10.1113/jphysiol.2006.121475

Noujaim, S. F., Stuckey, J. A., Ponce-Balbuena, D., Ferrer-Villada, T., Lopez-Izquierdo, A., Pandit, S., et al. (2010). Specific residues of the cytoplasmic domains of cardiac inward rectifier potassium channels are effective antifibrillatory targets. *FASEB J.: Off. Publ. Fed. Am. Soc. Exp. Biol.* 24, 4302–4312. doi: 10.1096/fj.10-163246

Noujaim, S. F., Stuckey, J. A., Ponce-Balbuena, D., Ferrer-Villada, T., Lopez-Izquierdo, A., Pandit, S. V., et al. (2011). Structural bases for the different anti-fibrillatory effects of chloroquine and quinidine. *Cardiovasc. Res.* 89, 862–869. doi: 10.1093/cvr/cvr008

Olshansky, B. (2004). Combining ablation of atrial fibrillation with ablation of atrial flutter: are we there yet? *J. Am. Coll. Cardiol.* 43, 2063–2065. doi: 10.1016/j.jacc.2004.03.020

Pegan, S., Arrabit, C., Zhou, W., Kwiatkowski, W., Collins, A., Slesinger, P. A., et al. (2005). Cytoplasmic domain structures of Kir2.1 and Kir3.1 show sites for modulating gating and rectification. *Nat. Neurosci.* 8, 279–287. doi: 10.1038/nn1411

Podd, S. J., Freemantle, N., Furniss, S. S., and Sulke, N. (2016). First clinical trial of specific IKACh blocker shows no reduction in atrial fibrillation burden in patients with paroxysmal atrial fibrillation: pacemaker assessment of BMS 914392 in patients with paroxysmal atrial fibrillation. *Eur.: Eur. Pacing Arrhythmias Cardiac Electrophysiol.: J. Working Groups Cardiac Pacing Arrhythmias Cardiac Cell. Electrophysiol. Eur. Soc. Cardiol.* 18, 340–346. doi: 10.1093/europace/euv263

Pond, A. L., Scheve, B. K., Benedict, A. T., Petrecca, K., Van Wagoner, D. R., Shrier, A., et al. (2000). Expression of distinct ERG proteins in rat, mouse, and human heart. *Relat. Funct. I(Kr) Channels J. Biol. Chem.* 275, 5997–6006. doi: 10.1074/jbc.275.8.5997

Rienstra, M., Van Veldhuisen, D. J., Hagens, V. E., Ranchor, A. V., Veeger, N. J., Crijns, H. J., et al. (2005). Gender-related differences in rhythm control treatment in persistent atrial fibrillation: data of the Rate Control Versus Electrical Cardioversion (RACE) study. *J. Am. Coll. Cardiol.* 46, 1298–1306. doi: 10.1016/j.jacc.2005.05.078

Rietbrock, S., Heeley, E., Plumb, J., and van Staa, T. (2008). Chronic atrial fibrillation: Incidence, prevalence, and prediction of stroke using the Congestive heart failure, Hypertension, Age >75, Diabetes mellitus, and prior Stroke or transient ischemic attack (CHADS2) risk stratification scheme. *Am. Heart J.* 156, 57–64. doi: 10.1016/j.ahj.2008.03.010

Riou, B., Barriot, P., Rimailho, A., and Baud, F. J. (1988). Treatment of severe chloroquine poisoning. *New Engl. J. Med.* 318, 1–6. doi: 10.1056/NEJM198801073180101

Rodriguez-Menchaca, A. A., Navarro-Polanco, R. A., Ferrer-Villada, T., Rupp, J., Sachse, F. B., Tristani-Firouzi, M., et al. (2008). The molecular basis of chloroquine block of the inward rectifier Kir2.1 channel. *Proc. Natl. Acad. Sci. U. States America* 105, 1364–1368. doi: 10.1073/pnas.0708153105

Ryu, K., Sahadevan, J., Khrestian, C. M., Stambler, B. S., and Waldo, A. L. (2006). Use of fast fourier transform analysis of atrial electrograms for rapid characterization of atrial activation-implications for delineating possible mechanisms of atrial tachyarrhythmias. *J. Cardiovasc. Electrophysiol.* 17, 198–206. doi: 10.1111/j.1540-8167.2005.00320.x

Sanchez-Chapula, J. A., Salinas-Stefanon, E., Torres-Jacome, J., Benavides-Haro, D. E., and Navarro-Polanco, R. A. (2001). Blockade of currents by the antimalarial drug chloroquine in feline ventricular myocytes. *J. Pharmacol. Exp. Ther.* 297, 437–445.

Sanchez-Chapula, J. A., Navarro-Polanco, R. A., Culberson, C., Chen, J., and Sanguinetti, M. C. (2002). Molecular determinants of voltage-dependent human ether-a-go-go related gene (HERG) K+ channel block. *J. Biol. Chem.* 277, 23587–23595. doi: 10.1074/jbc.M200448200

Sastry, G. M., Adzhigirey, M., Day, T., Annabhimoju, R., and Sherman, W. (2013). Protein and ligand preparation: parameters, protocols, and influence on virtual screening enrichments. *J. Computer-aided Mol. Design* 27, 221–234. doi: 10.1007/s10822-013-9644-8

Schotten, U., Greiser, M., Benke, D., Buerkel, K., Ehrenteidt, B., Stellbrink, C., et al. (2002). Atrial fibrillation-induced atrial contractile dysfunction: a tachycardiomyopathy of a different sort. *Cardiovasc. Res.* 53, 192–201. doi: 10.1016/S0008-6363(01)00453-9

Shelley, J. C., Cholleti, A., Frye, L. L., Greenwood, J. R., Timlin, M. R., and Uchimaya, M. (2007). Epik: a software program for pK(a) prediction and protonation state generation for drug-like molecules. *J. Computer-aided Mol. Design* 21, 681–691. doi: 10.1007/s10822-007-9133-z

Shivakumar, D., Williams, J., Wu, Y., Damm, W., Shelley, J., and Sherman, W. (2010). Prediction of Absolute Solvation Free Energies using Molecular Dynamics Free Energy Perturbation and the OPLS Force Field. *J. Chem. Theory Comput.* 6, 1509–1519. doi: 10.1021/ct900587b

Shukla, A., and Curtis, A. B. (2014). Avoiding permanent atrial fibrillation: treatment approaches to prevent disease progression. *Vasc. Health Risk Manage.* 10, 1–12. doi: 10.2147/VHRM.S49334

Singh-Manoux, A., Fayosse, A., Sabia, S., Canonico, M., Bobak, M., Elbaz, A., et al. (2017). Atrial fibrillation as a risk factor for cognitive decline and dementia. *Eur. Heart J.* 38, 2612–2618. doi: 10.1093/eurheartj/ehx208

Skibsbye, L., Jespersen, T., Christ, T., Maleckar, M. M., van den Brink, J., Tavi, P., et al. (2016). Refractoriness in human atria: Time and voltage dependence of sodium channel availability. *J. Mol. Cell. Cardiol.* 101, 26–34. doi: 10.1016/j.yjmcc.2016.10.009

Stas, P., Faes, D., and Noyens, P. (2008). Conduction disorder and QT prolongation secondary to long-term treatment with chloroquine. *Int. J. Cardiol.* 127, e80–e82. doi: 10.1016/j.ijcard.2007.04.055

Takemoto, Y., Slough, D. P., Meinke, G., Katnik, C., Graziano, Z. A., Chidipi, B., et al. (2018). Structural basis for the antiarrhythmic blockade of a potassium channel with a small molecule. *FASEB J.: Off. Publ. Fed. Am. Soc. Exp. Biol.* 32, 1778–1793. doi: 10.1096/fj.201700349R

Teixeira, R. A., Borba, E. F., Pedrosa, A., Nishioka, S., Viana, V. S., Ramires, J. A., et al. (2014). Evidence for cardiac safety and antiarrhythmic potential of chloroquine in systemic lupus erythematosus. *Eur.: Eur. Pacing Arrhythmias Cardiac Electrophysiol.: J. Working Groups Cardiac Pacing Arrhythmias Cardiac Cell. Electrophysiol. Eur. Soc. Cardiol.* 16, 887–892. doi: 10.1093/europace/eut290

Tobon, C., Ruiz-Villa, C. A., Heidenreich, E., Romero, L., Hornero, F., and Saiz, J. (2013). A three-dimensional human atrial model with fiber orientation. *Electrograms Arrhythmic Activation Patterns Relat. PloS One* 8, e50883. doi: 10.1371/journal.pone.0050883

Traebert, M., Dumotier, B., Meister, L., Hoffmann, P., Dominguez-Estevez, M., and Suter, W. (2004). Inhibition of hERG K+ currents by antimalarial drugs in stably transfected HEK293 cells. *Eur. J. Pharmacol.* 484, 41–48. doi: 10.1016/j.ejphar.2003.11.003

Van Wagoner, D. R. (2003). Electrophysiological remodeling in human atrial fibrillation. *Pacing Clin. Electrophysiol. : PACE* 26, 1572–1575. doi: 10.1046/j.1460-9592.2003.t01-1-00234.x

Vest, J. A., Wehrens, X. H., Reiken, S. R., Lehnart, S. E., Dobrev, D., Chandra, P., et al. (2005). Defective cardiac ryanodine receptor regulation during atrial fibrillation. *Circulation* 111, 2025–2032. doi: 10.1161/01.CIR.0000162461.67140.4C

Voigt, N., Friedrich, A., Bock, M., Wettwer, E., Christ, T., Knaut, M., et al. (2007). Differential phosphorylation-dependent regulation of constitutively active and muscarinic receptor-activated IK,ACh channels in patients with chronic atrial fibrillation. *Cardiovasc. Res.* 74, 426–437. doi: 10.1016/j.cardiores.2007.02.009

Voigt, N., Trausch, A., Knaut, M., Matschke, K., Varro, A., Van Wagoner, D. R., et al. (2010). Left-to-right atrial inward rectifier potassium current gradients in patients with paroxysmal versus chronic atrial fibrillation. *Circ. Arrhythmia Electrophysiol.* 3, 472–480. doi: 10.1161/CIRCEP.110.954636

Volkova, M., Garg, R., Dick, S., and Boheler, K. R. (2005). Aging-associated changes in cardiac gene expression. *Cardiovasc. Res.* 66, 194–204. doi: 10.1016/j.cardiores.2004.11.016

Walfridsson, H., Anfinsen, O. G., Berggren, A., Frison, L., Jensen, S., Linhardt, G., et al. (2015). Is the acetylcholine-regulated inwardly rectifying potassium current a viable antiarrhythmic target? Translational discrepancies of AZD2927 and A7071 in dogs and humans. *Eur. : Eur. Pacing Arrhythmias Cardiac Electrophysiol. : J. Working Groups Cardiac Pacing Arrhythmias Cardiac Cell. Electrophysiol. Eur. Soc. Cardiol.* 17, 473–482. doi: 10.1093/europace/euu192

White, N. J. (2007). Cardiotoxicity of antimalarial drugs. *Lancet Infect. Dis.* 7, 549–558. doi: 10.1016/S1473-3099(07)70187-1

Wishart, D. S., Knox, C., Guo, A. C., Cheng, D., Shrivastava, S., Tzur, D., et al. (2008). DrugBank: a knowledgebase for drugs, drug actions and drug targets. *Nucleic Acids Res.* 36, D901–D906. doi: 10.1093/nar/gkm958

Wolf, P. A., Abbott, R. D., and Kannel, W. B. (1991). Atrial fibrillation as an independent risk factor for stroke: the Framingham Study. *Stroke; J. Cereb. Circ.* 22, 983–988. doi: 10.1161/01.STR.22.8.983

Workman, A. J., Kane, K. A., and Rankin, A. C. (2001). The contribution of ionic currents to changes in refractoriness of human atrial myocytes associated with chronic atrial fibrillation. *Cardiovasc. Res.* 52, 226–235. doi: 10.1016/S0008-6363(01)00380-7

Wozniacka, A., Cygankiewicz, I., Chudzik, M., Sysa-Jedrzejowska, A., and Wranicz, J. K. (2006). The cardiac safety of chloroquine phosphate treatment in patients with systemic lupus erythematosus: the influence on arrhythmia, heart rate variability and repolarization parameters. *Lupus* 15, 521–525. doi: 10.1191/0961203306lu2345oa

Zimetbaum, P. (2012). Antiarrhythmic drug therapy for atrial fibrillation. *Circulation* 125, 381–389. doi: 10.1161/CIRCULATIONAHA.111.019927

Zlochiver, S., Yamazaki, M., Kalifa, J., and Berenfeld, O. (2008). Rotor meandering contributes to irregularity in electrograms during atrial fibrillation. *Heart Rhythm. : Off. J. Heart Rhythm. Soc.* 5, 846–854. doi: 10.1016/j.hrthm.2008.03.010

13

ArrhythmoGeno Pharma Co-Therapy

*Arpad Tosaki**

Department of Pharmacology, School of Pharmacy, University of Debrecen, Debrecen, Hungary

Correspondence:
Arpad Tosaki
tosaki.arpad@pharm.unideb.hu

This review is focusing on the understanding of various factors and components governing and controlling the occurrence of ventricular arrhythmias including (i) the role of various ion channel-related changes in the action potential (AP), (ii) electrocardiograms (ECGs), (iii) some important arrhythmogenic mediators of reperfusion, and pharmacological approaches to their attenuation. The transmembrane potential in myocardial cells is depending on the cellular concentrations of several ions including sodium, calcium, and potassium on both sides of the cell membrane and active or inactive stages of ion channels. The movements of Na^+, K^+, and Ca^{2+} *via* cell membranes produce various currents that provoke AP, determining the cardiac cycle and heart function. A specific channel has its own type of gate, and it is opening and closing under specific transmembrane voltage, ionic, or metabolic conditions. APs of sinoatrial (SA) node, atrioventricular (AV) node, and Purkinje cells determine the pacemaker activity (depolarization phase 4) of the heart, leading to the surface manifestation, registration, and evaluation of ECG waves in both animal models and humans. AP and ECG changes are key factors in arrhythmogenesis, and the analysis of these changes serve for the clarification of the mechanisms of antiarrhythmic drugs. The classification of antiarrhythmic drugs may be based on their electrophysiological properties emphasizing the connection between basic electrophysiological activities and antiarrhythmic properties. The review also summarizes some important mechanisms of ventricular arrhythmias in the ischemic/reperfused myocardium and permits an assessment of antiarrhythmic potential of drugs used for pharmacotherapy under experimental and clinical conditions.

Keywords: genetics, ischemia—reperfusion, electrocardiogram (ECG), arrhythmia < cardiovascular, therapy -, action potential (AP)

THE HEART AND ARRHYTHMIAS

The heart is the key center of the blood circulation in fish, reptiles, birds, and mammals, an organ contracts autonomously and rhythmically, and functioning in conjunction with an extensive network of blood vessels to supply all cells and organs with oxygen and nutrients for serving their physiological function. Do we really need another review on cardiac arrhythmias in a special issue, someone may ask as you browse through several publications in cardiovascular journals. The answer is yes, and the mission of the current review is to present a short and comprehensive analysis of what is currently known about ischemia- and reperfusion-induced arrhythmias and their mechanisms, focusing on changes in shapes and waves in action potential (AP) and electrocardiogram (ECG), respectively, in animal models and human beings. The human heart produces left ventricular contraction about 70 times in a minute under physiological conditions.

The duration and shape of APs are controlled and determined by the function and activity of various ion channels and genes in an individual cardiac cell. In various myocardial cell types, the duration of AP is varied from species to species and the beat-to-beat variability for the AP duration is an important arrhythmogenic predictor, determining the intensity of cell-to-cell coupling (Magyar et al., 2016; Nanasi et al., 2017).

Various techniques for AP recordings and ion current measurements started about 70 years ago and became more sophisticated decade by decade, including the use of monophasic, two-electrode voltage clamp, and whole cell configuration of patch clamp. The recording of resting membrane potential and AP duration have initially been reported by Woodbury et al. (Woodbury et al., 1950), Burgen and Terroux (Burgen and Terroux, 1953), Coraboeuf and Weidmann (Coraboeuf and Weidmann, 1954), and Vaughan Williams (Vaughan Williams, 1959) in cardiac muscle fiber under *in vitro* conditions. Particularly, ion movements *via* voltage-regulated ion channels and pore-regulated proteins across cardiac cell membranes primarily determine the morphology and the duration of the AP in myocardial cells (Sankaranarayanan et al., 2017; Smith and Eisner, 2019). The resting transmembrane potential in an intact cardiac cell is about 85–90 mV negative to the exterior, and the move of Na^+ into the resting cell leads to the change of the membrane potential and the propagation of the cellular AP. Thus, this movement of Na^+ determines Ca^{2+} and K^+ release and exchange mechanisms *via* outer and inner cell membranes and organelles.

Ventricular arrhythmias are the leading cause of sudden cardiac death during and/or following an ischemic episode, acute heart failure, and recovery from myocardial infarction. Life threatening arrhythmias are very common and unpredictable in the failing myocardium; thus, the primary objective of their prevention is to eliminate various environmental risk factors, following the application of appropriate pharmacotherapies or nonpharmacological interventions. Heart failure and sudden ventricular arrhythmia caused deaths are likely to occur before an intervention can be implemented (Ramirez et al., 2014; Ramirez et al., 2017). The tool used for the detection and diagnosis of cardiac arrhythmias is the ECG, thus, the aim of antiarrhythmic therapy could be considered for acute termination or long-term treatment to prevent recurrence of various types of arrhythmias. However, antiarrhythmic drugs have multiple effects on the generation of AP and the waves of ECG, and their mechanisms are very complex (Alvarez et al., 2019; Paar et al., 2019). In addition, an antiarrhythmic agent could modulate other targets and tissues in the different parts of the myocardium in comparison with its primary site of action. In other words, an arrhythmia type and its origin could result from multiple underlying mechanisms at the same time, which may result in either from increased or decreased various types of K^+, Na^+, and Ca^{2+} currents *via* cell membranes and cell organelles. Thus, pharmacological therapies of cardiac arrhythmias should be focused on the most relevant underlying mechanism of arrhythmias, where it's known, and interventions may be antiarrhythmic by suppressing the initiating arrhythmogenic mechanism. Atrial fibrillation (AF) is caused by various mechanisms and one of the most common cardiac rhythm disturbances (Chua et al., 2019; Sutanto et al., 2019) associated with increased risk of heart failure, stroke (Kostopoulou et al., 2019), and death. More than dozens of genetic loci have been associated with AF, but the current review does not attempt to focus on these genetic mechanisms (Kalsto et al., 2019) and clinical management (Sutanto et al., 2019) of AF in detail.

THE ACTION POTENTIAL

Ion currents through cell membranes critically determine the shape of the AP and the waves of the ECG, which serve for the recognition and diagnosis of various types of cardiac arrhythmias. Namely, Na^+ currents, L- and T-type Ca^{2+} currents, transient outward currents, inward rectifier and pacemaker currents, *delayed rectifier K^+ currents,* Na^+–Ca^{2+}-exchanger (NCX), and Na^+–K^+-ATPase pump are the basic components of the AP development. In each AP, Na^+ entry and K^+ efflux and exchanges are the initial processes for determining of other ion concentrations and functions inside the cardiac cell. The ATP-depending exchange mechanism, called Na^+–K^+-pump, serves to determine and maintain intracellular ion homeostasis, which is electrogenic, and generating a net K^+ current. Under physiological conditions, intracellular Ca^{2+} is maintained at very low level in cardiac cells, and the entry of Ca^{2+} during AP *via* L-type Ca^{2+} channels is the primary signal to the sarcoplasmic reticulum (SR) to release Ca^{2+} ions from its store, leading to the initiation of Ca^{2+}-dependent contraction termed excitation–contraction coupling. Ca^{2+} efflux from SR into the cytoplasm happens *via* ryanodine receptor release channels (RyRc), and the subsequent elimination of intracellular Ca^{2+} from cytoplasm occurs by SERCA, which pumps Ca^{2+} ions back to the SR. In the meantime, the electrogenic NCX located on the cardiac cell membrane surface exchanges three Na^+ from the exterior for each Ca^{2+} ion extruded. During the past three decades, intensive investigation focused on the ion currents in AP phases, which were connected to specific channel-controlled genes, encoding the major pore-regulated proteins.

THE AP, ION CHANNELS, AND GENES

The identification of specific ion channels and their encoded proteins has contributed to a better understanding of the physiological and pathological APs and their changes, which affect the shape of ECG waves, leading to the mechanisms and diagnosis of various types of arrhythmias and discovery of potential new antiarrhythmic drug targets.

SCN5A

The primary gene (SCN5A) encodes the pore-forming alpha subunit of the primary Na^+ channel ($Na_{v1.5}$) in the human heart

(Lieve et al., 2017; Verkerk et al., 2018), and this so-called "gain-of-function mutation" determines the late Na^+ current (I_{Na}), which leads to (i) the development of one type of long-QT syndrome (LQTS), (ii) the prolongation of the duration of the AP, and (iii) the genesis of premature ventricular contractions in myocardial cells (Keating and Sanguinetti, 2001; Splawski et al., 2002; Wang et al., 2004; Amin et al., 2018). In addition, it was found that genetic mutations of SCN5A variants, including $Na_{v1.5}$, determine I_{Na} and the development of both the LQTS and Brugada syndromes (Tse et al., 2017; Li et al., 2018). Therefore, interventions, which inhibit the mutated gene's (SCN5A) function and/or the abnormal late Na^+ current (**Figure 1**) may prevent the development of LQTS. In contrast, drugs enhance the late Na^+ current may cause both atrial and ventricular arrhythmias; called proarrhythmic agents.

KCND2-D3

Transient outward potassium currents (KCND2-D3, Kv4.2, and Kv4.3) determine the development of the phases (0, 1, and 2) of the AP, however, the activation of KCND2 (Kv4.2) is rapidly terminated in the "notch" phase of the AP. It has been reported that KCND2 and KCND3 (Frank-Hansen et al., 2005), encoding of the voltage-gated potassium channel alpha subunits, Kv4.2 and Kv4.3, conducting the fast transient outward K^+ current ($I_{to,f}$) in the prolongation of AP duration, which may be associated with the development of LQTS in the myocardium. These authors (Frank-Hansen et al., 2005) concluded that mutations of KCND2 and KCND3 are not a frequent cause of LQTS, however, some variants of these two genes may play a significant role in the development of LQTS phenotype. In another study (Perrin et al., 2014), it was shown that KCND2 gene, as a susceptibility gene, contributes to the sudden cardiac death in an anterior J-wave ECG pattern in patients. The results of the aforementioned publication (Perrin et al., 2014) were the first to implicate KCND2 gene (Kv4.2) as a potential cause of an atypical J-wave pattern related to the sudden cardiac death. Considerable attention has been paid to the understanding of the roles of two functionally distinct K^+ channels; Kv4.2 and Kv4.3 subunits (Niwa and Nerbonne, 2010), which encode the fast transient outward potassium channels ($I_{to,f}$), while Kv1.4 (KCNA4) encodes the function of the slow potassium channels ($I_{to,s}$). Thus, it could be concluded that several signaling cascade mechanisms and regulatory proteins have been implicated in the control and regulation of $I_{to,f}$ and $I_{to,s}$ proteins/channels, regarding the mechanisms of arrhythmogenesis under physiological and various pathological conditions. Although cardiac $I_{to,f}$ and $I_{to,s}$ channels are differently expressed in various mammalian species and contribute to the heterogeneity of the AP and its waveforms, they have a potential importance in the genesis of cardiac arrhythmias. In addition, it has recently been demonstrated by Zhang et al. (2019a), that jingzhaotoxin-V (JZTX-V), a selective inhibitor of A-type potassium channel, plays a crucial role in the regulation of I_{to} potassium channels, supporting its use as a new potential and novel antiarrhythmic agent.

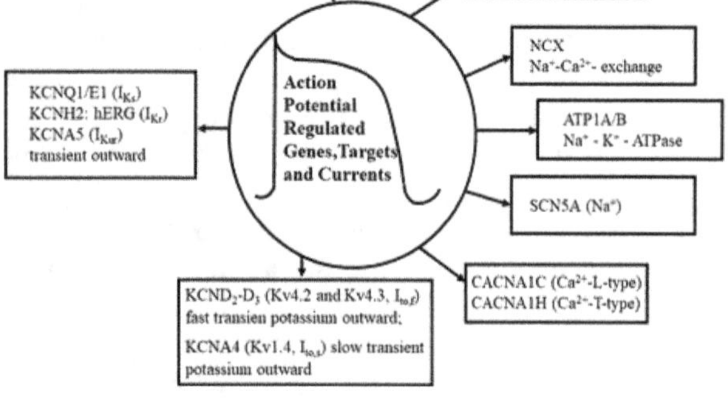

FIGURE 1 | Action potential (AP) genes and ion channels. The figure shows the summary of basic ion currents, genes and their targets in the AP. Various types of Ca^{2+} currents are shown, including L-type and T-type Ca^{2+} currents (CACNA1C, CACNA1H). KCND2-D3 genes (Kv4.2, Kv4.3), as voltage-gated fast transient outward potassium ($I_{to,f}$) and slow transient K^+ outward ($I_{to,s}$) channels are also shown. Additionally, Na^+ and K^+ channels and their pore-regulated proteins and voltage regulations are also depicted. The Na^+ current (SCN5A) is about 50 times lager as any other current during the depolarization phase (phase 1) of the AP, although its portion persists in the plateau phase. Several types of Ca^{2+} currents e.g., CACNA1C (L-type) and CACNA1H (T-type), are activated during the phases 0, 1, and 2 of the AP. Fast transient outward potassium currents (KCND2-D3, encoding Kv4.2-Kv4.3) are functioning in the phases of 0, 1, and 2 of the AP. The activation of KCDN2 is rapidly terminated in the "notch" phase, phase 1, of the AP. Rectifier potassium channels include I_{Ks} (KCNQ1, KCNE1), I_{Kr} (KCNH2, hERG), and I_{Kur} (KCNA5), which are also activated in the phases of 0, 1, and 2 of the AP. Inward rectifier current (KCNJ2), pacemaker current (HCN4, I_f), and Na^+–K^+-ATPase (ATP1A/B) are activated in the phase 4 of the AP. Na^+–Ca^{2+} exchange mechanism (NCX) is functioning in the phases of 1, 2, and 3 of the AP.

KCNQ1/E1 and KCNA5

K^+ currents so-called delayed rectifier currents, including slow (I_{Ks}) and ultrarapid (I_{Kur}) channels (Zareba et al., 2003), have been dissociated on the basis how quickly they are activated during the AP. However, cardiac KCNQ1/E1 encodes only slow delayed rectifier channels and does not I_{Kr} (rapid delayed rectifier K^+ current). These K^+ rectifier channel activations are increased with the time, whereas Ca^{2+} currents are inactivated, leading to the phase-3 (repolarization phase) of AP (**Figure 1**). It was described (Christophersen et al., 2013) that KCNA5 (I_{Kur}) has a high frequency of rare variants related to the development of AF, emphasizing that KCNA5 (**Figure 1**) is probably one of the most predominant genes to produce AF (Colman et al., 2017). KCNA5 also encodes hKv1.5, and this genetic alteration increases the electrical activity of cells, therefore, the controlling of hKv1.5 expression and function may result in a proper physiological electrical activity, suggesting that hKv1.5 may be a potential target for the treatment of AF (Xie et al., 2019). Thus, the selective inhibition of hKv1.5 function could be related to the prolongation of atrial AP without an increase in the duration of ventricular AP in human beings.

KCNH2

KCNH2, initially described and termed hERG, regulates I_{Kr} (rapid delayed rectifier K^+ channel) and the blocking of I_{Kr} still remains a major issue in the development of antiarrhythmic drugs (Chen et al., 2000; Mitcheson et al., 2000; Mehta et al., 2018) in connection with the pharmacotherapy of LQTS at genetic levels (Mehta et al., 2018; Yin et al., 2018; Cortez et al., 2019; Kerr et al., 2019). The voltage activated potassium channel (Kv11.1) is encoded by the humane-ether-a-go-go related gene (hERG), which predominantly contributes to the electrical activity of the myocardium (Vandenberg et al., 2012; Vasseur et al., 2019). This channel mediates I_{Kr} current (**Figure 1**) during the repolarization phase of the AP (Orvos et al., 2019) and its malfunction plays a critical role in the development of LQTS (Perissinotti et al., 2018; Ng et al., 2019). In an additional elegant study, Wu et al. (2019) described that KCNQ1 mutation interferes with intracellular hERG transport processes, leading to the development of the phenotype LQTS.

KCNJ2

It was published in an elegant review (Kubo et al., 2005) that inward rectifier K^+ channel (K_{ir}) subfamilies, based on their amino acid sequence alignments, play important roles in various human diseases, including arrhythmogenesis (**Figure 1**). Therefore, pharmacological aspects of K_{ir} channel mediated functions could be expected as therapeutic tools for the treatment of various cardiac arrhythmias. It was suggested that (Yue et al., 2011; Qi et al., 2015) myofibroblasts also play a critical role in arrhythmogenesis in chronic heart failure by increasing extracellular matrix protein production and having a direct electric interaction with myocytes. However, fibroblasts are not excitable cells electrically, but they are able to express various ion channels including I_{K1}, and having resting membrane potential about −40 mV (Kamkin et al., 2003). The study by Qi et al. (2015), demonstrated that KCNJ2 (inward rectifier potassium channel; I_{K1}) subunit is present in fibroblasts and cardiomyocytes as well. Thus, drug therapies, which alter the function of KCNJ2 ion channels in connection with Ca^{2+} entry may be an important target for the development of other new antiarrhythmic agents, as inward rectifier potassium channel blockers, in failing myocardium (Szuts et al., 2013).

HCN4, "Funny" Current

The pacemaker current (I_f or I_{Kf}) is called "funny" current or pacemaker channel, which is an electric current through the HCN4 and subtype genes regulated proteins in the myocardium (**Figure 1**). The "funny" current is a component of the electrical conduction system producing the natural pacemaker activity of the heart. The I_f was first described in Purkinje fibers and atrial cells, and has been extensively studied for several decades (Difrancesco and Ojeda, 1980; Mesirca et al., 2013; Mengesha et al., 2017; Monfredi et al., 2018), however, its function is not completely understood in arrhythmogenesis. HCN4 gene-related arrhythmias, including atrioventricular block and AF, have still an unexplored role in arrhythmogenesis, although HCN4 gene (cyclic nucleotide gated 4 channel) is generally accepted as a genetic marker in myocardial pacemaker tissues (Difrancesco, 2015). Thus, myocardial structural abnormalities could be closely associated with HCN4 mutations, leading to the development of cardiac arrhythmias *via* phosphatidyl-inositol 3,4,5-trisphosphate (PIP3) signal transduction mechanism; regulating the function of funny current, controlling the pacemaker activity and heart rate in the myocardium (Difrancesco, 2019). The term of "funny" refers to a mixed Na^+ and K^+ permeability through cell membranes and having a very slow physiological kinetic. In addition, an increase in the activation of I_f augments Na^+ influx in the cell, and paradoxically, in a "reverse mode," elevates intracellular Ca^{2+} accumulation leading to elevated systolic calcium transients. Consequently, the inhibition of I_f reduces intracellular Ca^{2+} rise, thus, alters several processes of ventricular remodeling and structural cardiac function, including apoptosis, cardiomyopathy, and arrhythmias (Yampolsky et al., 2019), which may have an important target in clinical managements of arrhythmogenesis.

NCX

The pharmacological inhibition of NCX protein expression could be a further target and may be an additional advantage for the therapy of heart failure and cardiac arrhythmias under both experimental and clinical conditions (Sipido et al., 2002; Jost et al., 2013; Schwartz et al., 2013; Bogeholz et al., 2016; Devalla et al., 2016; Kohajda et al., 2016; Javidanpour et al., 2018). During the period of diastole in the myocardium, cytosolic free Ca^{2+} is removed by both the reuptake of SERCA (Ca^{2+}-ATPase) and transmembrane extrusion by NCX (Voigt et al., 2012). The basic role of NCX has been recognized in two major types of triggered arrhythmias including delayed afterdepolarization (DAD) and early afterdepolarization (EAD). DAD is developed by Ca^{2+} release from the SR under cellular Ca^{2+} overload. The increased Ca^{2+} overload in the cytosol is removed by NCX, causing additional Na^+ influx and cell membrane depolarization, which leads to DAD. Thus, interventions, which are able to interfere with the NCX could be an effective antiarrhythmic pharmacotherapy in patients, showing DAD signs on AP and/or on ECG recordings. EAD interrupts AP in the phase of repolarization, and not only various Ca^{2+} channel-related intracellular Ca^{2+} overload but even other ion channels and transporters, particularly Na^+ and K^+ channels and exchangers, could also contribute to the development of EAD. Under clinical conditions, EAD triggering is a very common event in human, if the heart rate is reduced and extracellular K^+ concentration is low. Basically, the duration of AP is longer in Purkinje and endocardial cells than in epicardial tissues, therefore, EAD is more frequently induced in Purkinje and endocardial cells in comparison with epicardial cells. Cardiac arrhythmias showing the sign of EAD could be treated by antiarrhythmic drugs, which shorten the AP duration, e.g., antiarrhythmic agents belong to class IB (Vaughan Williams, 1992).

ATP1alpha/Beta (Na^+–K^+-ATP-ase, Na^+–K^+-Pump)

It is of interest to note that calcium channels include the structurally homologous family of voltage-gated ion channels, such as CACNA1C-encoded L-type calcium channel ($Ca_v1.2$, LTCC), which transports calcium ions into myocytes, regulating the excitation–contraction coupling process, and leading to the development of LQTS phenotype (Estes et al., 2019; Ye et al., 2019). The results of the aforementioned recent publications reveal that a new population of Ca^{2+} channels represents a new "pathological substrates" for LQTS-related arrhythmias. During each AP the cell gains intracellular Na^+ and loses intracellular K^+ content. At the end of each AP, for returning to the physiological membrane potential of −90 mV in the myocyte, the Na^+–K^+-ATP-ase serves the energy to extrude three Na^+ ions and enter two K^+ ions. This process is electrogenic, generating a net outward Na^+ current during the phases 3 and 4 of the AP. Several decades ago, it was measured and described, using the whole-cell patch-clamp technique that the aforementioned exchange mechanism is generated by the Na^+–K^+-pump, leading to the outward membrane current (I_P) in a single myocyte (Gadsby et al., 1985). Several groups published that peak I_P may be the clearing of excess of Na^+, which is accumulated close to the inner cardiac cell membrane leaflet, if the Na^+–K^+-pump is inhibited (Carmeliet, 1992; Aronsen et al., 2013; Garcia et al., 2016). Thus, a restricted Na^+ diffusion at a subsarcolemmal area in the cardiomyocyte may be a reasonable therapeutic implication (Han et al., 2010; Lu and Hilgemann, 2017) in the treatment of cardiac arrhythmias.

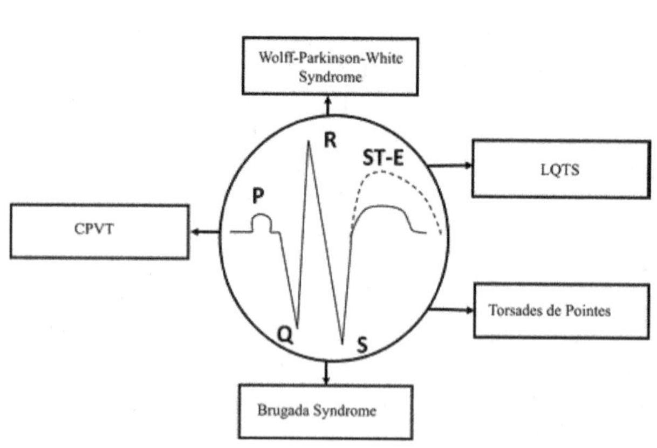

FIGURE 2 | Schematic representation of the ECG. Types of syndromes originated from various gene mutations. Gene mutation-related arrhythmias include long-QT and Brugada syndromes, catecholaminergic polymorphic ventricular tachycardia (CPVT), "torsade de pointes" arrhythmias, and Wolff–Parkinson–White (WPW) syndrome. ST-E, ST-segment elevation.

THE ECG AND INHERITED SYNDROMES

The duration of APs from different regions of the myocardium, including the sinus node, AV node, and His-Purkinje system, determines the coordinated ventricular contraction, and the electrical activation of the heart, which is normally represented by ECG recordings. In the ECG, P wave, QRS complex, and T wave show the physiological or pathological electrical activity of the myocardium. P wave represents the depolarization phase of the atria, QRS complex indicates the depolarization of the left and right ventricles, while T wave shows the repolarization phase of both ventricles in the ECG (**Figure 2**).

At least, four major inherited syndromes (**Figure 2**) are currently known, which may lead to sudden cardiac death without any structural myocardial diseases, including LQTS, catecholaminergic polymorphic ventricular tachycardia (CPVT), Brugada syndrome, and "torsades de pointes" arrhythmias (Savastano et al., 2014; Delise et al., 2018; Michowitz et al., 2019). However, Wolff–Parkinson–White (WPW) syndrome, which may also be an inherited cardiac disease and leads to reentry ventricular arrhythmias, has some significant structural changes in the myocardial conduction system. Although, these syndromes and sudden consequences were first published several decades ago, the investigation of their genetic origins started about only in the last decade of the twentieth century.

Sodium channels and cardiac structural abnormalities lead to changes in ECG signs and pathological cardiac consequences, which may be associated with SCN5A gene mutation in Brugada syndrome (Coronel et al., 2005). It was suggested that a reduced expression in the number of $Na_v1.5$ sodium channels may result in Brugada syndrome in myocardial cells and heterozygous patients (Mohler et al., 2004). Thus, interventions, which could increase the expression of $Na_v1.5$ channels in the myocardium may prevent the development of lethal arrhythmias in "Brugada patients," however, this mechanism should be further investigated.

The increased length of ventricular AP prolongs the QT interval on the ECG, which could be associated with the LQTS and the development of ventricular tachycardia. Four of the aforementioned syndromes (LQT, CPVT, Brugada syndrome, torsades de pointes) appear in patients who did not previously show any cardiac symptoms (Singh et al., 2019) or gross structural changes except syncope before the sudden cardiac death. The ventricular tachycardia with prolonged QT interval is termed "torsades de points" arrhythmia (Bossu et al., 2018). LQT and Brugada syndromes are the most common inherited arrhythmias, while CPVT occurs much rarely.

Dessertenne published (Dessertenne, 1966) initially several original articles about polymorphic ventricular tachycardia in the 1960s, and termed "torsades de pointes" arrhythmia based on ECG signs. Then, it has been the subject of debate for decades, whether "torsades de pointes" is a syndrome or an arrhythmia (Curtis, 1991), and it was concluded that this type of arrhythmia can be a type of arrhythmias and also a syndrome. The final outcomes of the "torsades de pointes" arrhythmia may be syncope, self-terminating, or ventricular fibrillation (VF) leading to sudden cardiac death. The QT interval's prolongation could be genetic origin or acquired (Thomas and Behr, 2016). It was also under extensive investigation (Naksuk et al., 2019) and published that LQTS is a type of arrhythmias, in which "torsades de pointes" arrhythmia causes ventricular tachycardia, VF, and sudden death by the mutation of various genes (KCNQ1/E1 and KCNH2/hERG) underlying potassium repolarization currents, including I_{Kr} and I_{Ks} (Anson et al., 2004; Nerbonne and Kass, 2005; Daubert et al., 2007; Vink et al., 2018;

Zhou et al., 2019). In conclusion, clinical management of "torsades de pointes" arrhythmia associated with prolonged QT interval can be pharmacologically treated with intravenous magnesium and potassium infusions for the correction of electrolyte imbalance, and administration of isoproterenol to increase heart rate (Narang and Ozcan, 2019). The application of antiarrhythmic drugs, which prolong the repolarization phase of AP in myocardial cells should be avoided.

The CPVT, which is relatively a rare disease in comparison with the appearance of Brugada and LQTS, applies to an autosomal inherited familial disorder characterized by exercise-induced adrenergic polymorphic ventricular tachycardia, leading to VF and sudden cardiac death (Marks et al., 2002). These "arrhythmogenic" genes are located to the region of genetic locus of chromosome 1q42–q43 as described by Marks et al. (2002), Swan et al. (1999), and Rampazzo et al. (1995). Genetic analyses and findings led to the conclusion that chromosomal area of 1q42–q43 genes is probably closely connected to the function of ryanodine receptor (RyR)–calcium-release channels in cardiac tissues (Priori et al., 2001; Marks et al., 2002). Based on these aforementioned publications, it was suggested that potential inhibitors of RyR, especially RyR2, could be an important antiarrhythmic target for the development of new therapeutic agents (Bongianino et al., 2017; Batiste et al., 2019).

WPW syndrome is defined as the prototype of reentry mechanism, having an accessory connection between the left atrium and left ventricle, and this connection results in a pathological characteristic in QRS complexes. WPW syndrome, based on ECG recordings, was described by these authors in details (Wolff et al., 1930) about ninety years ago. Gollob et al. (2001) first published the gene in familial WPW syndrome, which could be responsible for this type of arrhythmia and sudden cardiac deaths. The authors (Gollob et al., 2001) described a mutation in the encoding gene of gamma subunit of AMP-activated protein kinase in families, which is associated with WPW syndrome, since gamma subunit of AMP-activated protein kinase has a substantial impact in the phosphorylation of several metabolic pathways, including the control of energy substrates in myocardial tissues. Currently, relatively little information is available about the mechanism of AV conduction system and the role of gamma subunit of AMP-activated protein kinase on the control and regulation of various ion channels in familial WPW syndrome (Miyamoto, 2018), although the genetic origin of WPW syndrome and gamma subunit of AMP-activated protein kinase in connection with the reentry mechanism was supported by some recent publications (Bowles et al., 2015; Ben Jehuda et al., 2018). Thus, these findings suggest that gamma subunit of AMP-activated protein kinase and glycogen regulation could be a potent therapeutic target in the treatment of familial WPW syndrome.

Clinical Management of Prolonged QT interval

Several variations are clinically available for the management of QT prolongation-related arrhythmias (Antoniou et al., 2017). The acceleration of the electrical conduction system in both under experimental and clinical conditions is generally accepted for the management of arrhythmias with prolonged QT interval. Thus, interventions that modify the function of various ion channels, especially Na^+, K^+, Ca^{2+}, and Mg^{2+} and their exchange mechanisms, could be useful tools for pharmacotherapies of arrhythmias with prolonged QT interval. The QRS wave until the end of the T wave represents the ventricular depolarization and repolarization phases on the ECG. Abnormalities of electrolytes should be corrected with K^+ infusion monitored continuously, following by intravenous Mg^{2+} sulfate infusion to terminate the prolonged QT interval. In some case, if it is indicated, lidocaine and phenytoin as Na^+ channel blockers successfully can be also used for the management of LQTS. The beta1/beta2 nonselective adrenergic receptor agonist agent, isoproterenol, shortens QT interval, which could be an effective therapy in humans unresponsive to magnesium sulfate infusion. However, other antiarrhythmic agents initially classified by Vaughan Williams (1975), which are used in clinical therapy against hypoxia- or ischemia-induced arrhythmias e.g., beta adrenergic receptor blockers and calcium channel antagonists, should be avoided for the therapeutic management of arrhythmias with prolonged QT interval. A promising future approach, under experimental conditions to manage the CPVT-initiated QT prolongation, was published by Batiste et al. (2019) showing that an unnatural verticilide enantiomer inhibits the function of RyR2-mediated calcium leak, which inhibits QT prolongation, and prevents life threatening arrhythmias.

The left cardiac sympathetic denervation was also proposed as a useful therapy for LQTS including CPVT (De Ferrari et al., 2015; Desimone et al., 2015; Sgro et al., 2019) in addition to the application of anti-arrhythmic agents and implantable cardioverter defibrillators. Thus, the combination of these interventions can significantly improve the final outcome of the clinical management of LQTS including CPVT in patients, and the prevention of sudden cardiac death.

REPERFUSION-INDUCED INJURY AND ARRHYTHMIAS: MAJOR COMPONENTS

The response of the ischemic myocardium to reperfusion depends on the condition of the tissue at the time it is reperfused. The condition of the myocardium depends on the severity of the ischemia and the duration of the ischemic event. Substantially altered physiological processes in ultrastructural and metabolic changes during ischemia are required for the understanding of the myocardial function to reperfusion. The major ultrastructural and metabolic changes observed in the ischemic myocardium destined to die develop because of the lack of nutrition and oxygen supply and the depressed coronary flow. By definition, the myocardium is considered to be in VF, the most severe life-threatening arrhythmias, if an irregular undulating baseline is observed on the ECG (Walker et al., 1988). The term of "reperfusion-induced" injury caused by VF is originated from the definition itself of the "reperfusion". Thousands of basic and clinical studies revealed that electrophysiological changes of the ischemic/reperfused myocardium is a dysfunction of cellular homeostasis, which includes the depletion and/or accumulation of various biochemical substances, altering the function of various ion channels and cell-to-cell coupling. Reperfusion-induced arrhythmias include the ectopic beat, tachycardia and fibrillation. The incidence and severity of reperfusion-induced arrhythmias is more frequently occurred under experimental conditions in comparison with human beings (Jennings and Reimer, 1983; Manning and Hearse, 1984; Nakata et al., 1990; Kloner, 1993; Yellon and Hausenloy, 2007; Van Der Weg et al., 2019). Under clinical conditions, reperfusion-induced arrhythmias could mainly be observed during the process of thrombolysis following myocardial ischemia and infarction, after an insult of angina and percutaneous coronary intervention (Corr and Witkowski, 1983; Tzivoni et al., 1983; Tolg et al., 2006; Yu et al., 2017; Van Der Weg et al., 2019). Thrombolytic agents, including urokinase, ataplase, tissue plasminogen activator, are used to dissolve coronary thrombus during early hours of cardiac infarction. The basic arrhythmogenic or proarrhythmogenic role of different mediators, biochemical components, and chemical substances, which accumulate or decompose by virtue of several pathological processes during ischemia/reperfusion in the cellular milieu of the myocardium could be evaluated by various criteria. Therefore, it is important to prove that the antiarrhythmic effect of a drug is primarily originated from its receptor binding activities, and not secondary, e.g., by modifying the coronary blood flow rate. The mission of this chapter is to present a brief summary of what is currently known about the origin of reperfusion-induced arrhythmias, their most important mechanisms, and final outcomes preventing the processes of necrosis, apoptosis and autophagy caused cell deaths under experimental and clinical conditions. The potential importance of major arrhythmogenic components and mediators in reperfusion is shown in **Figure 3**.

The potential mechanisms underlying the genesis of reperfusion-induced arrhythmias have been extensively studied by thousands of investigators. The several pathological processes include the elevation of cAMP (Podzuweit et al., 1978; Oikawa et al., 2013), stimulation of adrenergic receptors (Sheridan et al., 1980; Amirahmadi et al., 2008; Robertson et al., 2014), abnormal lipid metabolism involving lysophosphatides' production (Akita et al., 1986; Axelsen et al., 2015), maldistribution of ionic components through cell membranes, particularly that of Na^+, Ca^{2+}, K^+, and Mg^{2+}, and the genesis of reactive oxygen species (ROS). While a huge variety of pathways may have separately been responsible for the reperfusion-induced arrhythmogenesis, it is reasonable to speculate that all of the aforementioned substances could be directly or indirectly connected to each other, and together they play a crucial final outcome, leading to irreversible arrhythmias, heart failure, and cardiac death.

K^+, Na^+, Ca^{2+}, and Mg^{2+}

If cardiac tissue is successfully reperfused in the early phase of reversible injury, its reaction is much different from that of the ischemia-induced injury. Myocytes explosively swell, thus, total tissue water content increases about by 20% following the first two min of reperfusion period (Whalen et al., 1974), and tissue electrolyte changes associate with the swelling are striking. As a consequence, there is a significant increase in cellular Na^+, Ca^{2+}, and Cl^-, while cellular K^+ and Mg^{2+} are substantially decreased (Whalen et al., 1974).

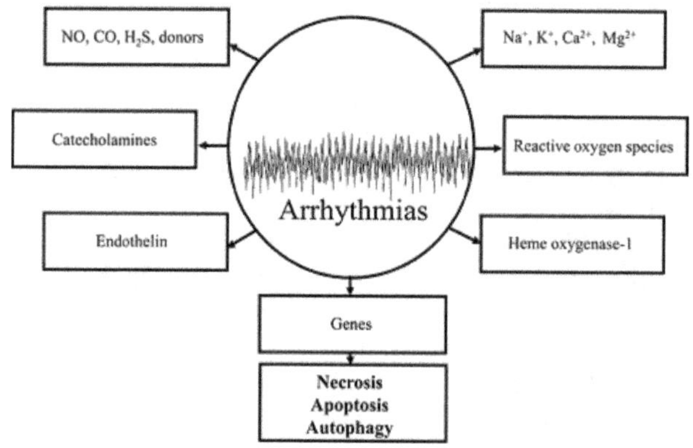

FIGURE 3 | Schematic representation of some important arrhythmogenic components and mediators in the genesis of reperfusion-induced arrhythmias. All of the depicted mechanisms are very complex and each of them significantly contributes to the maldistribution of Na^+, K^+, Ca^{2+} exchange mechanisms by virtue of causing damages in cell membranes and receptors leading to necrotic-, apoptotic-, and autophagic-induced cell deaths.

K^+

Ischemia causes functional disturbance in K^+ homeostasis in the myocardium and plays a critical role in the genesis of ischemia/reperfusion-induced ventricular arrhythmias (Harris et al., 1958; Tosaki et al., 1988; Curtis and Hearse, 1989). Various mechanisms of drugs by which cellular K^+ loss causes electrophysiological disturbances, including the function and expression of ATP-dependent K^+ channels, may involve the blocking and/or opening of these K^+ channels (Noma, 1983; Tosaki et al., 1995; Das and Sarkar, 2005; Kaya et al., 2019) at various degrees, which may aggravate or diminish the severity of ventricular arrhythmias in the ischemic/reperfused myocardium. Thus, the modification of the expression of K_{ATP} channels by K_{ATP} channel opener or blocker agents, respectively, can increase or decrease the incidence of ischemia/reperfusion-induced arrhythmias. The results of the papers cited above clearly show that interventions, which modify K^+ transport mechanisms *via* cell membranes, can even increase or reduce the incidence of ischemia/reperfusion-induced arrhythmias.

Na^+

The sodium ion plays a basic process determining the physiological or pathological shape of APs and ECGs in the myocardium. Several mechanisms are currently known, which lead to intracellular Na^+ accumulation under both physiological and pathological conditions, and the degree of the sodium channel blockade critically determines the membrane potential of the cell and the heart rate. Under pathological conditions, such as myocardial ischemia, the effects of Na^+/H^+, Na^+/K^+, and Na^+/

Ca^{2+} exchange mechanisms increase the intracellular Ca^{2+} entry, and as a consequence, the ischemic load with additional Ca^{2+} results in a further activation of Na^+/Ca^{2+} mechanism during reperfusion, leading to the development of reperfusion-induced arrhythmias (Tani and Neely, 1989; Belardinelli et al., 2006). At the early minutes of reperfusion, the substantial accumulation of intracellular Na^+ during ischemia contributes to a significant increase of cellular edema formation, heart failure, and ventricular arrhythmias. All of these complex mechanisms, without any pharmacological or nonpharmacological interventions, produce an excessive intracellular Ca^{2+} overload leading to necrotic, apoptotic, and autophagic cell deaths. Antiarrhythmic agents, which can modify these pathologic processes, including Na^+-induced Ca^{2+} overload (Wang et al., 2007), Na^+/H^+ exchange mechanism, and Na^+-induced K^+ loss could prevent the genesis of reperfusion-induced ventricular arrhythmias and sudden cardiac death. In this respect, the Na^+/H^+ exchange mechanism is extensively studied to prevent reperfusion-induced arrhythmias in a variety of experimental models (Karmazyn, 1996; Ravens and Himmel, 1999; Wirth et al., 2001; Woodcock et al., 2001; Ono et al., 2004; Yamada et al., 2005; Szepesi et al., 2015; Hegyi et al., 2018). It can be concluded that Na^+/H^+ exchange mechanism, which is not species specific, is a basic target for pharmacological prevention in the attenuation of ischemia/reperfusion-induced cardiac damage, and may emerge as an effective basic therapeutic strategy in human beings. Finally, it is of interest to note that a direct manipulation in extracellular Na^+ concentration in isolated buffer perfused hearts, a significant decrease in the incidence of reperfusion-induced VF and ventricular tachycardia was detected (Tosaki et al., 1989).

Ca^{2+}

Under physiological conditions, intracellular Ca^{2+} content is maintained at very low levels, less than 100 nmol. Upon reperfusion, the massive osmotic load in ischemic myocytes, which contain very low level of ATP to fuel the ion channel proteins and pumps results in explosive cell swelling with membrane disruption and myocyte death. Reperfusion-induced arrhythmias are associated with sudden ECG changes, in which there is a Ca^{2+} overload at sufficient level to produce an elevated oscillatory release of Ca^{2+}, reflecting in a significant ATP depletion (Coetzee et al., 1987; Coetzee et al., 1988). Thus, the preservation of cell membrane integrity includes maintenance of Ca^{2+} homeostasis, various types of ion exchange receptor-mediated mechanisms, osmotic control, and the preservation of the rich-energy phosphates. Therefore, interventions, e.g., Ca^{2+} channel antagonists (Tosaki et al., 1987a; Otani et al., 2013; Becerra et al., 2016), beta-adrenergic receptor blockers (Tosaki et al., 1987b; Winchester and Pepine, 2014; Gatzke et al., 2018), and several other newly discovered molecular structures and interventions (Wilder et al., 2016; Bukhari et al., 2018; Gatzke et al., 2018), which directly or indirectly contribute to the preservation of the aforementioned processes can diminish the incidence of reperfusion-induced arrhythmias, heart failure, and sudden cardiac death. In addition, during the past three decades several new mechanisms have been proved and implicated based on molecular biological studies, as endogenous mediators, into the pathways of ischemia/reperfusion-induced injury and arrhythmogenesis, including gaseous molecules; nitric monoxide, carbon dioxide, and hydrogen sulfide.

Mg^{2+}

Magnesium is a "natural" Ca^{2+} channel antagonists (Iseri and French, 1984), a potent cofactor for the function of several enzymes, and plays a crucial role in protein synthesis. Mg^{2+} is also necessary for the insertion of various proteins into cell membranes, and stabilizes the structure of ribosomes (Flatman, 1984). A variety of disorders including diabetes, hypertension, renal tubular disease, hyperthyroidism, steatorrhea, hepatic and cardiac failure may deplete Mg^{2+} stores causing severe ventricular arrhythmias (Iseri and French, 1984; Lazzerini et al., 2018). It was demonstrated about three decades ago by Tzivoni et al. (1988) that "torsade de pointes" ventricular arrhythmias, which were previously resistant to conventional antiarrhythmic therapies, were prevented and controlled by the infusion of magnesium sulfate. In addition, it was also published by other investigators (Tosaki et al., 1993b; Ying et al., 2007; Amoni et al., 2017) that application of Mg^{2+} is a useful tool for the prevention in the development of reperfusion-induced arrhythmias. Although, the precise mechanism of Mg^{2+}-induced antiarrhythmic effect is unclear, it has recently been supported that inhibition of the upregulation of P-selectin expression (Ying et al., 2007) and G-protein-coupled receptors (Ye et al., 2018) may be involved in Mg^{2+}-induced cardiac protection. The antiarrhythmic effect of Mg^{2+} may be related to the mediation of a number of cellular processes, including particularly the reduction of cellular K^+ loss, displacement of intracellular Ca^{2+}, and maintaining the physiological Mg^{2+} level in myocardial cells. In addition, the possibility that Mg^{2+} could reduce cellular Na^+ accumulation during ischemia and hence limit intracellular Ca^{2+} overload, could be of considerable importance to its antiarrhythmic effect (Tosaki et al., 1993b).

Reactive Oxygen Species

Studies focusing on the role of ROS in arrhythmogenesis were first published by Manning and Hearse (Manning and Hearse, 1984) and Woodward and Zakaria (Woodward and Zakaria, 1985). The authors described that ROS, which particularly derive from oxygen, cause ventricular tachycardia and VF during the first minute of the reperfusion period. The arrhythmogenic ROS may arise from several sources in the ischemic/reperfused myocardium including the degradation of catecholamines, the metabolism of arachidonic acid, mitochondrial electron transport processes, and the conversion of xanthine to hypoxanthine by xanthine oxidase. Direct evidence for the burst of ROS generation during the first few minutes of reperfusion has been initially proved by several investigators (Garlick et al., 1987; Zweier and Kuppusamy, 1988; Zweier et al., 1988; Blasig et al., 1990; Tosaki and Braquet, 1990; Samouilov et al., 2019), using electron paramagnetic resonance spectroscopy and its modification. The association between the role of sudden burst of ROS and arrhythmogenesis came also first from electrophysiological studies, proving that ROS generating systems can be potentially arrhythmogenic (Kusama et al., 1989).

The presented results strongly suggest that ROS generation plays a basic role in arrhythmogenesis in reperfusion, and the possibility also exists that ROS formation could interact with other potential pathological mechanisms to facilitate arrhythmogenesis during reperfusion. Therefore, several groups of natural and synthetic pharmacological agents could significantly diminish and/or suppress the incidence of reperfusion-induced arrhythmias. Thus, beta adrenergic receptor blockers (Manning and Hearse, 1984; Lujan et al., 2007; Kloner et al., 2011), calcium channel antagonists (Guc et al., 1993; Podesser et al., 1995; Kato et al., 2004; Bukhari et al., 2018), spin traps (Hearse and Tosaki, 1987; Tosaki et al., 1993a; Zuo et al., 2009; Pisarenko et al., 2019), and natural plants or their extracts (Tosaki et al., 1996; Shen et al., 1998; Broskova et al., 2013; Sedighi et al., 2018; Zhang et al., 2019b) alone, or in their combinations can significantly reduce the severity of ischemia/reperfusion-induced arrhythmias. Several natural products originated from plants, fruits, and/or vegetables showing antiarrhythmic activity by reducing the incidence of reperfusion-induced arrhythmias and preserving myocardial function, include mainly polyphenol and flavonoid molecular structures (Hung et al., 2000; Pataki et al., 2002; Bak et al., 2006; Broskova et al., 2013; Ma et al., 2014; Woodman et al., 2018; Kaya et al., 2019). Natural antioxidant activities and features of flavonoids/polyphenols are important examples of myocardial protection and preservation in ischemic/reperfused hearts, and being not merely a matter of various action mechanisms but showing that differences in molecular formulations may exist among them, even when they are of similar structures.

Heme Oxygenase-1 and Carbon Monoxide System

Heme oxygenase (HO) catalyzes the first step of heme degradation to carbon monoxide (CO) and biliverdin, and subsequently releases heme iron (Lee et al., 1997; Ryter et al., 1998). CO is an endogenous gaseous molecule and having an important role in hemodynamic regulation in vascular smooth muscle cells (Ishizaka and Griendling, 1997), thus, HO is able to modulate vessel tone, and regulate the changes in blood pressure *via* the increase of cellular cGMP contents by the activation of soluble guanylate cyclase (Johnson et al., 1995).

Two major isozymes of HO exist and produced by two distinct genes (Choi and Alam, 1996); HO-1 is inducible and can be found in various mammalian cells, and HO-2 is constitutively mainly expressed in neurons of the central nervous system. HO-1 expression or repression can be occurred in various disorders (Dulak and Jozkowicz, 2014; Loboda et al., 2016; Haines and Tosaki, 2018) and tissues subjected to oxidative and/or hemodynamic stress (Ottani et al., 2015; Cheng and Rong, 2017). Studies demonstrated that HO-1 expression can afford cellular protection *via* different mechanisms against oxidant stress under both *in vitro* (Lee et al., 1996) and *in vivo* (Nath et al., 1992; Waldman et al., 2019; Yu et al., 2019) conditions. It has been suggested that HO-1-mediated CO production, as a signal transduction molecule, prevents the development of reperfusion-induced VF (Csonka et al., 1999b; Pataki et al., 2001; Bak et al., 2003; Bak et al., 2010). Liang et al. (2014) published that CO prolongs the duration of AP by the inhibition of inward rectifying K^+ channels. These authors also demonstrated that CO inhibits the function of Kir2.2 and Kir2.3 inward rectifier channels in myocardial cells, and directly affects Kir2.3 function *via* the phosphatidylinositol (4,5)-bisphosphate system. The aforementioned findings show that the inhibition of Kir2.2 and Kir2.3 leads to a substantial prolongation of AP, which may be responsible for the development of reperfusion-induced VF. In addition, Ottani A et al. (Ottani et al., 2015) demonstrated the beneficial effect of NDP-α-MSH, which associated with the overexpression of HO-1 and Bcl-XL, reducing the incidence of arrhythmias and infarct size in the ischemic/reperfused myocardium. It was also shown that very low concentration of CO added directly to the perfusion buffer protects the ischemic/reperfused myocardium *via* cGMP signaling in isolated hearts (Bak et al., 2005). It is reasonable to believe that manipulation of various pathways with pharmacological interventions in the HO-1/CO system plays an important and preventive role in the genesis of the development of reperfusion-induced arrhythmias and myocardial cell death.

NO, CO, H_2S (Gaseous Molecules)

NO

Nitric oxide (NO) is an endogenous free-radical-type cell signaling molecule with several therapeutic applications. Under physiological conditions, NO is originated from the terminal nitrogen of L-arginine and produced by NO synthase, which has three different isozymes, including endothelial, neural, and inducible encoded by three different genes. NO activates guanylyl cyclase enzyme leading to the increase of cellular cGMP levels by the dephosphorylation of myosin light chains and reducing cytosolic Ca^{2+} concentration, thereby the relaxation of smooth muscles in a board range of organs in mammalians. Thus, NO as a soluble gas molecule is having several pharmacological potentials and therapeutic applications in various diseases including the central nervous and cardiovascular systems, treatment of pulmonary and arterial hypertension, vasospastic angina, and myocardial infarction. NO is able also to inhibit the aggregation of thrombocytes. The signaling and physiological importance of NO was recognized by the awarding of Nobel Prize in Medicine and Physiology to R. Furchgott, L. Ignaro, and F. Murad in 1998.

The role of NO was also intensively studied in ischemia/reperfusion-induced injury in the myocardium during the past two and half decades (Pabla and Curtis, 1995; Liu et al., 1997; Csonka et al., 1999a; Masini et al., 1999; Varga et al., 1999; Fauconnier et al., 2011; Bienvenu et al., 2017; Van Der Weg et al., 2019). The substantial role and investigation of precise mechanisms of NO, both under physiological or pathological conditions, are not a question of debate in cell signaling and myocardial function. A number of studies show that interventions contributed to NO production *via* different mechanisms significantly reduced the reperfusion-induced injury including the incidence of arrhythmias (Shen et al., 1998; Kawahara et al., 2003; Imaizumi et al., 2008; Egom et al., 2011; Kisvari et al., 2015; Enayati et al., 2018; Jones et al., 2018). Various protective NO-mediated signal mechanisms, including the mitoK-(ATP) (Kawahara et al., 2003), the nuclear factor erythroid 2-related factor (NrF2), the extracellular-signaling-regulated-kinase (ERK) (Imaizumi et al., 2008), and Pak1/Akt1 signaling cascade (Egom et al., 2011) have also been reported.

In addition, organic nitrates used for the therapy of myocardial ischemia as NO donors, activate the soluble guanylyl cyclase increasing cGMP and subsequently reducing the intracellular Ca^{2+} level, and prevent the genesis of ischemia and reperfusion-induced arrhythmias. This latest pharmacologically controlled NO-mediated mechanism by organic nitrates is currently probably one of the most important interventions in the clinical management of myocardial ischemia/reperfusion-induced damages. However, it is of also interest to note that other synthetic molecules, e.g., aspirin and molsidomine, which are currently used in clinical medication, and their modified molecular structures (Bertuglia et al., 2004; Szoke et al., 2019) could release NO, leading to cardiac protection in the ischemic/reperfused myocardium.

CO

CO is another vasoactive gaseous molecule in close connection with heme oxygenase-1 system discussed in one of the previous chapters, and having substantial toxicological and physiological importance in living subjects (Peers and Steele, 2012). Several tissues including cardiac myocytes express both HO-1 and HO-2 proteins, and HO-1 expression can be particularly increased by several stress factors (Ewing et al., 1994; Wu et al., 2011; Haines and Tosaki, 2018) including myocardial ischemia/reperfusion (Maulik et al., 1996; Lakkisto et al., 2002) as demonstrated at mRNA and protein levels. Interestingly, homozygote ($HO\text{-}1^{-/-}$) knockout mouse hearts subjected to ischemia/reperfusion period produced significantly higher cardiac damage and the incidence of VF in comparison with that of heterozygote ($HO\text{-}1^{+/-}$) and wild-type mice ($HO\text{-}1^{+/+}$) (Bak et al., 2010; Juhasz et al., 2011). Substantial scientific evidence suggests that several of the beneficial and harmful effects of CO arise from its ability, at dose-dependent manner, to modify signal transduction pathways and activities of ion channel proteins. It is apparent from these publications reviewed here that HO-1 and HO-1-mediated endogenous cellular CO levels have cardioprotective effects against myocardial ischemia/reperfusion-induced arrhythmias, and the pharmacological manipulation of HO-1 expression under severely controlled conditions may have clinical application as an antiarrhythmic agent.

H_2S

Hydrogen sulfide was initially considered as a toxic molecule due to its property to inhibit cytochrome-oxidase c in mitochondrial respiration processes. H_2S, like CO and NO, is endogenously generated gaseous molecule having substantial metabolic and physiological effects in various tissues including neuronal and myocardial cells. In mammalian tissues, three different enzymes encoded by three distinct genes produce H_2S: cystathionine-gamma-lyase, cystathionine-beta-synthase, and 3-mercaptopiruvate sulfur transferase. In most cells, cystathionine-gamma-lyase and cystathionine-beta-synthase utilize homocysteine and L-cysteine as substrates to liberate pyruvate, ammonium, and H_2S (Wang, 2002). A number of studies have reported the cardioprotective effect of H_2S in myocardial ischemia/reperfusion-induced injury *via* different actions, which include ATP-sensitive K^+-channel opening (Johansen et al., 2006), cGMP generation (Salloum et al., 2012), Akt-mTORC2 (Zhou et al., 2014), and microRNAs (Ren et al., 2019) mediated mechanisms, lead to the significant reduction of apoptotic and necrotic cellular deaths. Consequently, later on, it was also reported that pharmacological interventions serving as H_2S donors produced cardiac protection against ischemic/reperfused cellular deaths (Sun et al., 2017; Sun et al., 2018). Currently, relatively little is known about H_2S-mediated cardiac protection and remodeling against reperfusion-induced arrhythmias, however, growing evidence indicates that H_2S donors could play a role in the reduction of the incidence of reperfusion-induced arrhythmias (Sun et al., 2015; Testai et al., 2016). Thus, H_2S releasing molecules may particularly be also considered as potential pharmacological option in the prevention of the development of reperfusion-induced arrhythmias, and may have the ability to protect the myocardium against necrosis- and apoptosis-induced cell death.

CATECHOLAMINES

The role of catecholamines in arrhythmogenesis is not a question of debate, however, sometimes, depending on the experimental conditions, it can be controversial, and these endogenous mediators may have different effects in the genesis of ischemia-induced arrhythmias in comparison with reperfusion-induced rhythm disturbances (Opie and Coetzee, 1988; Kurz et al., 1991; Vanoli et al., 1994). The results of several published papers support the fact that stimulation of adrenergic receptors, especially alpha-1 and beta-1, is arrhythmogenic under ischemic/reperfused conditions (Sheridan et al., 1980; Bolli et al., 1984; Thandroyen et al., 1987; Tosaki et al., 1987b; Yasutake and Avkiran, 1995), and the alpha-1 adrenergic receptor stimulation could be due to the elevated transsarcolemmal Ca^{2+} influx and increased release of this ion from the SR (Thandroyen et al., 1987). Furthermore, the pharmacological blockade of alpha-1 adrenergic stimulation could mediate Na^+/H^+ exchange mechanism during reperfusion, leading to the reduction of the incidence of reperfusion-induced VF (Yasutake and Avkiran, 1995). Beta adrenergic receptor blockers could also be effective against arrhythmias by virtue of their ability to directly inhibit catecholamine-induced arrhythmogenesis on beta receptors (Ibanez et al., 2012; Winchester and Pepine, 2014). If this is so, the stimulation of beta adrenergic receptors and the concomitant activation of adenyl cyclase enzyme would appear be directly involved in the development of reperfusion-induced dysrhythmias. Therefore, these observations would suggest that stimulation of beta adrenergic receptors could be involved in the genesis of reperfusion-induced arrhythmias and the beta receptor blockade may be pharmacologically expected to be potentially protective.

ENDOTHELIN

Endothelin (ET) is one of numerous endogenous substances generating and accumulating in the ischemic/reperfused heart, or washed out during reperfusion periods, has been implicated as a potential arrhythmogenic factor. Thus, ET could function as an endogenous peptide-structure mediator in arrhythmogenesis, and has a potentially strong vascular action capable of exacerbating myocardial ischemia and heart failure. ET ("big endothelin," endothelin-1) was first isolated from aortic endothelial cells (Yanagisawa et al., 1988), and is a potent vasoconstrictor agent, which specifically binds to ET-1 receptors, modulating the function of sodium, calcium and potassium ion channels, leading to pathologic changes on the ECG (Curtis et al., 1993; Brunner and Kukovetz, 1996; Wang et al., 2002; Vago et al., 2004; Adlbrecht et al., 2014; Falk et al., 2018). Hundreds of antiarrhythmic mechanisms, synthetic and nonsynthetic pharmacological agents were proposed, with more or less success, to protect directly or indirectly the myocardium against ET-1-related cardiac dysfunction (Isaka et al., 2007; Na et al., 2007; Du et al., 2008; Chan et al., 2016; Lee et al., 2017). The aforementioned approaches of ET-elicited vascular activities lead to multiple theories without precise and very specific discrimination between mechanisms in terms of their importance in reperfusion-induced arrhythmogenesis. However, it is reasonable to suppose that the cardiac protection is probably originated from (i) the inhibition of ET synthesis (Ceylan et al., 2018), (ii) the direct pharmacological blockade of ET receptors (Wainwright et al., 2005; Kaoukis et al., 2013), (iii) downregulation of various microRNAs (Wang et al., 2019), and (iv) their multiple combinations (i–iii).

GENETIC ORIGIN OF REPERFUSION-INDUCED ARRHYTHMIAS

At the time of writing, there is no substantial scientific evidence available, opposite to ischemia-induced arrhythmias, about the direct genetic origin of reperfusion-induced arrhythmias, since their origin itself is the "reperfusion event," and such an approach has not been yet intensively investigated based on its genetic-mediated mechanisms (Szendrei et al., 2002; Kovacs et al., 2013; Ravingerova et al., 2013; Bienvenu et al., 2017; Paar et al., 2019). Therefore, it is reasonable to suppose that some gene encoded proteins and channels are already present upon reperfusion in their inactive forms in the myocardium, which may be immediately or quickly activated upon a reperfusion event, leading to the rapid maldistribution of ionic homeostasis, producing other arrhythmogenic components, and the genesis of reperfusion-induced arrhythmias. In majority of experimental studies, drugs and interventions were added prior to the induction of myocardial ischemia, thereby slowing the rate of ischemia-induced damages so that, less degree of cellular injury is present at the onset of reperfusion in the myocardium in drug-treated groups. Therefore, about a drug-afforded protection or a rapid activation of an inactive gene at the moment of reperfusion can only be obtained from observations, in which drug-induced ion channel activities or gene expression-related changes are immediately studied (or even later) at the onset of reperfusion. Therefore, it is important to consider all the possible inactive/active stages of various genes and function of ion channels at the onset of reperfusion, by which a drug induced cardiac protection might be successfully achieved.

CONCLUSION

Myocardial ischemia/reperfusion-induced alterations resulting in heart failure, conduction abnormalities and arrhythmias, in view of structural and electrical remodeling, which are important processes in the development various myocardial diseases. Multiple mechanisms responsible for the development of reperfusion-induced VF, which lead to the sudden cardiac death without pharmacological or nonpharmacological intervention in animal models and post-myocardial infarcted patients.

Potential mechanisms depicted in **Figure 3** show that reperfusion of the ischemic myocardium intensifies the incidence of reperfusion-induced arrhythmias, which are followed by necrosis-, apoptosis-, and autophagy-induced cell deaths (Osipov et al., 2009; Zhang et al., 2012; Chang et al., 2013; Czegledi et al., 2019; Gyongyosi et al., 2019; Yasuda et al., 2019). From a different point of view, autophagic processes may be even beneficial, depending on their intensity in reversible injured myocardial cells. However, necrosis-induced cell death could dominate and mask autophagic signal transduction processes and autophagy-induced cell death in myocardial tissues (Czegledi et al., 2019; Gyongyosi et al., 2019). Cellular biology and genetics have a real value and significant impact to try better to define the generation of cardiovascular diseases, including life threatening cardiac arrhythmias. Nowadays, the research direction and available modern techniques in cell biology are intensively productive, but should do much to clarify gaps between the basic molecular science and clinical relevance in arrhythmogenesis.

LIMITATION

Cardiac muscle contraction and relaxation are very complex and primarily determined by several intracellular processes that control the force activation and inactivation, which include Na^+, K^+, and Ca^{2+} exchange mechanisms, including the ATP-dependent rate and Ca^{2+} sequestration capacity of the SR. The immediate extrapolation of AP and ECG changes obtained under experimental conditions to an actual clinical situation must be viewed with some caution because of the presence or absence of the blood and its elements (e.g., leukocytes, platelets), signal transductions, and possible interspecies differences in cardiac metabolism. In addition, the duration and shape of APs are different in His-Purkinje cells, AV node, and ventricular tissues, and the refractoriness is basically determined by the voltage-dependent recovery of Na^+ channels from inactivation returning to activation in close connection with the function of calcium channels. Thus, the duration of effective refractory period is varied in different cells of the heart and the longest interval at which a premature stimuli fails to generate a propagated response, frequently is used to estimate drug effects in physiologically functioning cardiac tissues. Under physiological and pathological experimental conditions, to investigate the effect of an antiarrhythmic agent, the key aim is related to study various changes in the duration of the effective refractory period, which could modify the activation/inactivation stage of Na^+ channels in close connection with different types of Ca^{2+} channels and genes e.g., Na^+-induced Ca^{2+} release from the SR. Despite the limitation of several antiarrhythmic drugs can possess protective effects against LQTS and reperfusion-induced arrhythmias even some of them may be of particular concern. Additional experimental and clinical prospective studies powered to determine differences in ventricular APs in connection with ion channels and ECGs to confirm these observations are now warranted.

AUTHOR CONTRIBUTIONS

The author confirms being the sole contributor of this work and has approved it for publication.

FUNDING

This work was supported by grants of NKFIH-K-124719 and the European Union and the State of Hungary, co-financed by the European Social Fund in the framework of GINOP-2.3.2-15-2016-00043.

REFERENCES

Adlbrecht, C., Wurm, R., Pezawas, T., Andreas, M., Redwan, B., Distelmaier, K., et al. (2014). Effects of endothelin A receptor blockade in patients with ST-elevation acute coronary syndrome–a rhythmologic substudy. *Life Sci.* 118, 430–434. doi: 10.1016/j.lfs.2014.02.015

Akita, H., Creer, M. H., Yamada, K. A., Sobel, B. E., and Corr, P. B. (1986). Electrophysiologic effects of intracellular lysophosphoglycerides and their accumulation in cardiac lymph with myocardial ischemia in dogs. *J. Clin. Invest.* 78, 271–280. doi: 10.1172/JCI112561

Alvarez, C. K., Cronin, E., Baker, W. L., and Kluger, J. (2019). Heart failure as a substrate and trigger for ventricular tachycardia. *J. Interv Card Electrophysiol* 56, 229–247. doi: 10.1007/s10840-019-00623-x

Amin, A. S., Reckman, Y. J., Arbelo, E., Spanjaart, A. M., Postema, P. G., Tadros, R., et al. (2018). SCN5A mutation type and topology are associated with the risk of ventricular arrhythmia by sodium channel blockers. *Int. J. Cardiol.* 266, 128–132. doi: 10.1016/j.ijcard.2017.09.010

Amirahmadi, F., Turnbull, L., Du, X. J., Graham, R. M., and Woodcock, E. A. (2008). Heightened alpha1A-adrenergic receptor activity suppresses ischaemia/reperfusion-induced Ins(1,4,5)P3 generation in the mouse heart: a comparison with ischaemic preconditioning. *Clin. Sci. (Lond)* 114, 157–164. doi: 10.1042/CS20070110

Amoni, M., Kelly-Laubscher, R., Petersen, M., and Gwanyanya, A. (2017). Cardioprotective and Anti-arrhythmic Effects of Magnesium Pretreatment Against Ischaemia/Reperfusion Injury in Isoprenaline-Induced Hypertrophic Rat Heart. *Cardiovasc. Toxicol.* 17, 49–57. doi: 10.1007/s12012-015-9355-6

Anson, B. D., Ackerman, M. J., Tester, D. J., Will, M. L., Delisle, B. P., Anderson, C. L., et al. (2004). Molecular and functional characterization of common polymorphisms in HERG (KCNH2) potassium channels. *Am. J. Physiol. Heart Circ. Physiol.* 286, H2434–H2441. doi: 10.1152/ajpheart.00891.2003

Antoniou, C. K., Dilaveris, P., Manolakou, P., Galanakos, S., Magkas, N., Gatzoulis, K., et al. (2017). QT Prolongation and Malignant Arrhythmia: How Serious a Problem? *Eur. Cardiol.* 12, 112–120. doi: 10.15420/ecr.2017:16:1

Aronsen, J. M., Swift, F., and Sejersted, O. M. (2013). Cardiac sodium transport and excitation-contraction coupling. *J. Mol. Cell Cardiol.* 61, 11–19. doi: 10.1016/j.yjmcc.2013.06.003

Axelsen, L. N., Calloe, K., Braunstein, T. H., Riemann, M., Hofgaard, J. P., Liang, B., et al. (2015). Diet-induced pre-diabetes slows cardiac conductance and promotes arrhythmogenesis. *Cardiovasc. Diabetol.* 14, 87. doi: 10.1186/s12933-015-0246-8

Bak, I., Szendrei, L., Turoczi, T., Papp, G., Joo, F., Das, D. K., et al. (2003). Heme oxygenase-1-related carbon monoxide production and ventricular fibrillation in isolated ischemic/reperfused mouse myocardium. *FASEB J.* 17, 2133–2135. doi: 10.1096/fj.03-0032fje

Bak, I., Varadi, J., Nagy, N., Vecsernyes, M., and Tosaki, A. (2005). The role of exogenous carbon monoxide in the recovery of post-ischemic cardiac function in buffer perfused isolated rat hearts. *Cell Mol. Biol. (Noisy-le-grand)* 51, 453–459.

Bak, I., Lekli, I., Juhasz, B., Nagy, N., Varga, E., Varadi, J., et al. (2006). Cardioprotective mechanisms of Prunus cerasus (sour cherry) seed extract against ischemia-reperfusion-induced damage in isolated rat hearts. *Am. J. Physiol. Heart Circ. Physiol.* 291, H1329–H1336. doi: 10.1152/ajpheart.01243.2005

Bak, I., Czompa, A., Juhasz, B., Lekli, I., and Tosaki, A. (2010). Reduction of reperfusion-induced ventricular fibrillation and infarct size via heme oxygenase-1 overexpression in isolated mouse hearts. *J. Cell Mol. Med.* 14, 2268–2272. doi: 10.1111/j.1582-4934.2010.01142.x

Batiste, S. M., Blackwell, D. J., Kim, K., Kryshtal, D. O., Gomez-Hurtado, N., Rebbeck, R. T., et al. (2019). Unnatural verticilide enantiomer inhibits type 2 ryanodine receptor-mediated calcium leak and is antiarrhythmic. *Proc. Natl. Acad. Sci. U. S. A* 116, 4810–4815. doi: 10.1073/pnas.1816685116

Becerra, R., Roman, B., Di Carlo, M. N., Mariangelo, J. I., Salas, M., Sanchez, G., et al. (2016). Reversible redox modifications of ryanodine receptor ameliorate ventricular arrhythmias in the ischemic-reperfused heart. *Am. J. Physiol. Heart Circ. Physiol.* 311, H713–H724. doi: 10.1152/ajpheart.00142.2016

Belardinelli, L., Shryock, J. C., and Fraser, H. (2006). Inhibition of the late sodium current as a potential cardioprotective principle: effects of the late sodium current inhibitor ranolazine. *Heart* 92 Suppl 4, iv6–iv14. doi: 10.1136/hrt.2005.078790

Ben Jehuda, R., Eisen, B., Shemer, Y., Mekies, L. N., Szantai, A., Reiter, I., et al. (2018). CRISPR correction of the PRKAG2 gene mutation in the patient's induced pluripotent stem cell-derived cardiomyocytes eliminates electrophysiological and structural abnormalities. *Heart Rhythm.* 15, 267–276. doi: 10.1016/j.hrthm.2017.09.024

Bertuglia, S., Giusti, A., and Del Soldato, P. (2004). Antioxidant activity of nitro derivative of aspirin against ischemia-reperfusion in hamster cheek pouch microcirculation. *Am. J. Physiol. Gastrointest. Liver Physiol.* 286, G437–G443. doi: 10.1152/ajpgi.00339.2003

Bienvenu, L. A., Morgan, J., Reichelt, M. E., Delbridge, L. M. D., and Young, M. J. (2017). Chronic in vivo nitric oxide deficiency impairs cardiac functional recovery after ischemia in female (but not male) mice. *J. Mol. Cell Cardiol.* 112, 8–15. doi: 10.1016/j.yjmcc.2017.08.012

Blasig, I. E., Ebert, B., Hennig, C., Pali, T., and Tosaki, A. (1990). Inverse relationship between ESR spin trapping of oxyradicals and degree of functional recovery during myocardial reperfusion in isolated working rat heart. *Cardiovasc. Res.* 24, 263–270. doi: 10.1093/cvr/24.4.263

Bogeholz, N., Pauls, P., Kaese, S., Schulte, J. S., Lemoine, M. D., Dechering, D. G., et al. (2016). Triggered activity in atrial myocytes is influenced by Na(+)/Ca(2 +) exchanger activity in genetically altered mice. *J. Mol. Cell Cardiol.* 101, 106–115. doi: 10.1016/j.yjmcc.2016.11.004

Bolli, R., Fisher, D. J., Taylor, A. A., Young, J. B., and Miller, R. R. (1984). Effect of alpha-adrenergic blockade on arrhythmias induced by acute myocardial ischemia and reperfusion in the dog. *J. Mol. Cell Cardiol.* 16, 1101–1117. doi: 10.1016/S0022-2828(84)80037-1

Bongianino, R., Denegri, M., Mazzanti, A., Lodola, F., Vollero, A., Boncompagni, S., et al. (2017). Allele-Specific Silencing of Mutant mRNA Rescues Ultrastructural and Arrhythmic Phenotype in Mice Carriers of the R4496C Mutation in the Ryanodine Receptor Gene (RYR2). *Circ. Res.* 121, 525–536. doi: 10.1161/CIRCRESAHA.117.310882

Bossu, A., Houtman, M. J. C., Meijborg, V. M. F., Varkevisser, R., Beekman, H. D. M., Dunnink, A., et al. (2018). Selective late sodium current inhibitor GS-458967 suppresses Torsades de Pointes by mostly affecting perpetuation but not initiation of the arrhythmia. *Br. J. Pharmacol.* 175, 2470–2482. doi: 10.1111/bph.14217

Bowles, N. E., Jou, C. J., Arrington, C. B., Kennedy, B. J., Earl, A., Matsunami, N., et al. (2015). Exome analysis of a family with Wolff-Parkinson-White syndrome identifies a novel disease locus. *Am. J. Med. Genet. A* 167A, 2975–2984. doi: 10.1002/ajmg.a.37297

Broskova, Z., Drabikova, K., Sotnikova, R., Fialova, S., and Knezl, V. (2013). Effect of plant polyphenols on ischemia-reperfusion injury of the isolated rat heart and vessels. *Phytother. Res.* 27, 1018–1022. doi: 10.1002/ptr.4825

Brunner, F., and Kukovetz, W. R. (1996). Postischemic antiarrhythmic effects of angiotensin-converting enzyme inhibitors. Role of suppression of endogenous endothelin secretion. *Circulation* 94, 1752–1761. doi: 10.1161/01.cir.94.7.1752

Bukhari, I. A., Almotrefi, A. A., Mohamed, O. Y., Al-Masri, A. A., and Sheikh, S. A. (2018). Protective effect of fenofibrate against ischemia-/reperfusion-induced cardiac arrhythmias in isolated rat hearts. *Fundam. Clin. Pharmacol.* 32, 141–146. doi: 10.1111/fcp.12342

Burgen, A. S., and Terroux, K. G. (1953). The membrane resting and action potentials of the cat auricle. *J. Physiol.* 119, 139–152. doi: 10.1113/jphysiol.1953.sp004834

Carmeliet, E. (1992). A fuzzy subsarcolemmal space for intracellular Na+ in cardiac cells? *Cardiovasc. Res.* 26, 433–442. doi: 10.1093/cvr/26.5.433

Ceylan, A. F., Wang, S., Kandadi, M. R., Chen, J., Hua, Y., Pei, Z., et al. (2018). Cardiomyocyte-specific knockout of endothelin receptor a attenuates obesity cardiomyopathy. *Biochim. Biophys. Acta Mol. Basis. Dis.* 1864, 3339–3352. doi: 10.1016/j.bbadis.2018.07.020

Chan, E. A., Buckley, B., Farraj, A. K., and Thompson, L. C. (2016). The heart as an extravascular target of endothelin-1 in particulate matter-induced cardiac dysfunction. *Pharmacol. Ther.* 165, 63–78. doi: 10.1016/j.pharmthera.2016.05.006

Chang, R., Li, Y., Yang, X., Yue, Y., Dou, L., Wang, Y., et al. (2013). Protective role of deoxyschizandrin and schisantherin A against myocardial ischemia-reperfusion injury in rats. *PloS One* 8, e61590. doi: 10.1371/journal.pone.0061590

Chen, J., Mitcheson, J. S., Lin, M., and Sanguinetti, M. C. (2000). Functional roles of charged residues in the putative voltage sensor of the HCN2 pacemaker channel. *J. Biol. Chem.* 275, 36465–36471. doi: 10.1074/jbc.M007034200

Cheng, Y., and Rong, J. (2017). Therapeutic Potential of Heme Oxygenase-1/carbon Monoxide System Against Ischemia-Reperfusion Injury. *Curr. Pharm. Des.* 23, 3884–3898. doi: 10.2174/1381612823666170413122439

Choi, A. M., and Alam, J. (1996). Heme oxygenase-1: function, regulation, and implication of a novel stress-inducible protein in oxidant-induced lung injury. *Am. J. Respir. Cell Mol. Biol.* 15, 9–19. doi: 10.1165/ajrcmb.15.1.8679227

Christophersen, I. E., Olesen, M. S., Liang, B., Andersen, M. N., Larsen, A. P., Nielsen, J. B., et al. (2013). Genetic variation in KCNA5: impact on the atrial-specific potassium current IKur in patients with lone atrial fibrillation. *Eur. Heart J.* 34, 1517–1525. doi: 10.1093/eurheartj/ehs442

Chua, W., Easter, C. L., Guasch, E., Sitch, A., Casadei, B., Crijns, H., et al. (2019). Development and external validation of predictive models for prevalent and recurrent atrial fibrillation: a protocol for the analysis of the CATCH ME combined dataset. *BMC Cardiovasc. Disord.* 19, 120. doi: 10.1186/s12872-019-1105-4

Coetzee, W. A., Opie, L. H., and Saman, S. (1987). Proposed role of energy supply in the genesis of delayed afterdepolarizations–implications for ischemic or reperfusion arrhythmias. *J. Mol. Cell Cardiol.* 19 Suppl 5, 13–21. doi: 10.1016/S0022-2828(87)80606-5

Coetzee, W., Biermans, G., Callewaert, G., Vereecke, J., Opie, L. H., and Carmeliet, E. (1988). The effect of inhibition of mitochondrial energy metabolism on the transient inward current of isolated guinea-pig ventricular myocytes. *J. Mol. Cell Cardiol.* 20, 181–185. doi: 10.1016/S0022-2828(88)80051-8

Colman, M. A., Ni, H., Liang, B., Schmitt, N., and Zhang, H. (2017). In silico assessment of genetic variation in KCNA5 reveals multiple mechanisms of human atrial arrhythmogenesis. *PloS Comput. Biol.* 13, e1005587. doi: 10.1371/journal.pcbi.1005587

Coraboeuf, E., and Weidmann, S. (1954). Temperature effects on the electrical activity of Purkinje fibres. *Helv. Physiol. Pharmacol. Acta* 12, 32–41.

Coronel, R., Casini, S., Koopmann, T. T., Wilms-Schopman, F. J., Verkerk, A. O., De Groot, J. R., et al. (2005). Right ventricular fibrosis and conduction delay in a patient with clinical signs of Brugada syndrome: a combined electrophysiological, genetic, histopathologic, and computational study. *Circulation* 112, 2769–2777. doi: 10.1161/CIRCULATIONAHA.105.532614

Corr, P. B., and Witkowski, F. X. (1983). Potential electrophysiologic mechanisms responsible for dysrhythmias associated with reperfusion of ischemic myocardium. *Circulation* 68, I16–I24. doi: -. 6305533.

Cortez, D., Zareba, W., Mcnitt, S., Polonsky, B., Rosero, S. Z., and Platonov, P. G. (2019). Quantitative T-wave morphology assessment from surface ECG is linked with cardiac events risk in genotype-positive KCNH2 mutation carriers with normal QTc values. *J. Cardiovasc. Electrophysiol* 30, 2907–2913. doi: 10.1111/jce.14210

Csonka, C., Szilvassy, Z., Fulop, F., Pali, T., Blasig, I. E., Tosaki, A., et al. (1999a). Classic preconditioning decreases the harmful accumulation of nitric oxide during ischemia and reperfusion in rat hearts. *Circulation* 100, 2260–2266. doi: 10.1161/01.cir.100.22.2260

Csonka, C., Varga, E., Kovacs, P., Ferdinandy, P., Blasig, I. E., Szilvassy, Z., et al. (1999b). Heme oxygenase and cardiac function in ischemic/reperfused rat hearts. *Free Radic. Biol. Med.* 27, 119–126. doi: 10.1016/S0891-5849(99)00077-5. 10443928.

Curtis, M. J., and Hearse, D. J. (1989). Ischaemia-induced and reperfusion-induced arrhythmias differ in their sensitivity to potassium: implications for mechanisms of initiation and maintenance of ventricular fibrillation. *J. Mol. Cell Cardiol.* 21, 21–40. doi: 10.1016/0022-2828(89)91490-9

Curtis, M. J., Pugsley, M. K., and Walker, M. J. (1993). Endogenous chemical mediators of ventricular arrhythmias in ischaemic heart disease. *Cardiovasc. Res.* 27, 703–719. doi: 10.1093/cvr/27.5.703

Curtis, M. J. (1991). Torsades de pointes: arrhythmia, syndrome, or chimera? A perspective in the light of the Lambeth Conventions. *Cardiovasc. Drugs Ther.* 5, 191–200. doi: 10.1007/BF03029820

Czegledi, A., Tosaki, A., Gyongyosi, A., Zilinyi, R., Tosaki, A., and Lekli, I. (2019). Electrically-Induced Ventricular Fibrillation Alters Cardiovascular Function and Expression of Apoptotic and Autophagic Proteins in Rat Hearts. *Int. J. Mol. Sci.* 20, 1628. doi: 10.3390/ijms20071628

Das, B., and Sarkar, C. (2005). Is the sarcolemmal or mitochondrial K(ATP) channel activation important in the antiarrhythmic and cardioprotective effects during acute ischemia/reperfusion in the intact anesthetized rabbit model? *Life Sci.* 77, 1226–1248. doi: 10.1016/j.lfs.2004.12.042

Daubert, J. P., Zareba, W., Rosero, S. Z., Budzikowski, A., Robinson, J. L., and Moss, A. J. (2007). Role of implantable cardioverter defibrillator therapy in patients with long QT syndrome. *Am. Heart J.* 153, 53–58. doi: 10.1016/j.ahj.2007.01.025

De Ferrari, G. M., Dusi, V., Spazzolini, C., Bos, J. M., Abrams, D. J., Berul, C. I., et al. (2015). Clinical Management of Catecholaminergic Polymorphic Ventricular Tachycardia: The Role of Left Cardiac Sympathetic Denervation. *Circulation* 131, 2185–2193. doi: 10.1161/CIRCULATIONAHA.115.015731

Delise, P., Allocca, G., Sitta, N., Migliore, F., Dagradi, F., Spazzolini, C., et al. (2018). Cardiac arrest and Brugada syndrome: Is drug-induced type 1 ECG pattern always a marker of low risk? *Int. J. Cardiol.* 254, 142–145. doi: 10.1016/j.ijcard.2017.10.118

Desimone, C. V., Bos, J. M., Bos, K. M., Liang, J. J., Patel, N. A., Hodge, D. O., et al. (2015). Effects on repolarization using dynamic QT interval monitoring in long-QT patients following left cardiac sympathetic denervation. *J. Cardiovasc. Electrophysiol* 26, 434–439. doi: 10.1111/jce.12609

Dessertenne, F. (1966). [Ventricular tachycardia with 2 variable opposing foci]. *Arch. Mal. Coeur Vaiss* 59, 263–272.

Devalla, H. D., Gelinas, R., Aburawi, E. H., Beqqali, A., Goyette, P., Freund, C., et al. (2016). TECRL, a new life-threatening inherited arrhythmia gene associated with overlapping clinical features of both LQTS and CPVT. *EMBO Mol. Med.* 8, 1390–1408. doi: 10.15252/emmm.201505719

Difrancesco, D., and Ojeda, C. (1980). Properties of the current if in the sino-atrial node of the rabbit compared with those of the current iK, in Purkinje fibres. *J. Physiol.* 308, 353–367. doi: 10.1113/jphysiol.1980.sp013475

Difrancesco, D. (2015). HCN4, Sinus Bradycardia and Atrial Fibrillation. *Arrhythm. Electrophysiol Rev.* 4, 9–13. doi: 10.15420/aer.2015.4.1.9

Difrancesco, D. (2019). Comparing pathways for long-term heart rate modulation by the funny current. *J. Gen. Physiol.* 151, 1066–1069. doi: 10.1085/jgp.201912409

Du, R. H., Yi, H. W., Dai, D. Z., Tang, W. H., and Dai, Y. (2008). Inflammatory factors that contribute to upregulation of ERG and cardiac arrhythmias are suppressed by CPU86017, a class III antiarrhythmic agent. *J. Pharm. Pharmacol.* 60, 1089–1095. doi: 10.1211/jpp.60.8.0015

Dulak, J., and Jozkowicz, A. (2014). Novel faces of heme oxygenase-1: mechanisms and therapeutic potentials. *Antioxid. Redox Signal* 20, 1673–1676. doi: 10.1089/ars.2013.5761

Egom, E. E., Mohamed, T. M., Mamas, M. A., Shi, Y., Liu, W., Chirico, D., et al. (2011). Activation of Pak1/Akt/eNOS signaling following sphingosine-1-phosphate release as part of a mechanism protecting cardiomyocytes against ischemic cell injury. *Am. J. Physiol. Heart Circ. Physiol.* 301, H1487–H1495. doi: 10.1152/ajpheart.01003.2010

Enayati, A., Yassa, N., Mazaheri, Z., Rajaei, M., Pourabouk, M., Ghorghanlu, S., et al. (2018). Cardioprotective and anti-apoptotic effects of Potentilla reptans L. root via Nrf2 pathway in an isolated rat heart ischemia/reperfusion model. *Life Sci.* 215, 216–226. doi: 10.1016/j.lfs.2018.11.021

Estes, S. I., Ye, D., Zhou, W., Dotzler, S. M., Tester, D. J., Bos, J. M., et al. (2019). Characterization of the CACNA1C-R518C Missense Mutation in the Pathobiology of Long-QT Syndrome Using Human Induced Pluripotent Stem Cell Cardiomyocytes Shows Action Potential Prolongation and L-Type Calcium Channel Perturbation. *Circ. Genom. Precis Med.* 12, e002534. doi: 10.1161/CIRCGEN.119.002534

Ewing, J. F., Raju, V. S., and Maines, M. D. (1994). Induction of heart heme oxygenase-1 (HSP32) by hyperthermia: possible role in stress-mediated elevation of cyclic 3':5'-guanosine monophosphate. *J. Pharmacol. Exp. Ther.* 271, 408–414. doi: 10.1006/abbi.1997.0169

Falk, M., Huhn, R., Behmenburg, F., Ritz-Timme, S., and Mayer, F. (2018). Biomechanical stress in myocardial infarctions: can endothelin-1 and growth differentiation factor 15 serve as immunohistochemical markers? *Int. J. Legal. Med.* 132, 509–518. doi: 10.1007/s00414-017-1726-z

Fauconnier, J., Meli, A. C., Thireau, J., Roberge, S., Shan, J., Sassi, Y., et al. (2011). Ryanodine receptor leak mediated by caspase-8 activation leads to left ventricular injury after myocardial ischemia-reperfusion. *Proc. Natl. Acad. Sci. U. S. A* 108, 13258–13263. doi: 10.1073/pnas.1100286108

Flatman, P. W. (1984). Magnesium transport across cell membranes. *J. Membr. Biol.* 80, 1–14. doi: 10.1007/BF01868686

Frank-Hansen, R., Larsen, L. A., Andersen, P., Jespersgaard, C., and Christiansen, M. (2005). Mutations in the genes KCND2 and KCND3 encoding the ion channels Kv4.2 and Kv4.3, conducting the cardiac fast transient outward current (ITO,f), are not a frequent cause of long QT syndrome. *Clin. Chim. Acta* 351, 95–100. doi: 10.1016/j.cccn.2004.08.017

Gadsby, D. C., Kimura, J., and Noma, A. (1985). Voltage dependence of Na/K pump current in isolated heart cells. *Nature* 315, 63–65. doi: 10.1038/315063a0

Garcia, A., Liu, C. C., Cornelius, F., Clarke, R. J., and Rasmussen, H. H. (2016). Glutathionylation-Dependence of Na(+)-K(+)-Pump Currents Can Mimic Reduced Subsarcolemmal Na(+) Diffusion. *Biophys. J.* 110, 1099–1109. doi: 10.1016/j.bpj.2016.01.014

Garlick, P. B., Davies, M. J., Hearse, D. J., and Slater, T. F. (1987). Direct detection of free radicals in the reperfused rat heart using electron spin resonance spectroscopy. *Circ. Res.* 61, 757–760. doi: 10.1161/01.res.61.5.757

Gatzke, N., Guc, N., Hillmeister, P., Dulsner, A., Le Noble, F., Buschmann, E. E., et al. (2018). Cardiovascular drugs attenuated myocardial resistance against ischaemia-induced and reperfusion-induced injury in a rat model of repetitive occlusion. *Open Heart* 5, e000889. doi: 10.1136/openhrt-2018-000889

Gollob, M. H., Green, M. S., Tang, A. S., Gollob, T., Karibe, A., Ali Hassan, A. S., et al. (2001). Identification of a gene responsible for familial Wolff-Parkinson-White syndrome. *N. Engl. J. Med.* 344, 1823–1831. doi: 10.1056/NEJM200106143442403

Guc, M. O., Boachie-Ansah, G., Kane, K. A., and Wadsworth, R. M. (1993). Comparison of antiarrhythmic and electrophysiologic effects of diltiazem and its analogue siratiazem. *J. Cardiovasc. Pharmacol.* 22, 681–686. doi: 10.1097/00005344-199311000-00002

Gyongyosi, A., Zilinyi, R., Czegledi, A., Tosaki, A., Tosaki, A., and Lekli, I. (2019). The role of autophagy and death pathways in dose-dependent isoproterenol-induced cardiotoxicity. *Curr. Pharm. Des.* 25 (19), 2192–2198. doi: 10.2174/1381612825666190619145025

Haines, D. D., and Tosaki, A. (2018). Role of Heme Oxygenases in Cardiovascular Syndromes and Co-morbidities. *Curr. Pharm. Des.* 24, 2322–2325. doi: 10.2174/1381612824666180727110353

Han, F., Bossuyt, J., Martin, J. L., Despa, S., and Bers, D. M. (2010). Role of phospholemman phosphorylation sites in mediating kinase-dependent regulation of the Na+-K+-ATPase. *Am. J. Physiol. Cell Physiol.* 299, C1363–C1369. doi: 10.1152/ajpcell.00027.2010

Harris, A. S., Toth, L. A., and Tan, E. H. (1958). Arrhythmic and antiarrhythmic effects of sodium, potassium, and calcium salts and of glucose injected into coronary arteries of infarcted and normal hearts. *Circ. Res.* 6, 570–579. doi: 10.1161/01.res.6.5.570

Hearse, D. J., and Tosaki, A. (1987). Free radicals and reperfusion-induced arrhythmias: protection by spin trap agent PBN in the rat heart. *Circ. Res.* 60, 375–383. doi: 10.1161/01.res.60.3.375

Hegyi, B., Bossuyt, J., Griffiths, L. G., Shimkunas, R., Coulibaly, Z., Jian, Z., et al. (2018). Complex electrophysiological remodeling in postinfarction ischemic heart failure. *Proc. Natl. Acad. Sci. U. S. A* 115, E3036–E3044. doi: 10.1073/pnas.1718211115

Hung, L. M., Chen, J. K., Huang, S. S., Lee, R. S., and Su, M. J. (2000). Cardioprotective effect of resveratrol, a natural antioxidant derived from grapes. *Cardiovasc. Res.* 47, 549–555. doi: 10.1016/s0008-6363(00)00102-4

Ibanez, B., Fuster, V., Macaya, C., Sanchez-Brunete, V., Pizarro, G., Lopez-Romero, P., et al. (2012). Study design for the "effect of METOprolol in CARDioproteCtioN during an acute myocardial InfarCtion" (METOCARD-CNIC): a randomized, controlled parallel-group, observer-blinded clinical trial of early pre-reperfusion metoprolol administration in ST-segment elevation myocardial infarction. *Am. Heart J.* 164, 473–480 e475. doi: 10.1016/j.ahj.2012.07.020

Imaizumi, S., Miura, S., Nakamura, K., Kiya, Y., Uehara, Y., Zhang, B., et al. (2008). Antiarrhythmogenic effect of reconstituted high-density lipoprotein against ischemia/reperfusion in rats. *J. Am. Coll. Cardiol.* 51, 1604–1612. doi: 10.1016/j.jacc.2007.12.040

Isaka, M., Kudo, A., Imamura, M., Kawakami, H., and Yasuda, K. (2007). Endothelin receptors, localized in sympathetic nerve terminals of the heart, modulate norepinephrine release and reperfusion arrhythmias. *Basic Res. Cardiol.* 102, 154–162. doi: 10.1007/s00395-006-0623-2

Iseri, L. T., and French, J. H. (1984). Magnesium: nature's physiologic calcium blocker. *Am. Heart J.* 108, 188–193. doi: 10.1016/0002-8703(84)90572-6

Ishizaka, N., and Griendling, K. K. (1997). Heme oxygenase-1 is regulated by angiotensin II in rat vascular smooth muscle cells. *Hypertension* 29, 790–795. doi: 10.1161/01.HYP.29.3.790

Javidanpour, S., Dianat, M., Badavi, M., and Mard, S. A. (2018). The inhibitory effect of rosmarinic acid on overexpression of NCX1 and stretch- induced arrhythmias after acute myocardial infarction in rats. *Biomed. Pharmacother.* 102, 884–893. doi: 10.1016/j.biopha.2018.03.103

Jennings, R. B., and Reimer, K. A. (1983). Factors involved in salvaging ischemic myocardium: effect of reperfusion of arterial blood. *Circulation* 68, I25–I36.

Johansen, D., Ytrehus, K., and Baxter, G. F. (2006). Exogenous hydrogen sulfide (H2S) protects against regional myocardial ischemia-reperfusion injury–

Evidence for a role of K ATP channels. *Basic Res. Cardiol.* 101, 53–60. doi: 10.1007/s00395-005-0569-9

Johnson, R. A., Lavesa, M., Askari, B., Abraham, N. G., and Nasjletti, A. (1995). A heme oxygenase product, presumably carbon monoxide, mediates a vasodepressor function in rats. *Hypertension* 25, 166–169. doi: 10.1161/01.HYP.25.2.166

Jones, D. A., Rathod, K. S., Williamson, A., Harrington, D., Andiapen, M., Van Eijl, S., et al. (2018). The effect of intracoronary sodium nitrite on the burden of ventricular arrhythmias following primary percutaneous coronary intervention for acute myocardial infarction. *Int. J. Cardiol.* 266, 1–6. doi: 10.1016/j.ijcard.2018.01.029

Jost, N., Nagy, N., Corici, C., Kohajda, Z., Horvath, A., Acsai, K., et al. (2013). ORM-10103, a novel specific inhibitor of the Na+/Ca2+ exchanger, decreases early and delayed afterdepolarizations in the canine heart. *Br. J. Pharmacol.* 170, 768–778. doi: 10.1111/bph.12228

Juhasz, B., Varga, B., Czompa, A., Bak, I., Lekli, I., Gesztelyi, R., et al. (2011). Postischemic cardiac recovery in heme oxygenase-1 transgenic ischemic/reperfused mouse myocardium. *J. Cell Mol. Med.* 15, 1973–1982. doi: 10.1111/j.1582-4934.2010.01153.x

Kalsto, S. M., Siland, J. E., Rienstra, M., and Christophersen, I. E. (2019). Atrial Fibrillation Genetics Update: Toward Clinical Implementation. *Front. Cardiovasc. Med.* 6, 127. doi: 10.3389/fcvm.2019.00127

Kamkin, A., Kiseleva, I., and Isenberg, G. (2003). Activation and inactivation of a non-selective cation conductance by local mechanical deformation of acutely isolated cardiac fibroblasts. *Cardiovasc. Res.* 57, 793–803. doi: 10.1016/s0008-6363(02)00775-7

Kaoukis, A., Deftereos, S., Raisakis, K., Giannopoulos, G., Bouras, G., Panagopoulou, V., et al. (2013). The role of endothelin system in cardiovascular disease and the potential therapeutic perspectives of its inhibition. *Curr. Top. Med. Chem.* 13, 95–114. doi: 10.2174/1568026611313020003

Karmazyn, M. (1996). The sodium-hydrogen exchange system in the heart: its role in ischemic and reperfusion injury and therapeutic implications. *Can. J. Cardiol.* 12, 1074–1082.

Kato, M., Dote, K., Sasaki, S., Takemoto, H., Habara, S., and Hasegawa, D. (2004). Intracoronary verapamil rapidly terminates reperfusion tachyarrhythmias in acute myocardial infarction. *Chest* 126, 702–708. doi: 10.1378/chest.126.3.702

Kawahara, K., Takase, M., and Yamauchi, Y. (2003). Increased vulnerability to ischemia/reperfusion-induced ventricular tachyarrhythmias by pre-ischemic inhibition of nitric oxide synthase in isolated rat hearts. *Cardiovasc. Pathol.* 12, 49–56. doi: 10.1016/S1054-8807(02)00155-2

Kaya, S. T., Bozdogan, O., Ozarslan, T. O., Taskin, E., Eksioglu, D., Erim, F., et al. (2019). The protection of resveratrol and its combination with glibenclamide, but not berberine on the diabetic hearts against reperfusion-induced arrhythmias: the role of myocardial KATP channel. *Arch. Physiol. Biochem.* 125, 114–121. doi: 10.1080/13813455.2018.1440409

Keating, M. T., and Sanguinetti, M. C. (2001). Molecular and cellular mechanisms of cardiac arrhythmias. *Cell* 104, 569–580. doi: 10.1016/s0092-8674(01)00243-4

Kerr, S. M., Klaric, L., Halachev, M., Hayward, C., Boutin, T. S., Meynert, A. M., et al. (2019). An actionable KCNH2 Long QT Syndrome variant detected by sequence and haplotype analysis in a population research cohort. *Sci. Rep.* 9, 10964. doi: 10.1038/s41598-019-47436-6

Kisvari, G., Kovacs, M., Seprenyi, G., and Vegh, A. (2015). The activation of PI 3-kinase/Akt pathway is involved in the acute effects of simvastatin against ischaemia and reperfusion-induced arrhythmias in anaesthetised dogs. *Eur. J. Pharmacol.* 769, 185–194. doi: 10.1016/j.ejphar.2015.11.016

Kloner, R. A., Dow, J. S., and Bhandari, A. (2011). First direct comparison of the late sodium current blocker ranolazine to established antiarrhythmic agents in an ischemia/reperfusion model. *J. Cardiovasc. Pharmacol. Ther.* 16, 192–196. doi: 10.1177/1074248410386485

Kloner, R. A. (1993). Does reperfusion injury exist in humans? *J. Am. Coll. Cardiol.* 21, 537–545. doi: 10.1016/0735-1097(93)90700-b

Kohajda, Z., Farkas-Morvay, N., Jost, N., Nagy, N., Geramipour, A., Horvath, A., et al. (2016). The Effect of a Novel Highly Selective Inhibitor of the Sodium/Calcium Exchanger (NCX) on Cardiac Arrhythmias in In Vitro and In Vivo Experiments. *PloS One* 11, e0166041. doi: 10.1371/journal.pone.0166041. PMC5104402 Pharma, have been involved in the development of ORM-10962. Other authors have nothing to declare. The commercial adherence of the Orion Pharma does not alter our adherence to PLOS ONE policies on sharing data and materials.

Kostopoulou, A., Zeljko, H. M., Bogossian, H., Ciudin, R., Costa, F., Heijman, J., et al. (2019). Atrial fibrillation-related stroke in women: Evidence and inequalities in epidemiology, mechanisms, clinical presentation, and management. *Clin. Cardiol.* 43 (1), 14–23. doi: 10.1002/clc.23284

Kovacs, M., Gonczi, M., Kovacs, E., and Vegh, A. (2013). Time course analysis of cardiac pacing-induced gene expression changes in the canine heart. *Mol. Cell Biochem.* 372, 257–266. doi: 10.1007/s11010-012-1467-8

Kubo, Y., Adelman, J. P., Clapham, D. E., Jan, L. Y., Karschin, A., Kurachi, Y., et al. (2005). International Union of Pharmacology. LIV. Nomenclature and molecular relationships of inwardly rectifying potassium channels. *Pharmacol. Rev.* 57, 509–526. doi: 10.1124/pr.57.4.11

Kurz, T., Yamada, K. A., Datorre, S. D., and Corr, P. B. (1991). Alpha 1-adrenergic system and arrhythmias in ischaemic heart disease. *Eur. Heart J.* 12 Suppl F, 88–98. doi: 10.1093/eurheartj/12.suppl_f.88

Kusama, Y., Bernier, M., and Hearse, D. J. (1989). Singlet oxygen-induced arrhythmias. Dose- and light-response studies for photoactivation of rose bengal in the rat heart. *Circulation* 80, 1432–1448. doi: 10.1161/01.cir.80.5.1432

Lakkisto, P., Palojoki, E., Backlund, T., Saraste, A., Tikkanen, I., Voipio-Pulkki, L. M., et al. (2002). Expression of heme oxygenase-1 in response to myocardial infarction in rats. *J. Mol. Cell Cardiol.* 34, 1357–1365. doi: 10.1006/jmcc.2002.2094

Lazzerini, P. E., Bertolozzi, I., Finizola, F., Acampa, M., Natale, M., Vanni, F., et al. (2018). Proton Pump Inhibitors and Serum Magnesium Levels in Patients With Torsades de Pointes. *Front. Pharmacol.* 9, 363. doi: 10.3389/fphar.2018.00363

Lee, P. J., Alam, J., Wiegand, G. W., and Choi, A. M. (1996). Overexpression of heme oxygenase-1 in human pulmonary epithelial cells results in cell growth arrest and increased resistance to hyperoxia. *Proc. Natl. Acad. Sci. U. S. A* 93, 10393–10398. doi: 10.1073/pnas.93.19.10393

Lee, P. J., Jiang, B. H., Chin, B. Y., Iyer, N. V., Alam, J., Semenza, G. L., et al. (1997). Hypoxia-inducible factor-1 mediates transcriptional activation of the heme oxygenase-1 gene in response to hypoxia. *J. Biol. Chem.* 272, 5375–5381. doi: 10.1074/jbc.272.9.5375

Lee, T. M., Chang, N. C., and Lin, S. Z. (2017). Inhibition of infarction-induced sympathetic innervation with endothelin receptor antagonism via a PI3K/GSK-3beta-dependent pathway. *Lab. Invest.* 97, 243–255. doi: 10.1038/labinvest.2016.138

Li, W., Yin, L., Shen, C., Hu, K., Ge, J., and Sun, A. (2018). SCN5A Variants: Association With Cardiac Disorders. *Front. Physiol.* 9, 1372. doi: 10.3389/fphys.2018.01372

Liang, S., Wang, Q., Zhang, W., Zhang, H., Tan, S., Ahmed, A., et al. (2014). Carbon monoxide inhibits inward rectifier potassium channels in cardiomyocytes. *Nat. Commun.* 5, 4676. doi: 10.1038/ncomms5676

Lieve, K. V., Verkerk, A. O., Podliesna, S., Van Der Werf, C., Tanck, M. W., Hofman, N., et al. (2017). Gain-of-function mutation in SCN5A causes ventricular arrhythmias and early onset atrial fibrillation. *Int. J. Cardiol.* 236, 187–193. doi: 10.1016/j.ijcard.2017.01.113

Liu, P., Hock, C. E., Nagele, R., and Wong, P. Y. (1997). Formation of nitric oxide, superoxide, and peroxynitrite in myocardial ischemia-reperfusion injury in rats. *Am. J. Physiol.* 272, H2327–H2336. doi: 10.1152/ajpheart.1997.272.5.H2327

Loboda, A., Damulewicz, M., Pyza, E., Jozkowicz, A., and Dulak, J. (2016). Role of Nrf2/HO-1 system in development, oxidative stress response and diseases: an evolutionarily conserved mechanism. *Cell Mol. Life Sci.* 73, 3221–3247. doi: 10.1007/s00018-016-2223-0

Lu, F. M., and Hilgemann, D. W. (2017). Na/K pump inactivation, subsarcolemmal Na measurements, and cytoplasmic ion turnover kinetics contradict restricted Na spaces in murine cardiac myocytes. *J. Gen. Physiol.* 149, 727–749. doi: 10.1085/jgp.201711780

Lujan, H. L., Kramer, V. J., and Dicarlo, S. E. (2007). Sex influences the susceptibility to reperfusion-induced sustained ventricular tachycardia and beta-adrenergic receptor blockade in conscious rats. *Am. J. Physiol. Heart Circ. Physiol.* 293, H2799–H2808. doi: 10.1152/ajpheart.00596.2007

Ma, Y., Wang, Y., Gao, Y., Fu, Y., and Li, J. (2014). Total flavonoids from Ganshanbian (Herba Hyperici Attenuati) effect the expression of CaL-alpha1C and K(ATP)-Kir6.1 mRNA of the myocardial cell membrane in myocardial ischemia-reperfusion arrhythmia rats. *J. Tradit. Chin. Med.* 34, 357–361. doi: 10.1016/S0254-6272(14)60102-3

Magyar, J., Kistamas, K., Vaczi, K., Hegyi, B., Horvath, B., Banyasz, T., et al. (2016). Concept of relative variability of cardiac action potential duration and its test under various experimental conditions. *Gen. Physiol. Biophys.* 35, 55–62. doi: 10.4149/gpb_2015019

Manning, A. S., and Hearse, D. J. (1984). Reperfusion-induced arrhythmias: mechanisms and prevention. *J. Mol. Cell Cardiol.* 16, 497–518. doi: 10.1016/S0022-2828(84)80638-0

Marks, A. R., Priori, S., Memmi, M., Kontula, K., and Laitinen, P. J. (2002). Involvement of the cardiac ryanodine receptor/calcium release channel in catecholaminergic polymorphic ventricular tachycardia. *J. Cell Physiol.* 190, 1–6. doi: 10.1002/jcp.10031

Masini, E., Salvemini, D., Ndisang, J. F., Gai, P., Berni, L., Moncini, M., et al. (1999). Cardioprotective activity of endogenous and exogenous nitric oxide on ischaemia reperfusion injury in isolated guinea pig hearts. *Inflamm. Res.* 48, 561–568. doi: 10.1007/s000110050504

Maulik, N., Sharma, H. S., and Das, D. K. (1996). Induction of the haem oxygenase gene expression during the reperfusion of ischemic rat myocardium. *J. Mol. Cell Cardiol.* 28, 1261–1270. doi: 10.1006/jmcc.1996.0116

Mehta, A., Ramachandra, C. J. A., Singh, P., Chitre, A., Lua, C. H., Mura, M., et al. (2018). Identification of a targeted and testable antiarrhythmic therapy for long-QT syndrome type 2 using a patient-specific cellular model. *Eur. Heart J.* 39, 1446–1455. doi: 10.1093/eurheartj/ehx394

Mengesha, H. G., Tafesse, T. B., and Bule, M. H. (2017). If Channel as an Emerging Therapeutic Target for Cardiovascular Diseases: A Review of Current Evidence and Controversies. *Front. Pharmacol.* 8, 874. doi: 10.3389/fphar.2017.00874

Mesirca, P., Marger, L., Toyoda, F., Rizzetto, R., Audoubert, M., Dubel, S., et al. (2013). The G-protein-gated K+ channel, IKACh, is required for regulation of pacemaker activity and recovery of resting heart rate after sympathetic stimulation. *J. Gen. Physiol.* 142, 113–126. doi: 10.1085/jgp.201310996

Michowitz, Y., Milman, A., Andorin, A., Sarquella-Brugada, G., Gonzalez Corcia, M. C., Gourraud, J. B., et al. (2019). Characterization and Management of Arrhythmic Events in Young Patients With Brugada Syndrome. *J. Am. Coll. Cardiol.* 73, 1756–1765. doi: 10.1016/j.jacc.2019.01.048

Mitcheson, J. S., Chen, J., Lin, M., Culberson, C., and Sanguinetti, M. C. (2000). A structural basis for drug-induced long QT syndrome. *Proc. Natl. Acad. Sci. U. S. A.* 97, 12329–12333. doi: 10.1073/pnas.210244497

Miyamoto, L. (2018). Molecular Pathogenesis of Familial Wolff-Parkinson-White Syndrome. *J. Med. Invest.* 65, 1–8. doi: 10.2152/jmi.65.1

Mohler, P. J., Rivolta, I., Napolitano, C., Lemaillet, G., Lambert, S., Priori, S. G., et al. (2004). Nav1.5 E1053K mutation causing Brugada syndrome blocks binding to ankyrin-G and expression of Nav1.5 on the surface of cardiomyocytes. *Proc. Natl. Acad. Sci. U. S. A* 101, 17533–17538. doi: 10.1073/pnas.0403711101

Monfredi, O., Tsutsui, K., Ziman, B., Stern, M. D., Lakatta, E. G., and Maltsev, V. A. (2018). Electrophysiological heterogeneity of pacemaker cells in the rabbit intercaval region, including the SA node: insights from recording multiple ion currents in each cell. *Am. J. Physiol. Heart Circ. Physiol.* 314, H403–H414. doi: 10.1152/ajpheart.00253.2016

Na, T., Huang, Z. J., Dai, D. Z., Zhang, Y., and Dai, Y. (2007). Abrupt changes in FKBP12.6 and SERCA2a expression contribute to sudden occurrence of ventricular fibrillation on reperfusion and are prevented by CPU86017. *Acta Pharmacol. Sin.* 28, 773–782. doi: 10.1111/j.1745-7254.2007.00580.x

Nakata, T., Hearse, D. J., and Curtis, M. J. (1990). Are reperfusion-induced arrhythmias caused by disinhibition of an arrhythmogenic component of ischemia? *J. Mol. Cell Cardiol.* 22, 843–858. doi: 10.1016/0022-2828(90)90116-J

Naksuk, N., Sugrue, A. M., Padmanabhan, D., Kella, D., Desimone, C. V., Kapa, S., et al. (2019). Potentially modifiable factors of dofetilide-associated risk of torsades de pointes among hospitalized patients with atrial fibrillation. *J. Interv. Card. Electrophysiol.* 54, 189–196. doi: 10.1007/s10840-018-0476-2

Nanasi, P. P., Magyar, J., Varro, A., and Ordog, B. (2017). Beat-to-beat variability of cardiac action potential duration: underlying mechanism and clinical implications. *Can. J. Physiol. Pharmacol.* 95, 1230–1235. doi: 10.1139/cjpp-2016-0597

Narang, A., and Ozcan, C. (2019). Severe Torsades de Pointes with acquired QT prolongation. *Eur. Heart J. Acute Cardiovasc. Care* 8, 775–776. doi: 10.1177/2048872616649473

Nath, K. A., Balla, G., Vercellotti, G. M., Balla, J., Jacob, H. S., Levitt, M. D., et al. (1992). Induction of heme oxygenase is a rapid, protective response in rhabdomyolysis in the rat. *J. Clin. Invest.* 90, 267–270. doi: 10.1172/JCI115847

Nerbonne, J. M., and Kass, R. S. (2005). Molecular physiology of cardiac repolarization. *Physiol. Rev.* 85, 1205–1253. doi: 10.1152/physrev.00002.2005

Ng, C. A., Perry, M. D., Liang, W., Smith, N. J., Foo, B., Shrier, A., et al. (2019). High-throughput phenotyping of heteromeric human ether-a-go-go-related gene potassium channel variants can discriminate pathogenic from rare benign variants. *Heart Rhythm.* 17 (3), 492–500. doi: 10.1016/j.hrthm.2019.09.020

Niwa, N., and Nerbonne, J. M. (2010). Molecular determinants of cardiac transient outward potassium current (I(to)) expression and regulation. *J. Mol. Cell Cardiol.* 48, 12–25. doi: 10.1016/j.yjmcc.2009.07.013

Noma, A. (1983). ATP-regulated K+ channels in cardiac muscle. *Nature* 305, 147–148. doi: 10.1038/305147a0

Oikawa, M., Wu, M., Lim, S., Knight, W. E., Miller, C. L., Cai, Y., et al. (2013). Cyclic nucleotide phosphodiesterase 3A1 protects the heart against ischemia-reperfusion injury. *J. Mol. Cell Cardiol.* 64, 11–19. doi: 10.1016/j.yjmcc.2013.08.003

Ono, M., Nakamura, M., and Koga, Y. (2004). KB-R9032, newly developed Na (+)/H(+) exchange inhibitor, attenuates reperfusion-induced arrhythmias in isolated perfused rat heart. *J. Anesth.* 18, 196–202. doi: 10.1007/s00540-004-0232-x

Opie, L. H., and Coetzee, W. A. (1988). Role of calcium ions in reperfusion arrhythmias: relevance to pharmacologic intervention. *Cardiovasc. Drugs Ther.* 2, 623–636. doi: 10.1007/BF00054202

Orvos, P., Kohajda, Z., Szlovák, J., Gazdag, P., Árpádffy-Lovas, T., Tóth, D., et al. (2019). Evaluation of Possible Proarrhythmic Potency: Comparison of the Effect of Dofetilide, Cisapride, Sotalol, Terfenadine, and Verapamil on hERG and Native IKr Currents and on Cardiac Action Potential. *Toxicol. Sci.* 168 (2), 365–380. doi: 10.1093/toxsci/kfy299

Osipov, R. M., Bianchi, C., Feng, J., Clements, R. T., Liu, Y., Robich, M. P., et al. (2009). Effect of hypercholesterolemia on myocardial necrosis and apoptosis in the setting of ischemia-reperfusion. *Circulation* 120, S22–S30. doi: 10.1161/CIRCULATIONAHA.108.842724

Otani, N., Matsuda, R., Oda, K., Nishino, S., Inoue, T., and Kaneko, N. (2013). Protective effect of K201 on isoproterenol-induced and ischemic-reperfusion-induced ventricular arrhythmias in the rat: comparison with diltiazem. *J. Cardiovasc. Pharmacol. Ther.* 18, 184–190. doi: 10.1177/1074248412465489

Ottani, A., Giuliani, D., Neri, L., Calevro, A., Canalini, F., Vandini, E., et al. (2015). NDP-alpha-MSH attenuates heart and liver responses to myocardial reperfusion via the vagus nerve and JAK/ERK/STAT signaling. *Eur. J. Pharmacol.* 769, 22–32. doi: 10.1016/j.ejphar.2015.10.022

Paar, V., Jirak, P., Larbig, R., Zagidullin, N. S., Brandt, M. C., Lichtenauer, M., et al. (2019). Pathophysiology of Calcium Mediated Ventricular Arrhythmias and Novel Therapeutic Options with Focus on Gene Therapy. *Int. J. Mol. Sci.* 20, 5304. doi: 10.3390/ijms20215304

Pabla, R., and Curtis, M. J. (1995). Effects of NO modulation on cardiac arrhythmias in the rat isolated heart. *Circ. Res.* 77, 984–992. doi: 10.1161/01.res.77.5.984

Pataki, T., Bak, I., Csonka, C., Kovacs, P., Varga, E., Blasig, I. E., et al. (2001). Regulation of ventricular fibrillation by heme oxygenase in ischemic/reperfused hearts. *Antioxid. Redox Signal* 3, 125–134. doi: 10.1089/152308601750100623

Pataki, T., Bak, I., Kovacs, P., Bagchi, D., Das, D. K., and Tosaki, A. (2002). Grape seed proanthocyanidins improved cardiac recovery during reperfusion after ischemia in isolated rat hearts. *Am. J. Clin. Nutr.* 75, 894–899. doi: 10.1093/ajcn/75.5.894

Peers, C., and Steele, D. S. (2012). Carbon monoxide: a vital signalling molecule and potent toxin in the myocardium. *J. Mol. Cell Cardiol.* 52, 359–365. doi: 10.1016/j.yjmcc.2011.05.013

Perissinotti, L. L., De Biase, P. M., Guo, J., Yang, P. C., Lee, M. C., Clancy, C. E., et al. (2018). Determinants of Isoform-Specific Gating Kinetics of hERG1 Channel: Combined Experimental and Simulation Study. *Front. Physiol.* 9, 207. doi: 10.3389/fphys.2018.00207

Perrin, M. J., Adler, A., Green, S., Al-Zoughool, F., Doroshenko, P., Orr, N., et al. (2014). Evaluation of genes encoding for the transient outward current (Ito) identifies the KCND2 gene as a cause of J-wave syndrome associated with sudden cardiac death. *Circ. Cardiovasc. Genet.* 7, 782–789. doi: 10.1161/CIRCGENETICS.114.000623

Pisarenko, O., Studneva, I., Timoshin, A., and Veselova, O. (2019). Protective efficacy of dinitrosyl iron complexes with reduced glutathione in cardioplegia and reperfusion. *Pflugers. Arch.* 471, 583–593. doi: 10.1007/s00424-018-02251-2

Podesser, B. K., Schwarzacher, S., Zwoelfer, W., Binder, T. M., Wolner, E., and Seitelberger, R. (1995). Comparison of perioperative myocardial protection with nifedipine versus nifedipine and metoprolol in patients undergoing elective coronary artery bypass grafting. *J. Thorac. Cardiovasc. Surg.* 110, 1461–1469. doi: 10.1016/S0022-5223(95)70069-2

Podzuweit, T., Dalby, A. J., Cherry, G. W., and Opie, L. H. (1978). Cyclic AMP levels in ischaemic and non-ischaemic myocardium following coronary artery ligation: relation to ventricular fibrillation. *J. Mol. Cell Cardiol.* 10, 81–94. doi: 10.1016/0022-2828(78)90008-1

Priori, S. G., Napolitano, C., Tiso, N., Memmi, M., Vignati, G., Bloise, R., et al. (2001). Mutations in the cardiac ryanodine receptor gene (hRyR2) underlie catecholaminergic polymorphic ventricular tachycardia. *Circulation* 103, 196–200. doi: 10.1161/01.cir.103.2.196

Qi, X. Y., Huang, H., Ordog, B., Luo, X., Naud, P., Sun, Y., et al. (2015). Fibroblast inward-rectifier potassium current upregulation in profibrillatory atrial remodeling. *Circ. Res.* 116, 836–845. doi: 10.1161/CIRCRESAHA.116.305326

Ramirez, J., Laguna, P., Bayes De Luna, A., Malik, M., and Pueyo, E. (2014). QT/RR and T-peak-to-end/RR curvatures and slopes in chronic heart failure: relation to sudden cardiac death. *J. Electrocardiol.* 47, 842–848. doi: 10.1016/j.jelectrocard.2014.08.013

Ramirez, J., Orini, M., Minchole, A., Monasterio, V., Cygankiewicz, I., Bayes De Luna, A., et al. (2017). Sudden cardiac death and pump failure death prediction in chronic heart failure by combining ECG and clinical markers in an integrated risk model. *PloS One* 12, e0186152. doi: 10.1371/journal.pone.0186152

Rampazzo, A., Nava, A., Erne, P., Eberhard, M., Vian, E., Slomp, P., et al. (1995). A new locus for arrhythmogenic right ventricular cardiomyopathy (ARVD2) maps to chromosome 1q42-q43. *Hum. Mol. Genet.* 4, 2151–2154. doi: 10.1093/hmg/4.11.2151

Ravens, U., and Himmel, H. M. (1999). Drugs preventing Na+ and Ca2+ overload. *Pharmacol. Res.* 39, 167–174. doi: 10.1006/phrs.1998.0416

Ravingerova, T., Carnicka, S., Ledvenyiova, V., Barlaka, E., Galatou, E., Chytilova, A., et al. (2013). Upregulation of genes involved in cardiac metabolism enhances myocardial resistance to ischemia/reperfusion in the rat heart. *Physiol. Res.* 62 Suppl 1, S151–S163.

Ren, L., Wang, Q., Chen, Y., Ma, Y., and Wang, D. (2019). Involvement of MicroRNA-133a in the Protective Effect of Hydrogen Sulfide against Ischemia/Reperfusion-Induced Endoplasmic Reticulum Stress and Cardiomyocyte Apoptosis. *Pharmacology* 103, 1–9. doi: 10.1159/000492969

Robertson, S., Thomson, A. L., Carter, R., Stott, H. R., Shaw, C. A., Hadoke, P. W., et al. (2014). Pulmonary diesel particulate increases susceptibility to myocardial ischemia/reperfusion injury via activation of sensory TRPV1 and beta1 adrenoreceptors. *Part. Fibre Toxicol.* 11, 12. doi: 10.1186/1743-8977-11-12

Ryter, S., Kvam, E., Richman, L., Hartmann, F., and Tyrrell, R. M. (1998). A chromatographic assay for heme oxygenase activity in cultured human cells: application to artificial heme oxygenase overexpression. *Free Radic. Biol. Med.* 24, 959–971. doi: 10.1016/S0891-5849(97)00380-8

Salloum, F. N., Das, A., Samidurai, A., Hoke, N. N., Chau, V. Q., Ockaili, R. A., et al. (2012). Cinaciguat, a novel activator of soluble guanylate cyclase, protects against ischemia/reperfusion injury: role of hydrogen sulfide. *Am. J. Physiol. Heart Circ. Physiol.* 302, H1347–H1354. doi: 10.1152/ajpheart.00544.2011

Samouilov, A., Ahmad, R., Boslett, J., Liu, X., Petryakov, S., and Zweier, J. L. (2019). Development of a fast-scan EPR imaging system for highly accelerated free radical imaging. *Magn. Reson. Med.* 82, 842–853. doi: 10.1002/mrm.27759

Sankaranarayanan, R., Kistamas, K., Greensmith, D. J., Venetucci, L. A., and Eisner, D. A. (2017). Systolic [Ca(2+)]i regulates diastolic levels in rat ventricular myocytes. *J. Physiol.* 595, 5545–5555. doi: 10.1113/JP274366

Savastano, S., Rordorf, R., Vicentini, A., Petracci, B., Taravelli, E., Castelletti, S., et al. (2014). A comprehensive electrocardiographic, molecular, and echocardiographic study of Brugada syndrome: validation of the 2013 diagnostic criteria. *Heart Rhythm.* 11, 1176–1183. doi: 10.1016/j.hrthm.2014.04.010

Schwartz, P. J., Ackerman, M. J., George, A. L.Jr., and Wilde, A. A. M. (2013). Impact of genetics on the clinical management of channelopathies. *J. Am. Coll. Cardiol.* 62, 169–180. doi: 10.1016/j.jacc.2013.04.044

Sedighi, M., Nazari, A., Faghihi, M., Rafieian-Kopaei, M., Karimi, A., Moghimian, M., et al. (2018). Protective effects of cinnamon bark extract against ischemia-reperfusion injury and arrhythmias in rat. *Phytother. Res.* 32, 1983–1991. doi: 10.1002/ptr.6127

Sgro, A., Drake, T. M., Lopez-Ayala, P., and Phan, K. (2019). Left cardiac sympathetic denervation in the management of long QT syndrome and catecholaminergic polymorphic ventricular tachycardia: A meta-regression. *Congenit. Heart Dis.* 14 (6), 1102–1112. doi: 10.1111/chd.12855

Shen, J., Wang, J., Zhao, B., Hou, J., Gao, T., and Xin, W. (1998). Effects of EGb 761 on nitric oxide and oxygen free radicals, myocardial damage and arrhythmia in ischemia-reperfusion injury in vivo. *Biochim. Biophys. Acta* 1406, 228–236. doi: 10.1016/s0925-4439(98)00007-6

Sheridan, D. J., Penkoske, P. A., Sobel, B. E., and Corr, P. B. (1980). Alpha adrenergic contributions to dysrhythmia during myocardial ischemia and reperfusion in cats. *J. Clin. Invest.* 65, 161–171. doi: 10.1172/JCI109647

Singh, M., Morin, D. P., and Link, M. S. (2019). Sudden cardiac death in Long QT syndrome (LQTS), Brugada syndrome, and catecholaminergic polymorphic ventricular tachycardia (CPVT). *Prog. Cardiovasc. Dis.* 62, 227–234. doi: 10.1016/j.pcad.2019.05.006

Sipido, K. R., Volders, P. G., Vos, M. A., and Verdonck, F. (2002). Altered Na/Ca exchange activity in cardiac hypertrophy and heart failure: a new target for therapy? *Cardiovasc. Res.* 53, 782–805. doi: 10.1016/s0008-6363(01)00470-9

Smith, G. L., and Eisner, D. A. (2019). Calcium Buffering in the Heart in Health and Disease. *Circulation* 139, 2358–2371. doi: 10.1161/CIRCULATIONAHA.118.039329

Splawski, I., Timothy, K. W., Tateyama, M., Clancy, C. E., Malhotra, A., Beggs, A. H., et al. (2002). Variant of SCN5A sodium channel implicated in risk of cardiac arrhythmia. *Science* 297, 1333–1336. doi: 10.1126/science.1073569

Sun, Y. G., Wang, X. Y., Chen, X., Shen, C. X., and Li, Y. G. (2015). Hydrogen sulfide improves cardiomyocytes electrical remodeling post ischemia/reperfusion injury in rats. *Int. J. Clin. Exp. Pathol.* 8, 474–481.

Sun, X., Wang, W., Dai, J., Jin, S., Huang, J., Guo, C., et al. (2017). A Long-Term and Slow-Releasing Hydrogen Sulfide Donor Protects against Myocardial Ischemia/Reperfusion Injury. *Sci. Rep.* 7, 3541. doi: 10.1038/s41598-017-03941-0

Sun, X., Wang, W., Dai, J., Huang, J., Shi, M., Chu, X., et al. (2018). Donor heart preservation with a novel long-term and slow-releasing hydrogen sulfide system. *Nitric. Oxide* 81, 1–10. doi: 10.1016/j.niox.2018.09.001

Sutanto, H., Laudy, L., Clerx, M., Dobrev, D., Crijns, H., and Heijman, J. (2019). Maastricht antiarrhythmic drug evaluator (MANTA): A computational tool for better understanding of antiarrhythmic drugs. *Pharmacol. Res.* 148, 104444. doi: 10.1016/j.phrs.2019.104444

Swan, H., Piippo, K., Viitasalo, M., Heikkila, P., Paavonen, T., Kainulainen, K., et al. (1999). Arrhythmic disorder mapped to chromosome 1q42-q43 causes malignant polymorphic ventricular tachycardia in structurally normal hearts. *J. Am. Coll. Cardiol.* 34, 2035–2042. doi: 10.1016/s0735-1097(99)00461-1

Szendrei, L., Turoczi, T., Kovacs, P., Vecsernyes, M., Das, D. K., and Tosaki, A. (2002). Mitochondrial gene expression and ventricular fibrillation in ischemic/reperfused nondiabetic and diabetic myocardium. *Biochem. Pharmacol.* 63, 543–552. doi: 10.1016/s0006-2952(01)00913-3

Szepesi, J., Acsai, K., Sebok, Z., Prorok, J., Pollesello, P., Levijoki, J., et al. (2015). Comparison of the efficiency of Na+/Ca2+ exchanger or Na+/H+ exchanger inhibition and their combination in reducing coronary reperfusion-induced arrhythmias. *J. Physiol. Pharmacol.* 66, 215–226.

Szoke, K., Czompa, A., Lekli, I., Szabados-Furjesi, P., Herczeg, M., Csavas, M., et al. (2019). A new, vasoactive hybrid aspirin containing nitrogen monoxide-releasing molsidomine moiety. *Eur. J. Pharm. Sci.* 131, 159–166. doi: 10.1016/j.ejps.2019.02.020

Szuts, V., Menesi, D., Varga-Orvos, Z., Zvara, A., Houshmand, N., Bitay, M., et al. (2013). Altered expression of genes for Kir ion channels in dilated cardiomyopathy. *Can. J. Physiol. Pharmacol.* 91, 648–656. doi: 10.1139/cjpp-2012-0413

Tani, M., and Neely, J. R. (1989). Role of intracellular Na+ in Ca2+ overload and depressed recovery of ventricular function of reperfused ischemic rat hearts. Possible involvement of H+-Na+ and Na+-Ca2+ exchange. *Circ. Res.* 65, 1045–1056. doi: 10.1161/01.res.65.4.1045

Testai, L., Marino, A., Piano, I., Brancaleone, V., Tomita, K., Di Cesare Mannelli, L., et al. (2016). The novel H2S-donor 4-carboxyphenyl isothiocyanate promotes cardioprotective effects against ischemia/reperfusion injury through activation of mitoKATP channels and reduction of oxidative stress. *Pharmacol. Res.* 113, 290–299. doi: 10.1016/j.phrs.2016.09.006

Thandroyen, F. T., Flint, N. S., Worthington, M. G., and Opie, L. H. (1987). Arrhythmogenic action of alpha 1-adrenoceptor stimulation in normoxic rat ventricular myocardium: influence of nisoldipine, reduced extracellular Ca2+ and ryanodine. *J. Mol. Cell Cardiol.* 19, 841–851. doi: 10.1016/S0022-2828(87)80613-2

Thomas, S. H., and Behr, E. R. (2016). Pharmacological treatment of acquired QT prolongation and torsades de pointes. *Br. J. Clin. Pharmacol.* 81, 420–427. doi: 10.1111/bcp.12726

Tolg, R., Witt, M., Schwarz, B., Kurz, T., Kurowski, V., Hartmann, F., et al. (2006). Comparison of carvedilol and metoprolol in patients with acute myocardial infarction undergoing primary coronary intervention–the PASSAT Study. *Clin. Res. Cardiol.* 95, 31–41. doi: 10.1007/s00392-006-0317-7

Tosaki, A., and Braquet, P. (1990). DMPO and reperfusion injury: arrhythmia, heart function, electron spin resonance, and nuclear magnetic resonance studies in isolated working guinea pig hearts. *Am. Heart J.* 120, 819–830. doi: 10.1016/0002-8703(90)90197-6

Tosaki, A., Szekeres, L., and Hearse, D. J. (1987a). Diltiazem and the reduction of reperfusion-induced arrhythmias in the rat: protection is secondary to modification of ischemic injury and heart rate. *J. Mol. Cell Cardiol.* 19, 441–451. doi: 10.1016/S0022-2828(87)80396-6

Tosaki, A., Szekeres, L., and Hearse, D. J. (1987b). Metoprolol reduces reperfusion-induced fibrillation in the isolated rat heart: protection is secondary to bradycardia. *J. Cardiovasc. Pharmacol.* 10, 489–497. doi: 10.1097/00005344-198711000-00001

Tosaki, A., Balint, S., and Szekeres, L. (1988). Protective effect of lidocaine against ischemia and reperfusion-induced arrhythmias and shifts of myocardial sodium, potassium, and calcium content. *J. Cardiovasc. Pharmacol.* 12, 621–628. doi: 10.1097/00005344-198812000-00001

Tosaki, A., Koltai, M., and Braquet, P. (1989). Effects of low extracellular sodium concentration on reperfusion induced arrhythmias: changes in the myocardial sodium, potassium and calcium contents in isolated guinea pig hearts. *Cardiovasc. Res.* 23, 993–1000. doi: 10.1093/cvr/23.12.993

Tosaki, A., Bagchi, D., Pali, T., Cordis, G. A., and Das, D. K. (1993a). Comparisons of ESR and HPLC methods for the detection of OH. radicals in ischemic/reperfused hearts. A relationship between the genesis of free radicals and reperfusion arrhythmias. *Biochem. Pharmacol.* 45, 961–969. doi: 10.1016/0006-2952(93)90182-v

Tosaki, A., Szerdahelyi, P., Engelman, R. M., and Das, D. K. (1993b). Effects of extracellular magnesium manipulation on reperfusion-induced arrhythmias and myocardial ion shifts in isolated ischemic reperfused rat hearts. *J. Pharmacol. Exp. Ther.* 267, 1045–1053.

Tosaki, A., Engelman, D. T., Engelman, R. M., and Das, D. K. (1995). Diabetes and ATP-sensitive potassium channel openers and blockers in isolated ischemic/reperfused hearts. *J. Pharmacol. Exp. Ther.* 275, 1115–1123.

Tosaki, A., Pali, T., and Droy-Lefaix, M. T. (1996). Effects of Ginkgo biloba extract and preconditioning on the diabetic rat myocardium. *Diabetologia* 39, 1255–1262. doi: 10.1007/s001250050567

Tse, G., Chan, Y. W., Keung, W., and Yan, B. P. (2017). Electrophysiological mechanisms of long and short QT syndromes. *Int. J. Cardiol. Heart Vasc.* 14, 8–13. doi: 10.1016/j.ijcha.2016.11.006

Tzivoni, D., Keren, A., Granot, H., Gottlieb, S., Benhorin, J., and Stern, S. (1983). Ventricular fibrillation caused by myocardial reperfusion in Prinzmetal's angina. *Am. Heart J.* 105, 323–325. doi: 10.1016/0002-8703(83)90534-3

Tzivoni, D., Banai, S., Schuger, C., Benhorin, J., Keren, A., Gottlieb, S., et al. (1988). Treatment of torsade de pointes with magnesium sulfate. *Circulation* 77, 392–397. doi: 10.1161/01.cir.77.2.392

Vago, H., Soos, P., Zima, E., Geller, L., Keltai, K., Roka, A., et al. (2004). Changes of endothelin-1 and big endothelin-1 levels and action potential duration during myocardial ischemia-reperfusion in dogs with and without ventricular fibrillation. *J. Cardiovasc. Pharmacol.* 44 Suppl 1, S376–S379. doi: 10.1097/01.fjc.0000166299.10443.0c

Van Der Weg, K., Prinzen, F. W., and Gorgels, A. P. (2019). Editor's Choice-Reperfusion cardiac arrhythmias and their relation to reperfusion-induced cell death. *Eur. Heart J. Acute Cardiovasc. Care* 8, 142–152. doi: 10.1177/2048872618812148

Vandenberg, J. I., Perry, M. D., Perrin, M. J., Mann, S. A., Ke, Y., and Hill, A. P. (2012). hERG K(+) channels: structure, function, and clinical significance. *Physiol. Rev.* 92, 1393–1478. doi: 10.1152/physrev.00036.2011

Vanoli, E., Hull, S. S.Jr., Foreman, R. D., Ferrari, A., and Schwartz, P. J. (1994). Alpha 1-adrenergic blockade and sudden cardiac death. *J. Cardiovasc. Electrophysiol.* 5, 76–89. doi: 10.1111/j.1540-8167.1994.tb01116.x

Varga, E., Bodi, A., Ferdinandy, P., Droy-Lefaix, M. T., Blasig, I. E., and Tosaki, A. (1999). The protective effect of EGb 761 in isolated ischemic/reperfused rat hearts: a link between cardiac function and nitric oxide production. *J. Cardiovasc. Pharmacol.* 34, 711–717. doi: 10.1097/00005344-199911000-00013

Vasseur, L., Cens, T., Wagner, R., Saint, N., Kugler, V., Chavanieu, A., et al. (2019). Importance of the Choice of a Recombinant System to Produce Large Amounts of Functional Membrane Protein hERG. *Int. J. Mol. Sci.* 20, 3181. doi: 10.3390/ijms20133181

Vaughan Williams, E. M. (1959). Relation of extracellular to intracellular potential records from single cardiac muscle fibres. *Nature* 183, 1341–1342. doi: 10.1038/1831341a0

Vaughan Williams, E. M. (1975). Classification of antidysrhythmic drugs. *Pharmacol. Ther. B* 1, 115–138. doi: 10.1016/0306-039x(75)90019-7

Vaughan Williams, E. M. (1992). Classifying antiarrhythmic actions: by facts or speculation. *J. Clin. Pharmacol.* 32, 964–977. doi: 10.1002/j.1552-4604.1992.tb03797.x

Verkerk, A. O., Amin, A. S., and Remme, C. A. (2018). Disease Modifiers of Inherited SCN5A Channelopathy. *Front. Cardiovasc. Med.* 5, 137. doi: 10.3389/fcvm.2018.00137

Vink, A. S., Neumann, B., Lieve, K. V. V., Sinner, M. F., Hofman, N., El Kadi, S., et al. (2018). Determination and Interpretation of the QT Interval. *Circulation* 138, 2345–2358. doi: 10.1161/CIRCULATIONAHA.118.033943

Voigt, N., Li, N., Wang, Q., Wang, W., Trafford, A. W., Abu-Taha, I., et al. (2012). Enhanced sarcoplasmic reticulum Ca2+ leak and increased Na+-Ca2+ exchanger function underlie delayed afterdepolarizations in patients with chronic atrial fibrillation. *Circulation* 125, 2059–2070. doi: 10.1161/CIRCULATIONAHA.111.067306

Wainwright, C. L., Mccabe, C., and Kane, K. A. (2005). Endothelin and the ischaemic heart. *Curr. Vasc. Pharmacol.* 3, 333–341. doi: 10.2174/157016105774329417

Waldman, M., Nudelman, V., Shainberg, A., Zemel, R., Kornwoski, R., Aravot, D., et al. (2019). The Role of Heme Oxygenase 1 in the Protective Effect of Caloric Restriction against Diabetic Cardiomyopathy. *Int. J. Mol. Sci.* 20, 2427. doi: 10.3390/ijms20102427

Walker, M. J., Curtis, M. J., Hearse, D. J., Campbell, R. W., Janse, M. J., Yellon, D. M., et al. (1988). The Lambeth Conventions: guidelines for the study of arrhythmias in ischaemia infarction, and reperfusion. *Cardiovasc. Res.* 22, 447–455. doi: 10.1093/cvr/22.7.447

Wang, Q. D., Pernow, J., Sjoquist, P. O., and Ryden, L. (2002). Pharmacological possibilities for protection against myocardial reperfusion injury. *Cardiovasc. Res.* 55, 25–37. doi: 10.1016/s0008-6363(02)00261-4

Wang, Q., Chen, S., Chen, Q., Wan, X., Shen, J., Hoeltge, G. A., et al. (2004). The common SCN5A mutation R1193Q causes LQTS-type electrophysiological alterations of the cardiac sodium channel. *J. Med. Genet.* 41, e66. doi: 10.1136/jmg.2003.013300

Wang, S., Radhakrishnan, J., Ayoub, I. M., Kolarova, J. D., Taglieri, D. M., and Gazmuri, R. J. (2007). Limiting sarcolemmal Na+ entry during resuscitation from ventricular fibrillation prevents excess mitochondrial Ca2+ accumulation and attenuates myocardial injury. *J. Appl. Physiol. (1985)* 103, 55–65. doi: 10.1152/japplphysiol.01167.2006

Wang, S., Guo, X., Long, C. L., Li, C., Zhang, Y. F., Wang, J., et al. (2019). SUR2B/Kir6.1 channel openers correct endothelial dysfunction in chronic heart failure via the miR-1-3p/ET-1 pathway. *Biomed. Pharmacother.* 110, 431–439. doi: 10.1016/j.biopha.2018.11.135

Wang, R. (2002). Two's company, three's a crowd: can H2S be the third endogenous gaseous transmitter? *FASEB J.* 16, 1792–1798. doi: 10.1096/fj.02-0211hyp

Whalen, D. A.Jr., Hamilton, D. G., Ganote, C. E., and Jennings, R. B. (1974). Effect of a transient period of ischemia on myocardial cells. I. Effects on cell volume regulation. *Am. J. Pathol.* 74, 381–397. doi: -. PMC1910794.

Wilder, C. D., Masoud, R., Yazar, D., O'brien, B. A., Eykyn, T. R., and Curtis, M. J. (2016). Contractile function assessment by intraventricular balloon alters the ability of regional ischaemia to evoke ventricular fibrillation. *Br. J. Pharmacol.* 173, 39–52. doi: 10.1111/bph.13332. PMC4813384.

Winchester, D. E., and Pepine, C. J. (2014). Usefulness of Beta blockade in contemporary management of patients with stable coronary heart disease. *Am. J. Cardiol.* 114, 1607–1612. doi: 10.1016/j.amjcard.2014.08.026

Wirth, K. J., Maier, T., and Busch, A. E. (2001). NHE1-inhibitor cariporide prevents the transient reperfusion-induced shortening of the monophasic action potential after coronary ischemia in pigs. *Basic Res. Cardiol.* 96, 192–197. doi: 10.1007/s003950170070

Wolff, L., Parkinson, J., and White, D. P. (1930). Bundle-branch block with short P-R interval in healthy young people prone to paroxysmal tachycardia. *Am. Heart J.* 5, 685–704. doi: 10.1016/S0002-8703(30)90086-5

Woodbury, L. A., Woodbury, J. W., and Hecht, H. H. (1950). Membrane resting and action potentials of single cardiac muscle fibers. *Circulation* 1, 264–266. doi: 10.1161/01.cir.1.2.264

Woodcock, E. A., Arthur, J. F., Harrison, S. N., Gao, X. M., and Du, X. J. (2001). Reperfusion-induced Ins(1,4,5)P(3) generation and arrhythmogenesis require activation of the Na(+)/Ca(2+) exchanger. *J. Mol. Cell Cardiol.* 33, 1861–1869. doi: 10.1006/jmcc.2001.1450

Woodman, O. L., Chin, K. Y., Thomas, C. J., Ng, D. C. H., and May, C. N. (2018). Flavonols and Flavones - Protecting Against Myocardial Ischemia/Reperfusion Injury by Targeting Protein Kinases. *Curr. Med. Chem.* 25, 4402–4415. doi: 10.2174/0929867325666180326161730

Woodward, B., and Zakaria, M. N. (1985). Effect of some free radical scavengers on reperfusion induced arrhythmias in the isolated rat heart. *J. Mol. Cell Cardiol.* 17, 485–493. doi: 10.1016/S0022-2828(85)80053-5

Wu, M. L., Ho, Y. C., and Yet, S. F. (2011). A central role of heme oxygenase-1 in cardiovascular protection. *Antioxid. Redox Signal* 15, 1835–1846. doi: 10.1089/ars.2010.3726

Wu, J., Sakaguchi, T., Takenaka, K., Toyoda, F., Tsuji, K., Matsuura, H., et al. (2019). A trafficking-deficient KCNQ1 mutation, T587M, causes a severe phenotype of long QT syndrome by interfering with intracellular hERG transport. *J. Cardiol.* 73, 343–350. doi: 10.1016/j.jjcc.2018.10.011

Xie, Y., Ding, W. G., Liu, Y., Yu, M., Sun, X., and Matsuura, H. (2019). Long-term 4-AP treatment facilitates functional expression of human Kv1.5 channel. *Eur. J. Pharmacol.* 844, 195–203. doi: 10.1016/j.ejphar.2018.12.022

Yamada, C., Xue, Y., Chino, D., and Hashimoto, K. (2005). Effects of KB-R9032, a new Na+/H+ exchange inhibitor, on canine coronary occlusion/reperfusion-induced ventricular arrhythmias. *J. Pharmacol. Sci.* 98, 404–410. doi: 10.1254/jphs.FP0050278

Yampolsky, P., Koenen, M., Mosqueira, M., Geschwill, P., Nauck, S., Witzenberger, M., et al. (2019). Augmentation of myocardial If dysregulates calcium homeostasis and causes adverse cardiac remodeling. *Nat. Commun.* 10, 3295. doi: 10.1038/s41467-019-11261-2

Yanagisawa, M., Kurihara, H., Kimura, S., Tomobe, Y., Kobayashi, M., Mitsui, Y., et al. (1988). A novel potent vasoconstrictor peptide produced by vascular endothelial cells. *Nature* 332, 411–415. doi: 10.1038/332411a0

Yasuda, J., Okada, M., and Yamawaki, H. (2019). Protective effect of T3 peptide, an active fragment of tumstatin, against ischemia/reperfusion injury in rat heart. *J. Pharmacol. Sci.* 139, 193–200. doi: 10.1016/j.jphs.2019.01.010

Yasutake, M., and Avkiran, M. (1995). Exacerbation of reperfusion arrhythmias by alpha 1 adrenergic stimulation: a potential role for receptor mediated activation of sarcolemmal sodium-hydrogen exchange. *Cardiovasc. Res.* 29, 222–230.

Ye, L., Neale, C., Sljoka, A., Lyda, B., Pichugin, D., Tsuchimura, N., et al. (2018). Mechanistic insights into allosteric regulation of the A2A adenosine G protein-coupled receptor by physiological cations. *Nat. Commun.* 9, 1372. doi: 10.1038/s41467-018-03314-9

Ye, D., Tester, D. J., Zhou, W., Papagiannis, J., and Ackerman, M. J. (2019). A pore-localizing CACNA1C-E1115K missense mutation, identified in a patient with idiopathic QT prolongation, bradycardia, and autism spectrum disorder, converts the L-type calcium channel into a hybrid nonselective monovalent cation channel. *Heart Rhythm.* 16, 270–278. doi: 10.1016/j.hrthm.2018.08.030

Yellon, D. M., and Hausenloy, D. J. (2007). Myocardial reperfusion injury. *N. Engl. J. Med.* 357, 1121–1135. doi: 10.1056/NEJMra071667

Yin, C., Zhang, P., Yang, J., and Zhang, L. (2018). Unique ECG presentations and clinical management of a symptomatic LQT2 female carrying a novel de novo KCNH2 mutation. *J. Electrocardiol.* 51, 111–116. doi: 10.1016/j.jelectrocard.2017.08.022

Ying, S. Q., Fang, L., Xiang, M. X., Xu, G., Shan, J., and Wang, J. A. (2007). Protective effects of magnesium against ischaemia-reperfusion injury through inhibition of P-selectin in rats. *Clin. Exp. Pharmacol. Physiol.* 34, 1234–1239. doi: 10.1111/j.1440-1681.2007.04697.x

Yu, L., Huang, B., Po, S. S., Tan, T., Wang, M., Zhou, L., et al. (2017). Low-Level Tragus Stimulation for the Treatment of Ischemia and Reperfusion Injury in Patients With ST-Segment Elevation Myocardial Infarction: A Proof-of-Concept Study. *JACC Cardiovasc. Interv.* 10, 1511–1520. doi: 10.1016/j.jcin.2017.04.036

Yu, L. M., Dong, X., Xue, X. D., Zhang, J., Li, Z., Wu, H. J., et al. (2019). Protection of the myocardium against ischemia/reperfusion injury by punicalagin through an SIRT1-NRF-2-HO-1-dependent mechanism. *Chem. Biol. Interact.* 306, 152–162. doi: 10.1016/j.cbi.2019.05.003

Yue, L., Xie, J., and Nattel, S. (2011). Molecular determinants of cardiac fibroblast electrical function and therapeutic implications for atrial fibrillation. *Cardiovasc. Res.* 89, 744–753. doi: 10.1093/cvr/cvq329

Zareba, W., Moss, A. J., Sheu, G., Kaufman, E. S., Priori, S., Vincent, G. M., et al. (2003). Location of mutation in the KCNQ1 and phenotypic presentation of long QT syndrome. *J. Cardiovasc. Electrophysiol.* 14, 1149–1153. doi: 10.1046/j.1540-8167.2003.03177.x. 14678125.

Zhang, T., Li, Z., Dang, H., Chen, R., Liaw, C., Tran, T. A., et al. (2012). Inhibition of Mas G-protein signaling improves coronary blood flow, reduces myocardial infarct size, and provides long-term cardioprotection. *Am. J. Physiol. Heart Circ. Physiol.* 302, H299–H311. doi: 10.1152/ajpheart.00723.2011

Zhang, Y., Luo, J., He, J., Rong, M., and Zeng, X. (2019a). JZTX-V Targets the Voltage Sensor in Kv4.2 to Inhibit Ito Potassium Channels in Cardiomyocytes. *Front. Pharmacol.* 10, 357. doi: 10.3389/fphar.2019.00357

Zhang, Y., Wu, J., Guo, S., Lin, W., Zhang, B., Chen, X., et al. (2019b). The clinical efficacy and safety of the Chinese herbal medicine Astragalus (Huangqi) preparation for the treatment of acute myocardial infarction: A systematic review of randomized controlled trials. *Med. (Baltimore)* 98, e15256. doi: 10.1097/MD.0000000000015256

Zhou, Y., Wang, D., Gao, X., Lew, K., Richards, A. M., and Wang, P. (2014). mTORC2 phosphorylation of Akt1: a possible mechanism for hydrogen sulfide-induced cardioprotection. *PloS One* 9, e99665. doi: 10.1371/journal.pone.0099665

Zhou, X., Bueno-Orovio, A., Schilling, R. J., Kirkby, C., Denning, C., Rajamohan, D., et al. (2019). Investigating the Complex Arrhythmic Phenotype Caused by the Gain-of-Function Mutation KCNQ1-G229D. *Front. Physiol.* 10, 259. doi: 10.3389/fphys.2019.00259

Zuo, L., Chen, Y. R., Reyes, L. A., Lee, H. L., Chen, C. L., Villamena, F. A., et al. (2009). The radical trap 5,5-dimethyl-1-pyrroline N-oxide exerts dose-dependent protection against myocardial ischemia-reperfusion injury through preservation of mitochondrial electron transport. *J. Pharmacol. Exp. Ther.* 329, 515–523. doi: 10.1124/jpet.108.143479

Zweier, J. L., and Kuppusamy, P. (1988). Electron paramagnetic resonance measurements of free radicals in the intact beating heart: a technique for detection and characterization of free radicals in whole biological tissues. *Proc. Natl. Acad. Sci. U. S. A* 85, 5703–5707. doi: 10.1073/pnas.85.15.5703

Zweier, J. L., Kuppusamy, P., and Lutty, G. A. (1988). Measurement of endothelial cell free radical generation: evidence for a central mechanism of free radical injury in postischemic tissues. *Proc. Natl. Acad. Sci. U. S. A* 85, 4046–4050. doi: 10.1073/pnas.85.11.4046

14

The Cardiac Pacemaker Story—Fundamental Role of the Na^+/Ca^{2+} Exchanger in Spontaneous Automaticity

Zsófia Kohajda[1,2†], Axel Loewe[3†], Noémi Tóth[2], András Varró[1,2] and Norbert Nagy[1,2]*

[1] *MTA-SZTE Research Group of Cardiovascular Pharmacology, Hungarian Academy of Sciences, Szeged, Hungary,*
[2] *Department of Pharmacology and Pharmacotherapy, Faculty of Medicine, University of Szeged, Szeged, Hungary,*
[3] *Institute of Biomedical Engineering, Karlsruhe Institute of Technology (KIT), Karlsruhe, Germany*

Correspondence:
András Varró
varro.andras@med.u-szeged.hu

†These authors have contributed equally to this work

The electrophysiological mechanism of the sinus node automaticity was previously considered exclusively regulated by the so-called "funny current". However, parallel investigations increasingly emphasized the importance of the Ca^{2+}-homeostasis and Na^+/Ca^{2+} exchanger (NCX). Recently, increasing experimental evidence, as well as insight through mechanistic *in silico* modeling demonstrates the crucial role of the exchanger in sinus node pacemaking. NCX had a key role in the exciting story of discovery of sinus node pacemaking mechanisms, which recently settled with a consensus on the coupled-clock mechanism after decades of debate. This review focuses on the role of the Na^+/Ca^{2+} exchanger from the early results and concepts to recent advances and attempts to give a balanced summary of the characteristics of the local, spontaneous, and rhythmic Ca^{2+} releases, the molecular control of the NCX and its role in the fight-or-flight response. Transgenic animal models and pharmacological manipulation of intracellular Ca^{2+} concentration and/or NCX demonstrate the pivotal function of the exchanger in sinus node automaticity. We also highlight where specific hypotheses regarding NCX function have been derived from computational modeling and require experimental validation. Nonselectivity of NCX inhibitors and the complex interplay of processes involved in Ca^{2+} handling render the design and interpretation of these experiments challenging.

Keywords: Na^+/Ca^{2+} exchanger, pacemaking, sinus node, automaticity, Ca^{2+}-handling

Abbreviations: AP, action potential; APD, action potential duration; ATP, adenosine triphosphate; Ca^{2+}/CA, Ca^{2+}-cation antiporter; $Ca^{2+}{}_i$, intracellular Ca^{2+} concentration; CaM, calmodulin; CaMKII, Ca^{2+}/calmodulin-dependent protein kinase; cAMP, cyclic adenosine monophosphate; CICR, Ca^{2+}-induced Ca^{2+} release; CL, cycle length; CRU, Ca^{2+}- release unit; DD, diastolic depolarization; DDR, diastolic depolarization rate; EC50, half maximal effective concentration; E_{NCX}, NCX equilibrium potential; GPCR, G-protein coupled receptor; hESC-CM, human embryonic stem cell-derived cardiomyocyte; IC50, half maximal inhibitory concentration; I_{CaL}, L-type Ca^{2+}-current; I_{CaT}, T-type Ca^{2+}-current; I_f, funny-current; I_{K1}, inward rectifier potassium current; $I_{K(Ca)}$: small-conductance Ca^{2+}-activated K^+ current; I_{Kr}, rapid delayed rectifier potassium current; I_{Ks}, slow delayed rectifier potassium current; I_{to}, transient outward potassium current; LCR, local Ca^{2+} releases; LDCaE, late diastolic Ca^{2+} elevation; LLFS model, Loewe–Lutz–Fabbri–Severi model; M-clock, membrane clock; MDP, maximal diastolic potential; $Na^+{}_i$, intracellular Na^+ concentration; NCX, Na^+/Ca^{2+} exchanger; NO, nitrogen-monoxide; PDE, phosphodiesterase; PKA, protein kinase A; PKC, protein kinase C; PLB, phospholamban; PP1, protein phosphatase 1; PP2A, protein phosphatase 2; RyR, ryanodine receptor; SERCA, sarcoplasmic reticulum Ca^{2+} ATPase; SN, sinus node; SNC, sinus node cell; SR, sarcoplasmic reticulum; V_m, transmembrane potential.

INTRODUCTION

Few areas of cardiac cellular electrophysiology had more intense debate over the years than 'what makes our hearts beat'—the electrophysiology of the sinus node (SN). In the last two decades, we could witness the struggle of two competing oscillator concepts explaining SN automaticity: in essence, the funny-current (I_f) and the Ca^{2+}-induced depolarization of the membrane potential (V_m) *via* Na^+/Ca^{2+} exchanger (NCX, I_{NaCa}). Year by year, several studies were published supporting both theories. Thus, the exciting exploration of SN pacemaking mechanisms has been full of debates for over a half century. Numerous mechanisms have been suggested, tested, refuted, accepted, tested, and retested again, updated and after intense point–counterpoint public debates finally settled at a delicate balance known as the coupled-clock mechanism that includes both membrane and sarcoplasmic reticulum (SR) linked contributions. The general field of SN pacemaking (Lakatta et al., 2010; Maltsev et al., 2014; DiFrancesco, 2020) and computational modeling thereof has been excellently reviewed elsewhere (Wilders, 2007; Li et al., 2013). In this review, we focus on the role of NCX function on SN pacemaking and aim to give a balanced view from the very early to recent experimental findings and accompanying computational models.

The SNCs show a characteristic slow diastolic depolarization (DD) starting from the maximal diastolic potential (MDP) and ending at the action potential (AP) threshold of about −40 mV. This threshold is called takeoff potential (Kharche et al., 2011). At the takeoff potential, the course of the AP changes qualitatively from slow DD to the AP upstroke (**Figure 1A**). I_f, NCX, and I_{CaT} (T-type Ca^{2+}-current) are mainly active before (at V_m more negative than the takeoff potential), whereas I_{CaL} (L-type Ca^{2+}-current) and I_{Kr} (rapid delayed rectifier potassium current) are mainly active thereafter (at more positive V_m), while NCX is active throughout the entire AP cycle. Early studies suggested a major role of a decaying delayed rectifier potassium current (I_{Kr}) (Noble, 1962) and the nonselective, cAMP-dependent and hyperpolarization activated current [funny-current, I_f, (DiFrancesco, 1991)] in the development of DD. This mechanism, governed by transmembrane ion channels with Hodgkin–Huxley kinetics was termed as "membrane-clock" (M-clock). Later studies identified rhythmic, spontaneous locally propagating subsarcolemmal Ca^{2+} releases (LCR) generated by the SR *via* ryanodine receptors (RYRs) during the DD (**Figure 1B**) (Huser et al., 2000; Bogdanov et al., 2001; Monfredi et al., 2013). The LCRs activate the forward mode of the Na^+/Ca^{2+} exchanger generating inward current that contributes to the DD (Bogdanov et al., 2001). Under certain experimental conditions,

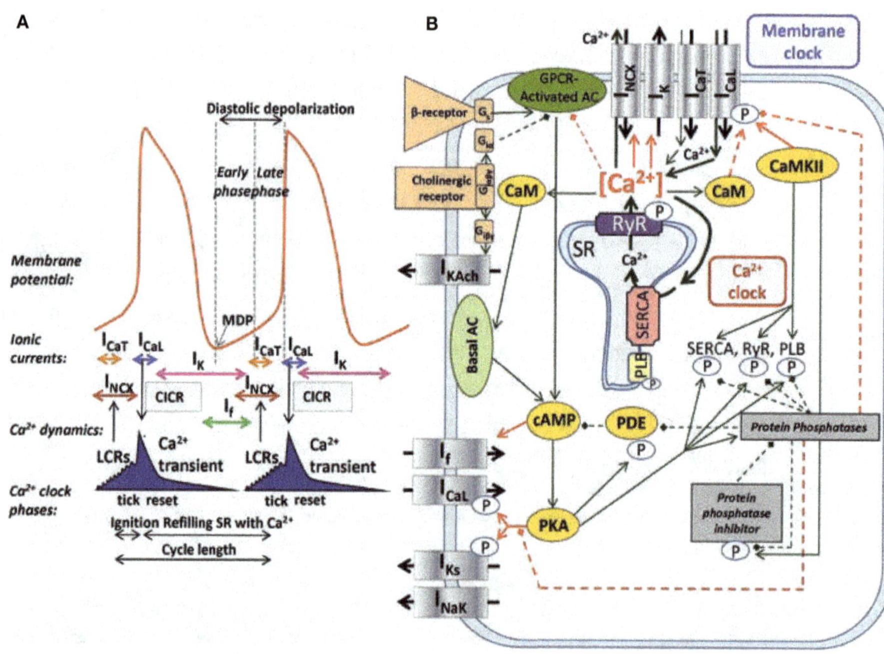

FIGURE 1 | The coupled-clock pacemaker system of the sinoatrial node. Schematic illustration of the currents and functional interactions between the two oscillator subsystem contributing to the SN AP **(A)**. The interplay of the regulatory molecules comprising the coupled-clock pacemaker system is illustrated in **(B)**. Membrane clock (M-clock) of sinoatrial node pacemaker cells comprises the major surface membrane currents: L-type Ca^{2+} channels (I_{CaL}), T-type Ca^{2+} channels (I_{CaT}), delayed rectifier K^+ channels (I_K), hyperpolarization activated funny channels (I_f), Na^+/Ca^{2+}exchanger (NCX), and Na^+/K^+ ATPase (I_{NaK}). Regulatory factors that affect the function of proteins of both clocks are indicated with different colors: molecules with red letters couple the Ca^{2+} clock to the M-clock; factors in orange regulate both the M-clock and Ca^{2+} clock *via* the GPCR pathway. Interrupted lines refer to inhibitory effects. AC, adenylate-cyclase; CaM, calmodulin; cAMP, cyclic adenosine monophosphate; CaMKII, Ca^{2+}/calmodulin-dependent protein kinase II; GPCR, G-protein coupled receptor; PDE, phosphodiesterase; PKA, protein kinase A; PLB, phospholamban; RyR, ryanodine receptor; SERCA, sarcoplasmic reticulum Ca^{2+} ATPase 2a.

and at least temporarily, this mechanism can operate independently of the M-clock, therefore it was termed as "Ca^{2+}-clock" (Maltsev et al., 2006). Many of the effects of the LCRs can be represented by their influence on the Ca^{2+} concentrations in the different compartments of the cell as done in most computational models of SNCs. After intense and long debate, several studies provided evidence that the M-clock and Ca^{2+}-clock are functionally coupled, converging to the concept of a coupled-clock system (**Figure 1B**). The coupling is based on numerous voltage-, time- and Ca^{2+}-dependent mechanisms (Maltsev and Lakatta, 2009; Lakatta et al., 2010) including an important role of the L-type Ca^{2+} current that "resets" and "refuels" the Ca^{2+}-clock (Maltsev and Lakatta, 2009) (**Figure 1**). Both I_{CaL} and NCX have important roles in the two clock-like subsystems, *i.e.* they contribute to both the membrane voltage-clock and the Ca^{2+}-clock (**Figure 1B**).

THE ROLE OF NCX IN THE Ca^{2+} FLUX BALANCE

Na^+/Ca^{2+} exchangers were identified as members of the Ca^{2+}/cation antiporters (CaCA) superfamily, as the exchanger carries three Na^+ in exchange for one Ca^{2+}. Thus, the exchanger is electrogenic and affects the transmembrane voltage. The first data regarding the exchange ratio of NCX was published by Reuter and Seitz describing the Na^+/Ca^{2+} exchange as neutral, *i.e.*, changing two Na^+ ions for one Ca^{2+} (Reuter and Seitz, 1968). Later, in squid axon experiments, it became clear that the NCX function is electrogenic, with a suggested stoichiometry of 4:1 (Mullins and Requena, 1979). Chapman and Tunstall (1980) suggested a 3:1 ratio in the heart muscle (Chapman and Tunstall, 1980). Nowadays, the 3:1 Na^+/Ca^{2+} stoichiometry is clearly supported by several experimental studies and generally accepted as the functional exchanger ratio (Bers and Ginsburg, 2007). The electrogenic operation of the Na^+/Ca^{2+} exchanger results in an ion current with one net elementary charge in each transport cycle. The mode in which the exchanger operates is defined by the relationship of V_m and the NCX equilibrium potential (E_{NCX}), where E_{NCX} is determined by the transmembrane Na^+ and Ca^{2+} gradients ($E_{NCX} = 3E_{Na} - 2E_{Ca}$). When the difference between V_m and the equilibrium potential is positive, the exchanger acts in the reverse mode; however Ca^{2+} extrusion is favored when V_m is more negative than the equilibrium potential (Bers, 2002). Depending on the mode of action (forward *vs.* reverse), the Na^+/Ca^{2+} exchanger can generate either inward or outward current, it can depolarize or repolarize the cell membrane, respectively.

The activity of the exchanger has complex intra- and extracellular regulatory molecules: Among the *intracellular factors*, the $Ca^{2+}{}_i$, ATP, phosphatidylinositol-di-phosphate-2 (PIP_2), NO and *extracellular factors* such as monovalent cations, PKC activators, and agents that induce proteolysis or protein phosphorylation can activate the exchanger (Ballard and Schaffer, 1996; Bers, 2001; Bers, 2008). Other *intracellular factors* like $Na^+{}_i$, H^+, bivalent and trivalent cations, and protein dephosphorylation are inhibitory factors of NCX function (Ballard and Schaffer, 1996; Bers, 2001; Bers, 2008). Modulatory proteins of NCX are PKA, PKC, PP1, and PP2A (Ballard and Schaffer, 1996; Bers, 2001; Bers, 2008). Based on previous experimental results, the modulatory effect of the cAMP-PKA pathway on the NCX function is controversial. Several studies have shown PKA-related activation of the Na^+/Ca^{2+} exchanger with forskolin and isoproterenol (Iwamoto et al., 1995; Iwamoto et al., 1996; Iwamoto et al., 1998); however, other studies do not demonstrate such effects. Latest studies concluded that the NCX function is not modified by PKA activation (Ginsburg and Bers, 2005).

Three mammalian NCX isoforms have been identified: NCX1 is expressed in the heart, kidney, and brain, having the most extended spectrum of expression among the isoforms, NCX2 is present in the brain, and NCX3 is expressed in the brain and skeletal muscle (Nicoll et al., 1990; Reilly and Shugrue, 1992; Kofuji et al., 1994; Li et al., 1994; Nicoll et al., 1996).

PHARMACOLOGY OF THE Na^+/Ca^{2+} EXCHANGER

Since NCX plays a crucial role under physiological circumstances in the maintenance of Ca^{2+} flux balance and SN pacemaking as well as in pathological settings, *e.g.*, in arrhythmia generation (delayed afterdepolarizations, Ca^{2+} overload), selective inhibition of the exchanger became one of the most intensive research areas demanding the development of properly selective agents. In this chapter, we summarize the NCX inhibitors from the early nonspecific substances to novel, highly selective agents.

Nonspecific Inhibitory Substances

Divalent (Co^{2+}, Sr^{2+}, Mg^{2+}, Cd^{2+}, Ba^{2+}, Mn^{2+}) and trivalent (La^{3+}, Nd^{3+}, Tm^{3+}, Y^{3+}) cations have a nonspecific inhibitory effect on the NCX current (Wakabayashi and Goshima, 1981; Trosper and Philipson, 1983) resulting from direct action on the NCX1 isoform or by replacing Ca^{2+} ions at the transport sites. It is important to note that these cations are nonselective blockers, even the most commonly used Ni^{2+} has nonspecific effects. Ni^{2+} is used in concentrations between 1 and 10 mM and inhibits the reverse mode rather than the forward mode of NCX.

"Selective" Benzyloxyphenyl Derivative Inhibitors

Some benzyloxyphenyl derivatives such as KB-R7943 (2-[2-[4-(4-nitrobenzyl-oxy)phenyl]ethyl]isothio-urea-methanesulfonate, carbamidothioic acid) were developed as novel NCX inhibitors with promising blocking potency; however experimental studies reported that KB-R7943 exerts complex nonspecific effects on other transmembrane ion currents including I_{CaL}, I_{Na}, I_{Kr}. The IC_{50} values of KB-R7943 are 3.35 ± 0.82 μM on the forward mode and 4.74 ± 0.69 μM on the reverse mode (Birinyi et al., 2005). SEA-0400 (2-(4-(2,5-difluorobenzyloxy)phenoxy)-5-ethoxy aniline) has improved selectivity compared to KB-R7943. However, an I_{CaL} inhibition of approximately 20% was reported (Birinyi et al., 2005). The reverse and forward modes were equally inhibited, having IC_{50} values of 108 ± 18 nM and 111 ± 43 nM, respectively (Birinyi et al., 2005).

Novel NCX Inhibitors With Increased Selectivity

Due to the lack of selective NCX inhibitors, the exact role of the exchanger in SN pacemaking, cardiac arrhythmogenesis, and Ca^{2+}-handling could not be investigated directly. Efforts were made continuously to develop a potent, selective inhibitor to clarify the role of this highly complex transport system in cardiac function. Recently, two novel NCX blocking compounds were identified: ORM-10103 and ORM-10962. The selectivity of both agents was intensively tested by (Jost et al., 2013) and (Kohajda et al., 2016). While ORM-10103 has improved selectivity compared to previous blockers, it still exhibits minor nonspecific effects of inhibiting I_{Kr} at 3 μM. The estimated EC_{50} values of ORM-10103 at 1 μM concentration for the forward and reverse modes of the NCX are 800 and 960 nM, respectively. In contrast, the EC_{50} values of ORM-10962 on the inward and outward NCX current are 55 and 67 nM, respectively. The inhibitory effect of ORM-10962 is highly selective with high efficacy on the NCX current and no effect on the L-type Ca^{2+} current, peak and late sodium current, sodium-potassium pump, and all the repolarizing potassium currents (I_{Kr}, I_{Ks}, I_{to} (transient outward potassium current), I_{K1} (inward rectifier potassium current)) (Kohajda et al., 2016). The effect of selective NCX-inhibition on SN pacemaking by using 1 μM ORM-10962 was also investigated recently (Kohajda et al., 2020).

NCX Activators

Probably the most important activating factor for NCX is Ca^{2+} itself. The activation is strongly promoted by elevated Na^+_i and increased by higher pacing frequency (Ginsburg et al., 2013). Pharmacological selective activation of the forward NCX mode is expected to facilitate Ca^{2+} extrusion. The utility of a possible NCX activator compound is controversial, since the facilitation of the forward NCX function could be useful under Ca^{2+} overload; however the arrhythmogenic inward current would also be increased, especially in ventricular cells. A possible increase of the reverse mode, at the same time, could largely modulate this effect. In SNCs, activation of the forward NCX mode may accelerate the firing rate without β-adrenergic activation and may decrease intracellular Ca^{2+}. However, currently there is no selective NCX activator compound available. Li^+ is known to stimulate NCX, but its effect on NCX1 is markedly smaller than on NCX2 and NCX3 (Nicoll et al., 1990; Iwamoto et al., 1998). Several papers also claimed that NCX1 is sensitive to redox agents (Reeves et al., 1986) (Amoroso et al., 2000; Santacruz-Toloza et al., 2000). A combination of a reductant (GSH, DTT, Fe^{2+}) and an oxidant (Fe^{3+}, H_2O_2) factor is required to enhance NCX. Diethylpyrocarbonate increased Na^+-dependent Ca^{2+} uptake (Ottolia et al., 2002). Several peptides (concanavalin-A and insulin) were also shown to activate the exchanger (Gupta et al., 1986; Makino et al., 1988).

DISCOVERY AND CHARACTERIZATION OF THE ROLE OF NCX IN SN PACEMAKING

Pioneer Studies Regarding the Role of NCX in SN Pacemaking

The first experimental results regarding NCX function in SNCs were published by Brown et al. (Brown et al., 1984). They suggested that the slow inward current is composed of two different types of inward currents: a fast component, which they attributed to a channel-gated mechanism ($I_{Ca,f}$) and a slow component: NCX triggered by the release of stored intracellular Ca^{2+} (I_{NaCa}). Satoh et al. (Satoh, 1993) provided experimental evidence that caffeine applied in the bath solution at concentrations of 1 to 10 mM caused a frequency decrease and arrhythmias in isolated rabbit cells. This work did not discuss the ionic currents (*e.g.*, NCX) in detail but demonstrated that cellular Ca^{2+} overload was induced during exposure of SNCs to caffeine (Satoh, 1993). However, considering the complex effects of caffeine especially if it is applied in the bath solution makes the interpretation extremely difficult. In the same year, Zhou and Lipsius strengthened the initial suggestions of NCX's role in SN automaticity by using latent pacemaker cells isolated from cat atrium (Zhou and Lipsius, 1993). They demonstrated that 1 μM ryanodine notably decreased the spontaneous pacemaking activity but did not stop automaticity, which led to the conclusion that a ryanodine sensitive component contributes to but is not essential for pacemaking. In line with these results, Rigg and Terrar (1996) found that 2 μM ryanodine and 100 μM CPA applied to guinea pig SNCs substantially decreased the spontaneous firing rate (29 ± 2% and 37 ± 6% respectively). They concluded that both agents markedly reduce the transient amplitude and the diastolic Ca^{2+} levels causing various changes in the Ca^{2+} dependent mechanisms and could affect the contribution of NCX. Similar conclusions were drawn one year later by Li et al. (1997) using ryanodine on rabbit isolated SNCs.

The first computational pacemaking model of mammalian SNCs including NCX was proposed by Noble and; Noble (1984) and later extended by Wilders et al. (1991) (Noble and Noble, 1984; Wilders et al., 1991). Another early SN model comprising NCX was proposed by Rasmusson et al. in 1990 (Rasmusson et al., 1990) for bullfrog SNCs. However, in their model parametrization, NCX was small and while modulating the MDP, it had little influence on the AP, which they attributed to Ca^{2+} buffering by myoplasmic proteins. In contrast, the Demir et al. (1994) rabbit model comprised a larger inward NCX (peak −96 pA) during the first third of the pacemaker potential, which then declined slowly through the remainder of the cycle (Demir et al., 1994). The model by Dokos et al. (1996) was mainly driven by an inward background Na^+ current (Dokos et al., 1996). Upon complete block of their NCX formulation, which reproduced the saturation characteristics at high Ca^{2+}_i and negative potential low Ca^{2+}_i, automaticity ceased. The Dokos et al. NCX formulation was later on integrated in a rabbit SNC model by Kurata et al. (2002) in which it contributed significantly to DD (Kurata et al., 2002). However,

NCX current amplitude decreases during DD in the Kurata et al. model (**Figure 2E**) in contrast to later models introduced below [*e.g.*, (Maltsev and Lakatta, 2009)] where I_{NaCa} increases before I_{CaL} is strongly activated. The NCX time course during the spontaneous APs of different early SNC models is shown in **Figure 2**. For the models available in the CellML repository, **Figure 2** also shows their response to complete NCX block (red lines). The Demir et al. model exhibited CLs as during control after 5 s, *i.e.*, continued to spontaneously generate APs in the absence of NCX (data not shown), the Dokos et al. and Kurata et al. models did not exhibit sustained pacemaking behavior upon complete NCX block. The effect of clamping the intracellular (and in the Kurata et al. model also the subspace) Ca^{2+} concentration to the initial value (*i.e.*, value during early DD) is shown in **Figure 2** as well (yellow lines). Under these conditions, pacemaking ceased in the Dokos et al. model; the CL was shortened in the Demir et al. model, whereas it was prolonged in the Kurata et al. model. **Table 1** compares all SN models comprising a NCX formulation mentioned in this paper. Almost all NCX formulations originate from either DiFrancesco and Noble (1985) or Matsuoka and Hilgemann (1992).

In 1998, Ju and Allen (1998) studied the potential role of Ca_i^{2+}-dynamics in the spontaneous firing rate of APs in sinus venosus of cane toad and provided quantitative data regarding the magnitude of the NCX current during the SN AP. They measured 20–27 pA NCX current in early diastole ($Ca^{2+}{}_i$: 250–300 nM) and 12 pA ($Ca^{2+}{}_i$: 200 nM) in late diastole in toad isolated sinus venosus cells. The authors emphasized that the net inward current (*i.e.*, total current) required during DD to generate a pacemaker potential is less than 1 pA (DiFrancesco, 1993):

$$I = C_m \cdot \frac{dV_m}{dt} = 0.02\frac{V}{s} \cdot 35\ pF = 0.7\ pA \quad (1)$$

Therefore, quite small relative changes of NCX current (as a response of $Ca^{2+}{}_i$ change) can cause substantial changes in the firing rate. Hagiwara and Irisawa (1989) reported 1 pA/pF NCX current density at V_m of −40 mV in the presence of 500 nM $Ca^{2+}{}_i$ (Hagiwara and Irisawa, 1989). Wilders et al. (1991), in a numerical model, demonstrated that the NCX current had an amplitude of 0.64 pA/pF under similar conditions (Wilders et al., 1991). However, one should keep in mind that the absolute value of NCX current amplitude *per se* does not exclusively define the contribution of the exchanger to DD. The current integral, *i.e.* the total charge transferred through the membrane and its relation to other, concurrently active currents, determines the role for pacemaking, meaning that larger NCX current amplitude does not necessarily imply larger contribution (*cf.* **Figure 3**).

Ju and Allen (1998) also reported that BAPTA and ryanodine (2 μM) caused frequency reduction until the cells stopped beating. However, this happened after 30 min when other nonspecific actions and spontaneous current decline could not be ruled out. They also demonstrated that decrease of external Na^+ caused a rise of $Ca^{2+}{}_i$ due to reverse mode NCX. Application of Na^+-free solution resulted in a rapid rise in $Ca^{2+}{}_i$ that exceeded the preceding systolic $Ca^{2+}{}_i$ level. This rapid rise of $Ca^{2+}{}_i$ and the generation of an inward current when intracellular $[Ca^{2+}]$ is elevated are characteristics of the activation of Na^+/Ca^{2+} exchange (Allen et al., 1983; Ju and Allen, 1998). The authors also demonstrated that the exchanger current seemed to be close to a linear function of $Ca^{2+}{}_i$. *Bufo marinus* pacemaker cells do

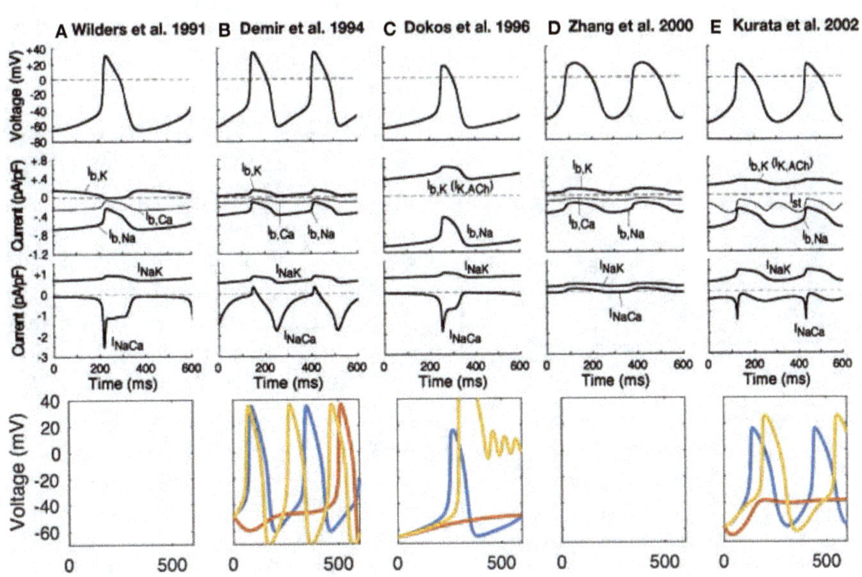

FIGURE 2 | Time-independent background and transporter currents including NCX during spontaneous pacemaking in early SN models: (Wilders et al., 1991) **(A)**, (Demir et al., 1994) **(B)**, (Dokos et al., 1996) **(C)**, (Zhang et al., 2000) [**(D)**; central model], and (Kurata et al., 2002) **(E)**. Top 3 rows reproduced from Kurata et al. (2002) with permission. Bottom row: effect of complete NCX block (red line) and clamping intracellular Ca^{2+} to the initial value (yellow line). As the Kurata et al. model comprised a separate subspace Ca^{2+} concentration, this was clamped as well. The Wilders et al. model was not available in the CellML repository, the Zhang model did not exhibit sustained pacemaking behavior in the version deposited in the CellML repository.

TABLE 1 | Comparison of model features for the 21 SNC models described in this review. Only studies that introduced new models or markedly advanced existing models are listed.

Model	Species	NCX formulation	Dynamic intracellular sodium/calcium concentrations	Separate subscarcolemmal space formulation	I_f	I_{Ks}
Noble and Noble, 1984	mammalian	DiFrancesco and Noble, 1985	no/yes	no	yes	no
Rasmusson et al., 1990	bullfrog	Fischmeister and Vassort, 1981	yes/yes	yes	no	no
Wilders et al., 1991	rabbit	Noble and Noble, 1984	yes/yes	no	yes	no
Demir et al., 1994	rabbit	DiFrancesco and Noble, 1985	yes/yes	yes	yes	no
Dokos et al., 1996	mammalian	Matsuoka and Hilgemann, 1992	yes/yes	no	yes	no
Zhang et al., 2000	rabbit	Demir et al., 1994	no/no	no	yes	yes
Kurata et al., 2002	rabbit	Dokos et al., 1996	yes/yes	yes	yes	yes
Garny et al., 2003	rabbit	Zhang et al., 2000	no/no	no	yes	yes
Silva and Rudy, 2003	derived from guinea pig ventricular cells	Luo and Rudy, 1994	yes/yes	no	no	no
Maltsev et al., 2004	rabbit	Kurata et al., 2002	yes/yes	yes	yes	yes
Kurata et al., 2005	derived from human ventricular cells	Priebe and Beuckelmann, 1998	yes/yes	no	no	yes
Maltsev and Lakatta, 2009	rabbit	Kurata et al., 2002	no/yes	yes	yes	no
Chandler et al., 2009	human	Courtemanche et al., 1998	yes/yes	no	yes	yes
Imtiaz et al., 2010	rabbit	Kurata et al., 2002	yes/yes	yes	yes	yes
Kharche et al., 2011	mouse	Kurata et al., 2002	yes/yes	yes	yes	yes
Severi et al., 2012	rabbit	Kurata et al., 2002	yes/yes	yes	yes	yes
Maltsev and Lakatta, 2013	rabbit/human-like	Maltsev and Lakatta, 2009	no/yes	yes	yes	no
Yaniv et al., 2013b	rabbit	Maltsev and Lakatta, 2009	no/yes	yes	yes	no
Stern et al., 2014	rabbit	Maltsev and Lakatta, 2009	no/yes	3D	yes	no
Fabbri et al., 2017	human	Severi et al., 2012	no/yes	yes	yes	yes
Lyashkov et al., 2018	rabbit	Maltsev and Lakatta, 2009	no/yes	yes	yes	yes

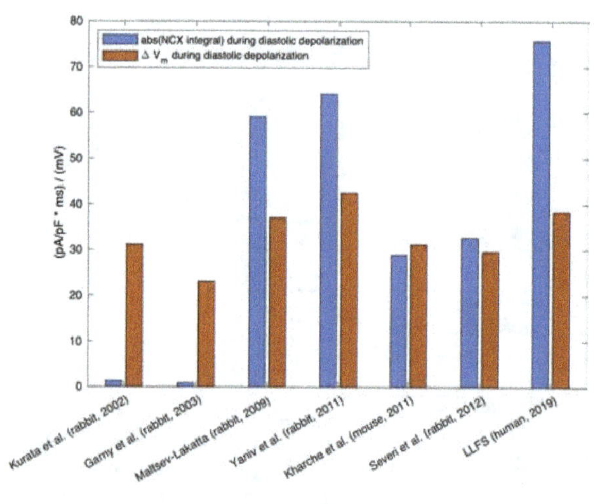

FIGURE 3 | Absolute value of the integral of signed NCX during the DD (MDP to AP takeoff) (blue, unit: ms * pA/pF ≡ mV), in relation to the difference in maximum diastolic V_m and takeoff potential for computational models of different species: rabbit (Kurata et al., 2002; Garny et al., 2003; Maltsev and Lakatta, 2009; Yaniv et al., 2011; Severi et al., 2012), mouse (Kharche et al., 2011), and the human Loewe–Lutz–Fabbri–Severi (LLFS) model (Loewe et al., 2019a; Loewe et al., 2019b).

not contain any I_f (Ju et al., 1995). Therefore, I_f decrease can be ruled out as a contamination of the experiments. They conclude that NCX has a crucial role in setting the resting heart rate, and the actual level of $Ca^{2+}{}_i$ has great importance for indirectly setting the AP firing rate.

Discovery and Characterization of Local Ca^{2+} Release (LCR) Events: The Role of NCX in SN Automaticity

A seminal study was published by Huser et al. in 2000 (Huser et al., 2000). By using voltage clamp and confocal fluorescence microscopy in cat atrial spontaneously beating cells, they discovered an increase of $Ca^{2+}{}_i$ in the last third of DD just before the action potential depolarization, due to local release of Ca^{2+} from the SR. As small dose (25–50 μM) of $NiCl_2$ suppressed the local release, thus they suggested the T-type Ca^{2+} channels triggered subsarcolemmal Ca^{2+} sparks, which in turn stimulated the inward NCX to depolarize the pacemaker potential to threshold.

One year later, the Lakatta group (Bogdanov et al., 2001) further analyzed the spontaneous Ca^{2+} releases (local Ca^{2+} releases, LCR, **Figure 4**) in isolated rabbit sinoatrial cells. Their findings indicate that the pre-AP releases are locally propagating Ca^{2+} waves, resulting from ryanodine-sensitive Ca^{2+}-induced

Ca^{2+} release (CICR). In turn, the negative chronotropic effect of ryanodine is the result of disappearance of localized pre-AP Ca^{2+} releases. Substituting Na^+ for Li^+ to inhibit NCX caused sinus arrest leading to the conclusion that Ca^{2+} release-NCX cross-talk has crucial importance in pacemaking. The authors provided a possible scenario for the current interactions underlying spontaneous automaticity: after reaching the maximal diastolic potential, I_f activates to depolarize the membrane and activates I_{CaT} and I_{CaL} causing LCR from the SR, which in turn activates NCX and the inward current augments to activate the remaining L-type Ca^{2+} channels. These results were interpreted such that SR Ca^{2+} release has a pivotal impact in defining the actual firing rate and inactivation of either the RyR or NCX activity lead to frequency slowing or abolishment.

The pivotal role of the strong interaction between the Ca^{2+} concentration in the subspace and V_m *via* NCX for spontaneous depolarizations in SNCs was numerically reproduced and mechanistically underpinned by Maltsev et al. (2004) in a biophysical modeling study in 2004 based on an extension of the Kurata et al. (2002) model (Kurata et al., 2002). In 2009, Maltsev and Lakatta proposed a coupled oscillator model incorporating aspects of both a membrane and a Ca^{2+} clock, which yielded rhythmic spontaneous depolarization over a wider range of parameters of the currents involved in the M-clock (I_{CaL}, I_f) (Maltsev and Lakatta, 2009). By modulating SR Ca^{2+} pumping rate, the coupled-clock yielded robust pacemaking in the range of 1.8 to 4.6 Hz, which is wider than could be achieved by modulation of M-clock properties alone. Kurata et al. (2012) performed stability and bifurcation analyses on this coupled-clock model and found that the most important model parameters for generation of cyclic depolarization (equilibrium point instability) are the SR Ca^{2+} pumping rate, NCX density as well as I_{CaL} conductance (Kurata et al., 2012). However, the model system does not exhibit cyclic intracellular Ca^{2+} oscillations when V_m is clamped (independent of the clamped value), *i.e.*, arguing against an independent Ca^{2+} clock, thus underlining the coupled nature of the pacemaking mechanism. In line with this finding, Maltsev and Lakatta (2009) observed damped oscillations when clamping the transmembrane voltage to −65 mV (at P_{up} = 20 mM/s) (Maltsev and Lakatta, 2009). However, sustained oscillations were observed at P_{up} = 40 mM/s. The NCX was a major contributor to the observed equilibrium point in the study by Kurata et al. (2012).

Vinogradova et al. explored in 2004 whether the LCRs require previous membrane depolarization as was suggested so far (Vinogradova et al., 2004). Experimental measurements on isolated rabbit SNCs as well as numerical modeling revealed three findings i) the LCRs during the DD do not require previous membrane depolarization; ii) the LCRs are rhythmic and generate rhythmic inward current movements; iii) the LCR periods are highly correlated with the spontaneous CLs.

In contrast to the increasing body of evidence, Sanders et al. claimed in 2006 that the contribution of NCX to spontaneous depolarization does not exclusively depend on the intact SR function in guinea pig SNCs (Sanders et al., 2006). They demonstrated that low Na^+ solution abolished spontaneous firing in the presence of CPA, an inhibitor of SR uptake. On the other hand, if NCX would be entirely a consequence of SR Ca^{2+} release, the CPA should have a similar effect as a low Na^+ solution. However, the SR inhibition only slowed the heart rate, while low Na^+ abolished spontaneous pacemaking within one beat, with concomitant decrease of $Ca^{2+}{}_i$. However, considering

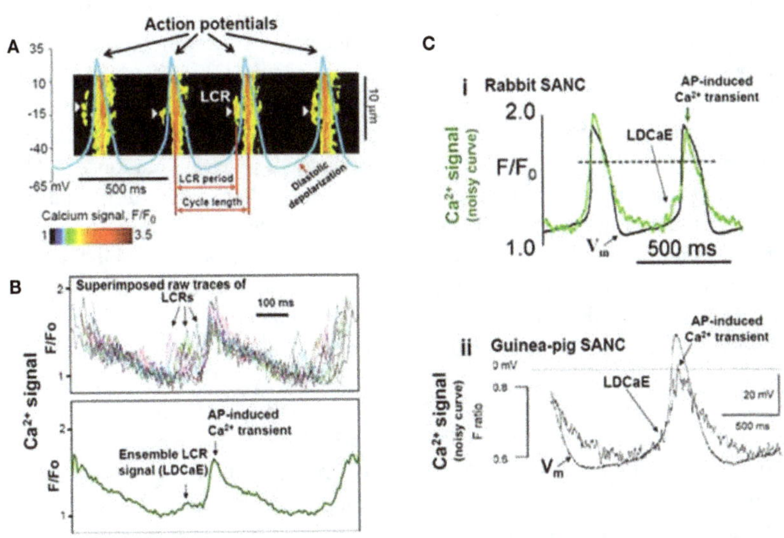

FIGURE 4 | Confocal line scanning image of Ca^{2+}-signal with superimposed spontaneous AP traces recorded in rabbit SNCs show DD, distribution of LCRs (white arrows), LCR period, and CL **(A)**. Confocal microscopic image of LCRs are depicted in [**(B)**, upper panel], ensemble LCR signal or Late Diastolic Ca^{2+} Elevation (LDCaE) that precedes Ca^{2+}-transient are created from temporal average of LCRs [**(B)**, lower panel]. LDCaE in single SNC of rabbit [**(C)**, panel i] and guinea-pig [**(C)**, panel ii] is shown. LCR: local Ca^{2+} release. From (Maltsev et al., 2014) with permission.

the rather complex effects of reduced Na^+ solution, the results could not unequivocally support the authors' hypothesis. The application of KB-R7943 to inhibit NCX has to be considered problematic because of its nonselectivity.

Using high-speed Ca^{2+} imaging, Yaniv et al. (2013) could show that the coupled clocks also control beat-to-beat regulation of the spontaneous beating rate (Yaniv et al., 2013b). Acute application of low concentrations of caffeine (2 to 4 mM) caused Ca^{2+} release from the SR and subsequently led to increased spontaneous beating rates *via* membrane depolarization caused by increased NCX activation. This effect could be reproduced mechanistically in an extended version of the Maltsev–Lakatta computational model (Yaniv et al., 2013b). Toward this end, Severi et al. (2012) proposed an update of the Maltsev–Lakatta rabbit SNC model incorporating a coupled-clock with Ca^{2+}-handling (including NCX) and refined current formulations based on more recent experimental data (Severi et al., 2012). On the other hand, the Severi et al. model could not predict the effect of acute caffeine injection described above and complete block of I_f lead to cessation of spontaneous activity. Simulations including the effects of 1 μM isoproterenol [causing, among other, a 25% increase of SR Ca^{2+} pumping as in Maltsev and Lakatta (2010) (Maltsev and Lakatta, 2010)], yielded a 28.2% rate increase in the Severi et al. model in good agreement with the experimentally observed increase of 26.3 ± 5.4% by Bucchi et al. (2007b).

In 2013, Sirenko et al. confirmed the presence of LCR in SNCs (Sirenko et al., 2013). The authors compared the spontaneous Ca^{2+} releases in permeabilized (*i.e.*, in the absence of functional ion channels) rabbit SN *vs.* ventricular cells. They found that in the presence of similar physiological Ca^{2+} concentrations, the SNCs generate large rhythmic spontaneous Ca^{2+} releases in contrast to ventricular cells in which they found Ca^{2+} sparks with small amplitude and stochastic nature, as was originally described (Cheng et al., 1993). This ability of SNCs was associated with more abundant SERCA, reduced extent of phospholamban (PLB), and increased Ca^{2+}-dependent phosphorylation of PLB and RyR.

In 2013, Yaniv et al. found new evidence regarding the membrane and Ca^{2+} clock coupling (Yaniv et al., 2013a). Application of the I_f-inhibitor ivabradine (3 μM) reduced the AP firing rate, partially by inhibiting I_f and by decreasing the SR Ca^{2+} content in isolated SNCs. This means that despite the fact that ivabradine has no direct effect on intracellular Ca^{2+} cycling and does not exert effects on surface membrane channels other than I_f, it still suppresses the SR Ca^{2+} load and the LCR events. These novel findings further supported the hypothesis that cross-talk between the membrane and Ca^{2+} clock regulates SN automaticity.

Sirenko et al. (2016) analyzed in detail the electrochemical Na^+/Ca^{2+} gradients in the pacemaker function of the NCX (Sirenko et al., 2016). They used a combination of numerical modeling and experimental rabbit approaches (by using the Na/K inhibitor digoxigenin) to determine how the coupling of Na^+ and Ca^{2+} electrochemical gradients regulates pacemaking. Minimal increase of Na^+_i (5%) enhanced the LCRs, shortened the CL, which was interpreted as an extension of normal chronotropic response. Further increase of Na^+_i by up to 15 mM caused reduction of LCRs, large CL variability as a consequence of V_m-Ca^{2+} clock uncoupling. In parallel with the biphasic CL changes, the NCX current also showed biphasic alterations: initially the I_{NCX} increased due to the high amplitude LCRs, then declined as E_{NCX} reduced. The authors claimed that E_{Na}, E_{Ca}, and E_{NCX} tightly regulate the SN automaticity *via* influencing several ion channels and components of the SN clocks.

Stern et al. (2014) proposed a computational model with subcellular spatial resolution that allows studying intracellular Ca^{2+} release propagation patterns that was employed in Maltsev et al. (2017) to classify LCRs and provide insight into mechanisms increasing robustness of pacemaking at various SERCA pumping rates. Consistent with previous studies, they found a major role of NCX in the fight-or-flight response: faster SR Ca^{2+} pumping prepared the cell for stronger (higher amplitude) and more synchronous LCRs (more subcellular Ca^{2+} wave collisions) in the next cycle, which elicited a higher NCX current.

Torrente et al. in 2016 studied the role of the predominant isoform of L-type Ca^{2+} channels ($Ca_v1.3$) in the generation of the LCRs and Ca^{2+}_i dynamics in SNCs from wild-type and $Ca_v1.3$ knockout mice (Torrente et al., 2016). This work challenged the results of previous experimental work (under voltage-clamp conditions with V_m below the activation of $Ca_v1.3$ (Vinogradova et al., 2004) and in membrane-permeabilized SNCs, without the influence of any plasma membrane ion channels (Sirenko et al., 2013) claiming that LCRs are clearly spontaneous in nature and entirely independent from the M-clock. $Ca_v1.3$ deficiency significantly impaired Ca^{2+}_i dynamics by reducing the frequency of LCR events and preventing synchronization. The results of Torrente et al. suggest that the local increase of Ca^{2+}_i generated by $Ca_v1.3$ Ca^{2+} current induces RyR opening, thus supporting the coupling between membrane depolarization and SR Ca^{2+} release. Thus $Ca_v1.3$ channels can be inducers of LCR generation in the late DD. Considering this mechanism, $Ca_v1.3$ could stimulate the NCX-mediated depolarizing current to reach the threshold potential necessary to trigger an AP. Although LCRs are likely triggered by $Ca_v1.3$-mediated I_{CaL} release in mouse SNCs (Torrente et al., 2016), LCR generation has different mechanisms in pacemaker cells of various species. As mentioned before, Vinogradova et al. showed that LCRs in rabbit SNCs do not require a change of V_m (Vinogradova et al., 2004). Instead, LCRs are spontaneous in nature and occur in permeabilized SNCs. Takimoto et al. showed that the α_{1D} Ca^{2+} channel mRNA is expressed in rat atrium (Takimoto et al., 1997). This observation was confirmed in mouse and human cells by Mangoni et al. (Mangoni et al., 2003). However, it remains unclear whether α_{1D} Ca^{2+} channels are present and functional in rabbit SNCs since expression at the protein level has not been verified (Qu et al., 2005).

Huser et al. found that T-type Ca^{2+} channels can also have a role in the generation of LCRs since in cat atrial pacemaker cells, LCRs are triggered by voltage-dependent activation of T-type Ca^{2+} channels (Huser et al., 2000).

The Role of Phosphorylation in SN Pacemaking and the Fight-or-Flight Response

A crucial feature of the SN is the capability of adapting the firing rate to the momentary requirements of the body. β-adrenergic activation stimulates the cAMP-PKA cascade and phosphorylates several components of the Ca^{2+} handling machinery and transmembrane ion channels. As a consequence, higher frequency and magnitude of LCRs provide enhanced drive for NCX, thus accelerating DD (Vinogradova et al., 2005; Vinogradova and Lakatta, 2009).

CaMKII

In 2000, Vinogradova et al. reported a crucial role of CaMKII in SN pacemaking (Vinogradova et al., 2000). Selective inhibition of CaMKII activity (by autocamtide 2-inhibitory peptide, and KN-93/KN-92) reduced the pacemaker frequency in rabbit SNCs, furthermore, larger doses of the compounds completely terminated SN automaticity. The authors also demonstrated that CaMKII activity is driven by subsarcolemmal Ca^{2+} movements and located in the vicinity of L-type Ca^{2+} channels. Therefore, the vital role of CaMKII could be based on the modulation of I_{CaL} *via* subsarcolemmal Ca^{2+} changes (Vinogradova et al., 2000).

In 2011, Gao and Anderson showed that CaMKII can support heart rate increase independent of β-adrenergic stimulation (Gao et al., 2011). Furthermore, CaMKII is required for β-adrenergic response and Ca^{2+}-based mechanism of pacemaking.

Li et al. demonstrated that CaMKII inhibition reduced phosphorylation of RyR and PLB, decreased the LCR size, and increased the LCR period (Li et al., 2016). As a consequence, SN firing rate was reduced. These results led the authors to the conclusion that high basal CaMKII activation ultimately regulates the pacemaker function *via* phosphorylation of Ca^{2+} handling proteins.

cAMP-PKA-PDE

The Lakatta group in 2008 demonstrated considerably high basal activity of phosphodiesterase (PDE) enzyme, which restricts local RyR Ca^{2+} release during DD *via* reduction of cAMP PKA-dependent protein phosphorylation to keep the basal spontaneous SNC firing under control (Vinogradova et al., 2008). Also in 2008, Younes et al. demonstrated in isolated SNCs that the adenylate-cyclase is activated in the entire physiological concentration range of intracellular Ca^{2+} and the cAMP-PKA axis activation drives SR Ca^{2+} release, which in turn activates AC (Younes et al., 2008). This feed-forward "fail-safe" system has a crucial role in maintaining the normal rhythm of SNCs.

In 2011, Liu et al. studied the role of the AC-cAMP-PKA-Ca^{2+} signaling cascade in mouse SNCs, and they demonstrated that the Ca^{2+} handling proteins are abundantly expressed, and LCRs were also detected in skinned cells. They showed that inhibition of intrinsic PKA activity reduces PLB phosphorylation and prolongs the LCR period causing reduction in the SNCs firing rate. The PDE inhibition resulted in the opposite effects: increased PLB phosphorylation, shortened LCR period, and accelerated firing. In the same study the authors also demonstrated that β-adrenergic activation requires intact Ca^{2+} handling, indicating a pivotal role of AC-cAMP-PKA-Ca^{2+} signaling cascade in maintaining the normal automaticity in mouse SNCs (Liu et al., 2011).

Vinogradova et al. provided data regarding the synergistic role of PDE3/PDE4 activity in rabbit SNCs in 2018. Individual inhibition of PDE3 or PDE4 caused a moderate increase in the beating rate (20 *vs.* 5%, respectively) (Vinogradova et al., 2018a). However, parallel block of both caused a 45% increase of pacemaking rate, indicating a synergistic effect. Furthermore, dual inhibition enhanced the LCR numbers and size, reduced the SR refilling time and LCR period due to decrease of cAMP/PKA phosphorylation (Vinogradova et al., 2018b). An amplification of local RyR Ca^{2+} release activates augmented NCX current at earlier times leading to an increase in the DD rate and spontaneous SANC beating rate. When RyRs were disabled by ryanodine, PDE inhibition failed to amplify local Ca^{2+} releases and increase NCX current. As a result, there was no increase in the DDR and spontaneous SN beating rate (Vinogradova et al., 2018b). In this context, Vinogradova et al. showed in the same year that PDE3/PDE4 modulation of SNCs is self-adaptive, *i.e.*, full functional effect is achieved only when both PDEs are inhibited. Such inhibition will lead to an elevation of the local level of cAMP and PKA phosphorylation. The authors claimed that local cAMP signals may have greater importance in the regulation of spontaneous automaticity in SNCs than the 'global cAMP' (Vinogradova et al., 2018a).

Autonomic Modulation

In 2002, Vinogradova et al. elucidated the Ca^{2+} release during DD as the specific link between β-adrenergic stimulation and increased firing rate in rabbit SNCs (Vinogradova et al., 2002). They demonstrated that 3 μM ryanodine abolished the effect of 0.1 μM isoproterenol. In the presence of ryanodine, the β-adrenergic stimulation failed to alter the slope of DD, firing rate, and subsarcolemmal Ca^{2+} releases, whereas the I_{CaL} amplitude exerted clear β-adrenergic stimulation-induced increase. In 2006, Bogdanov et al. described how application of agents affecting the timing or amplitude of LCRs (ryanodine, BAPTA, nifedipine or isoproterenol) caused immediate changes of spontaneous beating rate, which could be traced back to changes of local NCX using mechanistic computational modeling (Bogdanov et al., 2006). Similarly, PKA-dependent phosphorylation affected LCR spatiotemporal synchronization and therefore modulated beating rate mediated by altered NCX (Vinogradova et al., 2006).

Himeno et al. (2008) studied β1-adrenergic stimulation in a computational model of guinea pig SNCs with large I_{Ks} in which they described the role of NCX (Himeno et al., 2008). While activation of I_{Ks} during the AP preceding the β1-adrenergic stimulation was negligibly small, I_{Ks} counterbalanced the increase in I_{CaL} and NCX, which otherwise compromised the positive chronotropic effect of the β1-adrenergic stimulation by elongating the APD in their model.

Lyashkov et al. (2009) investigated the mechanism of muscarinic-receptor stimulation on heart rate reduction (Lyashkov et al., 2009). They found that carbachol (at IC_{50}) reduced the number and size of LCRs and lengthened the LCR period with concomitant decrease of the beating rate. Numerical modeling indicated that cholinergic-modulation of the beating rate is integrated into the Ca^{2+} cycling *via* LCR-mediated function of the NCX. The authors concluded that in the presence of low doses of carbachol, the muscarinic activation induced beating rate reduction is mediated by suppression of cAMP-PKA-Ca^{2+} signaling, while $I_{K(Ach)}$ activation contributes only under higher carbachol concentrations.

In the same year, Maltsev and Lakatta (2010) published a modeling study demonstrating how G protein-coupled receptor modulation of spontaneous SNC beating rate is not only mediated by effects on membrane currents but also by effects on the SR Ca^{2+} pumping rate, which in turn affect diastolic NCX (Maltsev and Lakatta, 2010). Also in 2010, Gao et al. demonstrated in healthy canine hearts that complete or almost complete I_f block attenuated but did not eliminate the positive chronotropy of isoproterenol suggesting that I_f is not the only target of the β-adrenergic response (Gao et al., 2010). Their results also support the notion of spontaneous Ca^{2+} releases during late DD, which was sensitive to isoproterenol. In their experiments, 2 μM ryanodine caused a 14% decrease in pacemaker frequency but dramatically decreased the effect of isoproterenol. They also provided evidence that ryanodine has no direct effect on I_f. The authors concluded that both voltage and Ca^{2+} dynamics have a role in the pacemaker mechanism.

In the same year, Vinogradova and Lakatta demonstrated that the LCR period and the spontaneous SN cycle is tightly regulated by the SR refilling time in rabbit SNCs (Vinogradova et al., 2010). Therefore, phosphorylation/dephosphorylation of the SERCA regulator protein PLB has also critical roles in setting the actual CL of the SN automaticity especially during β-adrenergic stimulation.

In a theoretical analysis of the relative importance of the membrane and Ca^{2+} oscillators, Imtiaz et al. (2010) could show that increased SR Ca^{2+} uptake leads to i) hyperpolarized MDP *via* a reduction of NCX due to lower $Ca^{2+}{}_i$ (Imtiaz et al., 2010). This means that due to lower Ca^{2+} the smaller inward current through NCX enables more negative MDP. ii) The more negative V_m increases the magnitude of I_f and I_{CaT} during early diastole. iii) The enhanced Ca^{2+} entry during DD increases intracellular Ca^{2+} and CICR causing a higher NCX current.

Transgenic Modifications of NCX

In 2013, several studies using transgenic NCX knockout mice were published. First, Gao et al. used cardiac specific, *incomplete* NCX1 knockout mice where the baseline sinus frequency was completely identical between control and NCX1-deleted mutants (Gao et al., 2013). However, they found that NCX1 deletion only partially impaired the isoproterenol effect indicating that I_f is also required. The authors concluded that the NCX has a minor role in maintaining the normal heart rate but NCX1 deletion dramatically enhanced the effects of ivabradine on isoproterenol-induced automaticity indicating that NCX and I_f mutually contribute in the fight-or-flight response. Since the genetic knockout of NCX was incomplete, one cannot rule out the possibility that the remaining NCX may be able to provide enough current to fulfill its role in maintaining the Ca^{2+} balance.

In response to that paper, Maltsev et al. in 2013 provided rabbit SN numerical simulations (Maltsev et al., 2013) to address some unanswered questions by Gao et al. (2013). The authors extended their simulation with new stabilization of NCX *via* local control of CICR. They argued that the Ca^{2+} released from the RyR is able to recruit the neighboring RyRs producing Ca^{2+} wavelets (LCRs) having amplitudes larger than the Ca^{2+} sparks and smaller than global Ca^{2+} transients. Since the NCX extrudes Ca^{2+} from the vicinity of RyRs it attenuates the spread of Ca^{2+} leading to weaker recruitment. However, when NCX is genetically decreased (*i.e.* incomplete NCX1 knockout), the Ca^{2+} spread and recruitment are enhanced providing larger Ca^{2+} and driving force for the remaining NCX molecules. These results indicate that NCX has a crucial role under the normal heart rate, and a small fraction (*i.e.* 20%) of NCX is able to produce sufficient current under DD. However, when NCX expression is low, its capacity is fully used for Ca^{2+} extrusion under rest and there is no more support for frequency increase under β-adrenergic response.

Herrmann et al. in 2013 used inducible and SN specific Cre transgenic mice lacking NCX1 selectively in SN pacemaking cells (Herrmann et al., 2013). The NCX1 was genetically ablated in a temporally controlled and tissue selective manner. The animals exerted severe bradycardia and large variability with arrhythmias leading to the conclusion that NCX has a role to maintain normal rhythm. The caffeine induced transient decay was markedly slowed (3.6% of control) in cpNCXKO cells indicating that in SNCs, almost the entire trans-sarcolemmal Ca^{2+} extrusion is carried by NCX. At the same time, it is an interesting finding that the Ca^{2+} transient amplitude was decreased and the decay was slowed while the SR Ca^{2+} content was unaffected. The authors claimed that the NCX1 deleted cells are not able to compensate the NCX1 deletion. They argue for a fundamental role of NCX in pacemaking even under resting conditions, and the normal pacemaking function is not possible without proper NCX function.

Groenke et al. found that in NCX1 knockout mice (Cre/LoxP system), there is no indication of spontaneous atrial depolarizations on the ECG and the animals exerted junctional escape rhythm (Groenke et al., 2013). Furthermore, isolated cells did not show spontaneous automaticity despite the presence of I_f and intact Ca^{2+} stores. They claim that NCX has a crucial role in normal pacemaking. They observed LCRs but no Ca^{2+} transients in NCX deleted cells. They also conclude that I_f is not sufficient to depolarize the cell membrane if NCX is completely lacking, interestingly not even if isoproterenol was added. Torrente et al. in 2015 created an atrial-specific NCX knockout mouse where NCX was totally eliminated from the atria including the SN (Torrente et al., 2015). These cells lacked spontaneous APs despite intact I_f. In contrast, the intact tissue showed spontaneous burst–pause type depolarizations. The authors conclude that in the absence of NCX-mediated depolarizations, I_{CaL} and I_f are able to initiate AP burst where Ca^{2+} is gradually accumulated and finally terminated burst activity *via* Ca^{2+}-dependent inactivation or by other Ca^{2+} activated processes such as small-conductance Ca^{2+}-activated K^+ currents (Torrente et al., 2017).

In 2016, Choi et al. observed regular oscillations of inward currents in voltage-clamped human embryonic stem cell-derived cardiomyocytes, which exhibit spontaneous APs when not being voltage clamped (Choi et al., 2016). The oscillatory Ca^{2+} releases could be eliminated by blocking NCX (with 1 μM SN-6 and 10 μM KB-R7943) but not by blocking I_f (with 3 mM ivabradine). Their observations suggest that in these hESC-CMs, the M-clock and the voltage clock act as two redundant pacemaker mechanisms which can work independently.

Kaese et al. (2017) used a homozygously overexpressed NCX mouse model and found that the basal heart rate is not affected, suggesting that NCX is not a crucial factor in setting the resting heart rate (Kaese et al., 2017). In contrast, β-adrenergic stimulation elicited higher heart rates in NCX-overexpressing mice, suggesting more inward NCX current which enhances the speed of DD.

Between 2003 and 2011 several genetically manipulated mice studies with deficient I_f function were published where autonomic rate modulation was preserved (Ludwig et al., 2003; Herrmann et al., 2007; Harzheim et al., 2008; Hoesl et al., 2008; Baruscotti et al., 2011). These results further indicate the lack of an essential and irreplaceable role of I_f in SN pacemaking and emphasize that I_f works together with its "teammates" within the coupled-clock system (Lakatta and Maltsev, 2012)

AP Ignition Model as the Most Current SN Pacemaking Mechanism

In 2018, a new model was proposed by the Lakatta group extending SN electrophysiology by an integrated regulatory mechanism including close interactions of LCRs, NCX, and I_{CaL} coupled by a positive feedback *via* diastolic CICR and DD acceleration (Lyashkov et al., 2018). In contrast to previous theories arguing for a role of LCRs during the late DD, the AP ignition model suggests that early LCRs (I_{CaL}-independent) activate inward NCX, which defines the ignition onset. I_f, and I_{CaT} also contribute to early depolarization to reach the I_{CaL} threshold. The physiological role of the low-voltage activation threshold L-type Ca^{2+} channel isoform ($Ca_v1.3$) may have more importance to regulate the early ignition phase. However, the details of the specific contribution of $Ca_v1.3$ require further investigation. The I_{CaL}-mediated Ca^{2+}-influx recruits more LCRs *via* diastolic CICR, and this positive feedback further increases NCX. It was also shown that I_{CaT} also has a role in the diastolic CICR, similarly as early results suggested (Huser et al., 2000). However, previously ivabradine and ryanodine were considered to cause AP CL lengthening by different mechanisms (*i.e.* ivabradine by I_f inhibition and ryanodine by takeoff potential depolarization). The underlying mechanism of ryanodine induced decrease in the firing rate could be driven by the marked decrease in DDR, which was observed in isolated rabbit sinoatrial node cells by Vinogradova et al. (2002). The AP ignition model brings them common ground: regardless of whether the M-clock (in case of ivabradine) or the Ca^{2+}-clock (in case of ryanodine) is perturbed, it will indirectly affect the other clock *via* the coupling mechanism. As a coupling, similar responses happened, the ignition potential become depolarized, and time-to-ignition phase becomes longer. This provides delay in clock-coupling by CICR delay.

The Role of NCX in Human SNCs in Comparison to Other Species

In contrast to the significant amount of experimental data on the role of NCX in pacemaking derived from animal experiments (mostly isolated rabbit SNCs), data from human SNCs or tissue are scarce. Considering the vast difference in the main quantity of interest, the beating rate, between commonly used laboratory animals and humans (mouse: 500 bpm, rabbit: 300 bpm, dog: 100 bpm, human: 60 bpm), it however cannot be assumed that the details of pacemaking mechanisms and most importantly the delicate balance of competing effects can be transferred from animal models to human in general. Indeed, it has been shown that computational models of SNCs of different species (mouse, rabbit, human) react markedly different to changes of *e.g.* extracellular Ca^{2+} concentration (Loewe et al., 2019b). Given the potential relevance of this alteration regarding sudden bradycardic death in dialysis patients (Loewe et al., 2019a), species-dependent investigations are desirable. As a particular example of interspecies differences, I_{Kr} has been reported to be absent in porcine SNCs and IKs to be negligibly small in rabbit SNCs during rest, while both are present in guinea pig SNCs (Satoh, 2003). Moreover, SN AP duration is markedly different between species (mouse: 80 ms, rabbit: 200 ms, human: 300 ms; approximate values) as are other electrophysiological parameters such as AP upstroke velocity, MDP, and DDR (Opthof, 2001). Regarding the role of NCX, its importance in terms of relative contribution to Ca^{2+} extrusion differs between species as well: 28% in rabbit compared to 7% in rat, *i.e.*, a 4-fold difference (Bers, 2002).

One of the few experiments using human SNCs was performed by Tsutsui et al. (2018). The authors show that similarly to animal models, spontaneous rhythmic LCRs generated by the Ca^{2+} clock are coupled to electrogenic surface membrane molecules to initiate rhythmic APs, and that Ca^{2+}-cAMP-protein kinase A (PKA) signaling has a regulatory role in the clock coupling in human SNCs (Tsutsui et al., 2018). In the absence of strong coupling between the oscillator subsystems, it was shown that SNCs fail to trigger spontaneous APs and only exhibit disorganized LCRs that were unable to activate the M-clock (Tsutsui et al., 2018). In summary, the study by Tsutsui et al. provides evidence that also in humans it is the coupled-clock mechanism that fundamentally drives SNC pacemaking and provides hints for mechanisms underlying SN dysfunction (Tsutsui et al., 2018).

To highlight interspecies differences and provide an overview of the characteristics of the role of NCX in different models, basic *in silico* experiments were performed.

Figure 5 shows the time courses of V_m, $Ca^{2+}{}_i$, total membrane current and NCX for several computational models of different species. Magnitude and temporal dynamics of NCX vary markedly between models and species. While NCX does not play a major role in the Garny et al. and Kurata et al. *rabbit* models, there is some early diastolic NCX in the Severi et al., Kharche et al. and Loewe–Lutz–Fabbri–Severi (LLFS) models, which becomes more pronounced only slightly before AP ignition. In the Yaniv et al. and Maltsev–Lakatta models in contrast, NCX is apparent markedly earlier. A current integral reflects the total charge transported across the membrane during a specific period of time. For a current normalized to the membrane capacitance (pA/pF), the integral is identical to the potential difference caused by the charge accumulated on the capacitive membrane due to the current (units: ms * pA/pF ≡ mV) is a measure of how much of the DD (in terms of mV) can be attributed to NCX. To quantify the role of NCX to DD in the models of different species, we computed the NCX integral during DD:

$$\left|\int_{t_{MDP}}^{t_{takeoff}} I_{NaCa}(t)dt\right|, \qquad (2)$$

where $t_{takeoff}$ was defined as the first time step for which d^2V_m/dt^2 exceeded 15% of the maximum d^2V_m/dt^2 in the time interval between MDP and $\max(V_m)$. The curvature based measure was inspired by the shape of the SN APs with the threshold empirically chosen to strike a balance between a detection early in the upstroke and robustness to minor increases of d^2V_m/dt^2 during DD. **Figure 3** compares the NCX integral in relation to the total rise in V_m during DD and gives an idea about how much of the total DD can be attributed to NCX in each of the models across different species. Under the simplifying assumption of independent currents, almost the entire DD can be attributed to NCX in the Severi et al. rabbit and Kharche et al. mouse model. In the Yaniv et al., LLFS, and Maltsev–Lakatta models, NCX alone would cause more DD than the net ΔV_m observed, *i.e.*, outward currents partly compensate the NCX-induced depolarization whereas the role of NCX is almost negligible in the Garny et al. and Kurata et al. rabbit models.

To further illustrate interspecies differences in the role of NCX in SN pacemaking, we evaluated how the models of different species respond to gradual block of NCX. **Figure 6** shows that the Garny et al. model exhibits an almost linear relation between NCX block and CL prolongation, however with a limited overall effect of +29.6 ms upon complete elimination of NCX. All other models required a certain amount of remaining NCX for reliable pacemaking (between 10% and 50%). In the Yaniv et al. model, 60% NCX block already terminated stable pacemaking. Instead, blocks of two subsequent APs followed by low amplitude V_m oscillations for several seconds were observed (compare **Figure 7**). The Yaniv et al. and Maltsev–Lakatta models showed a monotonic relation with CL prolongation for all degrees of block. In contrast, the Severi et al., Kharche et al., and LLFS models exhibited a biphasic relation with CL shortening up to a certain degree of block (80%, 50%, 50% block, respectively) and pronounced CL prolongation beyond (up to +420 ms in the LLFS model).

To identify the drivers for these CL changes across species, we evaluated the effects on APD as well as early and late depolarization with the following metrics:

$$t_{dia,early} = \frac{V_{takeoff} - MDP}{DDR_{early}}, \quad t_{dia,late} = t_{takeoff} - t_{dia,early}, \qquad (3)$$

where DDR_{early} was defined as a first order approximation of the DDR during the first 35 ms for the small animal models and

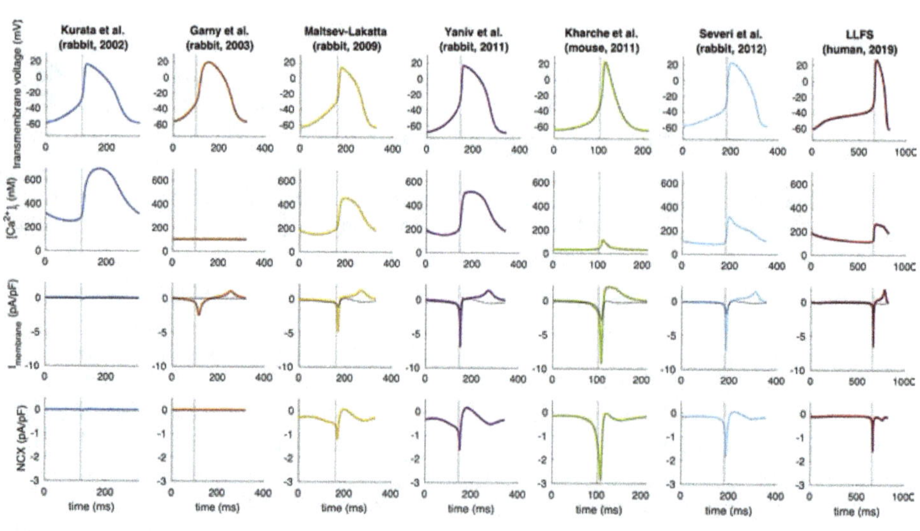

FIGURE 5 | Spontaneous APs, Ca^{2+} transients, total membrane currents, and NCX in computational models of different species (compare **Figure 3**). Note the different time axes as a result of the markedly different spontaneous beating rates. The vertical gray line indicates the time of AP takeoff. For comparison, NCX is plotted in gray in the total membrane current panels.

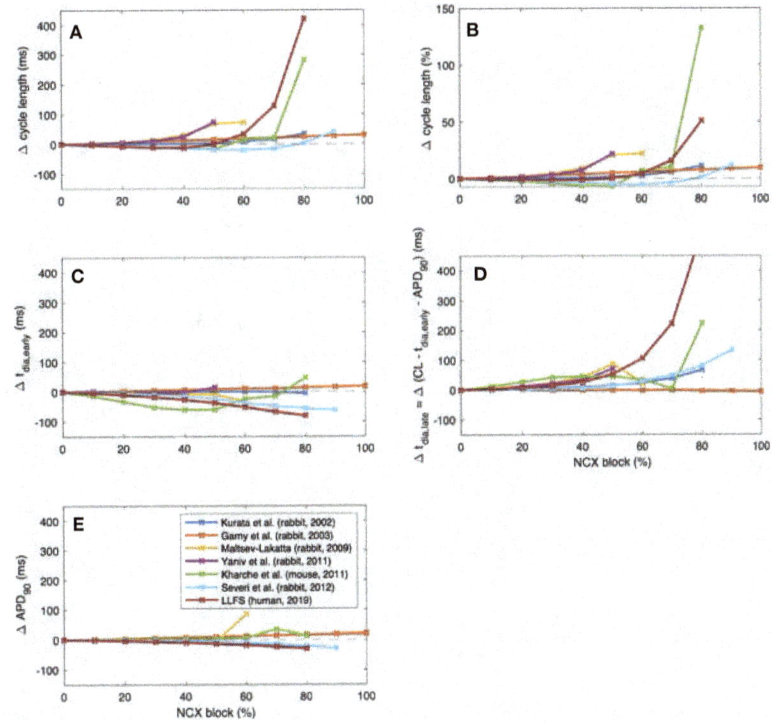

FIGURE 6 | Change of CL [absolute **(A)** and relative **(B)**], $t_{dia,early}$ **(C)**, $t_{dia,late}$ **(D)** and APD **(E)** of computational models of different species (compare **Figure 4**) in response to gradual NCX block.

the first 100 ms for the *human* LLFS model. APD shortening was responsible for the initial CL shortening in the Severi et al. rabbit and LLFS human models in combination with a reduction of $t_{dia,early}$, which also affected the CL of the Kharche et al. model for degrees of block ≤70%. The superlinear CL prolongation for high degrees of block was mainly driven by changes in $t_{dia,late}$, *i.e.*, changes that could not be attributed to APD, $V_{takeoff}$, or changes in early DDR. Absolute values of CL, overshoot potential, MDP, APD_{90}, DDR_{early}, and dV_m/dt_{max} upon NCX block of different degrees are shown in **Figure 8**. In addition to the effects included in the integral measures in **Figure 6**, a monotonic reduction of AP upstroke velocity could be observed in all but the Garny et al. rabbit model. As models of the same species (such as the Severi et al., Garny et al., and Yaniv et al. rabbit models presented here) sometimes exhibit different properties, it cannot be clearly pinned down which of the effects are truly species-dependent and which are simply model-dependent. Future studies should address this issue to identify which of the insights derived from animal experiments can be transferred to the human setting in which ways.

To study the biophysical identity of human SNCs, Chandler et al. (2009) performed an mRNA and protein expression analysis of human SNCs suggesting similar NCX1 in SN and atrial cells (Chandler et al., 2009). Based on their experimental findings, they derived one of the first computational models of human SNCs by adapting the atrial Courtemanche et al. (1998) model (Courtemanche et al., 1998) based on their experimental findings where NCX was scaled down by 26%. Allah et al. (2011) found rabbit SN NCX1 mRNA expression levels to be 78% of that of right atrial and 69% of that of left ventricular myocytes, respectively (Allah et al., 2011). Based on these two studies and I_f recordings in human SNCs, Verkerk et al. presented another early human SNC model (Verkerk et al., 2007; Verkerk et al., 2013). Compared to rabbit cells, their model of human SN cells had smaller absolute NCX, smaller absolute I_f, and a less pronounced Ca^{2+} transient. When comparing to the net diastolic membrane current, NCX was of similar magnitude between human and rabbit cells whereas I_f remained smaller in human cells.

The first human SNC model originating from a SNC model rather that an atrial model was presented by Fabbri et al. (2017). Their model is based on the Severi et al. rabbit model (Severi et al., 2012) and considered human data wherever available (Fabbri et al., 2017). The NCX formulation was adopted from the parent model and goes back to Kurata et al. (2002) (Kurata et al., 2002). As a result of the model parameter fitting to experimental data on the AP and Ca^{2+} transient level, the maximal NCX current was reduced by 53% (3.34 nA) compared to the parent model. Interestingly, NCX block experiments caused an increase in beating rate in the Fabbri et al. model. (50% block: 83 bpm [+12.2%]; 75% block: 93 bpm [+25.7%]) mediated by a synergistic acceleration of DD caused by elevated $Ca^{2+}{}_i$, shortening of APD and less negative maximum diastolic potential. Upon 90% NCX block, automaticity ceased.

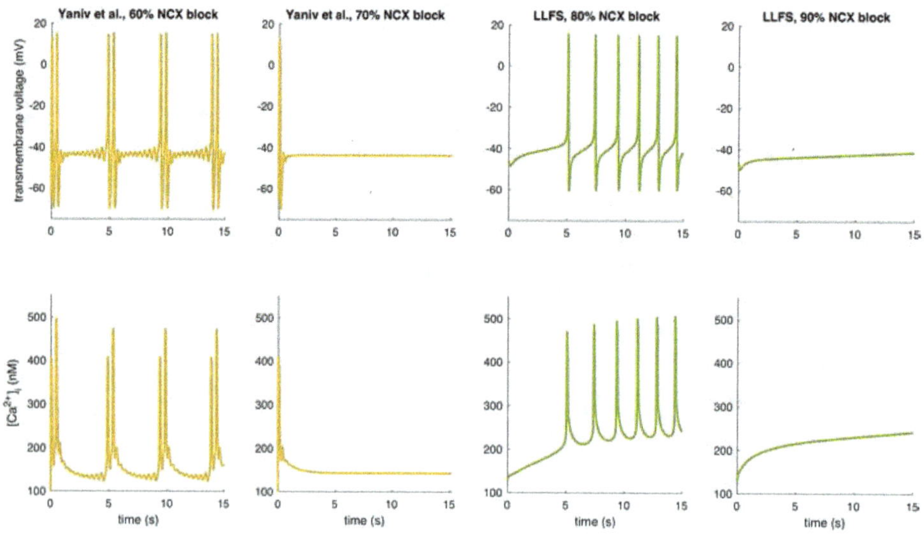

FIGURE 7 | APs and Ca^{2+} transients of the Yaniv et al. and LLFS models for NCX block degrees slightly below and above the threshold for cessation of automaticity.

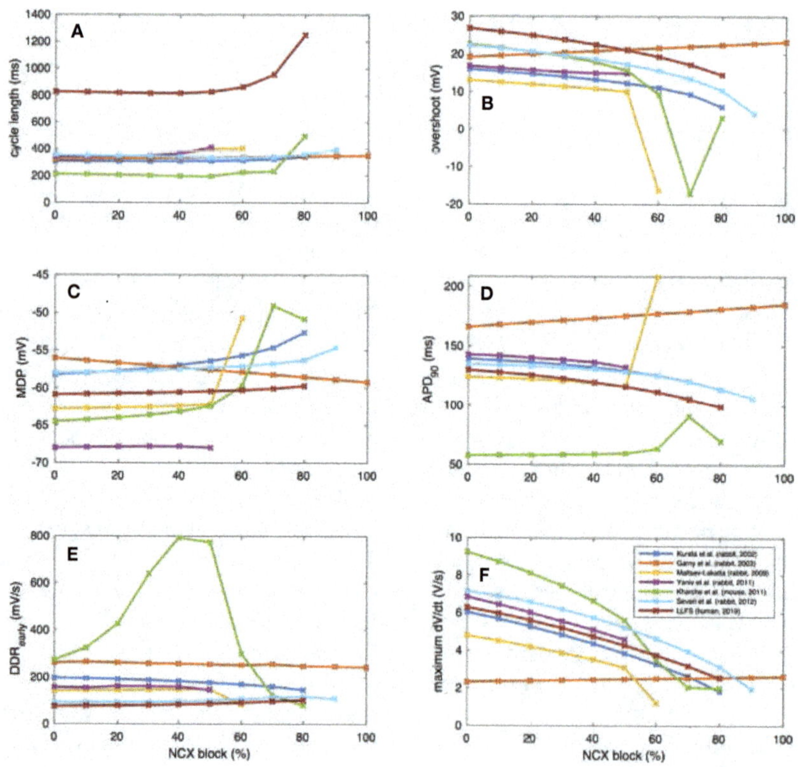

FIGURE 8 | AP properties of computational models of different species (compare **Figure 3**) in response to gradual NCX block: CL **(A)**, overshoot **(B)**, MDP **(C)**, APD **(D)**, early DDR **(E)**, $(dV_m/dt)_{max}$ **(F)**.

The β-adrenergic rate modulation experiments by Fabbri et al. did not include any direct effects on NCX but the SR Ca^{2+} pumping was modeled as a target of isoproterenol. The application of 1 μM isoproterenol yielded a 27.9% increase in beating rate. If only SR Ca^{2+} pumping was modeled as a target of isoproterenol, this increase was markedly attenuated and even slightly reversed with a remaining effect of −0.4%. Loewe et al. proposed the Loewe–Lutz–Fabbri–Severi model (LLFS) (Loewe et al., 2019b) as an extension of the Fabbri et al. model which considers, among other improvements, the dynamics and transients of the intracellular sodium and potassium concentrations in contrast to the previously fixed concentrations, thus further constraining the model physiologically by requiring homeostasis across time spans of minutes (Loewe et al., 2019a). In the LLFS model, the response to complete I_f block (CL +25.9%) was in accordance with the available experimental *human* data [+26% reported by Verkerk et al. (2007)] (Verkerk et al., 2007).

LOCAL CONTROL OF NCX

Several studies suggested that in cardiac muscle (Lipp et al., 1990) and other cells such as squid axon (Mullins and Requena, 1979), pancreatic acinar cells (Osipchuk et al., 1990), and smooth muscle (Stehno-Bittel and Sturek, 1992) ionic concentrations close to the intracellular surface of the plasma membrane may be different from those in the cytoplasm. These concentration gradients are thought to result from transient net fluxes across the surface membrane and may crucially influence the transmembrane ion channels. In atrial cells, which lack a well-developed t-tubule system, a non-uniform distribution of Ca^{2+} within the cell following release from the SR has been found and the results were interpreted in terms of distinct release sites under different control mechanisms (Lipp et al., 1990). Trafford et al. in rat ventricular myocytes also demonstrated the existence of the submembrane "area" by using the NCX current as a reporter and found that $Ca^{2+}{}_i$ changes near the surface membrane can be considerably larger than those averaged over the cell. The differences can be explained by a diffusion barrier between the release site and the bulk cytosol (Trafford et al., 1995).

In SNCs, the diastolic NCX is not only regulated by V_m but also by the LCRs, which in turn depend on local cross-talk including Ca^{2+}-dependent functions of NCX, RyR, and SERCA (**Figure 1B**). This feedback mechanism between LCR and NCX can rapidly change NCX. It is known that RyRs are tightly organized in clusters, which are coupled with the L-type Ca^{2+} channels to form Ca^{2+} release units (CRU). RyRs are activated by an increase of local $Ca^{2+}{}_i$ resulting in Ca^{2+}-induced Ca^{2+} release (CICR). Each CRU generates small, temporal Ca^{2+} release events, called Ca^{2+} sparks which have a radius of 1.5 μm (Stern et al., 2013; Hoang-Trong et al., 2015). Therefore, a LCR (4–12 μm) involves several sparks fired by neighboring CRUs *via* fire-diffuse-fire propagation (Maltsev et al., 2011a; Stern et al., 2014). Spark characteristics can be modulated by β-adrenergic response *via* variation of single CRU Ca^{2+} currents (I_{spark}). The LCR controls SN chronotropy (acceleration and slowing) *via* changing the LCR size, amplitude, and number per cell surface area.

In 2011, Maltsev et al. demonstrated, by two-dimensional Ca^{2+} measurements on rabbit SNCs and *via* numerical modeling, that increasing the I_{spark} amplitude results in local synchronization of CRU firing yielding increasing LCR size, rhythmicity, and occurrence rate (Maltsev et al., 2011a). I_{spark} regulates both the time shift and the amplitude of the spontaneous release. Since the LCRs are directly coupled with NCX, this means that I_{spark} amplitude indirectly influences NCX during DD (**Figure 9**). In 2013, Maltsev et al. discovered a novel stabilization mechanism *via* local control of CICR (Maltsev et al., 2013). The Ca^{2+} released from the RyRs during DD is able to recruit the neighboring RyRs to release more Ca^{2+}. This local recruitment depends on the extent of released Ca^{2+} and its diffusion to the neighboring RyRs. Since NCX extrudes Ca^{2+} from the vicinity of RyRs, it restrains CICR because the Ca^{2+} occurrence to diffuse and activate neighboring RyRs is reduced. The diastolic NCX increase is described by:

$$NCX = n_{sparks} \times NCX_{spark}, \tag{4}$$

where n_{sparks} is the number of Ca^{2+} sparks and NCX_{spark} is the NCX current generated by one spark. This formula predicts that during NCX suppression the decreased NCX current (NCX_{spark}) in turn increases the number of sparks (n_{sparks}) since there is more Ca^{2+} available for diffusion and activation of additional RyRs. As the above formula predicts, the larger number of sparks tends to increase the NCX current, and finally, these opposite changes are able to largely compensate each other providing marginal change in the NCX. Stern et al. in 2014 provided three-dimensional SNC computational modeling including diffusion and buffering of Ca^{2+} in the cytosol and SR but omitted the submembrane space and inactivation of RyRs because of the lack of experimental validation data (Stern et al., 2014). Immunostaining experiments revealed that bridging RyR groups exist between large RyR clusters, organized in irregular networks. This architecture provides the basis for propagating LCR events. When a structure without bridges was incorporated in the model, the separated RyR clusters produced only isolated sparks, without LCRs and NCX activity. The model indicates that this hierarchical RyR clustering provides a pivotal adaptive mechanism and contributes to the β-adrenergic adaptation. Maltsev et al. (2017) characterized the complex spatiotemporal structure of LCRs in cardiac pacemaker cells (Maltsev et al., 2017). Using automatic classification of LCRs, they demonstrated that SR pumping controls LCRs and pacemaker rate *via* timely synchronized occurrence of LCRs creating a powerful ensemble signal to activate NCX. This also means that when SR pumping rate is low, the LCRs exert smaller amplitudes due to the lower SR Ca^{2+} load. However, the system compensates and maintains the NCX signal by increasing LCR size and duration. This mechanism ensures fail-safe pacemaker function within a wide range of pacing frequencies.

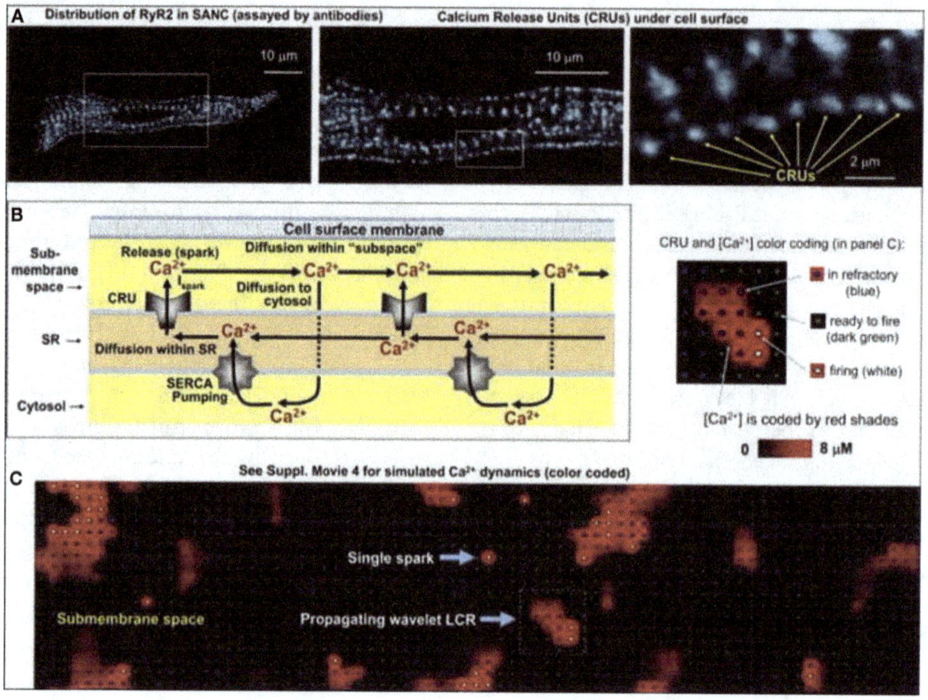

FIGURE 9 | Development of the numerical model of local Ca^{2+} dynamics in rabbit SNCs: Ca^{2+} release units (CRUs) and Ca^{2+} cycling. RyR clusters, *i.e.*, CRUs, are visualized in confocal images of immuno-fluorescence in rabbit SNCs under cell surface membrane **(A)**. Schematic drawing of local Ca^{2+} cycling through different cell compartments (submembrane space, SR, and cytosol) **(B)**. Local Ca^{2+} fluxes are depicted with arrows, Ca^{2+} waves travel from left to right. **(C)** Instantaneous distributions of local $[Ca^{2+}]$ in the submembrane space predicted by our model: single Ca^{2+} spark and a wavelet LCRs (propagating from *left* to *right*). Inset illustrates the color-coding for CRU states and $[Ca^{2+}]$ (from (Maltsev et al., 2011a) with permission).

HETEROGENEITY OF SNCS

Functionally and electrophysiologically, the SN has a heterogeneous structure [as excellently reviewed by Boyett et al. (2000) and Lancaster et al. (2004)]. During normal cardiac activation, the spontaneous AP is initiated from the center, the leading pacemaker site of the SN, and then the AP is conducted through the periphery to the surrounding atrial muscle of the crista terminalis (Bleeker et al., 1980). In response to different interventions, the leading pacemaker site can shift to the peripheral region causing major importance in the pacemaker function. In the center the cells are described being smaller compared to those in the periphery and contain fewer myofilaments (Bleeker et al., 1980; Masson-Pevet et al., 1984; Boyett et al., 2000). The possible differences in the AP characteristics and the expression of ion channels were intensively studied, and the question whether the expression levels of proteins depend on the cell size of the SNCs remains equivocal (Honjo et al., 1996; Boyett et al., 1998; Lyashkov et al., 2007). The majority of the studies report that the expression of the Ca^{2+} regulatory proteins differs between regions of the SN, which results in heterogeneity of intracellular Ca^{2+} handling and pacemaker activity between cells across the nodal tissue. Musa et al. showed that the density of I_{CaL} was significantly ($p < 0.001$) correlated with cell capacitance in rabbit sinoatrial node, and larger cells showed greater density (Musa et al., 2002). The authors also performed immunocytochemical labeling of L-type Ca^{2+} channel, RYR2, and SERCA2, showing in significantly higher density in cells from the periphery compared to the center of the SN (Musa et al., 2002). In line with this, larger cells exhibited greater systolic Ca^{2+}, diastolic Ca^{2+}, Ca^{2+} transient amplitude, and spontaneous rate compared with smaller, probably central cells (Lancaster et al., 2004). Sarcolemmal Ca^{2+} ATPase and NCX have a lower activity in central cells, and the exchanger is responsible for a larger proportion of sarcolemmal Ca^{2+} extrusion in those cells compared with larger, peripheral cells (Lancaster et al., 2004). In 2007, Lyashkov et al. determined the density and distribution of cRyR, NCX1, and SERCA2 in SNCs of different sizes from the rabbit SN tissue (Lyashkov et al., 2007). They found that both bigger and smaller SN cells have identical AP-induced Ca^{2+} transients and spontaneous localized Ca^{2+} release characteristics (Lyashkov et al., 2007). They provided evidence on robust NCX1 as well as SERCA2 and cRyR cellular labeling densities in SNCs and they found that the entire sinoatrial node—including the Cx43 negative primary pacemaker area—exhibits positive labeling for NCX1, cRyR, and SERCA2 (Lyashkov et al., 2007). Furthermore, submembrane colocalization of NCX1 and cardiac RyR was shown, which exceeds the degree observed in atrial or ventricular cells (Lyashkov et al., 2007). However, Tellez et al. examined the molecular basis of the ion currents in rabbit SN with measuring the abundance of messenger RNAs coding for ion channels and regulatory proteins of the SN tissue. Ca^{2+} handling proteins abundance showed variability between tissues from different parts of the SN (Tellez et al., 2006). The abundance of NCX1 mRNA was significantly lower in the periphery of the SN compared with other regions. In the transcript profile, an apparent isoform switch from the atrial muscle to the center of the SN was found: RYR2 to RYR3, $Na_v1.5$ to $Na_v1.1$, $Ca_v1.2$ to $Ca_v1.3$ and $K_v1.4$ to $K_v4.2$ (Tellez et al., 2006).

Maltsev and Lakatta in 2013, by using a numerical model, explored large variation of ensembles of electrogenic molecules to identify the minimum set of proteins that confer a robust (i.e. fail-safe) and flexible (i.e. adaptation to a given vegetative stimulus) pacemaker function (Maltsev and Lakatta, 2013). The minimal model was found to contain: I_{CaL}+ I_{Kr}+ NCX+ Ca^{2+} clock. The further addition of I_{CaT} and I_f decreased flexibility but increased robustness of the system. Therefore the higher balance of flexibility and robustness contains five parameters: I_{CaL} + I_{Kr} + NCX + Ca^{2+} clock + I_f. It is important to note that in the four parameter models, all model sets without NCX failed to generate rhythmic APs in at least one of the tests, confirming the fundamental importance of the exchanger in the pacemaking.

Monfredi et al. examined the major ionic currents in intercaval pacemaker cells (IPCs) obtained from rabbit heart and found marked electrophysiological heterogeneity in IPCs (Monfredi et al., 2018). Experiments and numerical simulations indicated that there is an IPC cell population with minimal or zero I_f, without correlation between I_f density and cell size. In the absence of I_f, the diastolic NCX in response to Ca^{2+} release (*i.e.*, the Ca^{2+} clock) could drive the pacemaking. Wide ranges of I_{CaL} and I_K densities were found in these cells. Functional heterogeneity of SNCs was recently described by Kim et al. (2018). Their experiments performed in guinea pigs demonstrated three types of SNCs: rhythmically firing, dysrhythmically beating, and dormant cells exerting no spontaneous activation. LCRs were present in all three types; however in the dysrhythmic and dormant cells only smaller, stochastic LCRs without spatial and temporal synchronization were observed. β-adrenergic stimulation synchronized LCRs in all dysrhythmic cells and in the 1/3 of the dormant cells. Furthermore, the dormant cells developed automaticity in response to β-adrenergic stimulation. These results indicate partial or complete uncoupling between Ca^{2+} and M-clocks in the dysrhythmic and dormant cells.

WHAT IS THE ROLE OF NCX IN PACEMAKING UNDER RESTING HEART RATE?

When active in forward mode, NCX generates inward current and at the same time represents the most important pathway for Ca^{2+} extrusion to maintain the Ca^{2+} flux balance (Bers, 2001). Since these two functions are not separable, profound (but incomplete) NCX inhibition may always have secondary effects by altering the intracellular Ca^{2+} levels. Considering the published results and the nature of NCX inhibition, it could be that pharmacological NCX inhibition (partial for all available agents) or incomplete transgenic knockout mutants are not able to unequivocally pin down NCX's function in pacemaking. Theoretically, partial NCX suppression (acute pharmacological, or incomplete transgenic models) may lead to 3 different outcomes, characterized by the intracellular Ca^{2+} concentration since NCX is the major pathway for Ca^{2+} extrusion:

i) NCX inhibition does not increase Ca^{2+}_i because of activation of other compensatory mechanisms (such as plasma membrane ATPase). In this fortunate case, all NCX inhibition is pure current inhibition with minimal secondary, indirect mechanisms through changes of Ca^{2+}_i. However, this scenario may have the lowest probability.

ii) NCX inhibition does not increase Ca^{2+}_i because the (potentially small) uninhibited fraction is able to remove the Ca^{2+}. This suggests a non-linear relationship between the degree of NCX inhibition and reduction of NCX function in terms of Ca^{2+} extrusion during the DD, making the interpretation difficult.

iii) NCX inhibition elevates Ca^{2+}_i. In this case, the Ca^{2+} gain will enhance the Ca^{2+}-dependent inactivation of the I_{CaL}, which may shorten the AP. However, also the AP threshold is expected to be higher, requiring more time to be reached. According to the ignition theory (Lyashkov et al., 2018), the decreased contribution of I_{CaL} also reduces the I_{CaL}-LCR-NCX interactions. Furthermore, the Ca^{2+} increase may activate other Ca^{2+}-dependent mechanisms such as $I_{K(Ca)}$. These indirect mechanisms may counteract the effect of NCX inhibition.

Groenke et al. demonstrated that NCX1 KO mice show no spontaneous atrial depolarization (Groenke et al., 2013); only junctional escape rhythm was observed. The cells did not show spontaneous automaticity despite the presence of I_f and intact Ca^{2+} stores. Current mechanistic models of both human (Loewe et al., 2019a) and rabbit (Yaniv et al., 2011) SNCs also support no spontaneous automaticity when NCX function is completely absent. Considering pharmacological data, it can be firmly stated that different maneuvers aiming to decrease the intracellular Ca^{2+} level such as ryanodine, CPA, BAPTA in all cases lead to a decrease of SN frequency to varying extents. However, the kinetics of Ca^{2+} currents also changes due to these interventions. Therefore, taking together the published results, it is doubtless that if NCX is largely inhibited or completely absent, the normal Ca^{2+} flux balance is considerably impaired which per se may influence spontaneous automaticity. These secondary shifts of Ca^{2+} balance make the experimental evaluation of the total NCX contribution during DD more difficult. At the same time, the available experimental data with manipulation of Ca^{2+}_i, modifications of second messengers (such as cAMP, PKA, PDE, CaMKII), transgenic animals and numerical modeling clearly indicate the fundamental role of NCX in maintaining the resting heart rate.

WHAT IS THE ROLE OF NCX IN THE FIGHT-OR-FLIGHT RESPONSE?

The β-adrenergic response involves the increase of intracellular cAMP and PKA, increases CaMKII activity and increases the intracellular Ca^{2+} load *via* phosphorylation of various channels (**Figure 1B**). A large body of evidence indicates that LCRs and therefore also NCX are under the influence and delicate control of several intracellular signaling molecules (such as CaMKII, PKA, cAMP, PDE), which are sensitive to β-adrenergic activation (see *The Role of Phosphorylation in SN Pacemaking and the Fight-or-Flight Response*). These results indicate a pivotal role of NCX not only in maintaining the basal SN automaticity but also in the sympathetic stimulus-mediated heart rate acceleration.

DOES THE REVERSE MODE OF NCX INFLUENCE SN PACEMAKING?

Currently, a transport-selective NCX inhibitor is not available. However, the KB-R7943 preferentially inhibits the reverse mode of NCX (Birinyi et al., 2005); it markedly influences I_{CaL} (Birinyi et al., 2005) making the interpretation difficult. The electrophysiological properties of the NCX predict functioning reverse mode when V_m is depolarized (more than 0 mV) and Na^+_i is high. Experimental results as well as modeling data demonstrate that SN APs peak around 20 mV, which could be considered high enough to "switch on" reverse mode; however the time at depolarized levels is very short. During normal Na^+_i, mechanistic modeling predicts only marginal reverse mode at the beginning of the AP, thus the NCX current is mainly inward throughout the entire AP. The Yaniv et al. (Yaniv et al., 2013b) and LFSS model (Loewe et al., 2019a) predicted termination of beating when intracellular Na^+_i is elevated, suggesting that this is not a way to augment reverse NCX during SN automaticity.

Maltsev and Lakatta in 2013 (Maltsev and Lakatta, 2013) reported a notable reverse mode of the NCX that was lacked in the previously published models. Numerical calculations revealed 2.45 pC of Ca^{2+} influx *via* reverse mode that is comparable with I_{CaL}-mediated Ca^{2+} influx for one AP cycle. This means that reverse NCX contributes in "refueling" the Ca^{2+} clock almost equal to I_{CaL}.

CRITICISMS OF Ca^{2+}-THEORY

The role of Ca^{2+}_i in the SN pacemaker function has been challenged from the beginning. However, the importance of intact Ca^{2+} handling in normal SN automaticity was accepted in a relatively short time. In contrast, the dominance of I_f over NCX and *vice versa* was a recurrent and often appearing question (Lakatta and DiFrancesco, 2009). Since the funny-current was the first proposed mechanism underlying pacemaking, it is hardly surprising that the Ca^{2+} theory was challenged many times experimentally.

Ryanodine Effect

Serious criticisms have emerged regarding the frequency modulating effect of ryanodine. Authors often found a 15–30% frequency decrease after application of ryanodine which was attributed to the effect of indirectly reduced NCX activity. However, Bucchi and DiFrancesco in 2003 showed that the ryanodine mediated increase of CL is not the consequence of decreased DD slope but the positive shift of AP threshold (Bucchi et al., 2003). A further consistent finding was that ryanodine considerably reduces the frequency-increasing effect of β-adrenergic activation (Bucchi et al., 2003). The DiFrancesco group (Bucchi et al., 2003) demonstrated that ryanodine disrupts the normal signal transduction pathway of of β-adrenergic response, and the intracellularly used cAMP analogues were able to increase the frequency in the presence of 3 μM ryanodine to a similar extent as during control. The authors claim that the SR Ca^{2+} release may represent only a "safety mechanism" for the DD to reach the threshold level. Another paper of DiFrancesco group (Bucchi et al., 2007b) investigated "signatures" of rate changes caused by different pharmacological maneuvers. They found that agents modifying I_f such as ivabradine, isoproterenol, cAMP, and acetylcholine affect only the slope of DD while ryanodine-mediated bradycardia is caused by an increase of the take-off potential. They conclude that while other mechanisms could be important I_f appears to be the simplest and most direct contributor to rate modulation. While the reduction of pacing rate after ryanodine application is an unequivocal finding, the underlying mechanisms (change of take-off potential *vs.* slowed DDR) are a matter of debate. Vinogradova et al. showed that ryanodine has a marked effect on the DD by decreasing DDR, thus causing significant CL prolongation (Vinogradova et al., 2002). In another study, they also observed that in the presence of ryanodine, the ability of the cAMP analogue CPT-cAMP to increase the SNC beating rate was markedly reduced from ~35% (in control) to ~10% (Vinogradova et al., 2006). The different findings of this study and the previously mentioned study by Bucchi et al. (2003) could be partly due to different experimental approaches. DiFrancesco's group used clusters of SNCs with whole cell recordings of APs, while Lakatta's group used single SNCs with the perforated patch technique.

However, ryanodine may have a direct inhibitory effect on I_{CaT} channels, which would complicate the interpretation of such experimental data (Li et al., 1997).

Bucchi et al. and Vinogradova et al. (Vinogradova et al., 2002; Bucchi et al., 2003; Vinogradova et al., 2006) were not the only ones investigating the effects of RyR Ca^{2+} release suppression by ryanodine in the response of β-adrenergic stimulation. The influence of ryanodine on the modulation of the chronotropic effect of β-adrenoceptor stimulation has been extensively studied in a variety of different species. In guinea-pig SNCs exposed to 100 nmol/L isoprenaline, a decrease in firing rate and decrease in the amplitude of Ca^{2+} transients were observed after ryanodine application, supporting that ryanodine decreases the positive chronotropic effect of isoprenaline (Rigg et al., 2000). In isolated mouse SNCs, in the presence of ryanodine, the chronotropic effect of β-adrenoceptor stimulation was entirely suppressed and a reduction of spontaneous AP frequency was observed after isoprenaline application (Wu et al., 2009). Consistent with this finding, Joung et al. showed that the isoprenaline dose-dependent increase of heart rate was suppressed by ryanodine infusion and SR Ca^{2+} depletion with ryanodine prevented isoproterenol-induced LDCaE and blunted sinus rate acceleration in canine right atrium (Joung et al., 2009).

It is important to note that the ryanodine effect highly depends on the concentration and experiment time (Rousseau et al., 1987; Smith et al., 1988; Buck et al., 1992; Zimanyi et al., 1992; Fill and Copello, 2002). In low doses, it locks the RyR in a subconductance open state (Buck et al., 1992). Before the SR depletion, the Ca^{2+} flux increases the firing rate indicating the direct role of Ca^{2+} and NCX in pacemaking (Rubenstein and Lipsius, 1989). The AP ignition model (Lyashkov et al., 2018) predicts that ryanodine substantially depolarizes the ignition potential and prolongs both CL and time-to-ignition, but does not significantly affect the MDP. Additional simulations with Ca^{2+} dynamics showed that Ca^{2+} release continues in the presence of SR Ca^{2+} leak (the leaky SR model mimics ryanodine-dependent lock of RyRs in the subconductance state) but it becomes persistent. In this case, the diffusional resistance between the network and junctional SR limits intra-SR flux and preserves the Ca^{2+}-load of the network SR. This maintains SR Ca^{2+} load and drives persistent release flux (Lyashkov et al., 2018).

Ca^{2+}-Dependence of I_f

A possible Ca^{2+}-dependence of the funny current would raise serious questions since the maneuvers to alter $Ca^{2+}{}_i$ levels were generally considered to influence the SR-NCX axis only, without interfering with I_f. Hagiwara and Irisawa (1989) demonstrated Ca^{2+} dependent changes of I_f (Hagiwara and Irisawa, 1989). Later inside-out patch clamp experiments revealed that Ca^{2+} ions do not directly influence the I_f current (Zaza et al., 1991). However, a Ca^{2+}-activated adenylate-cyclase isoform was found in SNCs (Mattick et al., 2007), indicating that a Ca^{2+} rise after NCX inhibition will induce augmented funny current. This effect is also proposed to counterbalance the effect of NCX inhibition on the CL. Furthermore, it may be another link between Ca^{2+} homeostasis and V_m. The actual value of the MDP is mainly defined by the potassium conductance during repolarization. Therefore, potassium channels indirectly influence automaticity. The small conductance Ca^{2+} activated potassium current may provide a direct link between Ca^{2+} handling and repolarization. Even though no effect was found in ventricular myocardium (Nagy et al., 2009), a possible contribution for pacemaking was reported (Torrente et al., 2017; Saeki et al., 2019).

Intracellular Buffering

The forward mode of the NCX extrudes Ca^{2+} from the intracellular space while generating inward current that contributes to DD. Since the primary driver of NCX during DD is the Ca^{2+} concentration, buffering of intracellular Ca^{2+} affects the role of NCX and potentially attenuates or terminates spontaneous automaticity. Several authors challenged the role of SR release in setting the actual frequency of SN pacemaking by application of the rapid Ca^{2+} buffer BAPTA. The results are summarized in **Table 2**. The data clearly demonstrate the significant role of $Ca^{2+}{}_i$ in the SN pacemaking, *i.e.*, the function of the inward NCX during DD. A contradictory result was published by Himeno et al., where unaffected AP firing rate was demonstrated in the presence of high $Ca^{2+}{}_i$ buffering, thus challenging the Ca^{2+} hypothesis (Himeno et al., 2011). Their results were later interpreted by the Lakatta group (Maltsev et al., 2011b) as methodological problems, *i.e.* incomplete seal resistance. When rabbit cells were loaded with the caged Ca^{2+} buffer NP-EGTA, the firing rate was slow and dysrhythmic with low SR Ca^{2+} levels. Rapid photolysis induced Ca^{2+} increase, in turn, markedly increased the frequency (by about 50%), accelerated the DD, augmented the LCRs, and reduced the CL variability (Yaniv et al., 2011).

Pharmacological Problems

Important pharmacological problems arose regarding I_f and NCX inhibitors. The contribution of I_f was traditionally investigated using caesium or ivabradine. The heart rate lowering effects of these compounds varied within a large range (7–31%) and even 20 mM caesium was unable to terminate spontaneous SN beating (Sohn and Vassalle, 1995). Therefore, the pacemaking role of I_f was regularly challenged by considering its I–V relationship (small current in the DD range), slow activation kinetics, and moderate effects of inhibitors (DiFrancesco, 1995; Vassalle, 1995; Bucchi et al., 2007a; Lakatta and DiFrancesco, 2009). However, both $CsCl_2$ and ivabradine cause incomplete and voltage-dependent block. A further issue with ivabradine is the significant I_{Kr} block even at the widely used concentration of 3 μM (Koncz et al., 2011). Similar situations can be found with selective NCX inhibitors. Both ORM-10103 and ORM-10962 however, exert no influence on other currents and partially inhibit NCX, may also depend on Ca^{2+}. As discussed above (*What is the Role of NCX in Pacemaking Under Resting Heart Rate*)?, increased Ca^{2+} limits the effect of NCX inhibition *via* secondary effects and covers the exact role of NCX during DD. Taking together these results, it seems likely that

TABLE 2 | Effects of BAPTA on spontaneous firing rate of SNCs.

Species	Preparation	Concentration	Period(s) of application	Control (bpm)	After drug (bpm)	Rate reduction (%)	Reference
Toad	Single sinus venosus cells	10 μM BAPTA	5 and 8 min	31	15	51.6	Ju and Allen et al.
Rabbit	Single SNc	5 μM BAPTA	7–10 min	149	69	53.7	Bogdanov et al.
Rabbit	Cultured SNc	25 μM BAPTA	10 min	94	65	30.9	Li et al.
Rabbit	Single SNc	5 μM BAPTA	5 min	174	80	54	Vinogradova et al.
Rabbit	Single SNc	25 μM BAPTA	25 min	210	120	43	Lyashkov et al.
Rabbit	Single SNc	25 μM BAPTA	30 min			87	Younnes et al.
Guinea pig	Single SNc	10 μM BAPTA	3 min			100%	Sanders et al.
Guinea pig	Single SNc	10 mM BAPTA	30 s	153	141	7.8%	Himeno et al.

complete pharmacological inhibition of I_f or NCX is currently not feasible using the available compounds, impeding the identification of the role of NCX and I_f in SN pacemaking.

An indirect experiment was also published in 2015 by Szepesi et al. (2015) using 10 μM ORM-10103 as a selective NCX inhibitor (Jost et al., 2013) in Langendorff perfused rat hearts. The results exerted identical R-R intervals after application of selective NCX blockade.

In 2008, Farkas et al. investigated the possible antiarrhythmic effect of selective NCX inhibition against dofetilide-induced Torsades de pointes arrhythmia by using 1 μM SEA0400, a nonselective NCX inhibitor in rabbit and rat Langendorff-perfused hearts (Farkas et al., 2008). However, the measured R-R intervals indicated no effect on sinus function of NCX inhibition in both species. In contrast, by using the most selective available NCX inhibitor ORM-10962, Kohajda et al. showed a tendency to decrease the heart rate in guinea pig hearts *in vivo*, however within the experimental variance (Kohajda et al., 2016). 1 μM ORM-10962 exerted statistically significant, however marginal (8%) decrease in rabbit atrial tissue, while $Ca^{2+}{}_i$ was significantly increased in SNCs (Kohajda et al., 2020).

APPLICATIONS

Besides its fundamental role for pacemaking under physiological conditions, various applications of engineered NCX and potential roles in pathogenesis have been put forward. Silva and Rudy (2003) numerically replicated biological pacemakers derived from guinea pig ventricular cells (Silva and Rudy, 2003). Suppression of I_{K1} by 81% elicited rhythmic spontaneous depolarizations at a CL of 594 ms caused by NCX as the main pacemaking current. The role of NCX was underlined by a bifurcation analysis of biological pacemaking driven by an unstable equilibrium point *via* a saddle-node bifurcation by Kurata et al. (2005) using a modified Priebe-Beuckelmann model in which NCX was identified as the primary pacemaker current (Kurata et al., 2005). However, they found that NCX is not necessarily required for rhythmic spontaneous depolarizations and that equilibrium point instability as a prerequisite for stable pacemaking is caused by I_{CaL} but not NCX. Jones et al. (2012) identified NCX as one of the key determinants of pulmonary vein automaticity, *i.e.* pacemaking in non-SN cells, which is considered as one of the most important triggers initiating atrial fibrillation (Jones et al., 2012). Youm et al. (2006) modeled pacemaker activity in mouse small intestine, *i.e.*, noncardiac, cells and found a role of NCX for automaticity in these cells as well (Youm et al., 2006).

Loewe et al. investigated the effect of extracellular Ca^{2+} concentration changes on SN pacemaking in the LLFS computational model motivated by the observation that the heart rate of dialysis patients, who experience marked shifts of extracellular ion concentrations, drops to very low values before they suffer from sudden cardiac death with an unexplained high incidence (Loewe et al., 2019a). They found that Ca^{2+} changes markedly affected the beating rate (46 bpm/mM ionized Ca^{2+} without autonomic control). While this pronounced bradycardic effect of hypocalcemia was mediated primarily by I_{CaL}, NCX was subsequently attenuated due to the reduction of $Ca^{2+}{}_i$. Wolf et al. (2013) proposed a computational model of ankyrin-B syndrome SNCs in which alterations of I_{CaL} and NCX as well as I_{NaK} due to ankyrin-B dysfunction increase variability in SN automaticity (Wolf et al., 2013). Choudhury et al. (2018) overexpressed NCX1 in bradycardic rat subsidiary atrial pacemaker tissue and found that it did not accelerate the rate of spontaneous depolarizations in contrast to overexpression of TBX18, which increased rate as well as stability and rescued isoproterenol response (Choudhury et al., 2018).

CONCLUDING REMARKS

A large body of experimental evidence indicates and mechanistic *in silico* modeling supports the crucial role of NCX in SN automaticity both under normal heart rate as well as during *β*-adrenergic stimulation. However, SN automaticity probably could be one of the areas of experimental cardiology where concise hypotheses have been derived from computational modeling that call for experimental testing which is not yet on the horizon, especially in context of NCX function. The complex effects of drugs modulating the Ca^{2+} handling (CPA, ryanodine, isoproterenol), the shortcomings of transgenic animal models, and the nonselectivity and/or indirect effects of parallel Ca^{2+} increase of selective inhibitors indicate a clear demand of further experimental research to fully reveal the role of NCX in SN pacemaking.

AUTHOR CONTRIBUTIONS

AL—preparing the manuscript: in silico mechanistic modeling, preparing the figures. AV—supervising the study. NN—preparing the manuscript: experimental results of the NCX function in SN. ZK, NT—searching of relevant publications, preparing subchapters of the manuscript.

FUNDING

We declare that all sources of funding received is submitted.

ACKNOWLEDGMENTS

This work was supported by grants from the National Research Development and Innovation Office (NKFIH PD-125402 (for NN), FK-129117 (for NN), GINOP-2.3.2-15-2016-00006 and GINOP-2.3.2-15-2016-00012), the LIVE LONGER EFOP-3.6.2-16-2017-00006 project, the János Bolyai Research Scholarship of the Hungarian Academy of Sciences (for NN), the UNKP-18-4-SZTE-76 New National Excellence Program of the Ministry for Innovation and Technology (for NN), the EFOP 3.6.3 VEKOP-16-2017-00009 (for NT). AL gratefully acknowledges financial support by the Deutsche Forschungsgemeinschaft (DFG, German Research Foundation)—Project-ID 399 258734477—SFB 1173 and through Project-ID 391128822-LO 2093/1-1. University of Szeged Open Access Fund, No.: 4314.

REFERENCES

Allah, E. A., Tellez, J. O., Yanni, J., Nelson, T., Monfredi, O., Boyett, M. R., et al. (2011). Changes in the expression of ion channels, connexins and Ca2 +-handling proteins in the sino-atrial node during postnatal development. *Exp. Physiol.* 96 (4), 426–438. doi: 10.1113/expphysiol.2010.055780

Allen, D. G., Eisner, D. A., Lab, M. J., and Orchard, C. H. (1983). The effects of low sodium solutions on intracellular calcium concentration and tension in ferret ventricular muscle. *J. Physiol.* 345, 391–407. doi: 10.1113/jphysiol.1983.sp014984

Amoroso, S., Tortiglione, A., Secondo, A., Catalano, A., Montagnani, S., Di Renzo, G., et al. (2000). Sodium nitroprusside prevents chemical hypoxia-induced cell death through iron ions stimulating the activity of the Na+-Ca2+ exchanger in C6 glioma cells. *J. Neurochem.* 74 (4), 1505–1513. doi: 10.1046/j.1471-4159.2000.0741505.x

Ballard, C., and Schaffer, S. (1996). Stimulation of the Na+/Ca2+ exchanger by phenylephrine, angiotensin II and endothelin 1. *J. Mol. Cell Cardiol.* 28 (1), 11–17. doi: 10.1006/jmcc.1996.0002

Baruscotti, M., Bucchi, A., Viscomi, C., Mandelli, G., Consalez, G., Gnecchi-Rusconi, T., et al. (2011). Deep bradycardia and heart block caused by inducible cardiac-specific knockout of the pacemaker channel gene Hcn4. *Proc. Natl. Acad. Sci. U. S. A* 108 (4), 1705–1710. doi: 10.1073/pnas.1010122108

Bers, D. M., and Ginsburg, K. S. (2007). Na:Ca stoichiometry and cytosolic Ca-dependent activation of NCX in intact cardiomyocytes. *Ann. N. Y. Acad. Sci.* 1099, 326–338. doi: 10.1196/annals.1387.060

Bers, D. M. (2001). *Excitation-Contraction Coupling and Cardiac Contractile Force* (Netherlands: Springer). doi: 10.1007/978-94-010-0658-3

Bers, D. M. (2002). Cardiac excitation-contraction coupling. *Nature* 415 (6868), 198–205. doi: 10.1038/415198a

Bers, D. M. (2008). Calcium cycling and signaling in cardiac myocytes. *Annu. Rev. Physiol.* 70, 23–49. doi: 10.1146/annurev.physiol.70.113006.100455

Birinyi, P., Acsai, K., Banyasz, T., Toth, A., Horvath, B., Virag, L., et al. (2005). Effects of SEA0400 and KB-R7943 on Na+/Ca2+ exchange current and L-type Ca2+ current in canine ventricular cardiomyocytes. *Naunyn Schmiedebergs Arch. Pharmacol.* 372 (1), 63–70. doi: 10.1007/s00210-005-1079-x

Bleeker, W. K., Mackaay, A. J., Masson-Pevet, M., Bouman, L. N., and Becker, A. E. (1980). Functional and morphological organization of the rabbit sinus node. *Circ. Res.* 46 (1), 11–22. doi: 10.1161/01.res.46.1.11

Bogdanov, K. Y., Vinogradova, T. M., and Lakatta, E. G. (2001). Sinoatrial nodal cell ryanodine receptor and Na(+)-Ca(2+) exchanger: molecular partners in pacemaker regulation. *Circ. Res.* 88 (12), 1254–1258. doi: 10.1161/hh1201.092095

Bogdanov, K. Y., Maltsev, V. A., Vinogradova, T. M., Lyashkov, A. E., Spurgeon, H. A., Stern, M. D., et al. (2006). Membrane potential fluctuations resulting from submembrane Ca2+ releases in rabbit sinoatrial nodal cells impart an exponential phase to the late diastolic depolarization that controls their chronotropic state. *Circ. Res.* 99 (9), 979–987. doi: 10.1161/01.RES.0000247933.66532.0b

Boyett, M. R., Honjo, H., Yamamoto, M., Nikmaram, M. R., Niwa, R., and Kodama, I. (1998). Regional differences in effects of 4-aminopyridine within the sinoatrial node. *Am. J. Physiol.* 275 (4), H1158–H1168. doi: 10.1152/ajpheart.1998.275.4.H1158

Boyett, M. R., Honjo, H., and Kodama, I. (2000). The sinoatrial node, a heterogeneous pacemaker structure. *Cardiovasc. Res.* 47 (4), 658–687. doi: 10.1016/s0008-6363(00)00135-8

Brown, H. F., Kimura, J., Noble, D., Noble, S. J., and Taupignon, A. (1984). The slow inward current, isi, in the rabbit sino-atrial node investigated by voltage clamp and computer simulation. *Proc. R. Soc. Lond. B. Biol. Sci.* 222 (1228), 305–328. doi: 10.1098/rspb.1984.0066

Bucchi, A., Baruscotti, M., Robinson, R. B., and DiFrancesco, D. (2003). I(f)-dependent modulation of pacemaker rate mediated by cAMP in the presence of ryanodine in rabbit sino-atrial node cells. *J. Mol. Cell Cardiol.* 35 (8), 905–913. doi: 10.1016/S0022-2828(03)00150-0

Bucchi, A., Barbuti, A., Baruscotti, M., and DiFrancesco, D. (2007a). Heart rate reduction via selective 'funny' channel blockers. *Curr. Opin. Pharmacol.* 7 (2), 208–213. doi: 10.1016/j.coph.2006.09.005

Bucchi, A., Baruscotti, M., Robinson, R. B., and DiFrancesco, D. (2007b). Modulation of rate by autonomic agonists in SAN cells involves changes in diastolic depolarization and the pacemaker current. *J. Mol. Cell Cardiol.* 43 (1), 39–48. doi: 10.1016/j.yjmcc.2007.04.017

Buck, E., Zimanyi, I., Abramson, J. J., and Pessah, I. N. (1992). Ryanodine stabilizes multiple conformational states of the skeletal muscle calcium release channel. *J. Biol. Chem.* 267 (33), 23560–23567.

Chandler, N. J., Greener, I. D., Tellez, J. O., Inada, S., Musa, H., Molenaar, P., et al. (2009). Molecular architecture of the human sinus node: insights into the function of the cardiac pacemaker. *Circulation* 119 (12), 1562–1575. doi: 10.1161/CIRCULATIONAHA.108.804369

Chapman, R. A., and Tunstall, J. (1980). The interaction of sodium and calcium ions at the cell membrane and the control of contractile strength in frog atrial muscle. *J. Physiol.* 305, 109–123. doi: 10.1113/jphysiol.1980.sp013353

Cheng, H., Lederer, W. J., and Cannell, M. B. (1993). Calcium sparks: elementary events underlying excitation-contraction coupling in heart muscle. *Science* 262 (5134), 740–744. doi: 10.1126/science.8235594

Choi, S. W., Lee, H. A., Moon, S. H., Park, S. J., Kim, H. J., Kim, K. S., et al. (2016). Spontaneous inward currents reflecting oscillatory activation of Na(+)/Ca(2)(+) exchangers in human embryonic stem cell-derived cardiomyocytes. *Pflugers Arch.* 468 (4), 609–622. doi: 10.1007/s00424-015-1769-2

Choudhury, M., Black, N., Alghamdi, A., D'Souza, A., Wang, R., Yanni, J., et al. (2018). TBX18 overexpression enhances pacemaker function in a rat subsidiary atrial pacemaker model of sick sinus syndrome. *J. Physiol.* 596 (24), 6141–6155. doi: 10.1113/JP276508

Courtemanche, M., Ramirez, R. J., and Nattel, S. (1998). Ionic mechanisms underlying human atrial action potential properties: insights from a mathematical model. *Am. J. Physiol.* 275 (1), H301–H321. doi: 10.1152/ajpheart.1998.275.1.H301

Demir, S. S., Clark, J. W., Murphey, C. R., and Giles, W. R. (1994). A mathematical model of a rabbit sinoatrial node cell. *Am. J. Physiol.* 266 (3 Pt 1), C832–C852. doi: 10.1152/ajpcell.1994.266.3.C832

DiFrancesco, D., and Noble, D. (1985). A model of cardiac electrical activity incorporating ionic pumps and concentration changes. *Philos. Trans. R. Soc. Lond. B. Biol. Sci.* 307 (1133), 353–398. doi: 10.1098/rstb.1985.0001

DiFrancesco, D. (1991). The contribution of the 'pacemaker' current (if) to generation of spontaneous activity in rabbit sino-atrial node myocytes. *J. Physiol.* 434, 23–40. doi: 10.1113/jphysiol.1991.sp018457

DiFrancesco, D. (1993). Pacemaker mechanisms in cardiac tissue. *Annu. Rev. Physiol.* 55, 455–472. doi: 10.1146/annurev.ph.55.030193.002323

DiFrancesco, D. (1995). Cesium and the pacemaker current. *J. Cardiovasc. Electrophysiol.* 6 (12), 1152–1155. doi: 10.1111/j.1540-8167.1995.tb00394.x

DiFrancesco, D. (2020). A Brief History of Pacemaking. *Front. Physiol.* 10, 1599. doi: 10.3389/fphys.2019.01599

Dokos, S., Celler, B., and Lovell, N. (1996). Ion currents underlying sinoatrial node pacemaker activity: a new single cell mathematical model. *J. Theor. Biol.* 181 (3), 245–272. doi: 10.1006/jtbi.1996.0129

Fabbri, A., Fantini, M., Wilders, R., and Severi, S. (2017). Computational analysis of the human sinus node action potential: model development and effects of mutations. *J. Physiol.* 595 (7), 2365–2396. doi: 10.1113/JP273259

Farkas, A. S., Acsai, K., Nagy, N., Toth, A., Fulop, F., Seprenyi, G., et al. (2008). Na (+)/Ca(2+) exchanger inhibition exerts a positive inotropic effect in the rat heart, but fails to influence the contractility of the rabbit heart. *Br. J. Pharmacol.* 154 (1), 93–104. doi: 10.1038/bjp.2008.83

Fill, M., and Copello, J. A. (2002). Ryanodine receptor calcium release channels. *Physiol. Rev.* 82 (4), 893–922. doi: 10.1152/physrev.00013.2002

Fischmeister, R., and Vassort, G. (1981). The electrogenic Na-Ca exchange and the cardiac electrical activity. I-Simulation on Purkinje fibre action potential. *J Physiol (Paris)* 77 (6–7), 705–709.

Gao, Z., Chen, B., Joiner, M. L., Wu, Y., Guan, X., Koval, O. M., et al. (2010). I(f) and SR Ca(2+) release both contribute to pacemaker activity in canine sinoatrial node cells. *J. Mol. Cell Cardiol.* 49 (1), 33–40. doi: 10.1016/j.yjmcc.2010.03.019

Gao, Z., Singh, M. V., Hall, D. D., Koval, O. M., Luczak, E. D., Joiner, M. L., et al. (2011). Catecholamine-independent heart rate increases require Ca2 +/calmodulin-dependent protein kinase II. *Circ. Arrhythm. Electrophysiol.* 4 (3), 379–387. doi: 10.1161/CIRCEP.110.961771

Gao, Z., Rasmussen, T. P., Li, Y., Kutschke, W., Koval, O. M., Wu, Y., et al. (2013). Genetic inhibition of Na+-Ca2+ exchanger current disables fight or flight sinoatrial node activity without affecting resting heart rate. *Circ. Res.* 112 (2), 309–317. doi: 10.1161/CIRCRESAHA.111.300193

Garny, A., Kohl, P., Hunter, P. J., Boyett, M. R., and Noble, D. (2003). One-dimensional rabbit sinoatrial node models: benefits and limitations. *J. Cardiovasc. Electrophysiol.* 14 (10 Suppl.), S121–S132. doi: 10.1046/j.1540.8167.90301.x

Ginsburg, K. S., and Bers, D. M. (2005). Isoproterenol does not enhance Ca-dependent Na/Ca exchange current in intact rabbit ventricular myocytes. *J. Mol. Cell Cardiol.* 39 (6), 972–981. doi: 10.1016/j.yjmcc.2005.09.005

Ginsburg, K. S., Weber, C. R., and Bers, D. M. (2013). Cardiac Na+-Ca2+ exchanger: dynamics of Ca2+-dependent activation and deactivation in intact myocytes. *J. Physiol.* 591 (8), 2067–2086. doi: 10.1113/jphysiol.2013.252080

Groenke, S., Larson, E. D., Alber, S., Zhang, R., Lamp, S. T., Ren, X., et al. (2013). Complete atrial-specific knockout of sodium-calcium exchange eliminates sinoatrial node pacemaker activity. *PLoS One* 8 (11), e81633. doi: 10.1371/journal.pone.0081633

Gupta, M. P., Makino, N., Khatter, K., and Dhalla, N. S. (1986). Stimulation of Na+-Ca2+ exchange in heart sarcolemma by insulin. *Life Sci.* 39 (12), 1077–1083. doi: 10.1016/0024-3205(86)90199-2

Hagiwara, N., and Irisawa, H. (1989). Modulation by intracellular Ca2+ of the hyperpolarization-activated inward current in rabbit single sino-atrial node cells. *J. Physiol.* 409, 121–141. doi: 10.1113/jphysiol.1989.sp017488

Harzheim, D., Pfeiffer, K. H., Fabritz, L., Kremmer, E., Buch, T., Waisman, A., et al. (2008). Cardiac pacemaker function of HCN4 channels in mice is confined to embryonic development and requires cyclic AMP. *EMBO J.* 27 (4), 692–703. doi: 10.1038/emboj.2008.3

Herrmann, S., Stieber, J., Stockl, G., Hofmann, F., and Ludwig, A. (2007). HCN4 provides a 'depolarization reserve' and is not required for heart rate acceleration in mice. *EMBO J.* 26 (21), 4423–4432. doi: 10.1038/sj.emboj.7601868

Herrmann, S., Lipp, P., Wiesen, K., Stieber, J., Nguyen, H., Kaiser, E., et al. (2013). The cardiac sodium-calcium exchanger NCX1 is a key player in the initiation and maintenance of a stable heart rhythm. *Cardiovasc. Res.* 99 (4), 780–788. doi: 10.1093/cvr/cvt154

Himeno, Y., Sarai, N., Matsuoka, S., and Noma, A. (2008). Ionic mechanisms underlying the positive chronotropy induced by beta1-adrenergic stimulation in guinea pig sinoatrial node cells: a simulation study. *J. Physiol. Sci.* 58 (1), 53–65. doi: 10.2170/physiolsci.RP015207

Himeno, Y., Toyoda, F., Satoh, H., Amano, A., Cha, C. Y., Matsuura, H., et al. (2011). Minor contribution of cytosolic Ca2+ transients to the pacemaker rhythm in guinea pig sinoatrial node cells. *Am. J. Physiol. Heart Circ. Physiol.* 300 (1), H251 H261. doi: 10.1152/ajpheart.00764.2010

Hoang-Trong, T. M., Ullah, A., and Jafri, M. S. (2015). Calcium Sparks in the Heart: Dynamics and Regulation. *Res. Rep. Biol.* 6, 203–214. doi: 10.2147/RRB.S61495

Hoesl, E., Stieber, J., Herrmann, S., Feil, S., Tybl, E., Hofmann, F., et al. (2008). Tamoxifen-inducible gene deletion in the cardiac conduction system. *J. Mol. Cell Cardiol.* 45 (1), 62–69. doi: 10.1016/j.yjmcc.2008.04.008

Honjo, H., Boyett, M. R., Kodama, I., and Toyama, J. (1996). Correlation between electrical activity and the size of rabbit sino-atrial node cells. *J. Physiol.* 496 (Pt 3), 795–808. doi: 10.1113/jphysiol.1996.sp021728

Huser, J., Blatter, L. A., and Lipsius, S. L. (2000). Intracellular Ca2+ release contributes to automaticity in cat atrial pacemaker cells. *J. Physiol.* 524 Pt 2, 415–422. doi: 10.1111/j.1469-7793.2000.00415.x

Imtiaz, M. S., von der Weid, P. Y., Laver, D. R., and van Helden, D. F. (2010). SR Ca2+ store refill–a key factor in cardiac pacemaking. *J. Mol. Cell Cardiol.* 49 (3), 412–426. doi: 10.1016/j.yjmcc.2010.03.015

Iwamoto, T., Wakabayashi, S., and Shigekawa, M. (1995). Growth factor-induced phosphorylation and activation of aortic smooth muscle Na+/Ca2+ exchanger. *J. Biol. Chem.* 270 (15), 8996–9001. doi: 10.1074/jbc.270.15.8996

Iwamoto, T., Watano, T., and Shigekawa, M. (1996). A novel isothiourea derivative selectively inhibits the reverse mode of Na+/Ca2+ exchange in cells expressing NCX1. *J. Biol. Chem.* 271 (37), 22391–22397. doi: 10.1074/jbc.271.37.22391

Iwamoto, T., Pan, Y., Nakamura, T. Y., Wakabayashi, S., and Shigekawa, M. (1998). Protein kinase C-dependent regulation of Na+/Ca2+ exchanger isoforms NCX1 and NCX3 does not require their direct phosphorylation. *Biochemistry* 37 (49), 17230–17238. doi: 10.1021/bi981521q

Jones, G., Spencer, B. D., Adeniran, I., and Zhang, H. (2012). Development of biophysically detailed electrophysiological models for pacemaking and non-pacemaking human pulmonary vein cardiomyocytes. *Conf. Proc. IEEE Eng. Med. Biol. Soc.* 2012, 199–202. doi: 10.1109/EMBC.2012.6345905

Jost, N., Nagy, N., Corici, C., Kohajda, Z., Horvath, A., Acsai, K., et al. (2013). ORM-10103, a novel specific inhibitor of the Na+/Ca2+ exchanger, decreases early and delayed afterdepolarizations in the canine heart. *Br. J. Pharmacol.* 170 (4), 768–778. doi: 10.1111/bph.12228

Joung, B., Tang, L., Maruyama, M., Han, S., Chen, Z., Stucky, M., et al. (2009). Intracellular calcium dynamics and acceleration of sinus rhythm by beta-adrenergic stimulation. *Circulation* 119 (6), 788–796. doi: 10.1161/CIRCULATIONAHA.108.817379

Ju, Y. K., and Allen, D. G. (1998). Intracellular calcium and Na+-Ca2+ exchange current in isolated toad pacemaker cells. *J. Physiol.* 508 (Pt 1), 153–166. doi: 10.1111/j.1469-7793.1998.153br.x

Ju, Y. K., Saint, D. A., Hirst, G. D., and Gage, P. W. (1995). Sodium currents in toad cardiac pacemaker cells. *J. Membr. Biol.* 145 (2), 119–128. doi: 10.1007/bf00237370

Kaese, S., Bogeholz, N., Pauls, P., Dechering, D., Olligs, J., Kolker, K., et al. (2017). Increased sodium/calcium exchanger activity enhances beta-adrenergic-mediated increase in heart rate: Whole-heart study in a homozygous sodium/calcium exchanger overexpressor mouse model. *Heart Rhythm.* 14 (8), 1247–1253. doi: 10.1016/j.hrthm.2017.05.001

Kharche, S., Yu, J., Lei, M., and Zhang, H. (2011). A mathematical model of action potentials of mouse sinoatrial node cells with molecular bases. *Am. J. Physiol. Heart Circ. Physiol.* 301 (3), H945–H963. doi: 10.1152/ajpheart.00143.2010

Kim, M. S., Maltsev, A. V., Monfredi, O., Maltseva, L. A., Wirth, A., Florio, M. C., et al. (2018). Heterogeneity of calcium clock functions in dormant, dysrhythmically and rhythmically firing single pacemaker cells isolated from SA node. *Cell Calcium* 74, 168–179. doi: 10.1016/j.ceca.2018.07.002

Kofuji, P., Lederer, W. J., and Schulze, D. H. (1994). Mutually exclusive and cassette exons underlie alternatively spliced isoforms of the Na/Ca exchanger. *J. Biol. Chem.* 269 (7), 5145–5149.

Kohajda, Z., Farkas-Morvay, N., Jost, N., Nagy, N., Geramipour, A., Horvath, A., et al. (2016). The Effect of a Novel Highly Selective Inhibitor of the Sodium/Calcium Exchanger (NCX) on Cardiac Arrhythmias in In Vitro and In Vivo Experiments. *PLoS One* 11 (11), e0166041. doi: 10.1371/journal.pone.0166041

Kohajda, Z., Tóth, N., Szlovák, J., Loewe, A., Bitay, G., Gazdag, P., et al. (2020). Novel Na+/Ca2+ Exchanger Inhibitor ORM-10962 Supports Coupled Function of Funny-Current and Na+/Ca2+ Exchanger in Pacemaking of Rabbit Sinus Node Tissue. *Front. Pharmacol.* 10, 1632. doi: 10.3389/fphar.2019.01632

Koncz, I., Szel, T., Bitay, M., Cerbai, E., Jaeger, K., Fulop, F., et al. (2011). Electrophysiological effects of ivabradine in dog and human cardiac preparations: potential antiarrhythmic actions. *Eur. J. Pharmacol.* 668 (3), 419–426. doi: 10.1016/j.ejphar.2011.07.025

Kurata, Y., Hisatome, I., Imanishi, S., and Shibamoto, T. (2002). Dynamical description of sinoatrial node pacemaking: improved mathematical model for primary pacemaker cell. *Am. J. Physiol. Heart Circ. Physiol.* 283 (5), H2074–H2101. doi: 10.1152/ajpheart.00900.2001

Kurata, Y., Hisatome, I., Matsuda, H., and Shibamoto, T. (2005). Dynamical mechanisms of pacemaker generation in IK1-downregulated human ventricular myocytes: insights from bifurcation analyses of a mathematical model. *Biophys. J.* 89 (4), 2865–2887. doi: 10.1529/biophysj.105.060830

Kurata, Y., Hisatome, I., and Shibamoto, T. (2012). Roles of sarcoplasmic reticulum Ca2+ cycling and Na+/Ca2+ exchanger in sinoatrial node pacemaking: insights from bifurcation analysis of mathematical models. *Am. J. Physiol. Heart Circ. Physiol.* 302 (11), H2285–H2300. doi: 10.1152/ajpheart.00221.2011

Lakatta, E. G., and DiFrancesco, D. (2009). What keeps us ticking: a funny current, a calcium clock, or both? *J. Mol. Cell Cardiol.* 47 (2), 157–170. doi: 10.1016/j.yjmcc.2009.03.022

Lakatta, E. G., and Maltsev, V. A. (2012). Rebuttal: what I(f) the shoe doesn't fit? "The funny current has a major pacemaking role in the sinus node". *Heart Rhythm.* 9 (3), 459–460. doi: 10.1016/j.hrthm.2011.09.024

Lakatta, E. G., Maltsev, V. A., and Vinogradova, T. M. (2010). A coupled SYSTEM of intracellular Ca2+ clocks and surface membrane voltage clocks controls the timekeeping mechanism of the heart's pacemaker. *Circ. Res.* 106 (4), 659–673. doi: 10.1161/CIRCRESAHA.109.206078

Lancaster, M. K., Jones, S. A., Harrison, S. M., and Boyett, M. R. (2004). Intracellular Ca2+ and pacemaking within the rabbit sinoatrial node:

heterogeneity of role and control. *J. Physiol.* 556 (Pt 2), 481–494. doi: 10.1113/jphysiol.2003.057372

Li, Z., Matsuoka, S., Hryshko, L. V., Nicoll, D. A., Bersohn, M. M., Burke, E. P., et al. (1994). Cloning of the NCX2 isoform of the plasma membrane Na (+)-Ca2+ exchanger. *J. Biol. Chem.* 269 (26), 17434–17439.

Li, J., Qu, J., and Nathan, R. D. (1997). Ionic basis of ryanodine's negative chronotropic effect on pacemaker cells isolated from the sinoatrial node. *Am. J. Physiol.* 273 (5), H2481–H2489. doi: 10.1152/ajpheart.1997.273.5.H2481

Li, P., Lines, G., Maleckar, M., and Tveito, A. (2013). Mathematical models of cardiac pacemaking function. *Front. Phys.* 1, 20. doi: 10.3389/fphy.2013.00020

Li, Y., Sirenko, S., Riordon, D. R., Yang, D., Spurgeon, H., Lakatta, E. G., et al. (2016). CaMKII-dependent phosphorylation regulates basal cardiac pacemaker function via modulation of local Ca2+ releases. *Am. J. Physiol. Heart Circ. Physiol.* 311 (3), H532–H544. doi: 10.1152/ajpheart.00765.2015

Lipp, P., Pott, L., Callewaert, G., and Carmeliet, E. (1990). Simultaneous recording of Indo-1 fluorescence and Na+/Ca2+ exchange current reveals two components of Ca2(+)-release from sarcoplasmic reticulum of cardiac atrial myocytes. *FEBS Lett.* 275 (1-2), 181–184. doi: 10.1016/0014-5793(90)81467-3

Liu, J., Sirenko, S., Juhaszova, M., Ziman, B., Shetty, V., Rain, S., et al. (2011). A full range of mouse sinoatrial node AP firing rates requires protein kinase A-dependent calcium signaling. *J. Mol. Cell Cardiol.* 51 (5), 730–739. doi: 10.1016/j.yjmcc.2011.07.028

Loewe, A., Lutz, Y., Fabbri, A., and Severi, S. (2019a). Sinus Bradycardia Due to Electrolyte Changes as a Potential Pathomechanism of Sudden Cardiac Death in Hemodialysis Patients. *Biophys. J.* 116, 231a. doi: 10.1016/j.bpj.2018.11.1271

Loewe, A., Lutz, Y., Nagy, N., Fabbri, A., Schweda, C.,.Varró, A., et al. (2019b). Inter-Species Differences in the Response of Sinus Node Cellular Pacemaking to Changes of Extracellular Calcium, in: *2019 41st Annual International Conference of the IEEE Engineering in Medicine and Biology Society (EMBC).* 1875–1878. doi: 10.1109/EMBC.2019.8857573

Ludwig, ,. A., Budde, T., Stieber, J., Moosmang, S., Wahl, C., Holthoff, K., et al. (2003). Absence epilepsy and sinus dysrhythmia in mice lacking the pacemaker channel HCN2. *EMBO J.* 22 (2), 216–224. doi: 10.1093/emboj/cdg032

Luo, C. H., and Rudy, Y. (1994). A dynamic model of the cardiac ventricular action potential. I. Simulations of ionic currents and concentration changes. *Circ. Res.* 74 (6), 1071–96.

Lyashkov, A. E., Juhaszova, M., Dobrzynski, H., Vinogradova, T. M., Maltsev, V. A., Juhasz, O., et al. (2007). Calcium cycling protein density and functional importance to automaticity of isolated sinoatrial nodal cells are independent of cell size. *Circ. Res.* 100 (12), 1723–1731. doi: 10.1161/CIRCRESAHA.107.153676

Lyashkov, A. E., Vinogradova, T. M., Zahanich, I., Li, Y., Younes, A., Nuss, H. B., et al. (2009). Cholinergic receptor signaling modulates spontaneous firing of sinoatrial nodal cells via integrated effects on PKA-dependent Ca(2+) cycling and I(KACh). *Am. J. Physiol. Heart Circ. Physiol.* 297 (3), H949–H959. doi: 10.1152/ajpheart.01340.2008

Lyashkov, A. E., Behar, J., Lakatta, E. G., Yaniv, Y., and Maltsev, V. A. (2018). Positive Feedback Mechanisms among Local Ca Releases, NCX, and ICaL Ignite Pacemaker Action Potentials. *Biophys. J.* 114 (5), 1176–1189. doi: 10.1016/j.bpj.2017.12.043

Makino, N., Zhao, D., and Dhalla, N. S. (1988). Stimulation of heart sarcolemmal Na+-Ca2+ exchange by concanavalin A. *Biochem. Biophys. Res. Commun.* 154 (1), 245–251. doi: 10.1016/0006-291x(88)90676-6

Maltsev, V. A., and Lakatta, E. G. (2009). Synergism of coupled subsarcolemmal Ca2+ clocks and sarcolemmal voltage clocks confers robust and flexible pacemaker function in a novel pacemaker cell model. *Am. J. Physiol. Heart Circ. Physiol.* 296 (3), H594–H615. doi: 10.1152/ajpheart.01118.2008

Maltsev, V. A., and Lakatta, E. G. (2010). A novel quantitative explanation for the autonomic modulation of cardiac pacemaker cell automaticity via a dynamic system of sarcolemmal and intracellular proteins. *Am. J. Physiol. Heart Circ. Physiol.* 298 (6), H2010–H2023. doi: 10.1152/ajpheart.00783.2009

Maltsev, V. A., and Lakatta, E. G. (2013). Numerical models based on a minimal set of sarcolemmal electrogenic proteins and an intracellular Ca(2+) clock generate robust, flexible, and energy-efficient cardiac pacemaking. *J. Mol. Cell Cardiol.* 59, 181–195. doi: 10.1016/j.yjmcc.2013.03.004

Maltsev, V. A., Vinogradova, T. M., Bogdanov, K. Y., Lakatta, E. G., and Stern, M. D. (2004). Diastolic calcium release controls the beating rate of rabbit sinoatrial node cells: numerical modeling of the coupling process. *Biophys. J.* 86 (4), 2596–2605. doi: 10.1016/S0006-3495(04)74314-3

Maltsev, V. A., Vinogradova, T. M., and Lakatta, E. G. (2006). The emergence of a general theory of the initiation and strength of the heartbeat. *J. Pharmacol. Sci.* 100 (5), 338–369. doi: 10.1254/jphs.cr0060018

Maltsev, A. V., Maltsev, V. A., Mikheev, M., Maltseva, L. A., Sirenko, S. G., Lakatta, E. G., et al. (2011a). Synchronization of stochastic Ca(2)(+) release units creates a rhythmic Ca(2)(+) clock in cardiac pacemaker cells. *Biophys. J.* 100 (2), 271–283. doi: 10.1016/j.bpj.2010.11.081

Maltsev, V. A., Vinogradova, T. M., Stern, M. D., and Lakatta, E. G. (2011b). Letter to the editor: "Validating the requirement for beat-to-beat coupling of the Ca2 + clock and M clock in pacemaker cell normal automaticity". *Am. J. Physiol. Heart Circ. Physiol.* 300 (6), H2323–2324; author reply H2325-2326. doi: 10.1152/ajpheart.00110.2011

Maltsev, A. V., Yaniv, Y., Stern, M. D., Lakatta, E. G., and Maltsev, V. A. (2013). RyR-NCX-SERCA local cross-talk ensures pacemaker cell function at rest and during the fight-or-flight reflex. *Circ. Res.* 113 (10), e94–e100. doi: 10.1161/CIRCRESAHA.113.302465

Maltsev, V. A., Yaniv, Y., Maltsev, A. V., Stern, M. D., and Lakatta, E. G. (2014). Modern perspectives on numerical modeling of cardiac pacemaker cell. *J. Pharmacol. Sci.* 125 (1), 6–38. doi: 10.1254/jphs.13r04cr

Maltsev, A. V., Maltsev, V. A., and Stern, M. D. (2017). Stabilization of diastolic calcium signal via calcium pump regulation of complex local calcium releases and transient decay in a computational model of cardiac pacemaker cell with individual release channels. *PloS Comput. Biol.* 13 (8), e1005675. doi: 10.1371/journal.pcbi.1005675

Mangoni, M. E., Couette, B., Bourinet, E., Platzer, J., Reimer, D., Striessnig, J., et al. (2003). Functional role of L-type Cav1.3 Ca2+ channels in cardiac pacemaker activity. *Proc. Natl. Acad. Sci. U. S. A* 100 (9), 5543–5548. doi: 10.1073/pnas.0935295100

Masson-Pevet, M. A., Bleeker, W. K., Besselsen, E., Treytel, B. W., Jongsma, H. J., and Bouman, L. N. (1984). Pacemaker cell types in the rabbit sinus node: a correlative ultrastructural and electrophysiological study. *J. Mol. Cell Cardiol.* 16 (1), 53–63. doi: 10.1016/s0022-2828(84)80714-2

Matsuoka, S., and Hilgemann, D. W. (1992). Steady-state and dynamic properties of cardiac sodium-calcium exchange. Ion and voltage dependencies of the transport cycle. *J. Gen. Physiol.* 100 (6), 963–1001. doi: 10.1085/jgp.100.6.963

Mattick, P., Parrington, J., Odia, E., Simpson, A., Collins, T., and Terrar, D. (2007). Ca2+-stimulated adenylyl cyclase isoform AC1 is preferentially expressed in guinea-pig sino-atrial node cells and modulates the I(f) pacemaker current. *J. Physiol.* 582 (Pt 3), 1195–1203. doi: 10.1113/jphysiol.2007.133439

Monfredi, O., Maltseva, L. A., Spurgeon, H. A., Boyett, M. R., Lakatta, E. G., and Maltsev, V. A. (2013). Beat-to-Beat Variation in Periodicity of Local Calcium Releases Contributes to Intrinsic Variations of Spontaneous Cycle Length in Isolated Single Sinoatrial Node Cells. *PLoS One* 8 (6), e67247. doi: 10.1371/journal.pone.0067247

Monfredi, O., Tsutsui, K., Ziman, B., Stern, M. D., Lakatta, E. G., and Maltsev, V. A. (2018). Electrophysiological heterogeneity of pacemaker cells in the rabbit intercaval region, including the SA node: insights from recording multiple ion currents in each cell. *Am. J. Physiol. Heart Circ. Physiol.* 314 (3), H403–H414. doi: 10.1152/ajpheart.00253.2016

Mullins, L. J., and Requena, J. (1979). Calcium measurement in the periphery of an axon. *J. Gen. Physiol.* 74 (3), 393–413. doi: 10.1085/jgp.74.3.393

Musa, H., Lei, M., Honjo, H., Jones, S. A., Dobrzynski, H., Lancaster, M. K., et al. (2002). Heterogeneous expression of Ca(2+) handling proteins in rabbit sinoatrial node. *J. Histochem. Cytochem.* 50 (3), 311–324. doi: 10.1177/002215540205000303

Nagy, N., Szuts, V., Horvath, Z., Seprenyi, G., Farkas, A. S., Acsai, K., et al. (2009). Does small-conductance calcium-activated potassium channel contribute to cardiac repolarization? *J. Mol. Cell Cardiol.* 47 (5), 656–663. doi: 10.1016/j.yjmcc.2009.07.019

Nicoll, D. A., Longoni, S., and Philipson, K. D. (1990). Molecular cloning and functional expression of the cardiac sarcolemmal Na(+)-Ca2+ exchanger. *Science* 250 (4980), 562–565. doi: 10.1126/science.1700476

Nicoll, D. A., Quednau, B. D., Qui, Z., Xia, Y. R., Lusis, A. J., and Philipson, K. D. (1996). Cloning of a third mammalian Na+-Ca2+ exchanger, NCX3. *J. Biol. Chem.* 271 (40), 24914–24921. doi: 10.1074/jbc.271.40.24914

Noble, D., and Noble, S. J. (1984). A model of sino-atrial node electrical activity based on a modification of the DiFrancesco-Noble, (1984) equations. *Proc. R. Soc. Lond. B. Biol. Sci.* 222 (1228), 295–304. doi: 10.1098/rspb.1984.0065

Noble, D. (1962). A modification of the Hodgkin–Huxley equations applicable to Purkinje fibre action and pace-maker potentials. *J. Physiol.* 160, 317–352. doi: 10.1113/jphysiol.1962.sp006849

Opthof, T. (2001). Function and structure of the mouse sinus node: nothing you can see that isn't shown. *Cardiovasc. Res.* 52 (1), 1–4. doi: 10.1016/s0008-6363(01)00417-5

Osipchuk, Y. V., Wakui, M., Yule, D. I., Gallacher, D. V., and Petersen, O. H. (1990). Cytoplasmic Ca2+ oscillations evoked by receptor stimulation, G-protein activation, internal application of inositol trisphosphate or Ca2+: simultaneous microfluorimetry and Ca2+ dependent Cl- current recording in single pancreatic acinar cells. *EMBO J.* 9 (3), 697–704. doi: 10.1002/j.1460-2075.1990.tb08162.x

Ottolia, M., Schumann, S., Nicoll, D. A., and Philipson, K. D. (2002). Activation of the cardiac Na+/Ca2+ exchanger by DEPC. *Ann. N. Y. Acad. Sci.* 976, 85–88. doi: 10.1111/j.1749-6632.2002.tb04720.x

Priebe, L., and Beuckelmann, D. J. (1998). Simulation study of cellular electric properties in heart failure. *Circ. Res.* 82 (11), 1206–1223.

Qu, Y., Baroudi, G., Yue, Y., El-Sherif, N., and Boutjdir, M. (2005). Localization and modulation of {alpha}1D (Cav1.3) L-type Ca channel by protein kinase A. *Am. J. Physiol. Heart Circ. Physiol.* 288 (5), H2123–H2130. doi: 10.1152/ajpheart.01023.2004

Rasmusson, R. L., Clark, J. W., Giles, W. R., Robinson, K., Clark, R. B., Shibata, E. F., et al. (1990). A mathematical model of electrophysiological activity in a bullfrog atrial cell. *Am. J. Physiol.* 259 (2 Pt 2), H370–H389. doi: 10.1152/ajpheart.1990.259.2.H370

Reeves, J. P., Bailey, C. A., and Hale, C. C. (1986). Redox modification of sodium-calcium exchange activity in cardiac sarcolemmal vesicles. *J. Biol. Chem.* 261 (11), 4948–4955.

Reilly, R. F., and Shugrue, C. A. (1992). cDNA cloning of a renal Na(+)-Ca2+ exchanger. *Am. J. Physiol.* 262 (6 Pt 2), F1105–F1109. doi: 10.1152/ajprenal.1992.262.6.F1105

Reuter, H., and Seitz, N. (1968). The dependence of calcium efflux from cardiac muscle on temperature and external ion composition. *J. Physiol.* 195 (2), 451–470. doi: 10.1113/jphysiol.1968.sp008467

Rigg, L., and Terrar, D. A. (1996). Possible role of calcium release from the sarcoplasmic reticulum in pacemaking in guinea-pig sino-atrial node. *Exp. Physiol.* 81 (5), 877–880. doi: 10.1113/expphysiol.1996.sp003983

Rigg, L., Heath, B. M., Cui, Y., and Terrar, D. A. (2000). Localisation and functional significance of ryanodine receptors during beta-adrenoceptor stimulation in the guinea-pig sino-atrial node. *Cardiovasc. Res.* 48 (2), 254–264. doi: 10.1016/s0008-6363(00)00153-x

Rousseau, E., Smith, J. S., and Meissner, G. (1987). Ryanodine modifies conductance and gating behavior of single Ca2+ release channel. *Am. J. Physiol.* 253 (3 Pt 1), C364–C368. doi: 10.1152/ajpcell.1987.253.3.C364

Rubenstein, D. S., and Lipsius, S. L. (1989). Mechanisms of automaticity in subsidiary pacemakers from cat right atrium. *Circ. Res.* 64 (4), 648–657. doi: 10.1161/01.res.64.4.648

Saeki, T., Kimura, T., Hashidume, K., Murayama, T., Yamamura, H., Ohya, S., et al. (2019). Conversion of Ca(2+) oscillation into propagative electrical signals by Ca(2+)-activated ion channels and connexin as a reconstituted Ca (2+) clock model for the pacemaker activity. *Biochem. Biophys. Res. Commun.* 510 (2), 242–247. doi: 10.1016/j.bbrc.2019.01.080

Sanders, L., Rakovic, S., Lowe, M., Mattick, P. A., and Terrar, D. A. (2006). Fundamental importance of Na+-Ca2+ exchange for the pacemaking mechanism in guinea-pig sino-atrial node. *J. Physiol.* 571 (Pt 3), 639–649. doi: 10.1113/jphysiol.2005.100305

Santacruz-Toloza, L., Ottolia, M., Nicoll, D. A., and Philipson, K. D. (2000). Functional analysis of a disulfide bond in the cardiac Na(+)-Ca(2+) exchanger. *J. Biol. Chem.* 275 (1), 182–188. doi: 10.1074/jbc.275.1.182

Satoh, H. (1993). Caffeine depression of spontaneous activity in rabbit sino-atrial node cells. *Gen. Pharmacol.* 24 (3), 555–563. doi: 10.1016/0306-3623(93)90212-G

Satoh, H. (2003). Sino-Atrial Nodal Cells of Mammalian Hearts: Ionic Currents and Gene Expression of Pacemaker Ionic Channels. *J. Smooth Muscle Res.* 39 (5), 175–193. doi: 10.1540/jsmr.39.175

Severi, S., Fantini, M., Charawi, L. A., and DiFrancesco, D. (2012). An updated computational model of rabbit sinoatrial action potential to investigate the mechanisms of heart rate modulation. *J. Physiol.* 590 (18), 4483–4499. doi: 10.1113/jphysiol.2012.229435

Silva, J., and Rudy, Y. (2003). Mechanism of pacemaking in I(K1)-downregulated myocytes. *Circ. Res.* 92 (3), 261–263. doi: 10.1161/01.res.0000057996.20414.c6

Sirenko, S., Yang, D., Li, Y., Lyashkov, A. E., Lukyanenko, Y. O., Lakatta, E. G., et al. (2013). Ca(2)(+)-dependent phosphorylation of Ca(2)(+) cycling proteins generates robust rhythmic local Ca(2)(+) releases in cardiac pacemaker cells. *Sci. Signal* 6 (260), ra6. doi: 10.1126/scisignal.2003391

Sirenko, S. G., Maltsev, V. A., Yaniv, Y., Bychkov, R., Yaeger, D., Vinogradova, T., et al. (2016). Electrochemical Na+ and Ca2+ gradients drive coupled-clock regulation of automaticity of isolated rabbit sinoatrial nodal pacemaker cells. *Am. J. Physiol. Heart Circ. Physiol.* 311 (1), H251–H267. doi: 10.1152/ajpheart.00667.2015

Smith, J. S., Imagawa, T., Ma, J., Fill, M., Campbell, K. P., and Coronado, R. (1988). Purified ryanodine receptor from rabbit skeletal muscle is the calcium-release channel of sarcoplasmic reticulum. *J. Gen. Physiol.* 92 (1), 1–26. doi: 10.1085/jgp.92.1.1

Sohn, H. G., and Vassalle, M. (1995). Cesium effects on dual pacemaker mechanisms in guinea pig sinoatrial node. *J. Mol. Cell Cardiol.* 27 (1), 563–577. doi: 10.1016/s0022-2828(08)80051-x

Stehno-Bittel, L., and Sturek, M. (1992). Spontaneous sarcoplasmic reticulum calcium release and extrusion from bovine, not porcine, coronary artery smooth muscle. *J. Physiol.* 451, 49–78. doi: 10.1113/jphysiol.1992.sp019153

Stern, M. D., Rios, E., and Maltsev, V. A. (2013). Life and death of a cardiac calcium spark. *J. Gen. Physiol.* 142 (3), 257–274. doi: 10.1085/jgp.201311034

Stern, M. D., Maltseva, L. A., Juhaszova, M., Sollott, S. J., Lakatta, E. G., and Maltsev, V. A. (2014). Hierarchical clustering of ryanodine receptors enables emergence of a calcium clock in sinoatrial node cells. *J. Gen. Physiol.* 143 (5), 577–604. doi: 10.1085/jgp.201311123

Szepesi, J., Acsai, K., Sebok, Z., Prorok, J., Pollesello, P., Levijoki, J., et al. (2015). Comparison of the efficiency of Na+/Ca2+ exchanger or Na+/H+ exchanger inhibition and their combination in reducing coronary reperfusion-induced arrhythmias. *J. Physiol. Pharmacol.* 66 (2), 215–226.

Takimoto, K., Li, D., Nerbonne, J. M., and Levitan, E. S. (1997). Distribution, splicing and glucocorticoid-induced expression of cardiac alpha 1C and alpha 1D voltage-gated Ca2+ channel mRNAs. *J. Mol. Cell Cardiol.* 29 (11), 3035–3042. doi: 10.1006/jmcc.1997.0532

Tellez, J. O., Dobrzynski, H., Greener, I. D., Graham, G. M., Laing, E., Honjo, H., et al. (2006). Differential expression of ion channel transcripts in atrial muscle and sinoatrial node in rabbit. *Circ. Res.* 99 (12), 1384–1393. doi: 10.1161/01.RES.0000251717.98379.69

Torrente, A. G., Zhang, R., Zaini, A., Giani, J. F., Kang, J., Lamp, S. T., et al. (2015). Burst pacemaker activity of the sinoatrial node in sodium-calcium exchanger knockout mice. *Proc. Natl. Acad. Sci. U. S. A* 112 (31), 9769–9774. doi: 10.1073/pnas.1505670112

Torrente, A. G., Mesirca, P., Neco, P., Rizzetto, R., Dubel, S., Barrere, C., et al. (2016). L-type Cav1.3 channels regulate ryanodine receptor-dependent Ca2+ release during sino-atrial node pacemaker activity. *Cardiovasc. Res.* 109 (3), 451–461. doi: 10.1093/cvr/cvw006

Torrente, A. G., Zhang, R., Wang, H., Zaini, A., Kim, B., Yue, X., et al. (2017). Contribution of small conductance K(+) channels to sinoatrial node pacemaker activity: insights from atrial-specific Na(+) /Ca(2+) exchange knockout mice. *J. Physiol.* 595 (12), 3847–3865. doi: 10.1113/JP274249

Trafford, A. W., Diaz, M. E., O'Neill, S. C., and Eisner, D. A. (1995). Comparison of subsarcolemmal and bulk calcium concentration during spontaneous calcium release in rat ventricular myocytes. *J. Physiol.* 488 (Pt 3), 577–586. doi: 10.1113/jphysiol.1995.sp020991

Trosper, T. L., and Philipson, K. D. (1983). Effects of divalent and trivalent cations on Na+-Ca2+ exchange in cardiac sarcolemmal vesicles. *Biochim. Biophys. Acta* 731 (1), 63–68. doi: 10.1016/0005-2736(83)90398-x

Tsutsui, K., Monfredi, O. J., Sirenko-Tagirova, S. G., Maltseva, L. A., Bychkov, R., Kim, M. S., et al. (2018). A coupled-clock system drives the automaticity of human sinoatrial nodal pacemaker cells. *Sci. Signal* 11 (534), eaap7608. doi: 10.1126/scisignal.aap7608

Vassalle, M. (1995). The pacemaker current (I(f)) does not play an important role in regulating SA node pacemaker activity. *Cardiovasc. Res.* 30 (2), 309–310. doi: 10.1016/S0008-6363(95)00028-3

Verkerk, A. O., Wilders, R., van Borren, M. M., Peters, R. J., Broekhuis, E., Lam, K., et al. (2007). Pacemaker current (I(f)) in the human sinoatrial node. *Eur. Heart J.* 28 (20), 2472–2478. doi: 10.1093/eurheartj/ehm339

Verkerk, A. O., van Borren, M. M., and Wilders, R. (2013). Calcium transient and sodium-calcium exchange current in human versus rabbit sinoatrial node pacemaker cells. *ScientificWorldJournal* 2013, 507872. doi: 10.1155/2013/507872

Vinogradova, T. M., and Lakatta, E. G. (2009). Regulation of basal and reserve cardiac pacemaker function by interactions of cAMP-mediated PKA-dependent Ca2+ cycling with surface membrane channels. *J. Mol. Cell Cardiol.* 47 (4), 456–474. doi: 10.1016/j.yjmcc.2009.06.014

Vinogradova, T. M., Zhou, Y. Y., Bogdanov, K. Y., Yang, D., Kuschel, M., Cheng, H., et al. (2000). Sinoatrial node pacemaker activity requires Ca(2+)/calmodulin-dependent protein kinase II activation. *Circ. Res.* 87 (9), 760–767. doi: 10.1161/01.res.87.9.760

Vinogradova, T. M., Bogdanov, K. Y., and Lakatta, E. G. (2002). beta-Adrenergic stimulation modulates ryanodine receptor Ca(2+) release during diastolic depolarization to accelerate pacemaker activity in rabbit sinoatrial nodal cells. *Circ. Res.* 90 (1), 73–79. doi: 10.1161/hh0102.102271

Vinogradova, T. M., Zhou, Y. Y., Maltsev, V., Lyashkov, A., Stern, M., and Lakatta, E. G. (2004). Rhythmic ryanodine receptor Ca2+ releases during diastolic depolarization of sinoatrial pacemaker cells do not require membrane depolarization. *Circ. Res.* 94 (6), 802–809. doi: 10.1161/01.RES.0000122045.55331.0F

Vinogradova, T. M., Maltsev, V. A., Bogdanov, K. Y., Lyashkov, A. E., and Lakatta, E. G. (2005). Rhythmic Ca2+ oscillations drive sinoatrial nodal cell pacemaker function to make the heart tick. *Ann. N. Y. Acad. Sci.* 1047, 138–156. doi: 10.1196/annals.1341.013

Vinogradova, T. M., Lyashkov, A. E., Zhu, W., Ruknudin, A. M., Sirenko, S., Yang, D., et al. (2006). High basal protein kinase A-dependent phosphorylation drives rhythmic internal Ca2+ store oscillations and spontaneous beating of cardiac pacemaker cells. *Circ. Res.* 98 (4), 505–514. doi: 10.1161/01.RES.0000204575.94040.d1

Vinogradova, T. M., Sirenko, S., Lyashkov, A. E., Younes, A., Li, Y., Zhu, W., et al. (2008). Constitutive phosphodiesterase activity restricts spontaneous beating rate of cardiac pacemaker cells by suppressing local Ca2+ releases. *Circ. Res.* 102 (7), 761–769. doi: 10.1161/CIRCRESAHA.107.161679

Vinogradova, T. M., Brochet, D. X., Sirenko, S., Li, Y., Spurgeon, H., and Lakatta, E. G. (2010). Sarcoplasmic reticulum Ca2+ pumping kinetics regulates timing of local Ca2+ releases and spontaneous beating rate of rabbit sinoatrial node pacemaker cells. *Circ. Res.* 107 (6), 767–775. doi: 10.1161/CIRCRESAHA.110.220517

Vinogradova, T. M., Kobrinsky, E., and Lakatta, E. G. (2018a). Dual Activation of Phosphodiesterases 3 and 4 Regulates Basal Spontaneous Beating Rate of Cardiac Pacemaker Cells: Role of Compartmentalization? *Front. Physiol.* 9, 1301. doi: 10.3389/fphys.2018.01301

Vinogradova, T. M., Sirenko, S., Lukyanenko, Y. O., Yang, D., Tarasov, K. V., Lyashkov, A. E., et al. (2018b). Basal Spontaneous Firing of Rabbit Sinoatrial Node Cells Is Regulated by Dual Activation of PDEs (Phosphodiesterases) 3 and 4. *Circ. Arrhythm. Electrophysiol.* 11 (6), e005896. doi: 10.1161/CIRCEP.117.005896

Wakabayashi, S., and Goshima, K. (1981). Comparison of kinetic characteristics of Na+-Ca2+ exchange in sarcolemma vesicles and cultured cells from chick heart. *Biochim. Biophys. Acta* 645 (2), 311–317. doi: 10.1016/0005-2736(81)90202-9

Wilders, R., Jongsma, H. J., and van Ginneken, A. C. (1991). Pacemaker activity of the rabbit sinoatrial node. A comparison of mathematical models. *Biophys. J.* 60 (5), 1202–1216. doi: 10.1016/S0006-3495(91)82155-5

Wilders, R. (2007). Computer modelling of the sinoatrial node. *Med. Biol. Eng. Comput.* 45 (2), 189–207. doi: 10.1007/s11517-006-0127-0

Wolf, R. M., Glynn, P., Hashemi, S., Zarei, K., Mitchell, C. C., Anderson, M. E., et al. (2013). Atrial fibrillation and sinus node dysfunction in human ankyrin-B syndrome: a computational analysis. *Am. J. Physiol. Heart Circ. Physiol.* 304 (9), H1253–H1266. doi: 10.1152/ajpheart.00734.2012

Wu, Y., Gao, Z., Chen, B., Koval, O. M., Singh, M. V., Guan, X., et al. (2009). Calmodulin kinase II is required for fight or flight sinoatrial node physiology. *Proc. Natl. Acad. Sci. U. S. A* 106 (14), 5972–5977. doi: 10.1073/pnas.0806422106

Yaniv, Y., Maltsev, V. A., Escobar, A. L., Spurgeon, H. A., Ziman, B. D., Stern, M. D., et al. (2011). Beat-to-beat Ca(2+)-dependent regulation of sinoatrial nodal pacemaker cell rate and rhythm. *J. Mol. Cell Cardiol.* 51 (6), 902–905. doi: 10.1016/j.yjmcc.2011.08.029

Yaniv, Y., Sirenko, S., Ziman, B. D., Spurgeon, H. A., Maltsev, V. A., and Lakatta, E. G. (2013a). New evidence for coupled clock regulation of the normal automaticity of sinoatrial nodal pacemaker cells: bradycardic effects of ivabradine are linked to suppression of intracellular Ca(2)(+) cycling. *J. Mol. Cell Cardiol.* 62, 80–89. doi: 10.1016/j.yjmcc.2013.04.026

Yaniv, Y., Stern, M. D., Lakatta, E. G., and Maltsev, V. A. (2013b). Mechanisms of beat-to-beat regulation of cardiac pacemaker cell function by Ca(2)(+) cycling dynamics. *Biophys. J.* 105 (7), 1551–1561. doi: 10.1016/j.bpj.2013.08.024

Youm, J. B., Kim, N., Han, J., Kim, E., Joo, H., Leem, C. H., et al. (2006). A mathematical model of pacemaker activity recorded from mouse small intestine. *Philos. Trans. A Math. Phys. Eng. Sci.* 364 (1842), 1135–1154. doi: 10.1098/rsta.2006.1759

Younes, A., Lyashkov, A. E., Graham, D., Sheydina, A., Volkova, M. V., Mitsak, M., et al. (2008). Ca(2+) -stimulated basal adenylyl cyclase activity localization in membrane lipid microdomains of cardiac sinoatrial nodal pacemaker cells. *J. Biol. Chem.* 283 (21), 14461–14468. doi: 10.1074/jbc.M707540200

Zaza, A., Maccaferri, G., Mangoni, M., and DiFrancesco, D. (1991). Intracellular calcium does not directly modulate cardiac pacemaker (if) channels. *Pflugers Arch.* 419 (6), 662–664. doi: 10.1007/bf00370312

Zhang, H., Holden, A. V., Kodama, I., Honjo, H., Lei, M., Varghese, T., et al. (2000). Mathematical models of action potentials in the periphery and center of the rabbit sinoatrial node. *Am. J. Physiol. Heart Circ. Physiol.* 279 (1), H397–H421. doi: 10.1152/ajpheart.2000.279.1.H397

Zhou, Z., and Lipsius, S. L. (1993). Na(+)-Ca2+ exchange current in latent pacemaker cells isolated from cat right atrium. *J. Physiol.* 466, 263–285. doi: 10.1113/jphysiol.1993.sp019720

Zimanyi, I., Buck, E., Abramson, J. J., Mack, M. M., and Pessah, I. N. (1992). Ryanodine induces persistent inactivation of the Ca2+ release channel from skeletal muscle sarcoplasmic reticulum. *Mol. Pharmacol.* 42 (6), 1049–1057.

Permissions

All chapters in this book were first published by Frontiers; hereby published with permission under the Creative Commons Attribution License or equivalent. Every chapter published in this book has been scrutinized by our experts. Their significance has been extensively debated. The topics covered herein carry significant findings which will fuel the growth of the discipline. They may even be implemented as practical applications or may be referred to as a beginning point for another development.

The contributors of this book come from diverse backgrounds, making this book a truly international effort. This book will bring forth new frontiers with its revolutionizing research information and detailed analysis of the nascent developments around the world.

We would like to thank all the contributing authors for lending their expertise to make the book truly unique. They have played a crucial role in the development of this book. Without their invaluable contributions this book wouldn't have been possible. They have made vital efforts to compile up to date information on the varied aspects of this subject to make this book a valuable addition to the collection of many professionals and students.

This book was conceptualized with the vision of imparting up-to-date information and advanced data in this field. To ensure the same, a matchless editorial board was set up. Every individual on the board went through rigorous rounds of assessment to prove their worth. After which they invested a large part of their time researching and compiling the most relevant data for our readers.

The editorial board has been involved in producing this book since its inception. They have spent rigorous hours researching and exploring the diverse topics which have resulted in the successful publishing of this book. They have passed on their knowledge of decades through this book. To expedite this challenging task, the publisher supported the team at every step. A small team of assistant editors was also appointed to further simplify the editing procedure and attain best results for the readers.

Apart from the editorial board, the designing team has also invested a significant amount of their time in understanding the subject and creating the most relevant covers. They scrutinized every image to scout for the most suitable representation of the subject and create an appropriate cover for the book.

The publishing team has been an ardent support to the editorial, designing and production team. Their endless efforts to recruit the best for this project, has resulted in the accomplishment of this book. They are a veteran in the field of academics and their pool of knowledge is as vast as their experience in printing. Their expertise and guidance has proved useful at every step. Their uncompromising quality standards have made this book an exceptional effort. Their encouragement from time to time has been an inspiration for everyone.

The publisher and the editorial board hope that this book will prove to be a valuable piece of knowledge for researchers, students, practitioners and scholars across the globe.

List of Contributors

István Baczkó
Department of Pharmacology and Pharmacotherapy, University of Szeged, Szeged, Hungary

Tibor Hornyik
Department of Pharmacology and Pharmacotherapy, University of Szeged, Szeged, Hungary
Department of Cardiology and Angiology I, Heart Center, University of Freiburg, Freiburg, Germany
Faculty of Medicine, University of Freiburg, Freiburg, Germany

Michael Brunner
Department of Cardiology and Angiology I, Heart Center, University of Freiburg, Freiburg, Germany
Faculty of Medicine, University of Freiburg, Freiburg, Germany
Department of Cardiology and Medical Intensive Care, St. Josefskrankenhaus, Freiburg, Germany

Gideon Koren
Cardiovascular Research Center, Division of Cardiology, Rhode Island Hospital, Alpert Medical School of Brown University, Providence, RI, United States

Katja E. Odening
Faculty of Medicine, University of Freiburg, Freiburg, Germany
Department of Cardiology and Medical Intensive Care, St. Josefskrankenhaus, Freiburg, Germany
Translational Cardiology, Department of Cardiology, Inselspital, Bern University Hospital, Bern, Switzerland
Institute of Physiology, University of Bern, Bern, Switzerland

Balázs Horváth
Department of Physiology, Faculty of Medicine, University of Debrecen, Debrecen, Hungary
Faculty of Pharmacy, University of Debrecen, Debrecen, Hungary

Verena Charwat and Bérénice Charrez
Department of Bioengineering, College of Engineering, University of California, Berkeley, CA, United States

Kevin E. Healy
Department of Bioengineering, College of Engineering, University of California, Berkeley, CA, United States
Department of Materials Science and Engineering, College of Engineering, University of California, Berkeley, CA, United States

Zsófia Kohajda, Norbert Jost, Julius Gy. Papp, András Varró and Norbert Nagy
MTA-SZTE Research Group of Cardiovascular Pharmacology, Hungarian Academy of Sciences, Szeged, Hungary
Department of Pharmacology and Pharmacotherapy, Faculty of Medicine, University of Szeged, Szeged, Hungary

Noémi Tóth, Jozefina Szlovák, Gergö Bitay, Péter Gazdag and János Prorok
Department of Pharmacology and Pharmacotherapy, Faculty of Medicine, University of Szeged, Szeged, Hungary

Axel Loewe
Institute of Biomedical Engineering, Karlsruhe Institute of Technology (KIT), Karlsruhe, Germany

Jouko Levijoki and Piero Pollesello
Orion Pharma, Espoo, Finland

Tamás Hézsö, Dénes Kiss, Kornél Kistamás and Tamás Bányász
Department of Physiology, Faculty of Medicine, University of Debrecen, Debrecen, Hungary

János Magyar
Department of Physiology, Faculty of Medicine, University of Debrecen, Debrecen, Hungary
Division of Sport Physiology, University of Debrecen, Debrecen, Hungary

Karoline Horgmo Jæger, Henrik Finsberg, Mary M. Maleckar, Samuel Wall and Aslak Tveito
Department of Scientific Computing, Simula Research Laboratory, Oslo, Norway

Péter P. Nánási
Department of Dental Physiology and Pharmacology, Faculty of Dentistry, University of Debrecen, Debrecen, Hungary
Department of Physiology, Faculty of Medicine, University of Debrecen, Debrecen, Hungary
Department of Dental Physiology, Faculty of Dentistry, University of Debrecen, Debrecen, Hungary

Drew Nassal
The Frick Center for Heart Failure and Arrhythmia and Dorothy M. Davis Heart and Lung Research Institute, The Ohio State University Wexner Medical Center, Columbus, OH, United States

Daniel Gratz
The Frick Center for Heart Failure and Arrhythmia and Dorothy M. Davis Heart and Lung Research Institute, The Ohio State University Wexner Medical Center, Columbus, OH, United States
Department of Biomedical Engineering, College of Engineering, The Ohio State University, Columbus, OH, United States

Thomas J. Hund
The Frick Center for Heart Failure and Arrhythmia and Dorothy M. Davis Heart and Lung Research Institute, The Ohio State University Wexner Medical Center, Columbus, OH, United States
Department of Biomedical Engineering, College of Engineering, The Ohio State University, Columbus, OH, United States
Department of Internal Medicine, the Ohio State University Wexner Medical Center, Columbus, OH, United States

Zoltán Szabó
Department of Emergency Medicine, Faculty of Medicine, University of Debrecen, Debrecen, Hungary

Roland Veress
Department of Physiology, Faculty of Medicine, University of Debrecen, Debrecen, Hungary

Kornél Kistamás
Department of Physiology, Faculty of Medicine, University of Debrecen, Debrecen, Hungary
Division of Cardiovascular Sciences, School of Medical Sciences, University of Manchester, Manchester, United Kingdom

Ya Suo, Meng Yuan, Hongmin Li, Yue Zhang, Ying Li, Huaying Fu, Fei Han, Changhui Ma, Yuanyuan Wang, Qiankun Bao and Guangping Li
Tianjin Key Laboratory of Ionic-Molecular Function of Cardiovascular Disease, Department of Cardiology, Tianjin Institute of Cardiology, the Second Hospital of Tianjin Medical University, Tianjin, China

Xin Zhou, Elisa Passini, Alfonso Bueno-Orovio and Blanca Rodriguez
Department of Computer Science, British Heart Foundation Centre of Research Excellence, University of Oxford, Oxford, United Kingdom

Yusheng Qu and Hugo M. Vargas
SPARC, Amgen Research, Amgen Inc., Thousand Oaks, CA, United States

Yang Liu
GAU, Amgen Research, Amgen Inc., South San Francisco, CA, United States

Antonius Ratte, Felix Wiedmann, Manuel Kraft, Hugo A. Katus and Constanze Schmidt
Department of Cardiology, University of Heidelberg, Heidelberg, Germany
DZHK (German Centre for Cardiovascular Research), partner site Heidelberg/Mannheim, University of Heidelberg, Heidelberg, Germany
HCR, Heidelberg Centre for Heart Rhythm Disorders, University of Heidelberg, Heidelberg, Germany

Dóra Ujvárosy, Tamás Ötvös and Veronika Sebestyén
Department of Emergency Medicine, Faculty of Medicine, University of Debrecen, Debrecen, Hungary
Doctoral School of Health Sciences, Faculty of Public Health, University of Debrecen, Debrecen, Hungary

Beáta Baláti
Department of Pharmacology and Pharmacotherapy, Faculty of Medicine, University of Szeged, Szeged, Hungary

David A. Eisner
Division of Cardiovascular Sciences, School of Medical Sciences, University of Manchester, Manchester, United Kingdom

Tamás Árpádffy-Lovas, Istvań Baczkó and László Virág
Department of Pharmacology and Pharmacotherapy, Faculty of Medicine, University of Szeged, Szeged, Hungary
Department of Pharmacology and Pharmacotherapy, Interdisciplinary Excellence Centre, University of Szeged, Szeged, Hungary

Miklós Bitay
Department of Cardiac Surgery, Faculty of Medicine, University of Szeged, Szeged, Hungary

Norbert Nagy
Department of Pharmacology and Pharmacotherapy, Faculty of Medicine, University of Szeged, Szeged, Hungary
MTA-SZTE Research Group for Cardiovascular Pharmacology, Hungarian Academy of Sciences, Szeged, Hungary

Norbert Jost and András Varró
Department of Pharmacology and Pharmacotherapy, Faculty of Medicine, University of Szeged, Szeged, Hungary
Department of Pharmacology and Pharmacotherapy, Interdisciplinary Excellence Centre, University of Szeged, Szeged, Hungary
MTA-SZTE Research Group for Cardiovascular Pharmacology, Hungarian Academy of Sciences, Szeged, Hungary

Csaba Lengyel
First Department of Internal Medicine, University of Szeged, Szeged, Hungary

Catalina Tobón and Laura C. Palacio
MATBIOM, Universidad de Medellín, Medellín, Colombia

Bojjibabu Chidipi, Michelle Reiser and Sami Noujaim
Molecular Pharmacology and Physiology Department, University of South Florida Morsani College of Medicine, Tampa, FL, United States

Yu-Shan Lin
Department of Chemistry, Tufts University, Medford, MA, United States

Bengt Herweg, Dany Sayad, Thanh Tran and Nhi Tran
Cardiology Department, University of South Florida Morsani College of Medicine, Tampa, FL, United States

Javier Saiz
Ci2 B, Universitat Politècnica de València, Valencia, Spain

Arpad Tosaki
Department of Pharmacology, School of Pharmacy, University of Debrecen, Debrecen, Hungary

Zsófia Kohajda
MTA-SZTE Research Group of Cardiovascular Pharmacology, Hungarian Academy of Sciences, Szeged, Hungary
Department of Pharmacology and Pharmacotherapy, Faculty of Medicine, University of Szeged, Szeged, Hungary

Noémi Tóth
Department of Pharmacology and Pharmacotherapy, Faculty of Medicine, University of Szeged, Szeged, Hungary

Index

www.ingramcontent.com/pod-product-compliance
Lightning Source LLC
LaVergne TN
LVHW081032210926
848485LV00004B/1003

* 9 7 8 1 6 3 9 2 7 8 3 3 6 *